Rob & Smith's
Operative Surgery

Hepatobiliary and Pancreatic Surgery

Fifth edition

Edited by

Sir David Carter MD, FRCS(Ed), FRCS(Glas)
Regius Professor of Clinical Surgery, Royal Infirmary, Edinburgh, UK

R. C. G. Russell MS, FRCS
Consultant Surgeon, The Middlesex Hospital, London, UK

Henry A. Pitt MD
Professor and Vice Chairman, Department of Surgery, The Johns Hopkins Hospital, Baltimore, Maryland, USA

Henri Bismuth MD, FACS, FRCS(Ed)
Professor of Surgery and Chairman of the Hepatobiliary Centre, Paul Brousse Hospital, Villejuif, France

CHAPMAN & HALL MEDICAL
London · Weinheim · New York · Tokyo · Melbourne · Madras

Published by Chapman & Hall, 2–6 Boundary Row, London SE1 8HN

Chapman & Hall, 2–6 Boundary Row, London SE1 8HN, UK

Chapman & Hall GmbH, Pappelallee 3,
69469 Weinheim, Germany

Chapman & Hall USA, 115 Fifth Avenue, New York, NY 10003, USA

Chapman & Hall Japan, ITP-Japan, Kyowa Building, 3F, 2-2-1 Hirakawacho
Chiyoda-ku, Tokyo 102, Japan

Chapman & Hall Australia, 102 Dodds Street, South Melbourne, Victoria 3205, Australia

Chapman & Hall India, R. Seshadri, 32 Second Main Road, CIT East,
Madras 600 035, India

Typeset in 10/11 Garamond ITC by Genesis Typesetting, Laser Quay, Rochester, Kent

Printed in Great Britain by Hartnolls Ltd, Bodmin, Cornwall

ISBN 0 412 61930 X

A catalogue record for this book is available from the British Library

Library of Congress Catalog Card Number: 96-84459

∞ Printed on permanent acid-free text paper, manufactured in
accordance with ANSI/NISO Z39.48-1992 (Permanence of Paper).

Contributors

A. N. Adam FRCP, FRCR
Professor, Department of Interventional Radiology, Guy's Hospital, London SE1 9RT, UK

R. P. Altman MD
Surgeon-in-Chief, Babies' and Children's Hospital of New York, Columbia-Presbyterian Medical Center, 3959 Broadway, Room 204 North, New York, NY 10032, USA

A. Andrén-Sandberg MD, PhD
Associate Professor, Department of Surgery, University Hospital, S-221 85 Lund, Sweden

S. Attwood MCh, FRCS, FRCS(I)
Consultant Surgeon, Department of Surgery, Hope Hospital, Salford, Lancashire M6 8HD, UK

H. G. Beger MD, FACS
Professor of Surgery, Chairman and Head of the Department of General Surgery, University of Ulm, Steinhovelstrasse 9, 89075 Ulm, Germany

J. Belghiti MD
Professor of Surgery, Department of Surgery, Beaujon Hospital, 92118 Clichy, France

J. P. Benhamou MD
Professor of Medicine, Department of Hepatology, Beaujon Hospital, 92118 Clichy, France

I. S. Benjamin BSc, MD, FRCS
Professor, Academic Department of Surgery, King's College Hospital, London SE5 9RS, UK

H. Bismuth MD, FACS, FRCS(Ed)
Professor of Surgery and Chairman of the Hepatobiliary Centre, Paul Brousse Hospital, 94804 Villejuif, France

P. C. Bornman FRCS(Ed), MMed(Surg)
Professor of Surgery and Head of Surgical Gastroenterology, Groote Schuur Hospital, Observatory 7925, Cape Town, South Africa

K. L. Brayman MD, PhD
Assistant Professor of Surgery, Department of Surgery, Hospital of the University of Pennsylvania, Philadelphia, Pennsylvania 19104, USA

C. E. Broelsch MD, PhD, FACS
Professor and Chairman, Chirurgische Klinik, Universitäts Krannkenhaus Eppendorf, 20246 Hamburg, Germany

D. C. Carter MD, FRCS(Ed), FRCS(Glas), FRCS, FRSE
Regius Professor of Clinical Surgery, Royal Infirmary, Edinburgh EH3 9YW, UK

S. Cheslyn-Curtis MS, FRCS, FRCS(Gen)
Consultant Surgeon, Luton & Dunstable Hospital, Lewsey Road, Luton LU4 0DZ, UK

A. Cuschieri MD, ChM, FRCS, FRCS(Ed)
Professor and Head of Department, Department of Surgery, University of Dundee, Ninewells Hospital & Medical School, Dundee DD1 9SY, UK

S. T. Fan MS, FRCS(Glas), FACS
Professor, Department of Surgery, Queen Mary Hospital, Hong Kong

C. M. Ferguson MD
Assistant Professor of Surgery and Associate Visiting Surgeon, Massachusetts General Hospital, Harvard Medical School, Boston, Massachusetts 02114, USA

B.-H. Ferraz-Neto MD
Transplant Fellow, The Liver and Hepatobiliary Unit, The Queen Elizabeth Hospital, Edgbaston, Birmingham B15 2TH, UK

G. A. Fielding FRACS, FRCS
Visiting Surgeon, Royal Brisbane Hospital, Wesley Medical Centre, Auchenflower, Queensland 4066, Australia

C. F. Frey MD, FACS
Professor, Department of Surgery, University of California, Davis Medical Center, Sacramento, California 95817, USA

O. J. Garden BSc, MD, FRCS(Ed), FRCS(Glas)
Senior Lecturer and Honorary Consultant Hepatobiliary Surgeon, University Department of Surgery and Scottish Liver Transplantation Unit, Royal Infirmary, Edinburgh EH3 9YW, UK

Y. Gincherman MD
Assistant Instructor in Medicine, Department of Medicine, Hospital of the University of Pennsylvania, Philadelphia, Pennsylvania 19104, USA

D. Gough FRCS, FRCS(Ed), FRACS, DCH
Consultant Paediatric Surgeon, Department of Surgery, Royal Manchester Children's Hospital, Pendlebury, Salford, Lancashire, UK

D. W. R. Gray DPhil(Oxon), MRCP, FRCS
Clinical Reader and Consultant Surgeon, Department of Surgery, John Radcliffe Hospital, Headington, Oxford OX3 9DU, UK

A. R. W. Hatfield MD, FRCP
Consultant Gastroenterologist, The Middlesex Hospital, Mortimer Street, London W1N 8AA, UK

J. M. Henderson FRCS(Ed), FACS
Chairman, Department of General Surgery, The Cleveland Clinic, 9500 Euclid Avenue, Cleveland, Ohio 44195, USA

B. A. Hicks MD
Assistant Professor of Surgery, Division of Pediatric Surgery, The University of Texas Southwestern Medical Center, Dallas, Texas, USA

H. S. Ho MD
Assistant Professor, Department of Surgery, University of California, Davis Medical Center, Sacramento, California 95817, USA

E. R. Howard MS, FRCS, FRCS(Ed)
Consultant Hepatobiliary and Paediatric Surgeon, King's College Hospital, London SE5 9RS, UK

I. Ihse MD, PhD
Professor and Chairman, Department of Surgery, University Hospital, S-221 85 Lund, Sweden

M. H. Irving MD, ChM, FRCS
Professor of Surgery, University Department of Surgery, Hope Hospital, Salford M6 8HD, Lancashire, UK

T. Ismail MD, FRCS
Senior Registrar in Surgery, The Liver and Hepatobiliary Unit, The Queen Elizabeth Hospital, Edgbaston, Birmingham B15 2TH, UK

A. G. Johnson MCh, FRCS
Professor of Surgery, Department of Surgical and Anaesthetic Sciences, Royal Hallamshire Hospital, Sheffield S10 2JF, UK

G. W. Johnston MCh, FRCS
Honorary Professor, Queen's University, Belfast and Consultant Surgeon, Royal Victoria Hospital, Belfast BT12 6BA, UK

F. B. V. Keane MD, FRCS, FRCSI
Associate Professor of Surgery, Dublin University, Meath and Adelaide Hospitals, Dublin 8, Ireland

M. Kobari MD
Visiting Scientist, Department of Surgery, University Hospital, S-221 85 Lund, Sweden

J. E. J. Krige FRCS, FCS(SA)
Associate Professor, Department of Surgery, University of Cape Town, Observatory 7925, Cape Town, South Africa

A. Lanzini MD, PhD
Senior Registrar, Internal Medicine I, University of Brescia, Spedali Civili, Brescia, Italy

M. M. Levy MD
Assistant Instructor in Surgery, Department of Surgery, Hospital of the University of Pennsylvania, Philadelphia, Pennsylvania 19104, USA

K. D. Lillemoe MD
Associate Professor, Department of Surgery, The Johns Hopkins Medical Institutions, Blalock 603, 600 N Wolfe Street, Baltimore, Maryland 21287-4603, USA

C.-Y. Lo FRCS(Ed), FCS(HK)
Senior Registrar, Department of Surgery, The University of Hong Kong, Queen Mary Hospital, Hong Kong

C. S. McArdle MD, FRCS, FRCS(Glas), FRCS(Ed)
Consultant Surgeon, University Department of Surgery, Royal Infirmary, Glasgow G31 2ER, UK

P. McMaster MCh, FRCS
Consultant Surgeon, The Liver and Hepatobiliary Unit, The Queen Elizabeth Hospital, Edgbaston, Birmingham B15 2TH, UK

W. C. Meyers MD
Professor and Chairman, Department of Surgery, University of Massachusetts, Worcester, Massachusetts 01655, USA

A. Nakeeb MD
Surgical Resident, Department of Surgery, The Johns Hopkins Medical Institutions, Blalock 688, 600 N Wolfe Street, Baltimore, Maryland 21287-4688, USA

T. C. Northfield MA, MD, FRCP
Professor of Gastroenterology, St George's Hospital, London SW17 0RE, UK

R. Noun MD
Assistant of Surgery, Department of Surgery, Beaujon Hospital, 92118 Clichy, France

K. R. Palmer MD, FRCP(Ed)
Consultant Physician, Western General Hospital, Edinburgh EH4, UK

S. Paterson-Brown MS, MPhil, FRCS(Ed), FRCS
Consultant Surgeon, University Department of Surgery, Royal Infirmary, Edinburgh EH3 9YW, UK

H. A. Pitt MD
Professor and Vice Chairman, Department of Surgery, The Johns Hopkins Medical Institutions, Blalock 688, 600 N Wolfe Street, Baltimore, Maryland 21287-4688, USA

D. N. Redhead DMRD, FRCR
Consultant Radiologist, Department of Radiology, Edinburgh Royal Infirmary, Edinburgh EH3 9YW, UK

X. Rogiers MD
Assistant Professor, Universität Hamburg, Chirurgische Klinik, D-20246 Hamburg, Germany

R. C. G. Russell MS, FRCS
Consultant Surgeon, The Middlesex Hospital, London W1N 8AA, UK

P. R. Schauer MD
Assistant Professor, Department of Surgery, University of Pittsburg, Pittsburg, Pennsylvania, USA

M. H. Schoenberg MD
Department of General Surgery, University of Ulm, Steinhovelstrasse 9, 89075 Ulm, Germany

R. Shields MD, DSc, PRCS(Ed), FRCS(Eng), FACS, FRCPS, FCS(SA), FCSHK
Professor of Surgery, University of Liverpool, Liverpool L69 3BX, UK

D. E. R. Sutherland MD, PhD
Professor of Surgery, Department of Surgery, University of Minnesota Medical School, Box 280, 420 Delaware Street, Minneapolis, Minnesota 55455, USA

J. Terblanche ChM, FRCS, FCS(SA)
Professor and Head, Department of Surgery and Co-Director, MRC Liver Research Unit, University of Cape Town, Observatory 7925, South Africa

M. Trede MD, FRCS(Hon), FACS(Hon)
Professor and Chairman, Department of Surgery, Klinikum Mannheim, D-68167 Mannheim, Theodor-Kutzer-Ufer 1-3, Germany

D. Valla MD
Professor of Medicine, Department of Hepatology, Beaujon Hospital, 92118 Clichy, France

A. L. Warshaw MD
Harold and Ellen Danser Professor of Surgery, Massachusetts General Hospital, Wang Ambulatory Care Center 336, Boston, Massachusetts 02114, USA

R. C. N. Williamson MA, MD, MChir, FRCS
Professor and Head, Department of Surgery, Royal Postgraduate Medical School, Hammersmith Hospital, London W12 0HS, UK

J. Wong PhD, FRACS, FRCS(Ed), FACS
Professor and Head, Department of Surgery, Queen Mary Hospital, Hong Kong

J. A. van Heerden MS, FRCS(C), FACS, FCM(SA), FRCS(Ed), FRCS(Glas)
Fred C. Anderson Professor of Surgery, Department of Gastroenterologic and General Surgery, Rochester, Minnesota 55905, USA

Contributing Medical Artists

Angela Christie MMAA
14 West End Avenue, Pinner,
Middlesex HA5 1BJ , UK

Peter Cox RDD, MMAA, AIMI
Canon Frome Court,
Canon Frome, Ledbury,
Herefordshire HR8 2TD, UK

Patrick Elliott BA(Hons), ATC, MMAA, AIMI
46 Stone Delf,
Sheffield S10 3QX, UK

Sandy Hill BA(Hons)
Gillian Lee Illustrations,
15 Little Plucketts Way, Buckhurst Hill,
Essex IG9 5QU, UK

Diane Kinton BA(Hons)
Gillian Lee Illustrations,
15 Little Plucketts Way, Buckhurst Hill,
Essex IG9 5QU, UK

Gillian Lee FMAA, HonFIMI, AMI, RMIP
Gillian Lee Illustrations,
15 Little Plucketts Way, Buckhurst Hill,
Essex IG9 5QU, UK

Marks Creative Consultants
4 Harrison's Rise, Croydon,
Surrey CR0 4LA, UK

Gillian Oliver MMAA, AIMI
15 Bramble Road, Hatfield,
Hertfordshire AL10 9RZ, UK

Contents

Preface

The volume devoted to Hepatobiliary and Pancreatic Surgery in the 4th edition of Rob & Smith's Operative Surgery series was a relatively slim volume and was certainly the slimmest of the three volumes covering the Alimentary Tract and Abdominal Wall. The balance is now redressed with the emergence of the 5th edition and reflects the growth of the specialty of hepatobiliary and pancreatic surgery. There have been significant advances in our understanding of hepatobiliary anatomy, improvements in diagnosis and preoperative management, and significant expansion in the number of operations now being undertaken for disorders of the liver, biliary system and pancreas. The great impact of minimally invasive surgery is also fully recognized with particular reference to its role in the evaluation and management of disorders of the biliary system. As always, the Operative Surgery series has striven for excellence and the volume editors have recruited an internationally recognized team of experts in this challenging field. Great emphasis has been placed on clear depiction of operative detail, and the volume editors are particularly grateful to Gillian Lee and her specially recruited team of artists who have produced line drawings of great clarity. We trust that the volume will be useful to surgical trainees and established surgeons alike, and in a number of areas we have attempted to provide descriptions of alternative approaches to the given problem. More than 10 years have elapsed since the 4th edition of this volume came to the bookstands, and it is hoped that the 5th edition will rectify the deficit and reflect the numerous and continuing changes in hepatobiliary and pancreatic surgery.

D. C. Carter
R. C. G. Russell
H. A. Pitt
H. Bismuth

Anatomy of the liver

O. James Garden BSc, MD, FRCS(Ed), FRCS(Glas)
Senior Lecturer and Honorary Consultant Hepatobiliary Surgeon, University Department of Surgery and
Scottish Liver Transplantation Unit, Royal Infirmary, Edinburgh, UK

Henri Bismuth MD, FACS, FRCS(Ed)
Professor of Surgery and Chairman of the Hepatobiliary Centre, Paul Brousse Hospital, Villejuif, France

History

Complete anatomical descriptions of the mammalian liver were presented by Rex in 1888[1]. Cantlie was credited with the first detailed description of the interior anatomy of the liver as long ago as 1898[2]. These studies, based on anatomical dissection, established that the liver was a segmental organ and that the hepatic arteries, bile ducts and branches of the portal vein (Glissonian triad) had a definite segmental distribution.

Although other workers confirmed these earlier observations, it was Couinaud[3] who provided surgeons with the precise anatomical terminology on which modern hepatic resectional surgery is based[4].

Surgical anatomy

A precise knowledge of the surgical anatomy of the liver, its blood vessels and biliary drainage is essential for safe hepatic resection.

Peritoneal attachments

1 The liver is supported beneath the diaphragm by the reflections of its visceral peritoneum. Over the posterior surface of the liver and to the right of the midline, the peritoneum is reflected on to the diaphragm superiorly as the upper layer of the right coronary ligament. Near the inferior margin of the liver, the peritoneal covering is reflected on to the diaphragm and posterior abdominal wall as the lower layer of the right coronary ligament. The posterior surface of the liver between these two reflections is referred to as the bare area. On the left side, the superior and inferior peritoneal surfaces coalesce to form the left coronary ligament, the lateral end of which surrounds and merges with the tip of the liver to form the left triangular ligament.

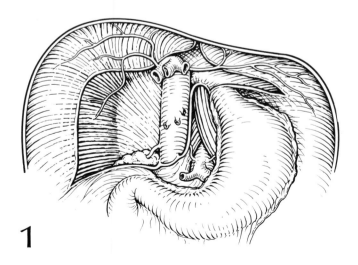

1

2 In the midline, the peritoneum is reflected as a double layer from the superior surface of the liver to form the falciform ligament. This ligament suspends the liver from the diaphragm and extends from the coronary ligaments on the superior surface of the liver to the umbilicus. The free margin of the falciform ligament contains the ligamentum teres which courses from the umbilicus to enter the falciform fissure on the inferior surface of the liver. The falciform ligament marks the boundary between the left and right lobes of the liver.

On the inferior surface of the liver, the area bounded by the ligamentum teres on the left, the gallbladder fossa on the right, and the porta hepatis posteriorly is commonly referred to as the quadrate lobe. This lobe, along with the left lobe, is supplied by the left branches of the hepatic artery and portal vein. The small portion of the liver bounded by the free edge of the lesser omentum on the left, the inferior cava and left hepatic vein posteriorly, and the porta hepatis anteriorly is referred to as the caudate lobe. On occasions, the right lobe of the liver contains a fissure which, on its inferior surface, often lies to the right of the gallbladder.

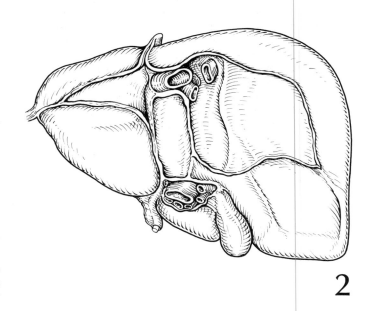

2

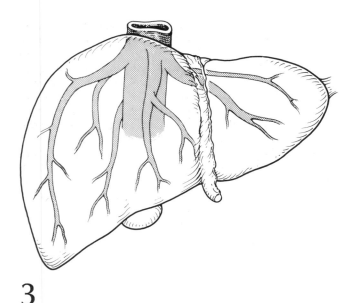

3

Segments of the liver

3 The right and left hemilivers are separated by a plane which runs from the gallbladder bed to the inferior vena cava above and posteriorly. Within this imaginary plane runs the middle hepatic vein which drains into the vena cava at a common confluence with the left hepatic vein. This confluence and the terminal portion of the right hepatic vein can only be clearly exposed by dividing the falciform and coronary ligaments and occasionally the veins enter the cava above and separate from the hepatic parenchyma. The left hepatic vein is most exposed on its lateral margin and can be damaged when the lesser omentum and left coronary ligament are divided. The right and left phrenic veins may enter the cava or hepatic veins directly and also have to be identified during mobilization of the liver from its peritoneal attachments. The caudate lobe of the liver drains directly into the vena cava through several short hepatic veins and, in 25% of individuals, a substantial accessory inferior right hepatic vein enters the vena cava at the level of the portal vein bifurcation. This and other small vessels draining blood directly into the vena cava must be carefully identified during hepatic mobilization and prior to hepatic resection.

4 Couinaud identified eight segments in the liver, each supplied by its own portal venous and hepatic arterial pedicle. The left hepatic vein divides the left lobe into the superiorly located segment II and the inferiorly placed segment III. These two segments are separated from segment IV on the anterior surface of the liver by the falciform ligament. Segment IV, the lateral boundary of which is marked superficially by the plane running between the gallbladder bed and the vena cava, is often referred to as having an inferior (IVa) and superior (IVb) portion.

The right hemiliver has an anterior and posterior sector which are separated by the right hepatic vein. The anterior sector comprises the inferiorly located segment V and superiorly situated segment VIII, whereas the posterior sector consists of segment VI inferiorly and segment VII superiorly.

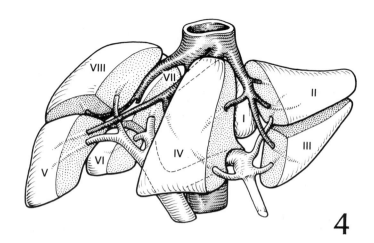

4

5 Each of the segments is drained by a single bile duct which accompanies the segmental branch of the hepatic artery and portal vein. Anatomical variations of the biliary tree are frequent but, in general, the anterior and posterior sectoral hepatic ducts of the right liver join to form a short intrahepatic right hepatic duct. The left hepatic duct emerges from the ligamentum teres fissure on the left to pursue a relatively long extrahepatic course beneath segment IV before its confluence with the right hepatic duct.

The portal vein and hepatic artery divide into their major right and left branches outwith the liver substance and below the hilus. The right branch of the portal vein is short, dividing into its anterior and posterior sectoral branches almost immediately within the liver. The posterior branch and any short vessels supplying the right portion of the caudate lobe are liable to damage during dissection at this point. The left branch of the portal vein turns almost horizontally to follow a long extrahepatic course before dividing into its numerous segmental branches. A variable number of small posterior branches to the caudate lobe must be identified if this structure is to be preserved during left hepatectomy. After entering the liver substance, the left branch of the portal vein divides within the ligamentum teres fissure into numerous segmental branches which lie superficially within the fissure and can often be identified after minimal dissection. The identification of the vessels and their ligation is a key manoeuvre in left lobectomy and extended right hepatectomy.

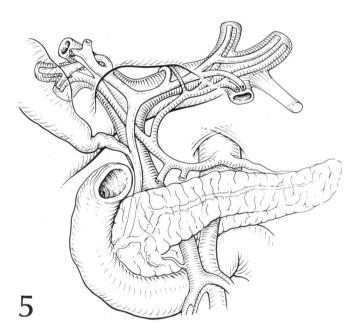

5

Nomenclature of hepatic resection

6 The confusion surrounding the nomenclature of hepatic resection has led to a general move on the part of hepatobiliary surgeons to employ Couinaud's segmental classification to define the type of hepatic resection accurately. According to this classification, left lobectomy comprises removal of all the liver to the left of the falciform ligament, including segments II and III. Left hepatectomy following division of the left branch of the portal vein and hepatic artery removes segments II, III and IV, although the caudate lobe (segment I) can be incorporated in this resection. Right hepatectomy removes all of the liver to the right of the plane running between the gallbladder bed and vena cava (segments V–VIII) and can be extended to include the quadrate lobe (segment IV) of the liver (extended right hepatectomy). Although this last type of resection can be termed 'right lobectomy', this term when used in the North American literature implies removal of only segments V–VIII. Similarly, the term 'right trisegmentectomy' should be avoided since this operation, popularized by Starzl, implies excision of three segments when, in fact, the five segments contained within three sectors are removed[5]. Similarly, the term 'lateral segmentectomy' should be avoided since, according to Couinaud's classification, this involves removal not of the left lobe (segments II and III), but of segment II alone.

Adoption of Couinaud's segmental anatomy by surgeons has also made possible the resection of small hepatic lesions contained within one or two segments, while at the same time preserving the maximum amount of functioning hepatic parenchyma. For example, a tumour arising in the gallbladder can be successfully excised along with segments IV and V (bisegmentectomy IV/V) without having to sacrifice the entire right lobe of the liver. Similarly, isolated small metastases in segment VIII can be removed by means of this segment alone (unisegmentectomy VIII).

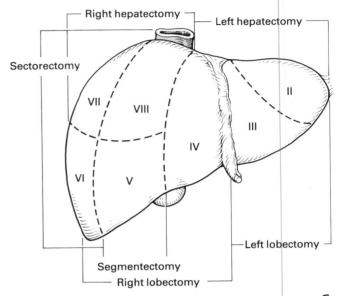

6

References

1. Rex H. Beiträge zur Morphologie der Säugerleber. *Morphol Jahrb* 1888; 14: 517–617.

2. Cantlie J. On a new arrangement of the right and left lobes of the liver. *J Anat Physiol (London)* 1898; 32: iv–ix.

3. Couinaud C. *Le Foie. Etudes Anatomique et Chirurgicales.* Paris: Masson, 1957.

4. Bismuth H. Surgical anatomy and anatomical surgery of the liver. *World J Surg* 1982; 6: 3–9.

5. Starzl TE, Bell RH, Beart RW, Putnum CW. Hepatic trisegmentectomy and other liver resections. *Surg Gynecol Obstet* 1975; 141: 429–37.

Preoperative evaluation of the liver including imaging

A. N. Adam FRCP, FRCR
Professor, Department of Interventional Radiology, Guy's and St Thomas' Hospital, London, UK

I. S. Benjamin BSc, MD, FRCS
Professor, Academic Department of Surgery, King's College Hospital, London, UK

A number of diagnostic techniques are now available to the hepatobiliary surgeon. In addition to clinical assessment and biochemical and haematological measurements, many imaging modalities are making an increasing contribution to the preoperative evaluation of potentially resectable liver tumours. The choice of procedure for each case depends on the availability of individual investigative modalities in each centre. However, it is important that a systematic approach is developed, particularly for the common clinical syndromes, in order to optimize the use of diagnostic facilities and to strike a balance between the goal of accurate preoperative diagnosis and the overuse of investigations which are often invasive and expensive. Accurate planning and good liaison between the surgeon and the hepatobiliary radiologist avoids the performance of unnecessary invasive radiological procedures. For example, if a patient is being investigated by percutaneous transhepatic cholangiography (PTC) it is important that the radiologist communicates with the surgeon before the patient leaves the fluoroscopy suite so that a decision can be taken regarding further management. If this involves the percutaneous introduction of a biliary endoprosthesis, this is best carried out immediately after the diagnostic cholangiogram rather than subjecting the patient to a second avoidable and unnecessary PTC before stenting.

Accurate preoperative imaging can help to establish the precise location of masses within the liver and the extent of ductal and vascular involvement. In many cases radiological investigations will determine that a particular mass is irresectable, whereas in others they will enable accurate planning of the operative approach. In cases of biliary obstruction, radiology can frequently demonstrate the cause of the obstruction. The choice of treatment in patients with obstructive jaundice will depend on the diagnosis and the clinical state of the patient. If surgery seems appropriate, accurate preoperative imaging will help to determine the best approach.

Definition of the nature of the disease is not the sole objective of radiology. It is also important to define the extent of the disease, the condition of the liver, the presence or absence of cirrhosis (or the atrophy/hyperplasia complex), and the patient's general condition with regard to nutritional status, sepsis and other potential risk factors. This complete diagnostic assessment is essential before surgery is undertaken for major biliary and hepatic disease.

Two categories of diagnostic problems are considered here: (1) biliary tract obstruction and (2) the intrahepatic mass.

Biliary obstruction

A careful history and thorough clinical examination may suggest a diagnosis in a proportion of patients and may direct the sequence of radiological investigations. In the case of patients presenting for the first time with jaundice, it is well established that progressive painless jaundice is frequently associated with malignant biliary obstruction. However, pain is common both with pancreatic cancer and with hilar biliary tumours[1], and also occurs frequently in patients with carcinoma of the gallbladder. Conversely, obstruction due to previously undetected gallstones may be painless. Nevertheless, a long history of symptoms consistent with biliary tract pain before the onset of obstructive jaundice is still strongly suggestive of benign biliary tract disease.

Clinical examination may reveal signs of respiratory and cardiovascular disease which make the patient unsuitable for major surgery. Stigmata of chronic hepatocellular failure (such as palmar erythema or spider naevi) may suggest the secondary effects of prolonged and severe biliary tract obstruction, but should also raise the suspicion of unrelated intrinsic parenchymal liver disease.

Standard biochemical testing is routine whenever biliary disease is suspected. Such tests are non-specific and may be of more value in following the course of a disease after treatment than in providing diagnostic information. However, minor changes in the liver enzymes, and in particular alkaline phosphatase, should not be ignored as they may be the only clue to continuing biliary tract disease in the absence of jaundice or other biochemical abnormalities. More complex serological tests, such as autoantibody estimations, are usually unnecessary unless there is a strong suspicion of intrinsic liver disease, although it is the authors' practice to carry out hepatitis B and C antigen screening routinely in all new referrals. This is particularly important in patients from overseas, especially those from areas where hepatitis is endemic.

In the initial biochemical screen, the patient's general condition is assessed by measuring renal function (by means of creatinine clearance) and by determining nutritional status. Nutritional status can be crudely assessed by haemoglobin and albumin values and, if these are abnormal, more sophisticated assessment may be indicated.

It is important whenever possible to gain some initial assessment of the presence of infection. Any external drainage from a tube or fistula should be cultured immediately for both aerobic and anaerobic organisms. Patients who are febrile should also have culture of the blood before any investigation or treatment, and at every episode of invasive radiology involving the biliary system, bile should be aspirated and cultured. The importance of having bacteriological information in advance of any septic episodes which may complicate the patient's course cannot be too strongly emphasized.

This will allow an informed choice of antibiotics when indicated for prophylaxis or the treatment of infective complications.

If the possibility of malignant disease is entertained but unproven, any aspirated bile is also sent for cytological examination. This has been found to be valuable before surgery in patients with hilar cholangio-carcinoma. The place of direct fine needle aspiration cytology in relation to individual clinical problems is considered below.

The nature and sequence of biliary imaging techniques and the decision to use angiography depends on the nature of the presentation and the presumed site of the problem within the biliary tract. The procedures available will be considered separately.

Jaundice

In the majority of patients presenting initially with jaundice a combination of clinical history and physical examination may reveal the diagnosis. The distinction between 'medical' and 'surgical' jaundice may be obvious in most cases, but it is in the difficult case that a carefully ordered approach to diagnosis is important. Most algorithmic schemes[2,3] rely on ultrasonography to detect the existence of dilated intrahepatic or extrahepatic bile ducts. While the classical sign of 'surgical' jaundice has long been dilatation of the intrahepatic ducts, biliary obstruction without ductal dilatation may be found in a significant proportion of patients – 16% in one series[4]. Thus, when the history and physical findings strongly suggest one of the variants of biliary obstruction, the finding of non-dilated intrahepatic ducts on ultrasonography does not exclude extrahepatic biliary obstruction. It should, on the other hand, alert the clinician to the possibility of severe secondary biliary fibrosis or concomitant hepatic disease. Conversely, gross ductal dilatation may occur in the presence of intermittent gallstone obstruction. However, ductal dilatation should not be accepted as a normal finding, and a subtle or intermittent cause of obstruction should always be sought in such cases.

Ultrasonographic scanning has long been the investigation of first choice for determining the obstructive nature of jaundice and has an accuracy of more than 90%[5,6]. The level of obstruction can also be defined in most patients (*Figure 1*), in 95% of 65 patients with biliary obstruction in one prospective study[7]. This is at least as good and probably superior to the performance of computed tomographic (CT) scanning with a prediction level of 90%. Moreover, ultrasonography produced valuable diagnostic information in the majority of cases and was able to distinguish with 88% accuracy between benign and malignant aetiology, again somewhat better than the performance of CT scanning

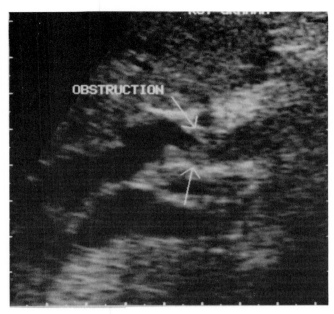

Figure 1 Ultrasonographic scan showing tapering of the common hepatic duct to the point of obstruction by a cholangiocarcinoma.

(63%). Ultrasonographic scanning is very reliable in the detection of cholelithiasis, although small bile duct stones, particularly those lying in the distal biliary tree, still pose difficulties.

Advances in ultrasonographic scanning techniques have raised the possibility that surgeons might be prepared to operate on the evidence of ultrasonography alone in the presence of obstructive jaundice. Eyre-Brook and colleagues[8] showed that the interpretation of ultrasonography was correct in 95% of 132 patients who underwent laparotomy for jaundice, concluding that it was safe to proceed directly to surgery only when an experienced ultrasonographer has demonstrated findings 'typical' of distal common bile duct obstruction due to gallstones or tumour. Duodenoscopy should also be performed before operation in order to detect unsuspected periampullary tumours. Full biliary imaging, particularly for cases of proximal obstruction, is of paramount importance. It is also important not to assume that biliary calculi demonstrated ultrasonographically are necessarily the cause of obstruction.

It is important to be cautious when assessing patients with possible obstruction of a surgically created biliary–enteric anastomosis. Wilson and Toi[9] suggested that ultrasonography accurately detects obstruction in such patients. In the authors' experience, ultrasonography usually shows dilated bile ducts in this setting but completely normal ultrasonographic scans have been seen by the authors in patients with significant anastomotic stenoses shown by cholangiography and proven at surgery (unpublished data).

If ultrasonography is unsatisfactory or incompletely diagnostic, the choice lies between endoscopic retrograde cholangiopancreatography (ERCP) and PTC as the next diagnostic test. PTC is generally preferred for cases of proximal bile duct obstruction and ERCP for cases with suspected distal obstruction. Controlled studies have compared the value of these two modalities[10, 11], but such comparisons are not particularly helpful in clinical practice. The tests are complementary and the order in which they are performed is usually dictated by the experience and expertise of the institution. PTC is contraindicated in patients with severely deranged coagulation, although in the authors' experience this has not been a major problem and can usually be overcome by the use of fresh frozen plasma and platelet infusion at the time of the investigation. In an experimental study[12] it was found that when performing fine needle aspiration biopsy of the liver – a procedure similar to PTC in its traumatic effects – the level of anticoagulation had no effect on the amount of bleeding. Gross ascites is a more important contraindication, particularly in the presence of biliary peritonitis. ERCP, on the other hand, may fail to demonstrate the proximal intrahepatic biliary tree fully, particularly when there is asymmetrical stricturing at the hilum. Some operators have used balloon catheters to overcome this problem, but the authors prefer the percutaneous route to evaluate the intrahepatic biliary tree completely in this situation. The chief advantage of ERCP is that it allows visualization of the periampullary region and provides a pancreatogram in most cases. This is particularly helpful when periampullary tumours or iatrogenic choledochoduodenal fistulae are suspected, and also when obstruction may be due to adenocarcinoma of the pancreas or to chronic pancreatitis.

Although the choice of route of biliary intubation usually depends on local practice and experience, there are now many centres at which both interventional radiology and interventional endoscopy are practised and, in certain situations, one is clearly superior to the other. For example, endoscopic papillotomy is an option for patients with choledocholithiasis and so ERCP is preferred in cases of gallstone obstruction. On the other hand, in patients with extensive hilar tumours infiltrating both lobes of the liver and in whom both sides need to be drained to recruit sufficient hepatocytes for palliation, the success rate of percutaneous drainage is significantly higher than that of endoscopic intubation so that PTC is preferred (*Figure 2*).

Recently magnetic resonance (MR) cholangiography has become feasible using fast-spin echo techniques[13, 14]. MR cholangiography can demonstrate both normal and dilated bile ducts but the anatomical detail provided is still inferior to that obtained by conventional cholangiographic techniques.

Angiography is of value in patients with biliary obstruction due to tumour. It is helpful in defining arterial anatomy and particularly in assessing tumour involvement, especially of the portal vein. Recent

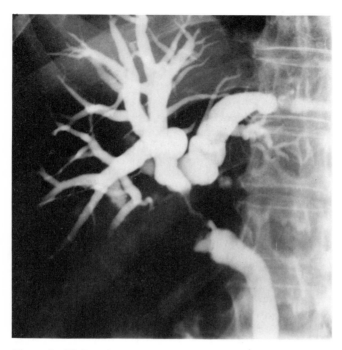

Figure 2   Tight stricture of the upper common hepatic duct in a patient with enlarged lymph nodes at the hilum of the liver shown on PTC.

advances have also made it possible to predict tumour involvement of the portal vein and its main branches by ultrasonography. Doppler ultrasound scanning allows positive identification of blood vessels and demonstrates the direction of blood flow. Colour-coded Doppler scanning has further increased the ability of radiologists to detect abnormalities of the hepatic and portal venous system[15]. In distally placed tumours, particularly those of the pancreatic head, irresectability may be inferred from arterial encasement as well as venous involvement[16]. Ultrasonography is less reliable at demonstrating tumour involvement of arteries than of large veins, so that arteriography may still be indicated.

Magnetic resonance angiography is making rapid advances as a means of assessing the portal venous system[17]. The presence or absence of portal vein occlusion, the direction of flow, and the presence of collateral vessels may be accurately demonstrated. This technique promises to replace angiography in many patients being considered for hepatic resection or transplantation.

In summary, in the authors' approach to the jaundiced patient detailed ultrasonography is the key to accurate diagnosis. When distal bile obstruction due to a clearly demonstrated pancreatic tumour or uncomplicated choledocholithiasis has been demonstrated, ultrasonography may be the only preoperative imaging required. However, this constitutes a minority of cases and direct biliary imaging is usually undertaken. The choice of

ERCP or PTC depends upon the probable site of the lesion, and on any contraindications that are present. If ultrasonography shows no evidence of biliary obstruction or any other suspicious pathology, and if the clinical history, physical examination and biochemical investigations are consistent with the possibility of a non-obstructive cause of the jaundice, percutaneous liver biopsy would then normally be performed. The use of needle biopsy of the liver without prior demonstration of non-dilated ducts on ultrasonography is regarded as a potentially hazardous procedure and is not recommended in this context[18, 19].

Hilar obstruction

Obstruction of the confluence of the hepatic ducts in the absence of previous surgery is commonly due to tumour arising in the bile ducts or gallbladder, or to tumour arising elsewhere within or outside the liver. When biliary obstruction at this level has been identified by ultrasonography, investigation is directed towards elucidating the nature and extent of a potentially malignant process. Ultrasonographic scanning defines adequately the level of the lesion and suggests its malignant nature in the majority of cases (*Figure 3*), but is not so effective in defining intrahepatic extension of tumour. Involvement of second order ducts in the intrahepatic biliary tree – an important indicator of irresectability – is frequently underestimated by ultrasonography[7, 20–22]. Thus, biliary contrast imaging is almost always required in hilar obstruction, and PTC is the preferred approach (*Figure 4*). When the obstruction is complete it may be necessary to use ERCP to define the lower end of the stricture, although in cases where ultrasonography has

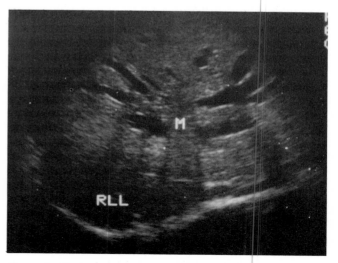

Figure 3   Cholangiocarcinoma of the hilum of the liver seen on ultrasonography. The mass (M) is slightly hypoechoic. Dilated intrahepatic ducts converge towards the lesion.

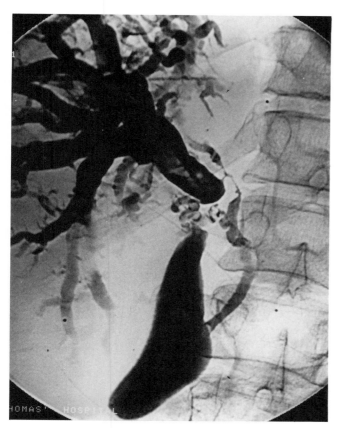

Figure 4   Hilar cholangiocarcinoma shown on PTC. Strictures of the right hepatic duct, left hepatic duct and the upper common hepatic duct are visible. The lower common hepatic duct and the common bile duct appear normal. The intrahepatic ducts are dilated.

been adequate this may not be essential. It is important to allow time to elapse and carry out delayed films with the patient tilted head up before accepting that there is a complete obstruction at the confluence. When there is no communication between the right and left hepatic ductal systems, separate punctures should be carried out to visualize the entire biliary tree.

In a significant number of patients with carcinoma of the gallbladder, neither CT nor ultrasonographic scanning reveal any abnormality of the gallbladder wall. The combination of these methods is more accurate than either alone and diffuse wall thickening or a mass is demonstrated in approximately 50% of patients. Carcinoma of the gallbladder causing hilar obstruction may produce specific subtle cholangiographic signs, particularly distortion of the intrahepatic bile ducts of segment V[23]. In patients with metastatic tumour or filling defects due to primary hepatocellular carcinoma, ultrasonographic scanning may demonstrate an extraductal hilar mass or loose tumour within the biliary system, while PTC may identify the rare cases of polypoid tumour within the hilar ductal system. The distinction may be important because of the possibility of local excision by

curettage with a relatively good prognosis[24]. At the time of PTC, bile should be aspirated for bacteriological and cytological examination. Exfoliative cytology is somewhat inferior to fine needle aspiration cytology (which yields positive results in 95% of cases, including both preoperative and operative specimens) and it may be valuable to perform PTC-guided or ultrasound-guided fine needle aspiration cytology in cases where a hilar mass is demonstrated[25].

Some workers, particularly in Japan, have made extensive use of cholangioscopy for diagnosis and staging of biliary tumours. This technique may be used following percutaneous transhepatic biliary drainage and has proved valuable in differentiating benign biliary strictures and polyps[26]. Nimura has used this technique in about two-thirds of patients undergoing diagnostic and staging procedures for hilar cholangiocarcinoma, and has used cholangioscopic biopsy following multiple segment percutaneous transhepatic biliary drainage to guide the extent of resection of intrahepatic ducts[27].

Angiography should be carried out in all cases of cholangiocarcinoma thought at initial ultrasonography and PTC to be potentially resectable. A combination of cholangiography and angiography is an accurate means of defining irresectability of hilar tumours. Preoperative diagnosis of tumour invasion of the portal venous wall would be extremely helpful in patients with hilar malignancy, but there is no completely satisfactory method for its detection. Although CT arterioportography (*Figure 5*) is routine in this situation, the technique delineates only the contrast medium-filled configuration of the vessel lumen and clarity is often poor. Also, given the anteroposterior projection of the ductal system, subtle infiltration or compression of the portal venous wall by cancer may not be defined. Similarly, other imaging modalities such as conventional ultrasonography, CT scanning and MRI do not reveal

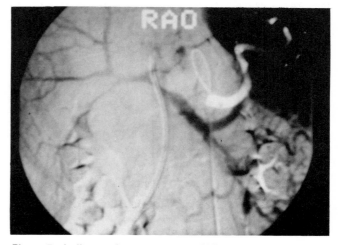

Figure 5   Indirect splenoportogram of hilar cholangiocarcinoma showing compression of the main portal vein at the liver hilum. An endoscopic stent can be seen in situ.

early invasion of the portal vein. Intraportal ultrasonography has recently been used to detect invasion of the portal vein wall. This involves inserting a catheter into an ileocolic venous branch exposed through a right lower pararectal incision. Under fluoroscopic guidance the catheter is advanced into the right or left portal vein through the main portal trunk. Real-time images are recorded on video tape using 20 MHz and 30 MHz transducers. As an alternative, percutaneous insertion of the catheter is possible using a transjugular or transhepatic approach. Preliminary results suggest that intraportal ultrasonography is helpful in detecting or excluding early invasion of the portal vein by bile duct cancer and may be useful when CT scanning or angiography fails to provide sufficient discrimination[28].

Another approach to portal venous imaging is percutaneous transhepatic portography, which some authors use in combination with PTC and biliary drainage. Nimura has also used transhepatic portal venous embolization in order to reduce the functional capacity of the hepatic parenchyma which will be resected, and so encourage contralateral hyperplasia in an effort to prevent postoperative hepatic failure[29].

In patients with hilar cholangiocarcinoma, CT scanning is valuable for demonstrating lobar or segmental atrophy of the liver (*Figure 6*), although this is often suggested on cholangiography. CT scanning is not as good as ultrasonography in demonstrating the cause and level of biliary obstruction. Contrast-enhanced CT scanning can define portal venous involvement by tumour but is less useful in demonstrating hepatic arterial encasement and cannot therefore replace angiography in the preoperative assessment of cholangiocarcinoma. Assessment of tumour involvement of the caudate lobe can be difficult. Intravascular ultrasonography via a probe mounted on a catheter

inserted in the inferior vena cava may help to resolve this problem (LH Blumgart *et al.*, 1992, personal communication).

Laparoscopy (and laparoscopic ultrasonography) is used increasingly in the diagnosis and staging of liver lesions. In the diagnosis of hepatocellular carcinoma it allows safe biopsy under direct vision, including biopsy of the non-tumorous liver, and there is evidence that this offers some advantage over 'blind' biopsies[30]. Although laparoscopy only allows visualization of about two-thirds of the liver surface, the assessment can now be extended by the use of laparoscopic ultrasonography[31]. Experience with the technique is limited and its true value is still being determined.

In summary, ultrasonographic scanning should be the first investigation in patients with hilar biliary obstruction, followed by PTC unless ultrasonography has demonstrated unequivocal evidence of irresectability. The whole of the biliary tree should be visualized, even if this requires several separate punctures. Bile must be obtained for culture and cytology and, in patients with hilar masses that are potentially resectable, fine needle aspiration cytology should be carried out. The presence or absence of vascular involvement should be established; if this cannot be achieved by high quality ultrasonography or contrast-enhanced CT scanning, angiography is indicated. It is important to be aware that a benign stricture may present as a possible hilar malignancy.

Distal obstruction

The first line investigation should be ultrasonography; this usually defines the level of obstruction although duodenal gas may limit the technical quality of the investigation. ERCP should be performed unless contraindicated on anatomical grounds or because or recent incompletely resolved pancreatitis. The ampulla of Vater should be inspected carefully, and biopsies and both brush and aspiration cytology (possibly after intravenous secretin administration) should be carried out if there is any suspicion of periampullary or pancreatic malignancy. Cholangiography should be as complete as possible, and a balloon catheter may be needed if the obstruction is higher than originally suspected. Pancreatography is obtained whenever possible as this is an accurate means of demonstrating pancreatic carcinoma or pancreatitis.

Ultrasonographic scanning and ERCP may adequately define a malignant obstruction of the common bile duct or may demonstrate clearly a benign cause such as cholelithiasis. Further investigation is indicated if the presence of malignancy cannot be confirmed or excluded, or when a malignant lesion has been shown which is potentially resectable. In such situations CT scanning is very valuable as it can demonstrate pancreatic carcinoma with an accuracy greater than 90%. CT-guided fine needle aspiration biopsy is very

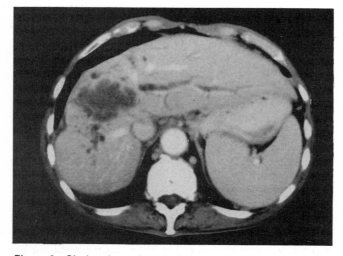

Figure 6   Cholangiocarcinoma shown on CT scan infiltrating mainly segment IV (the quadrate lobe) of the liver. Dilated intrahepatic ducts are evident in the right and left lobes. The right lobe is significantly atrophic.

useful in providing cytological proof of malignancy. Ultrasonography, ERCP and angiography are now most commonly used as adjunctive modalities when the CT diagnosis is equivocal[32]. Angiography may be valuable in demonstrating portal venous occlusion (which is non-specific and may occur with chronic pancreatitis) and arterial encasement (which rarely occurs in benign disease). It is not always possible to exclude malignancy with certainty, but if the history is consistent with obstruction due to chronic pancreatitis then a period of observation may be warranted provided any jaundice is resolving.

The assessment of resectability of pancreatic carcinoma depends on evidence of spread beyond the limits of normal resection margins or on the invasion of local structures, particularly the portal vein. A combination of ultrasonography, CT scanning and angiography will define the majority of such cases. In future intraportal ultrasonography may also be used if further information is needed. In patients with periampullary carcinoma, angiography is not normally performed since portal venous involvement is very rare.

The use of laparoscopy and laparoscopic ultrasonography has already been mentioned. It has proved valuable in the staging and planning of treatment for pancreatic cancer with distal bile duct obstruction[31,33]. Laparoscopy is certainly of benefit in demonstrating small peritoneal nodules which elude detection by ultrasonography and CT scanning and unnecessary laparotomy can be avoided in a number of patients.

In summary, ERCP is the preferred investigation in patients with distal biliary obstruction, and the objective is to define the presence of malignancy, preferably with cytological diagnosis. CT scanning is frequently sufficient for the definition of irresectability but, in selected cases, angiography may be required.

After cholecystectomy

Approximately 10–40% of patients have symptoms after cholecystectomy. In many cases these are unrelated to the biliary tract and only a few patients have symptoms caused by biliary tract obstruction. However, unless a positive diagnosis is achieved and implicates factors outside the biliary tract, the possibility of retained common bile duct stones, benign stricture formation, biliary–enteric fistula, one of the many periampullary problems, or an undisclosed biliary or periampullary tumour must be sought.

Ultrasonographic scanning should be the first investigation as it can rapidly provide information about the biliary tree and surrounding structures. If fistulae or indwelling biliary tubes are present, these should be used to obtain fistulograms or tubograms. Endoscopy is mandatory in the investigation of patients after cholecystectomy since a large proportion may have a lesion which can be identified by endoscopy alone. ERCP is the most useful investigation in this group of

patients. Care must be taken to exclude iatrogenic biliary–enteric fistula which may be responsible for persistent late symptoms[34]. If a benign iatrogenic bile duct stricture is encountered at ERCP, it may also be necessary to undertake PTC to obtain full cholangiography, although this is needed less frequently than in cases of biliary tumour.

Benign iatrogenic biliary injuries

Some patients present early in the postoperative phase after cholecystectomy with evidence of biliary injuries. The major modes of presentation are biliary peritonitis (either generalized or as a local collection of bile in the subhepatic space), an external biliary fistula with leakage of bile through a drain or through the abdominal wound, and early obstructive jaundice. The initial investigation in each case is ultrasonography, and in the case of a localized collection, percutaneous drainage under ultrasound guidance is often useful for diagnosis and as a temporizing measure. It may occasionally provide definitive management if the biliary leak has come from a small radicle in the gallbladder bed or from a slipped clip on the cystic duct. Early ERCP may be indicated, and may allow the placement of an endoscopic stent in cases of minor ductal leak or a leakage from the cystic duct stump.

However, many patients present some time after cholecystectomy and in such cases ERCP is performed early in the investigation. High strictures are not fully delineated by ERCP if there is a major disruption of the common bile duct and in such patients PTC should be carried out. All separately obstructed segments should be identified at PTC. Ultrasonography and CT scanning may be helpful in demonstrating the presence of lobar atrophy (*Figure* 7) or segmental obstruction over-

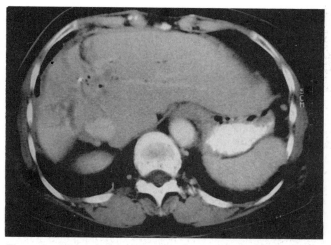

Figure 7   CT scan of a patient who had separate anastomoses of the right and left hepatic ducts to jejunum to repair a benign biliary stricture following cholecystectomy. Marked atrophy of the right lobe caused by longstanding obstruction is evident. Dilated intrahepatic ducts are seen in the atrophic lobe.

looked at PTC. These investigations will also help to demonstrate the portal vein and its branches. Portal venous collaterals and splenomegaly are usually obvious on the CT scan.

The use of angiography in patients with benign hilar strictures is restricted to the following groups of patients:

1. those with a history of major bleeding at the time of the initial operation, suggestive of vascular damage;
2. those with a history of gastrointestinal haemorrhage suggestive of portal hypertension with oesophageal varices;
3. patients with splenomegaly detected clinically or on scanning, or those with oesophagogastric varices seen on routine endoscopy;
4. those with established lobar atrophy on cholangiography or on ultrasonographic or CT scanning.

If there is any doubt regarding vascular injury and, in particular, if there is evidence of the atrophy/hypertrophy complex with rotation of the liver, angiography may be essential both for full diagnosis and as a guide to the best surgical approach. In a series of 130 patients in whom biliary strictures developed after cholecystectomy, angiography was performed selectively according to these criteria in 41 cases; vascular damage was unidentified in 28 of these (68%)[35].

Some patients with chronic incomplete bile duct strictures may also merit needle biopsy of the liver to define the degree of hepatic damage before undertaking surgery.

Intrahepatic mass

Patients may present with a mass in the epigastrium or right upper quadrant which is thought to arise from the liver. The mass may be the initial presenting feature but quite commonly it is found during investigation of known or suspected malignant disease elsewhere, and particularly in the gastrointestinal tract. As with the investigation of biliary tract obstruction, the diagnosis is evident in the majority of cases at an early stage, but there are numerous pitfalls and exceptions so that an ordered approach to investigation is advised. It is important to state at the outset that percutaneous needle biopsy of the liver mass is not recommended at an early stage of investigation. This point will be justified and emphasized below. In many non-specialist units, biopsy may be considered the most direct route to complete diagnosis. However, the biopsy of focal liver lesions is not only often unhelpful in the management, but carries the risk of serious and sometimes life-threatening complications and may jeopardize subsequent curative surgery.

Clinical assessment

Abdominal palpation will normally have already revealed the liver mass. The clinician should direct particular attention to the following points: jaundice, signs of hepatocellular insufficiency and collateral circulation, nutritional impairment, lymphadenopathy, abnormal chest signs, cutaneous or anorectal malignancies, or mucocutaneous angiomata. In the abdomen attention should be paid to the mass itself, determining whether it is regular or irregular, whether there is a palpable or ballottable gallbladder, separate masses within the abdomen, splenomegaly or ascites. A bruit may be audible in some cases of haemangioma, arteriovenous malformation or malignant liver tumour. It must be remembered that not all masses suspected of being intrahepatic on presentation and even on initial investigation prove to have arisen from the liver. We have seen duodenal, renal and adrenal tumours, as well as retroperitoneal sarcomas and leiomyosarcoma of the inferior vena cava, present in this manner. While it may not always be possible to identify these tumours clinically, a plane of cleavage can sometimes be palpated between the mass and the liver which moves with respiration. However, some masses which appear to be separate are, in fact, pedunculated liver tumours and arise from the lower margin of the liver (e.g. from the quadrate lobe, i.e. segment IV).

Biochemistry

Full initial screening of haematological and biochemical parameters is normally performed. Hepatitis B and C antigen screening is carried out as a routine, particularly in view of the association between primary hepatocellular carcinoma and hepatitis. More specialized tests reflect the previous experience and referral pattern of an individual unit. Serum tumour markers, including alpha-fetoprotein, carcinoembryonic antigen and CA19-9 are routinely measured. In appropriate cases, blood samples are also taken for hydatid serological testing, and fasting blood samples are obtained for measurement of hormone levels in case the lesion is a primary or secondary endocrine tumour. In addition, plasma neurotensin levels and serum vitamin B_{12} binding capacity are measured because these are useful tumour markers for the fibrolamellar variant of hepatocellular carcinoma[36]. It is not, of course, necessary to await the results of these specialized investigations before proceeding with further diagnostic evaluation.

Imaging investigations

Further investigation of the liver mass most usefully follows an algorithmic approach as illustrated in *Figures 8* and *9*. The procedures adopted depend on whether hepatic lesions are thought to be focal or multicentric,

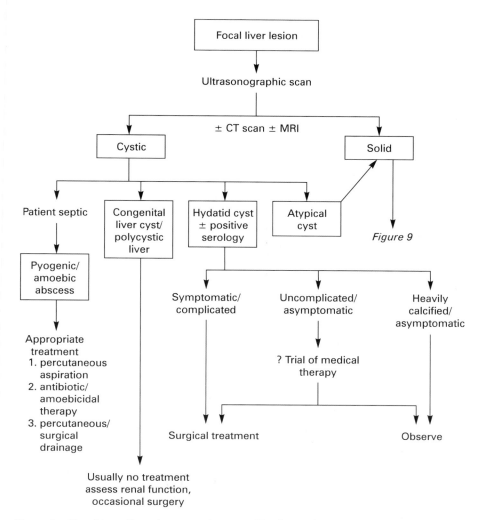

Figure 8   *Algorithm of imaging procedures used in diagnosing the cause of a cystic liver lesion.*

and whether they are cystic or solid (*Figure 10*). Thus, the first investigation is normally ultrasonography to allow early separation of cystic and solid lesions and also to exclude large bile duct obstruction. If ultrasonography shows multiple solid lesions suggesting tumour not amenable to surgical cure, a biopsy may be performed during the same session to obtain a pathological diagnosis. However, in most cases with solitary lesions the patient should have a CT scan. CT scanning performed with dynamic incremental bolus techniques is the acknowledged gold standard for liver tumour imaging[37,38]. Hepatic parenchymal enhancement reaches a plateau approximately 40 s after a bolus injection of contrast medium. Most metastases are hypovascular and appear as low attenuation lesions within the opacified parenchyma (*Figure 11*). Tumours that may be hypervascular in relation to normal hepatic parenchyma (e.g. primary hepatoma and metastases from pancreatic islet cell tumour, carcinoid and renal cell carcinoma) may become isodense during the non-equilibrium phase of maximum hepatic enhancement. Patients with suspected hypervascular tumours should have both a non-contrast and a dynamic contrast study.

Bolus dynamic contrast CT scanning ensures positive enhancement of the hepatic veins in addition to the portal veins, so that detected lesions can be located with respect to specific hepatic lobes and segments (*Figure 12*). Hepatic CT scanning usually requires 12–20 contiguous sections (average 16) and can almost always be achieved in less than 2 min when using a modern fast CT scanner.

Unfortunately, many centres still use infusion techniques in CT scanning of the liver. With these methods significant portions of the liver may not be examined until 5–10 min after the beginning of the infusion of contrast medium, and metastases may appear isodense with normal liver. In other cases the increase in

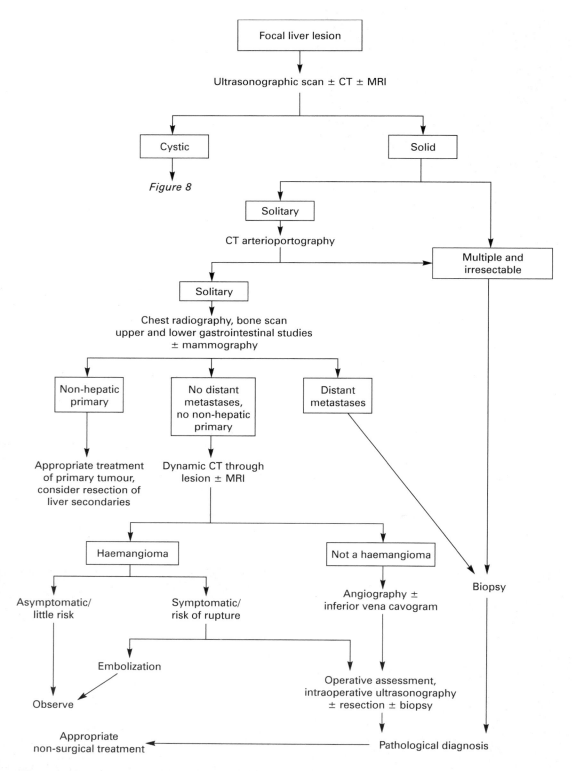

Figure 9   Algorithm of imaging procedures used in diagnosing the cause of a solid liver lesion.

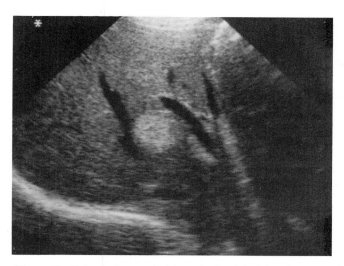

Figure 10   Echogenic rounded mass in the right lobe of the liver seen on ultrasonography. This was a metastasis from a colonic carcinoma.

attenuation of the hepatic parenchyma may be insufficient to reveal small lesions. Dynamic CT scanning of the liver should be the routine method. Compared with unenhanced CT scanning, dynamic sequential hepatic CT scanning does not markedly increase the number of patients correctly diagnosed as having liver metastases, but the number of lesions detected can be increased by as much as 40% and this is an important consideration in patients being considered for partial hepatic resection.

Helical CT scanning is an excellent method of dynamic CT scanning. Contrast medium (150 ml) is injected intravenously at the rate of 3 ml/s. Scanning begins 17 s after starting the injection. For routine evaluation of the liver 7 mm collimation is used and the entire liver is covered in approximately 21–25 s. Even if

5 mm collimation is used the entire liver can be scanned in 30 s in most patients. Because helical data are continuous, the location in which slices are reconstructed can be selected retrospectively by the radiologist. For small lesions in the liver it may be useful to reconstruct 10 mm 'thick' slices every 5 mm to reduce partial volume averaging. Reconstructing overlapping slices should make small haemangiomas and metastases more apparent.

Delayed hepatic CT scanning is a technique that uses contrast medium contained within hepatocytes and interstitial spaces some 4–6 h after the initial injection[39, 40]. This represents the small percentage of contrast medium 'vicariously' taken up and excreted by the liver, as well as contrast medium that remains in equilibrium with that circulating intravascularly. Provided that an adequate iodine load (at least 60 g) has been used initially, an increase of hepatic CT number of some 20 Hounsfield units (HU) is seen at 4–6 h. Delayed hepatic CT scanning is a very sensitive technique in the detection of hepatic metastases but few centres use it routinely because of the inconvenience of scheduling examinations 4–6 h after the initial injection of contrast medium.

CT arterioportography (CTAP) is the most sensitive preoperative method of investigation of a liver mass. It is a 'super' intravenous bolus contrast-enhanced CT study in which the contrast medium is delivered selectively into the portal venous supply without prior systemic distribution and dilution. This is achieved by selective catheterization of the superior mesenteric artery. The technique results in greater hepatic parenchymal enhancement and contrast differentiation between focal lesions and background. The basic principle of CTAP is that normal liver parenchyma is enhanced by contrast medium delivered selectively via the portal vein, whereas liver neoplasms receive their blood supply mainly from the hepatic artery and remain unenhanced

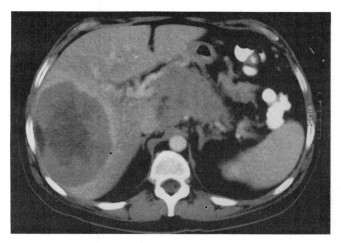

Figure 11   CT scan showing metastases from carcinoma of the colon. A large mass can be seen in the right lobe of the liver containing necrotic areas.

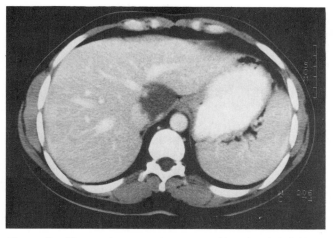

Figure 12   Metastatic tumour in segment I (caudate lobe). Note the clear demonstration of the right, middle and left hepatic veins converging towards the inferior vena cava.

during the portal and parenchymal phase of contrast distribution[30]. A recent study established that optimum parenchymal enhancement is achieved 18–67 s after injection of contrast material into the superior mesenteric artery[41]. To scan the liver within such a narrow time window a spiral technique is necessary. The authors use 150 ml of 60% contrast medium administered at a rate of 3 ml/s; the spiral CT sequence is started 20 s after the beginning of the injection. Parenchymal enhancement of 80–100 HU can be achieved compared with 50–70 HU after intravenous bolus injections. CTAP is an exquisitely sensitive technique for the detection of hepatic metastases[39, 42–44].

During CTAP perfusion, defects may be observed due to incomplete mixing of enhanced blood in the superior mesenteric vein with unenhanced blood in the splenic vein, resulting in hypoperfusion of the left hepatic lobe. In addition, central metastases may compress central portal vein branches resulting in hypoperfusion defects (*Figure 13*). Although non-tumorous attenuation differences are significantly more frequent with CTAP than with dynamic CT scanning, they are seldom a diagnostic problem because of their geographical pattern. In patients in whom it is unclear whether there is a hypoperfusion defect or a true focal lesion, it is advisable to perform a delayed hepatic CT study 4–6 h after CTAP. However, lesions may be missed in areas which have not opacified sufficiently and it is important not to interpret CTAP in isolation from a conventional dynamic study and, if appropriate, other examinations such as ultrasonography and MRI.

Lipiodol CT scanning has been advocated as a method of preoperative investigation, especially in patients with vascular tumours (*Figure 14*). Lipiodol injected selectively into the hepatic artery is taken up by tumours in a variety of patterns. Normal hepatic parenchyma also takes up lipiodol, but the contrast medium is cleared from the normal liver within approximately 1 week, whereas it is retained in tumours. In general, vascular tumours such as hepatomas take up lipiodol in a diffuse manner, whereas avascular lesions may not retain it or may demonstrate only peripheral uptake. It is thought that some abnormality of neoplastic vasculature encourages leakage of contrast medium into the tumour. Another explanation is that Kupffer cells clear lipiodol from the normal hepatic parenchyma, but these cells do

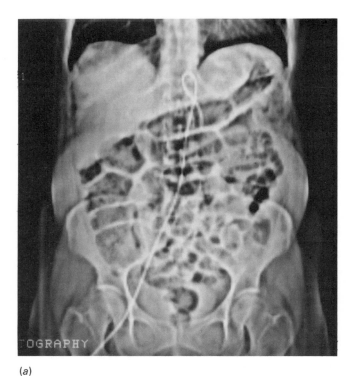

(a)

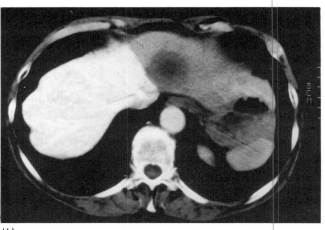

(b)

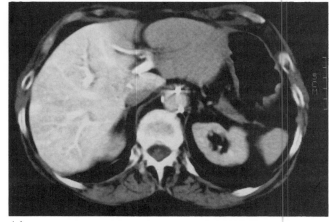

(c)

Figure 13 CT arterioportography. (a) Scout view showing a catheter in position; the tip of the catheter is in the superior mesenteric artery. (b) Metastasis in the left lobe of the liver. The right lobe is perfused whereas no perfusion is seen in the left lateral segments. (c) Lack of opacification of portal vein branches in the lateral segments (compressed by the metastasis shown in b).

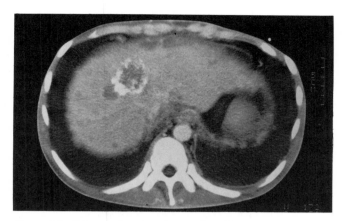

Figure 14   CT scan showing rim uptake of lipiodol around a metastasis from colorectal carcinoma. The lipiodol injection has been made several months before the CT examination. New metastases appear as low attenuation lesions without lipiodol uptake.

not exist within neoplastic tissue and lipiodol is retained within the latter. Usually about 10 ml lipiodol emulsion is injected into the hepatic artery and the CT scan is performed 7–10 days later, but both the contrast volume and the timing vary considerably from centre to centre. Residual lipiodol, particularly in the left lobe of the liver, may make it difficult to distinguish normal from diseased liver and, in one study, the technique did not contribute to decisions about surgical management in any of the 20 cases studied[45].

Magnetic resonance imaging (MRI) is a powerful tool in the evaluation of primary liver neoplasms. Determination of tumour extent and tissue characterization is provided with standard spin-echo T1- and T2-weighted imaging and is enhanced by the gradient-echo, fast spin-echo and fat suppression techniques. Intravenously administered contrast agents such as gadopentetate dimeglumine and superparamagnetic iron oxide provide additional opportunities for lesion characterization[46]. The major problem with the use of MRI in the upper abdomen is physiological movements, but this appears to have been solved by newly introduced fast-sequence and timing-parameter strategies. Short-TR/TE spin-echo sequences with extensive signal averaging and heavy T1 weighting produce images with exceptional anatomical detail and contrast differences between the liver tissue and tumour. MRI identified 14% more individual metastases and 3% more patients with liver cancer than CT scanning in a blinded comparative study of 142 patients undergoing both examinations. It also showed greater specificity (98%) than CT scanning (91%) in distinguishing patients without liver metastases. Differentiation of haemangioma from metastases was possible with more than 98% specificity by using heavily T2-weighted sequences[47]. On T2-weighted spin-echo images, intensity ratios between the lesion and liver tissue can be used

to distinguish hepatic cavernous haemangioma from malignant lesions with accuracy. However, since patients with focal liver lesions may also have diffuse liver disease, this relationship can be misleading. In doubtful cases the use of the intensity ratio between the lesion and fat tissue improves accuracy in the diagnosis of liver lesions. The combination of both ratios into a single diagnostic index in one study gave a correct classification of malignancy versus haemangioma in 92.3% of cases[48]. Superparamagnetic iron particles can be used as a tissue-specific MR contrast medium for the reticuloendothelial system. Contrast enhanced spin-echo sequences provide a marked contrast between the liver tissue and tumour, greater than the contrast values of T1- and T2-weighted images[49].

Despite advances in MRI of the liver, CT scanning remains the screening method of choice for focal liver lesions because (1) CT scanning is superior to MRI in the detection of extrahepatic disease; and (2) CTAP has a higher sensitivity than MRI in assessing liver lesions before surgery[39, 40]. However, accurate interpretation of CTAP requires the availability of a 'standard' bolus dynamic CT scan. If MRI is to replace CT as the routine screening method, a bolus dynamic CT study would have to be carried out before CTAP, thus increasing the cost and complexity of preoperative investigations.

Contact ultrasonography at the time of surgery is a very sensitive technique for detecting small lesions with a resolution of less than 0.5 cm. Used in combination with palpation, a hand-held probe in direct contact with the liver capsule allows both lobes of the liver to be fully assessed. Furthermore, the relationship of metastases to hepatic veins and bile ducts can be seen. This may influence the extent of the final resection at operation[50].

The use of preoperative laparoscopy and ultrasonography has already been mentioned[31]. There is early evidence that the technique may avoid unnecessary laparotomy in some patients with metastatic disease.

Patients must be routinely assessed for evidence of extrahepatic secondary tumours by clinical examination, chest radiography and, where appropriate, a radioisotopic bone scan. Upper and lower gastrointestinal endoscopy or barium studies, intravenous urography and mammography (in female patients) may be valuable in patients with a single liver secondary of unknown origin.

The major indication for angiography is a proven solitary solid lesion with no evidence of primary tumour elsewhere and no other sites of secondary spread. However, this is only necessary if the general condition of the patient suggests suitability for hepatic resection. In patients who proceed to angiography, multiple tumours not detected on ultrasonographic or CT scanning are occasionally found, or a mass may have the characteristic appearance of a haemangioma. In some patients with lesions close to the inferior vena cava, inferior vena cavography may also be performed at the time of angiography, since compression or invasion of the vena cava may be found. This information is of value at operation. However, MR angiography or contrast-enhanced spiral CT scanning with subsequent coronal and sagittal or three-dimensional reconstructions obviate the need for inferior vena cavography in most patients.

Biopsy

If a solitary liver lesion is amenable to surgical resection in an eligible patient, it is not normally necessary to obtain the formal tissue diagnosis before laparotomy. However, in certain circumstances with resectable lesions and where pathological confirmation is necessary in patients with a contraindication to resection, the choice lies between percutaneous fine needle aspiration cytology or Tru-Cut needle biopsy. These procedures are best performed under ultrasound or CT guidance, although in the case of obstructing biliary tumours fluoroscopic guidance during cholangiography is a rapid and accurate method (*Figure 15*). In patients with primary hepatocellular carcinoma it may be valuable to take a biopsy sample of the uninvolved liver to detect and determine the severity of parenchymal liver disease such as chronic hepatitis or cirrhosis, as this is a relative contraindication to major hepatic resection. There may be some advantages to taking a biopsy during angiography, since immediate embolization is then possible if major haemorrhage occurs. It is also now possible to perform direct embolization of a needle biopsy track[51, 52]. New automated biopsy devices utilizing relatively small calibre needles with a Tru-Cut action provide excellent specimens and probably reduce the risk of haemorrhage.

The complication rate of percutaneous liver biopsy varies from centre to centre and reflects the type of patients undergoing investigation. Complications are more frequent in biopsies performed for focal lesions than in those done predominantly for elucidation of cirrhosis or hepatocellular disorders, although it is difficult to acquire evidence from the literature to support this assumption. Biopsy is obviously contraindicated in those with an audible bruit and those who have highly vascular tumours on investigation, and in suspected hydatid disease. The risk of tumour dissemination by liver biopsy is small but finite[53]. Fine needle aspiration cytology appears to carry less risk than cutting needle biopsy[54], and the latter method should probably be used only when fine needle aspiration has failed to provide a diagnosis. False negatives may occur in up to one-third of cases of fine needle aspiration for focal liver lesion[55], and an experienced cytologist is required.

There are some potential benefits to performing a preoperative cytological and histological biopsy. Laparotomy may occasionally be avoided because of a firm diagnosis of a benign lesion such as focal nodular hyperplasia or liver cell adenoma, although even for these benign tumours direct inspection is often indicated and resection may sometimes be required.

Assessment of resectability

The criteria for resectability of solid hepatic tumours must be very carefully defined. Size alone is rarely a contraindication to attempted resection of a solitary primary or secondary liver tumour. Moreover, multiple colonic secondary deposits confined to one lobe do not contraindicate resection, and the criteria for potentially curative surgery have to be considered carefully in this light.

The management plans outlined in the algorithms in *Figures 8* and *9* have proved useful in a unit where the principal referral practice consists of potentially resectable tumours. The key to rational and successful management of these lesions is a complete and accurate preoperative assessment.

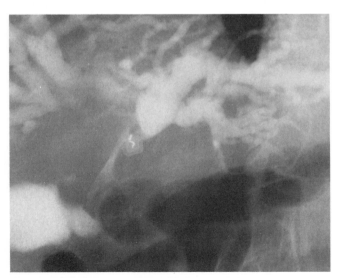

Figure 15 Fluoroscopically-guided biopsy of a hilar cholangiocarcinoma. A fine needle is guided immediately below the level of obstruction of the common hepatic duct.

References

1. Blumgart LH, Hadjis NS, Benjamin IS, Beazley RM. Surgical approaches to cholangiocarcinoma at the confluence of hepatic ducts. *Lancet* 1984; i: 66–70.

2. Benjamin IS, Allison ME, Moule B, Blumgart LH. The early use of fine needle percutaneous transhepatic cholangiography in an approach to the diagnosis of jaundice in a surgical unit. *Br J Surg* 1978; 65: 92–8.

3. Karran S, Dewbury KC, Wright R. Investigation of the jaundiced patient. In: Wright R, Alberti KGMM, Karran S, Milward-Sadler GDT, eds. *Liver and Biliary Disease: Pathophysiology, Diagnosis, Management*. 2nd edn. London: Baillière Tindall, 1994: 647–58.

4. Beinart C, Efremedis S, Cohen B, Mitty HA. Obstruction without dilation. Importance in evaluating jaundice. *JAMA* 1981; 245: 353–6.

5. Koenigsberg M, Wiener SN, Walzer A. The accuracy of sonography in the differential diagnosis of obstructive jaundice: a comparison with cholangiography. *Radiology* 1979; 133: 157–65.

6. Ferrucci JT, Adson MA, Mueller PR, Stanley RJ, Stewart ET. Advances in the radiology of jaundice: a symposium and review. *AJR* 1983; 141; 1–20.

7. Gibson RN, Yeung E, Thompson JN *et al*. Bile duct obstruction: radiologic evaluation of level, cause and tumour resectability. *Radiology* 1986; 160: 43–7.

8. Eyre-Brook IA, Ross, B, Johnson AG. Should surgeons operate on the evidence of ultrasound alone in jaundiced patients? *Br J Surg* 1983; 70: 587–9.

9. Wilson SR, Toi A. Sonography accurately detects biliary obstruction in patients with surgically created biliary-enteric anastomosis. *AJR* 1990; 155: 789–94.

10. Elias E, Hamlyn AN, Jain S *et al*. A randomized trial of percutaneous transhepatic cholangiography with the Chiba needle versus endoscopic retrograde cholangiography for bile duct visualization in jaundice. *Gastroenterology* 1976; 71: 439–43.

11. Matzen P, Malchow-Moller A, Lejerstofte J, Stage P, Juhl E. Endoscopic retrograde cholangiopancreatography and transhepatic cholangiography in patients with suspected obstructive jaundice. A randomized study. *Scand J Gastroenterol* 1982; 17: 731–5.

12. Gazelle GS, Haaga JR. Effect of needle gauge and level of anticoagulation on bleeding associated with biopsy of the liver. *Radiology* 1989; 173(P): 427.

13. Holland GH, Meakem TJ, Baeum RA, Schnall MD, Cope C, Kressell HY. MR cholangiography performed with fast SE technique. *Radiology* 1993; 189(P): 415.

14. Takehara Y, Ichijo K, Tooyama N *et al*. Breath-hold MR cholangiopancreatography performed with long-echo train, fast SE sequence and a surface coil in chronic pancreatitis. *Radiology* 1994; 192: 73–8.

15. Ralls PW. Color Doppler sonography of the hepatic artery and portal venous system. *AJR* 1990; 155: 517–25.

16. Appleton GV, Bathurst NC, Virjee J *et al*. The value of angiography in the surgical management of pancreatic disease. *Ann R Coll Surg Engl* 1989; 71: 92–6.

17. Finn JP, Eldelman RR, Longmaid HE, Jenkins RL, Lewis D. MR angiography. Prospective, blinded study with surgical validation in liver transplantation. *Radiology* 1990; 177(P): 92.

18. Benjamin IS, Imrie CW, Blumgart LH. Liver biopsy in 'difficult' jaundice. *BMJ* 1977; ii: 578.

19. Conn HO. Liver biopsies in extrahepatic biliary obstruction and other 'contraindicated' disorders. *Gastroenterology* 1975; 68: 817–21.

20. Smout JL, Bellemans MA, vanHerreweghe W. Klatskin tumours: radiological and imaging findings in eleven patients. *J Belge Radiol* 1991; 74: 177–81.

21. Looser C, Stain SC, Baer HU, Friller J, Blumgart LH. Staging of hilar cholangiocarcinoma by ultrasound and duplex sonography; a comparison with angiography and operative findings. *Br J Radiol* 1993; 65: 871–7.

22. Adam A, Benjamin IS. The staging of cholangiocarcinoma. *Clin Radiol* 1992; 46: 299–303.

23. Collier NA, Carr D, Hemmingway A, Blumgart LH. Preoperative diagnosis and its effect on the treatment of carcinoma of the gallbladder. *Surg Gynecol Obstet* 1984; 159: 465–70.

24. Gouma DJ, Mutum SS, Benjamin IS, Blumgart LH. Intrahepatic biliary papillomatosis. *Br J Surg* 1984; 71: 72–4.

25. Desa LA, Akosa AB, Lazzara S, Domizio P, Krausz T, Benjamin IS. Cytodiagnosis in the management of extrahepatic biliary stricture. *Gut* 1991; 32: 1188–91.

26. Nimura Y, Kamiya J, Hayakawa N, Shionoya S. Cholangioscopic differentiation of biliary strictures and polyps. *Endoscopy* 1989; 21 (Suppl 1): 351–6.

27. Nimura Y. Staging of biliary carcinoma: cholangiography and cholangioscopy. *Endoscopy* 1993; 25: 76–80.

28. Kaneko T, Nakoa A, Inoue S *et al*. Portal venous invasion by pancreatobiliary carcinoma: diagnosis by intraportal endovascular US. *Radiology* 1994; 192: 681–6.

29. Nagino M, Hayakawa N, Nimura Y, Dohke M, Kitagawa S. Percutaneous transheptic biliary drainage in patients with malignant biliary obstruction of the hepatic confluence. *Hepatogastroenterology* 1992; 39: 296–300.

30. Pagliaro L, Rinaldi F, Craxi A *et al*. Percutaneous blind biopsy versus laparoscopy with guided biopsy in diagnosis or cirrhosis. A prospective, randomized trial. *Dig Dis Sci* 1983; 28: 39–43.

31. Cuesta MA, Meijer S, Borgstein PJ *et al*. Laparoscopic ultrasonography for hepatobiliary and pancreatic malignancy. *Br J Surg* 1993; 80: 1571–4.

32. Freeny PC, Lunderquist A. The pancreas. In: Grainger RG, Allison DJ, eds. *Diagnostic Radiology.* Edinburgh: Churchill Livingstone, 1992: 1129–47.

33. Warshaw AL, Tepper JE, Shipley WU. Laparoscopy in the staging and planning of therapy for pancreatic cancer. *Am J Surg* 1986; 151: 76–80.

34. Hunt DR, Blumgart LH. Iatrogenic choledochoduodenal fistula: an unsuspected cause of postcholecystectomy symptoms. *Br J Surg* 1980; 67: 10–13.

35. Chapman WC, Halevy A, Blumgart LH, Benjamin IS. Post-cholecystectomy bile duct strictures: management and outcome in 130 patients. *Arch Surg* 1995; 130 (in press).

36. Collier NA, Weinbren K, Bloom SR, Lee YC, Hodgson HJF, Blumgart LH. Neurotensin secretion by fibrolamellar carcinoma of the liver. *Lancet* 1984; i: 538–40.

37. Foley WD. Dynamic hepatic CT. *Radiology* 1989; 170: 617–22.

38. Ferrucci JT. Liver tumour imaging: current concepts. *AJR* 1990; 155: 472–84.

39. Nelson RC, Chezmar JL, Sugarbaker PH, Murray DR, Bernadino ME. Preoperative localization of focal liver lesions to specific liver segments: utility of CT during arterial portography. *Radiology* 1990; 176: 89–94.

40. Heiken JP, Weyman PJ, Lee JLT et al. Detection of focal hepatic masses: prospective evaluation with CT, delayed CT, CT during arterial portography, and MR imaging. *Radiology* 1989; 171: 47–51.

41. Graf O, Dock WI, Lammer J et al. Determination of optimal time window for liver scanning with CT during arterial portography. *Radiology* 1994; 190: 43–7.

42. Matsui O, Takashima T, Kodoya M et al. Liver metastases from colorectal cancers: detection with CT during arterial portography. *Radiology* 1987; 165: 65–9.

43. Soyer P, Roche A, Gad M et al. Preoperative segmental localization of hepatic masses: utility of three-dimensional CT during arterial portography. *Radiology* 1991; 180: 653–8.

44. Soyer P, Levesque M, Elias D, Zeitoun G, Roche A. Preoperative assessment of resectability of hepatic metastases from colonic carcinoma: CT portography vs sonography and dynamic CT. *AJR* 1992; 159: 741–4.

45. Dawson P, Adam A, Banks L. Diagnostic iodized oil embolization of liver tumours – the Hammersmith experience. *Eur J Radiol* 1993; 16: 201–6.

46. Power C, Ros PR, Stoupis C, Johnson WK, Segel KH. Primary liver neoplasms: MR imaging with pathological correlation. *Radiographics* 1994; 14: 459–82.

47. Ferrucci JT. MR Imaging of the liver. *AJR* 1986; 147: 1103–16.

48. Marti-Bonmati L, Torrijo C, Vilar J, Ronchera C, Paniagua JC, Talens A. Lesion/fat intensity ratio in MR characterization of hepatic masses. *J Comput Assist Tomogr* 1991; 15: 539–41.

49. Ham B, Reichel M, Vogl T, Taupitz, Wolf KJ. Superparamagnetische eisenpartikel. Klinische ergebnisse in der MR-diagnostik von Lebermetastasen. *Rofo Fortschr Geb Rontgenstr Neuen Bildgeb Verfahr* 1994; 160: 52–8.

50. Hartley MN, Poston GJ. Treatment strategies for the patient with colorectal liver metastases. *Surgery* 1994; 12: 256–60.

51. Allison DJ, Adam A. Percutaneous liver biopsy and track embolization with steel coils. *Radiology* 1988; 169: 261–3.

52. Dawson P, Adam A, Edwards R. Technique for steel coil embolisation of liver biopsy tract for use with the 'Biopty' needle. *Br J Radiol* 1992; 65: 538–40.

53. Quaghebeur G, Thompson JN, Blumgart LH, Benjamin IS. Implantation of hepatocellular carcinoma after percutaneous needle biopsy. *J R Coll Surg Edinb* 1991; 36: 127.

54. Ferrucci JT, Wittenberg J, Mueller PR et al. Diagnosis of abdominal malignancy by radiologic fine-needle aspiration biopsy. *AJR* 1980; 134: 323–30.

55. Zornoza J, Wallace S, Ordonez N, Lukeman J. Fine-needle aspiration biopsy of the liver. *AJR* 1980; 134: 331–4.

Illustrations by Gillian Lee Illustrations

Perioperative evaluation of the liver including laparoscopic ultrasonography

O. James Garden BSc, MD, FRCS(Ed), FRCS(Glas)
Senior Lecturer and Honorary Consultant Hepatobiliary Surgeon, University Department of Surgery and Scottish Liver Transplantation Unit, Royal Infirmary, Edinburgh, UK

Principles and justification

The routine use of intraoperative ultrasound scanning of the liver was largely popularized in the East by Makuuchi[1] and in the West by Bismuth and his colleagues[2,3]. These workers showed that the technique consistently provides more information than conventional preoperative imaging[3,4]. The nature of the hepatic lesion can be confirmed and any tumour can be localized precisely with respect to the intrahepatic vessels. The presence of other lesions in the liver can be excluded, thereby avoiding inappropriate hepatic resection. The information obtained from the ultrasound scan may change the surgical approach and allow the rational use of adjuvant surgical techniques, such as those that employ local or total vascular exclusion[5,6].

As in the case of other forms of intra-abdominal malignancy, there has been considerable reluctance among surgeons to use diagnostic laparoscopy to assess hepatic involvement. The advent of laparoscopic ultrasonography may prove an important development in the assessment of hepatic malignancy since it combines the advantages of a minimal access approach to visualization of the liver with high resolution ultrasonographic scanning of the liver[7].

Laparotomy

1 Once access to the abdominal cavity has been achieved, the surgeon should confirm the nature of the underlying hepatic pathology and, in the case of hepatic malignancy, undertake a careful search for extrahepatic dissemination of disease. Palpation of the liver is a notoriously poor method of detecting deep intrahepatic lesions but allows the detection of subcapsular lesions. The presence of benign lesions such as hepatic cysts and biliary hamartomas may mislead the surgeon into believing that there is more widespread dissemination of hepatic malignancy and specimens of such lesions should be taken for confirmatory histological examination.

A careful search must be made for tumour dissemination to the peritoneal cavity and recurrence of the primary tumour must be excluded in patients undergoing laparotomy for the assessment and management of secondary tumour deposits. The regional lymphatic drainage of the liver must be carefully examined and portal and para-aortic nodes should be biopsied for histological confirmation of disease.

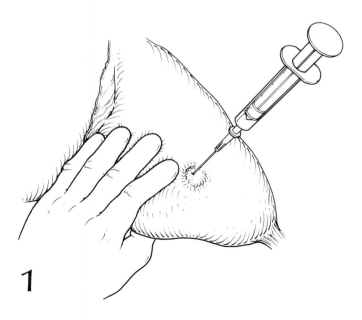

1

Intraoperative ultrasonography

2 Further evaluation of the liver is facilitated by the use of a high frequency (7.5 MHz) ultrasound transducer which does not require the same penetration of tissues as a transcutaneous ultrasound probe. The author prefers to employ a linear array transducer since this allows the surgeon to build a dynamic image of the hepatic lesion. Without mobilizing the liver the ultrasound transducer is placed directly on the anterior portion of the quadrate lobe (segment IV) without the need for an interposing fluid medium.

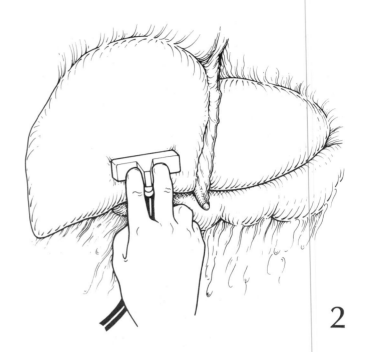

2

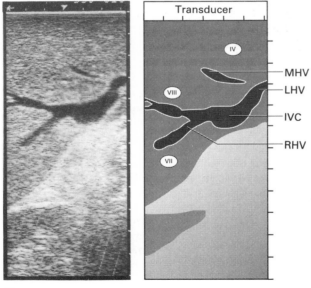

3

3 With the probe inclined superiorly, the hepatic veins can be readily recognized as they converge posteriorly to enter the inferior vena cava (IVC). The left (LHV), middle (MHV) and right (RHV) veins, which are characterized by their position and almost indistinct hyperechoic walls, can be used to identify the sectors and segments of the liver.

4   The portal vein and its right (RBPV) and left (LBPV) branches can be examined by inclining the transducer inferiorly on the inferior portion of the quadrate lobe (segment IV). The anterior (ASB) and posterior (PSB) sectoral branches of the right branch of the portal vein and their segmental divisions can be differentiated from the hepatic veins by their prominent hyperechoic walls and the right (RHA) and left (LHA) hepatic arteries and the intrahepatic ducts may be evident. The presence of a hyperechoic lesion with a hypoechoic rim (T) is characteristic of a hepatic metastasis, whereas a hypoechoic lesion with no obvious wall is characteristic of a hepatic cyst. Once the lesion is identified, its relationship to the intrahepatic vessels can be determined. The presence of other tumour deposits can be established by careful examination of the remaining liver. The clearance of tumour by the proposed hepatic resection can therefore be assessed before dissection of the liver proceeds.

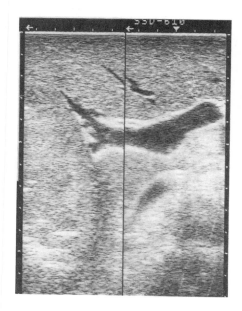
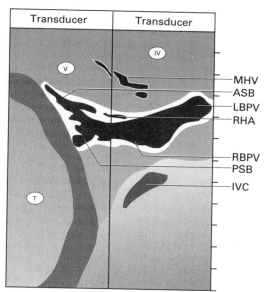

4

Laparoscopic ultrasonography

Early results with laparoscopic ultrasonography in the assessment of patients with potentially resectable liver tumours at the author's institution suggest that a substantial number of patients will benefit from this investigation since the additional information may avoid unnecessary laparotomy in those with advanced disease. In other centres, overall benefit depends on the accuracy of other available imaging modalities, the expertise of the laparoscopist, and the criteria employed by the surgeon to determine irresectability.

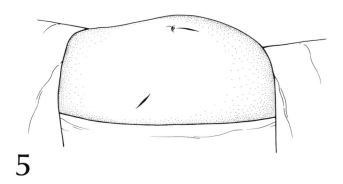

5

5 With the patient anaesthetized, peritoneal insufflation with carbon dioxide is undertaken following insertion of a 10 or 11-mm port using a cutdown technique at the umbilicus. A second 10 or 11-mm port is placed to the right of the first one in the midclavicular or anterior axillary line. It is preferable to use disposable ports to enable safe passage of the ultrasound probe, the surface of which may be inadvertently damaged by the metal spring valves of reusable metal ports. The laparoscope and laparoscopic ultrasound probe can be interchanged between the two ports to provide different views of the liver and allow the probe to be placed on different parts of the liver surface.

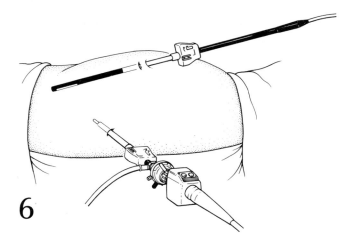

6

6 Displacement of the liver or the structures at the porta hepatis is best avoided at the outset of the examination, since gas in the tissue spaces may interfere with subsequent imaging of the structures at the porta hepatis. The use of a transducer with a flexible tip may improve contact with the liver and allows a transverse image of the liver to be readily obtained. However, the author prefers to use a rigid linear array transducer and to commence the examination by transferring the laparoscope from the umbilical to the right lateral port, and by passing the ultrasound probe through the umbilical cannula.

7a, b The 7.5 MHz transducer is placed under direct laparoscopic visualization on the anterior surface of segment IV and this enables the surgeon to visualize the portal vein and its bifurcation readily at the outset of the examination. The liver substance and the intrahepatic vessels can be explored from both the right and left sides of the liver. The depth of the liver substance can be further assessed by repositioning the transducer over another part of the liver capsule and obtaining tangential views.

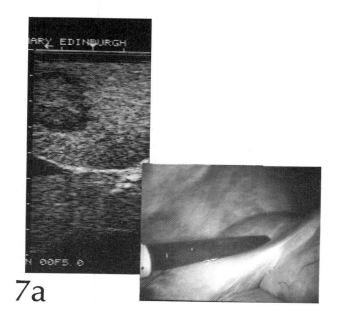

7a

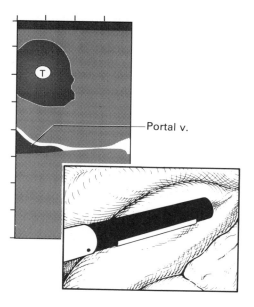

Portal v.

7b

8a, b The nature and position of any lesions can be determined from their appearance and by assessing their position relative to the intrahepatic vessels. A targeted biopsy can be undertaken by passing a Tru-cut needle through the anterior abdominal wall onto the surface of the liver. By carefully positioning the ultrasound transducer the course of the needle can be followed within the hepatic parenchyma and an accurate targeted biopsy taken. The tip of the biopsy needle can be better visualized on the ultrasound image if it is scored with a scalpel blade before passing it into the abdomen.

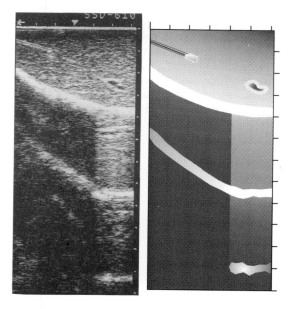

8a

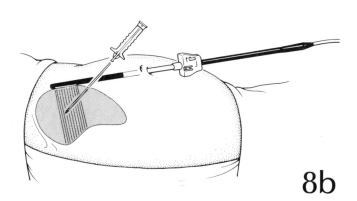

8b

Postoperative care

Ultrasonography is undertaken as part of the laparotomy or laparoscopy and is not associated with any specific complication. The postoperative care of the patient undergoing laparoscopic ultrasonography is identical to that of any other laparoscopic procedure. Infiltration of the abdominal wounds with bupivacaine 0.5% and avoidance of excessive opiate analgesia ensure rapid recovery so that the patient can be discharged following an overnight stay.

References

1. Makuuchi M, Hasegawa H, Yamazaki S, Takayasu K, Moriyama N. The use of operative ultrasound as an aid to liver resection in patients with hepatocellular carcinoma. *World J Surg* 1987; 11: 615–21.

2. Bismuth H, Castaing D. *Operative Ultrasound of the Liver and Biliary Ducts*. Berlin: Springer-Verlag, 1987.

3. Bismuth H, Castaing D, Garden OJ. The use of operative ultrasound in surgery of primary liver tumours. *World J Surg* 1987: 11: 610–14.

4. Lau WY, Leung KL, Lee TW, Li AK. Ultrasonography during liver resection for hepatocellular carcinoma. *Br J Surg* 1993; 80: 493–4.

5. Castaing D, Garden OJ, Bismuth H. Segmental liver resection using ultrasound-guided selective portal venous occlusion. *Ann Surg* 1989; 210: 20–3.

6. Bismuth H, Castaing D, Garden OJ. Major hepatic resection under total vascular exclusion. *Ann Surg* 1989; 210: 13–19.

7. John TG, Greig JD, Crosbie JL, Miles WF, Garden OJ. Superior staging of liver tumours with laparoscopy and laparoscopic ultrasound. *Ann Surg* 1994; 220: 711–19.

Further reading

Garden OJ, ed. *Intra-operative and Laparoscopic Ultrasonography*. Oxford: Blackwell Scientific, 1995.

Perioperative care of patients with hepatobiliary disease

O. James Garden BSc, MD, FRCS(Ed), FRCS(Glas)
Senior Lecturer and Honorary Consultant Hepatobiliary Surgeon, University Department of Surgery and Scottish Liver Transplantation Unit, Royal Infirmary, Edinburgh, UK

Perioperative care of patients with hepatobiliary disease should include assessment of risk to ensure that the patient receives the most appropriate management. If surgery is indicated, it is essential to identify factors that may be improved prior to surgical intervention so that operative risk may be reduced and outcome improved. Extensive hepatic resection may be well tolerated when the remaining liver has normal function, but even minor resection in cirrhotic patients may be poorly tolerated[1]. Surgical intervention directed at the obstructed biliary tree, and the increased blood loss associated with portal hypertension, carry a particularly high risk of hepatic decompensation in the postoperative period.

Preoperative evaluation

Existing liver disease and current medication

The patient with liver disease presenting for surgical intervention may benefit from specific medical manage-ment of the underlying liver disease. Surgery in the presence of active alcoholic hepatitis carries a substantial risk and abstinence for as little as 3 months will reduce this risk. The development of alcohol withdrawal syndrome during the perioperative period is best managed by the administration of alcohol rather than excessive doses of sedative drugs. Patients with active hepatitis who are on long-term steroid therapy may require an increase in steroid cover during the perioperative period.

Modified Child's grading

The use of clinical and biochemical parameters in the assessment of surgical risk in cirrhotic patients is well established (*Table 1*). The modified Child's classification correlates well with surgical risk and only the most urgent surgery should be contemplated in patients with modified Child's class C, in whom surgical mortality can exceed 50%[2-4].

Table 1 Modified Child's classification used to assess severity of liver disease in patients undergoing surgery (after Pugh *et al.*[2])

	1	*2*	*3*
Encephalopathy	Absent	Mild	Moderate to severe
Ascites	Absent	Minimal to moderate	Severe
Serum bilirubin (μmol/l)	< 34	34–51	> 51
Serum albumin (g/l)	> 35	28–35	< 28
Prolonged prothrombin time (s)	1–3	4–6	> 6

Child's grade A, 5 or 6 points; grade B, 7–9 points; grade C, 10–15 points.

Encephalopathy

The presence of even mild encephalopathy in the perioperative period is a significant adverse event and a number of factors, including the administration of sedative drugs, sepsis, bleeding and hypoxia can precipitate decompensation. Restriction of protein intake and the administration of enemas and lactulose in the preoperative period are required.

Ascites

Ascites increases the risk of wound breakdown and the development of incisional herniae. Spontaneous bacterial peritonitis should be excluded by diagnostic paracentesis and treated by prescribing appropriate antibiotics. Ascites should be controlled preoperatively by salt restriction and diuretic therapy (spironolactone). Aggressive paracentesis and intravenous administration of salt-poor albumin may be helpful in resistant ascites, but the need for such measures signifies the presence of severe hepatic disease.

Jaundice

Surgery for obstructive jaundice secondary to malignancy carries an increased risk of renal failure and has a high mortality when associated with preoperative anaemia. Preoperative relief of obstructive jaundice by endoscopic or percutaneous means may reduce operative risk but such manoeuvres may introduce infection and the benefit of preoperative stenting is now questioned. Renal failure is most likely to be prevented by adequate hydration throughout the perioperative period, but the precise role of mannitol and renal doses of dopamine remains uncertain.

Nutrition

It is extremely difficult to counter nutritional depletion in patients with severe liver disease. In the presence of ascites, weight may be a poor indicator of nutritional status and, since aggressive feeding may precipitate encephalopathy, suboptimal nutritional status may have to be accepted.

Coagulation

Preoperative administration of parenteral vitamin K should improve coagulation disorders secondary to poor nutrition and absence of luminal bile salts due to obstructive jaundice, but will not reverse coagulopathy secondary to hepatocellular dysfunction. Fresh frozen plasma should be administered to correct the prothrombin time to within 2 seconds of control before surgery if possible. Thrombocytopenia may not respond well to perioperative platelet transfusion, since this is usually secondary to hypersplenism, but platelet transfusion is indicated when the platelet count is less than $50 \times 10^9/l$. It should, however, be borne in mind that platelet function may be deranged and a normal platelet count does not preclude difficulties in controlling haemorrhage. Patients receiving aspirin therapy should have this discontinued for at least 3 weeks before surgical intervention.

Renal failure

Central venous pressure monitoring in the preoperative period may help to differentiate prerenal failure from the hepatorenal syndrome, since the former can be improved by appropriate fluid resuscitation. Associated hypoxia, sepsis, fluid imbalance, blood loss and drugs can contribute to renal failure in patients with liver dysfunction.

Intraoperative management

The quality of general anaesthesia and provision of intraoperative monitoring is crucially important in hepatic resectional surgery. Both hypocapnia and hypoxaemia reduce hepatic arterial flow and should be avoided during anaesthesia. Portal venous flow is sensitive to decreases in blood pressure and cardiac output, while spinal and epidural blocks are associated with a decrease in liver blood flow if hypotension occurs. Poor patient positioning on the operating table, increased intra-abdominal pressure, excessive surgical retraction and positive pressure ventilation can all reduce liver blood flow. These mechanical factors can be offset by increasing circulating blood volume.

Anaesthesia

Premedication

In the presence of severe liver disease, premedication is best omitted. Ranitidine may reduce the risk of gastric aspiration, but can reduce liver blood flow and is best avoided.

Induction and maintenance

All intravenous agents used to induce and maintain anaesthesia may lead to hypotension, but the risk is theoretically diminished if propofol is used.

All volatile anaesthetic agents reduce portal venous blood flow secondary to a decrease in cardiac output.

Isoflurane is the volatile agent of choice, since it is associated with preservation or an increase in hepatic arterial blood flow and carries a reduced risk of postoperative hepatic dysfunction. The efficacy of the neuromuscular blocking agents atracurium and rocuronium is not influenced by hepatic and renal failure.

The elimination of fentanyl is unchanged in cirrhosis and it is a suitable opioid analgesic. Regional analgesic techniques are commonly used after major surgery and may reduce the need for opioids. Regional anaesthesia can reduce the risk of precipitating encephalopathy, but coagulopathy is regarded as a contraindication to spinal and epidural anaesthesia.

Fluid replacement

Fluid losses should be replaced appropriately, with the proviso that large quantities of sodium-containing fluids may contribute to ascites in the postoperative period. Albumin solutions are useful in maintaining circulating volume and conserving liver and renal blood flow. Plasma volume is best maintained by giving fresh frozen plasma at an early stage. The development of significant coagulopathy in patients with liver disease who require blood transfusion should be anticipated, and aggressive maintenance of coagulation status will reduce postoperative bleeding complications and the need for blood products after surgery.

Monitoring

Monitoring and maintenance of body temperature is of prime importance during hepatobiliary surgery, since coagulopathy is compounded by hypothermia[5]. Body temperature can be maintained by adequate warming of all intravenous fluids, warming of inspired gases, provision of an adequate ambient temperature and the use of an effective warming blanket. In major hepatic resectional surgery it is the author's practice to site intra-arterial and internal jugular catheters to monitor arterial and central venous pressures.

Postoperative care

In the postoperative period, high dependency nursing or intensive care will be required to provide adequate observation of vital signs and conscious level and to detect ongoing blood losses. Monitoring includes regular measurement of heart rate, blood pressure, oxygen saturation, urine output, central venous pressure and conscious level, judged using a simple sedative scoring system combined with an assessment of pain control.

Patients undergoing major hepatic resection and those with poor preoperative liver function are at particular risk of developing postoperative hepatic decompensation. Maintenance of adequate liver function can be judged by regular assessment of conscious level, acid base status, blood glucose levels, blood lactate concentrations and prothrombin time.

References

1. Friedman LS. When patients with liver disease need surgery. *Int Med* 1993; 14: 25–34.

2. Pugh RN, Murray-Lyon IM, Dawson JL, Pietroni MC, Williams R. Transection of the oesophagus for bleeding oesophageal varices. *Br J Surg* 1973; 60: 646–9.

3. Garden OJ, Motyl H, Gilmour WH, Utley RJ, Carter DC. Prediction of outcome following acute variceal haemorrhage. *Br J Surg* 1985; 72: 91–5.

4. Brown RB. Anesthesia considerations in patients with liver disease. *Anesth Rev* 1993; 20: 213–20.

5. Rohrer MJ, Natale AM. Effect of hypothermia on the coagulation cascade. *Crit Care Med* 1992; 20: 1402–5.

Hepatic resection

O. James Garden BSc, MD, FRCS(Ed), FRCS(Glas)
Senior Lecturer and Honorary Consultant Hepatobiliary Surgeon, University Department of Surgery and Scottish Liver Transplantation Unit, Royal Infirmary, Edinburgh, UK

Henri Bismuth MD, FACS, FRCS(Ed)
Professor of Surgery and Chairman of the Hepatobiliary Centre, Paul Brousse Hospital, Villejuif, France

History

Although surgical removal of portions of the human liver was recorded in the 18th and 19th centuries, the first successful elective hepatic resection is credited to Langenbuch[1]. However, regular and extended hepatectomies to remove well defined anatomical portions of the liver have only been undertaken in the last few decades. Lortat-Jacob[2] and Tung and Quang[3] were among the pioneers of modern hepatic resection and were largely responsible for the evolution of classical hepatic resection techniques. The improved understanding of the segmental liver anatomy as described by Couinaud[4] subsequently provided the basis for the technique of segmental resection[5].

Principles and justification

Indications

The main indication for hepatic resection is primary or secondary hepatic malignancy, but the presence of benign lesions may also be an indication (*Table 1*).

Preoperative

Preoperative evaluation is aimed at determining the nature of the hepatic lesion and the potential for its resection. Patients with malignant hepatic tumours should be screened for extrahepatic metastases by chest radiography, and an abdominal and thoracic computed tomographic (CT) scan. Such preoperative evaluation may well require more advanced scanning techniques such as CT portography and nuclear magnetic resonance (NMR) imaging. The information obtained from such investigations is of paramount importance in planning the type of hepatic resection. The use of intraoperative ultrasonography is essential in defining intrahepatic anatomy and the boundaries of the tumours, and in facilitating resection.

Table 1   Indications for hepatic resection

Benign hepatic lesions:	Liver trauma
	Hepatic cyst
	Haemangioma
	Adenoma
	Fibronodular hyperplasia
Malignant hepatic lesions:	
Primary	Hepatocellular carcinoma (cirrhotic and non-cirrhotic liver)
	Cholangiocellular carcinoma
	Haemangiosarcoma
Metastases	Colorectal
	Leiomyosarcoma
Contiguous tumour	Gallbladder carcinoma
	Cholangiocarcinoma involving extrahepatic biliary tree
	Adrenal carcinoma

Operations

Perioperative morbidity and mortality can be kept to a minimum by adhering to a number of basic principles (*see* chapter on pp. 27–29). The key to successful hepatic resectional surgery is to undertake the procedure with adequate exposure and following full and appropriate mobilization of the liver. Before the hepatic parenchyma is transected, control of the appropriate supplying and draining vessels must be considered. Postoperative morbidity and mortality are diminished if the segmental anatomy of the liver is respected.

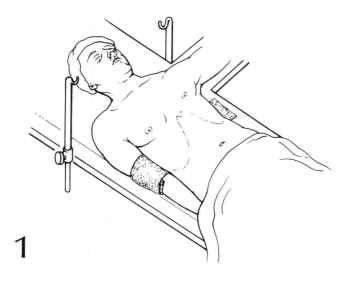

1

Position of the patient

1 The patient is positioned supine with the left arm extended at right angles to the body. The authors prefer to secure the patient's right arm to the side by means of a folded towel. This provides full access to the right hand side of the patient for the surgeon and assistant(s). It is unnecessary to place the patient in a lateral position, although placement of small sandbags or pillows beneath the right shoulder and right hip may improve access in patients undergoing resection of right-sided hepatic lesions. Tilting of the table can be used to improve exposure. ECG and monitoring leads should be kept clear of the lower chest and presternal area.

The abdomen and lower chest are prepared and draped, taking care to apply the drapes on the right side to the posterior axillary line. Two adjustable poles may be positioned beneath the upper drapes to facilitate attachment of subcostal retractors.

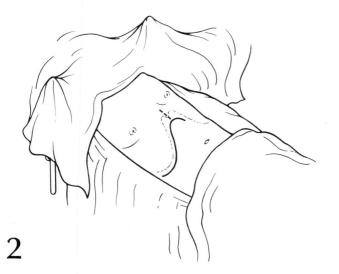

2

Incision

2 The initial incision depends upon the nature of the resection, but the surgeon should not hesitate to extend the wound to improve access. Although a midline incision may be employed for exploration of the abdomen in trauma patients, in elective resection the authors use a long S-shaped incision which follows the costal margin on the right side and can be extended on the left as appropriate. Exposure may be further improved in some patients with a narrow costal margin by extending the incision in the midline upwards to the xiphoid process. The authors have not found it necessary to extend the incision into the chest.

3 Once the abdomen is opened and a preliminary laparotomy has been undertaken, the ligamentum teres is divided between ties, one of which is left on the ligamentum teres and secured with a small forceps. The falciform ligament is incised using diathermy and separated from the anterior abdominal wall to facilitate placement of two large subcostal retractors. These are secured, in turn, by stout tapes applied to the two adjacent poles. The traction on the right subcostal retractor is best applied at the same height as the costal margin, although access to the liver is improved if traction to the left subcostal retractor is applied more vertically, approximately 8 cm above the level of the costal margin. Further retraction of intra-abdominal organs may be undertaken with carefully applied retractors, but the use of an additional fixed retractor system (Omnitract) frees the hands of the surgeon's assistant.

Exploration of the abdomen

In patients with hepatic malignancy, a thorough search is made of the peritoneum and regional lymph nodes to exclude extrahepatic dissemination of malignancy. The liver is carefully palpated and intraoperative ultrasonography is undertaken to confirm the position of the tumour and to assess its relationship with adjacent vascular structures. The presence of further lesions can be excluded using this technique. It may be necessary to take down any inflammatory adhesions, excising the parietal peritoneum if this is adherent to the hepatic tumour.

4 The right and left lobes are mobilized by first taking down any obvious capsular adhesions with diathermy. The falciform ligament is further incised using diathermy while gently retracting the liver inferiorly. Care is taken not to damage the suprahepatic cava and the hepatic veins which are identified by a combination of blunt and sharp dissection.

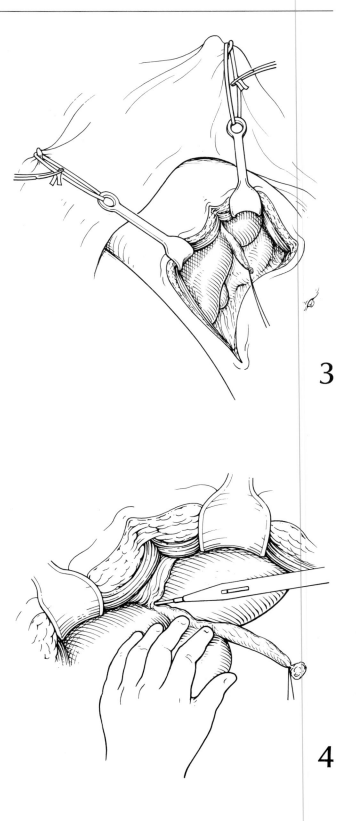

3

4

5 For left-sided lesions the left triangular ligament is incised with the diathermy, having previously placed a large pack over the stomach and oesophagus and beneath the left lobe of the liver. In this way the peritoneal attachment of the liver can be incised with diathermy, cutting down onto the pack below and so avoiding damage to the stomach and spleen. Care must be taken to avoid damage to the left hepatic vein as the left triangular ligament is freed close to the vena cava.

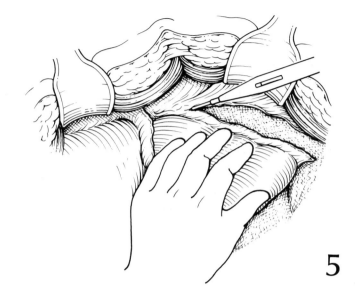

5

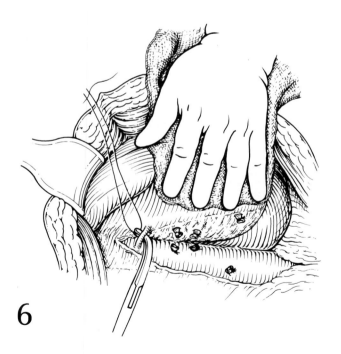

6

6 The right lobe can be similarly mobilized using diathermy to incise the anterior leaf of the coronary ligament and right triangular ligament as the liver is displaced inferiorly and across to the left of the abdomen by the assistant, whose hand retracts the right lobe of the liver using a gauze swab or pack. The dissection can be continued posteriorly, carefully separating the adhesions between the right adrenal gland and the bare area of the liver. In this way, the retrohepatic vena cava can be cleared downwards from its suprahepatic portion. When a lesion in the right liver is to be excised, it is useful to secure the short hepatic veins between the liver and vena cava. The authors prefer to divide these veins between Absolok clips or fine ties. In those patients with an accessory inferior right hepatic vein, formal ligature or oversewing of this vessel may be required. The short caudate veins can be similarly dealt with if excision of the caudate lobe is being considered.

7 As the vena cava is freed from the liver, the resection can continue superiorly to free the right hepatic vein from the overlying fibrous band of tissue which often tethers the right lobe to the vena cava superiorly. In this way, the right hepatic vein can be identified and encircled by means of a right angle forceps and Silastic sling. Any further attempts to secure this vessel are deferred until the inflow to the liver is secured. If troublesome bleeding is encountered at any stage during the freeing of the vena cava, a small swab or pack can be applied and the liver returned to the abdomen.

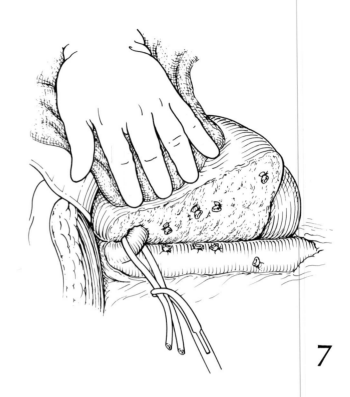

7

RIGHT HEPATECTOMY

8 Following thorough mobilization of the right lobe of the liver, the gallbladder is taken down from its bed using diathermy. The cystic duct and artery are exposed, ligated and divided. Division of the peritoneal reflection along the free edge of the lesser omentum and behind the common bile duct exposes the lateral side of the portal vein.

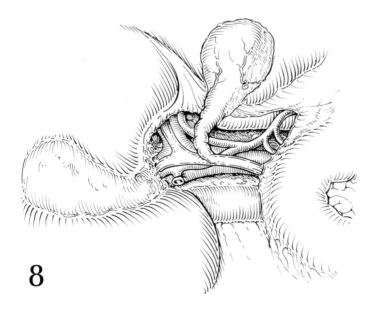

8

9 The portal vein is dissected free from the surrounding adventitial tissue by blunt dissection and, when traced upwards, its bifurcation is identified. The right branch of the portal vein is freed posteriorly, taking care to avoid inadvertent damage to any small caudate branches passing posteriorly. The right branch of the portal vein is secured with a Silastic sling.

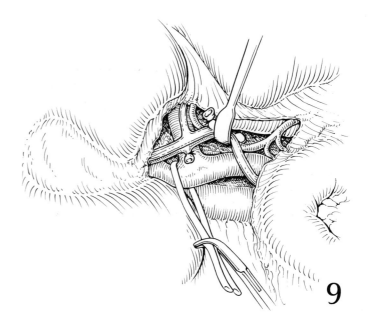

9

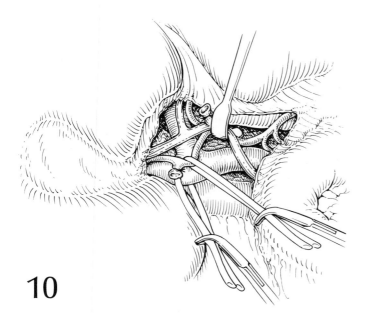

10

10 The right branch of the hepatic artery will normally be identified as it passes behind the common hepatic duct. This vessel is isolated and secured with a fine Silastic sling. No attempt is made at this stage to secure the right hepatic duct. Prolonged attempts at encircling the short right duct risk devascularizing it or ensnaring the left hepatic duct as it passes towards the midline.

11 The right branch of the portal vein is occluded by means of a straight bladed vascular clamp and the right hepatic artery is secured with a small bulldog clamp as the artery lies to the right or medial to the duct. A clear line of demarcation develops on the liver surface, running from the gallbladder fossa to the vena cava in the principal vascular plane. The capsule of the liver is incised with diathermy approximately 1 cm to the right of this line of demarcation. This avoids inadvertent dissection of the middle hepatic vein which is to be left intact on the residual liver. It is useful if the first assistant holds the quadrate lobe of the liver with a gauze swab secured in the left hand. Compression of the liver tissue will minimize blood loss.

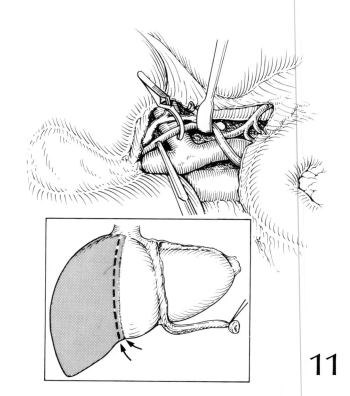

11

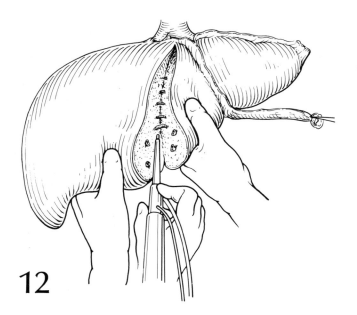

12

12 The liver dissection can be undertaken in a number of ways, but it is the authors' preference to employ a Cavitron ultrasonic surgical aspirator (CUSA) which skeletonizes the vessels within the hepatic parenchyma, allowing their identification before they are damaged and giving them an opportunity to retract into the liver substance. Small vessels (less than 2 mm) can be secured by diathermy before division with sharp scissors, although larger vessels and branches of the middle hepatic vein are best secured by ligation or application of Absolok clips.

13 The dissection is continued posteriorly along the entire length of the transected surface of the liver, taking care to avoid damage to the middle hepatic vein. The dissection is continued inferiorly, and the right portal pedicles are identified and dissected down onto the hilar plate using the Cavitron. The sectoral pedicles are isolated and divided between strong ligatures. In this way, the intrahepatic ducts are secured well away from the main confluence of the ducts at the hilus of the liver.

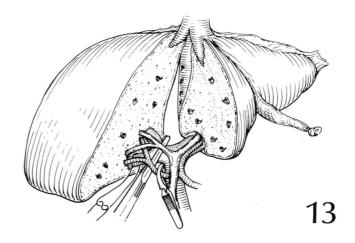

13

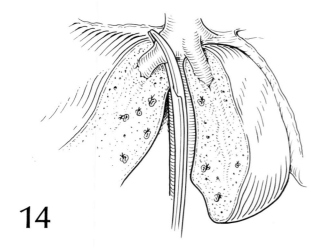

14

14 The dissection is continued posteriorly towards the vena cava. The dissection through the liver is better directed if the parenchyma to the right of the caudate lobe is opened inferiorly onto the vena cava which is protected by placement of the surgeon's left hand behind the right lobe of the liver. The dissection is continued superiorly to the right hepatic vein which, having previously been secured, is clamped and divided.

On delivery of the specimen from the operating field, the transected liver, vena cava and retroperitoneum are inspected carefully for bleeding points. These can be controlled by diathermy and an argon beam coagulator can be used to avoid removal of the coagulum which may be dislodged by conventional diathermy.

15 The right hepatic vein is secured by a running 4/0 polypropylene (Prolene) suture before removal of the clamp. The clamps on the right branch of the portal vein and right hepatic artery can be removed before confirming haemostasis at the porta hepatis. Bile leaks should be secured by careful placement of interrupted 4/0 polydioxanone (PDS) sutures. The transected surface of the liver can be sprayed with thrombin glue. Although this may not significantly reduce postoperative loss of blood, there is some evidence that it reduces the incidence of postoperative bile leakage. Large liver sutures or liver buffers should not be used to improve haemostasis since this is likely to promote necrosis of the liver and may risk damaging the intrahepatic ducts.

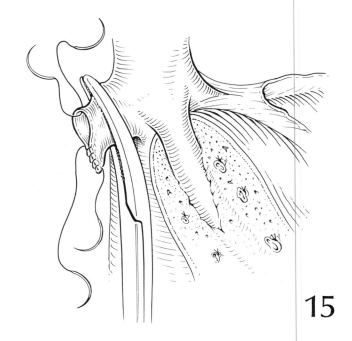

15

Wound closure and drainage

16 Two large bore drains are placed through separate stab incisions and connected to a closed drainage system. The tips of the drains are placed into the right subphrenic space and to the porta hepatis.

The wound is closed in layers using looped 1/0 polydioxanone sutures to the muscle layers and staples to the skin.

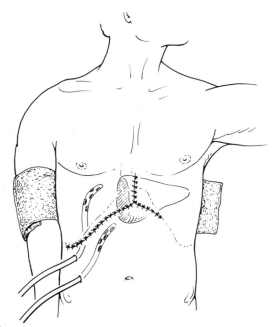

16

LEFT HEPATECTOMY

Access to the liver is the same as for a right hepatectomy. The left lobe is freed by dividing the falciform ligament towards the vena cava posteriorly and by dividing the left triangular ligament.

17 At the porta hepatis the left branch of the hepatic artery is identified and the left branch of the portal vein cleared at its bifurcation from the main portal vein trunk. When this vessel is encircled, care must be taken to avoid damage to the short posteriorly situated caudate branches. If the caudate lobe is to be left intact, the left branch of the portal vein is encircled distal to their origin. The left hepatic artery and left branch of the portal vein are secured with vascular clamps and this produces a clear line of demarcation between the right and left hemilivers. The gallbladder is normally dissected free from its bed by diathermy and the cystic duct and artery are divided between ties.

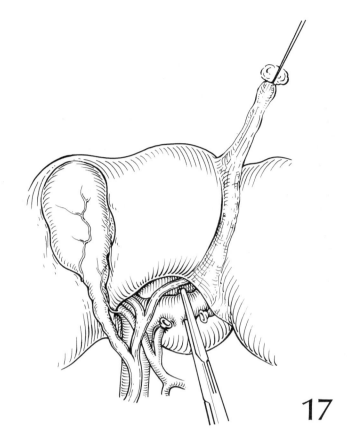

17

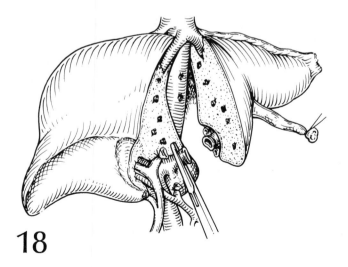

18

18 The capsule of the liver is incised about 0.5 cm to the left of the main scissura, running from the left border of the vena cava down to the gallbladder bed and hilus of the liver. The hepatic parenchyma is dissected with the Cavitron aspirator as for a right hepatectomy, but the middle hepatic vein on the right hemiliver is preserved. Once the dissection proceeds to the hilus, the left branch of the hepatic artery and the left hepatic ducts are ligated and divided distal to the hilar clamp. The anterior aspect of the hilus is then opened and the left branch of the portal vein is exposed, divided and oversewn with continuous 4/0 polypropylene. The left branch is generally smaller than the right branch of the portal vein, but it is still preferable to clamp and suture the divided vessel.

19 The liver transection is continued posteriorly, preserving the caudate lobe (segment I) along the well defined plane that extends from the left of the liver hilus. As the inferior vena cava is reached, the left hepatic vein is identified and secured with a vascular clamp within the liver substance. This vein is divided and the specimen delivered before oversewing the left branch of the portal vein with continuous 4/0 polypropylene.

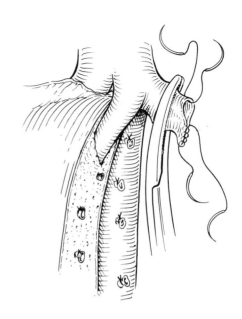

19

LEFT LOBECTOMY

Left lobectomy is the most straightforward of the classic hepatic resections since the left lobe is morphologically separate from the rest of the liver parenchyma. The positioning of the patient and the incision are as for the previously described hepatectomies, although this is one of the few hepatic resections that can be safely undertaken through an upper midline incision.

20 The left lobe is freed by division of the falciform and left triangular ligaments. The lesser omentum is opened with diathermy, taking care to identify any aberrant left hepatic artery. The falciform ligament and obliterated umbilical vein are retracted upwards by a secured tie and any bridge of liver parenchyma between the right and left lobes of the liver is divided by diathermy and the Cavitron aspirator.

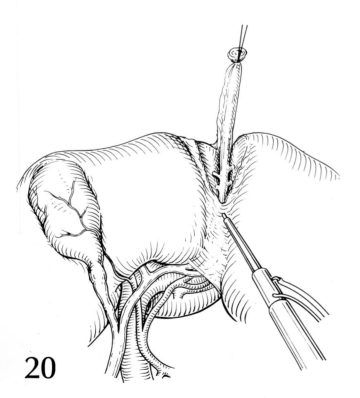

20

21 The arterial and portal venous branches to segments II and III are easily identified and can be encircled following incision of the overlying peritoneum. These vessels are divided between ligatures. The pedicle to segment II is situated more posteriorly at the junction of the vertical portion of the round ligament and the horizontal left hilar branches. These vessels are similarly divided between ligatures, although it may be necessary to oversew any more substantial vessels to avoid bleeding following further mobilization of the left lobe.

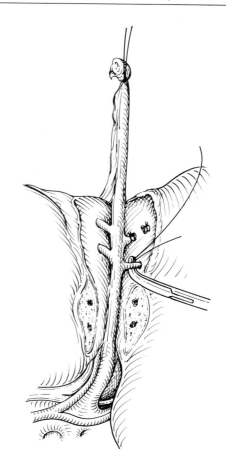

21

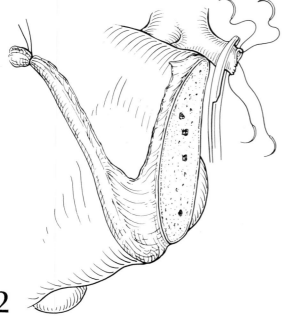

22

22 A clear line of demarcation will be observed to the left of the falciform ligament and the liver capsule is incised on its superior aspect about 0.5 cm to the left of the falciform ligament. The hepatic parenchyma is opened along its bloodless plane using the Cavitron aspirator and any further small vascular or biliary pedicles can be secured by fine ligatures. The left hepatic vein is identified posteriorly, clamped at its origin, divided and oversewn with continuous 4/0 polypropylene.

On delivery of the specimen, the transected liver surface is examined for bleeding or bile leakage. A single tube drain is normally passed through a separate stab incision down to the resected margin.

EXTENDED RIGHT HEPATECTOMY

The principles of extended right hepatectomy are drawn from those of right hepatectomy and left lobectomy.

23 The initial mobilization of the right liver and the preliminary hilar dissection are identical to those of right hepatectomy. The portal and arterial pedicles to segment IV are identified to the right of the round ligament following division of the overlying bridge of hepatic parenchyma if this is present. As the divided ligamentum teres is retracted upwards, the pedicles to segment IV are visualized and will require division between ligatures.

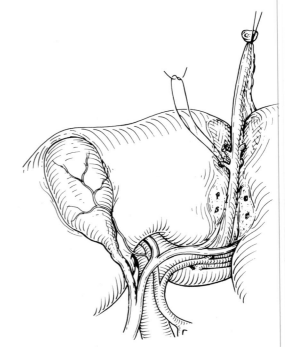

23

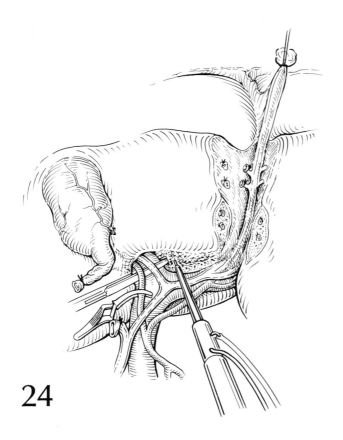

24

24 As the pedicles to segment IV are divided, the dissection proceeds with the Cavitron beneath the retracted undersurface of segment IV (quadrate lobe) and the left hepatic duct. There are often one or two small arterial branches present which may require division between ligatures. The dissection is continued to the cystic duct and artery which are divided between ligatures. This manoeuvre exposes the right hepatic artery and right branch of the portal vein which are dealt with in the same manner as for right hepatectomy. With the division of the segment IV branches and placement of clamps on the right hepatic artery and right portal pedicle, a clear line of demarcation develops between the devascularized right lobe of the liver and the left lobe to the right of the falciform ligament.

25 The hepatic parenchyma is incised approximately 0.5 cm to the left of this line of demarcation and the dissection is continued into the hepatic parenchyma using the Cavitron. Any further small vessels can be divided between ties, but the absence of substantial hepatic venous branches in the plane of dissection ensures a relatively bloodless operating field. Once the liver has been opened to the hilus of the liver and the posterior border of the quadrate lobe has been raised, the portal pedicle can be approached in the same way as for a right hepatectomy. The vessels are ligated and divided distal to the clamps and the dissection can continue posteriorly in the direction of the inferior vena cava, skirting and preserving the caudate lobe. The plane of this dissection passes to the right border of the inferior vena cava. The middle hepatic vein is clamped before being divided and oversewn with continuous 4/0 polypropylene. If the right hepatic vein has not previously been secured, the dissection continues onto the vena cava and the right hepatic vein is dealt with in the same manner as for the right hepatectomy.

If segment I is to be removed with this resection, the small vascular pedicles that pass from the portal vein are ligated. It is preferable for the small caudate veins which drain into the vena cava to have been divided between ties during the preliminary mobilization of the liver, but if this has not been possible, the posterior dissection should continue following division of the middle hepatic vein to the left border of the inferior vena cava. When this is done, the small caudate vessels can be isolated and divided between ligatures.

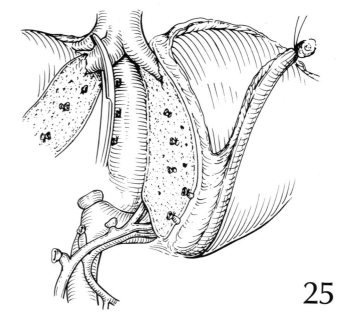

25

EXTENDED LEFT HEPATECTOMY

Left hepatectomy can be extended to include resection of segments I, V and VIII. The liver is mobilized from its peritoneal attachments as described for left hepatectomy. The boundary between the anterior and posterior sectors of the right hemiliver is situated along a plane 4 cm to the right and parallel to the main hepatic scissura, but peroperative ultrasonography may be used to localize the right hepatic vein and the right anterior sectoral vessels.

26 The liver is mobilized from its peritoneal attachments as described for left hepatectomy. The gallbladder is dissected from the liver bed and the left hepatic artery and left branch of the portal vein are isolated at the porta hepatis. In this resection, the left hepatic duct is best divided at an early stage and this facilitates mobilization of segment IV from the porta hepatis. The Cavitron is used to skeletonize the right portal pedicle which is traced along its length to enable the anterior sectoral pedicle to be encircled with a Silastic sling. This pedicle is clamped to produce a line of demarction between the right posterior sector and the anterior sector. The liver capsule is incised with diathermy approximately 1 cm anterior to this line of demarcation and the Cavitron is used to open up the plane of dissection, preserving the right hepatic vein on the posterior sector.

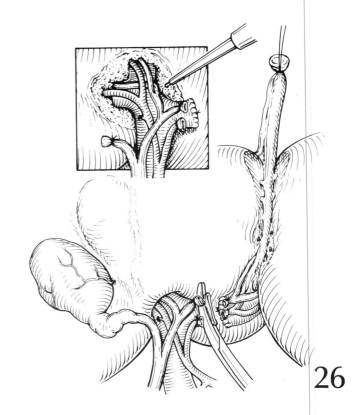

26

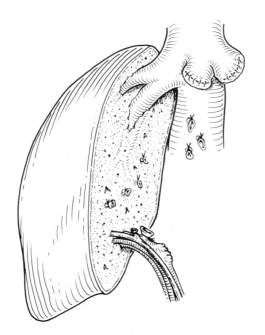

27

27 The resection is continued superiorly and enables isolation of the confluence of the middle and left hepatic veins which are divided once secured by a vascular clamp. These vessels are oversewn with 4/0 continuous polypropylene.

On delivering the specimen, haemostasis is secured and the absence of a bile leak confirmed. The right anterior sectoral pedicle is suture ligated.

Postoperative care

In the recovery room the blood pressure, pulse, temperature and urinary output are monitored continuously. If the central venous pressure has been maintained at a low level peroperatively to minimize venous bleeding, the patient may require an additional infusion of colloid or crystalloid solution. Serum concentrations of urea, electrolytes, potassium and blood sugar are measured immediately in the postoperative period and 6-hourly BMstix are undertaken in the first 48 h until it is clear that hypoglycaemia no longer poses a risk.

Complications

If haemostasis was satisfactory during operation it is unlikely that postoperative bleeding will be a significant problem, but drainage should be monitored for excessive blood loss and/or bile leakage. Disordered liver function tests are inevitable following major hepatic resection, but jaundice is usually mild if blood replacement has not been required and if a less major resection has been undertaken. In major liver resection, monitoring of serum lactate concentration, blood gases and prothrombin time will better reflect liver function. Correction of coagulation defects should only be undertaken by administration of blood products and vitamin K if there is evidence of haemorrhage. The major complications relating to hepatic resection are the development of jaundice and liver failure. The latter complication is more likely to arise if there has been hypoperfusion of the liver during surgery or extensive resection of normal liver. The risk is greatest in the cirrhotic patient and can only be minimized by careful preoperative selection.

Wound infection and intra-abdominal sepsis are now rare complications of major hepatic resectional surgery. Such collections can be managed by percutaneous drainage techniques and re-exploration is not usually required. More general complications inlcude atelectasis and chest infection.

References

1. Langenbuch C. Einfall von resection eines linksseitigen schnurlappens der leber. *Berl Klin Wochenschr* 1888; 25: 37–8.

2. Lortat-Jacob JL, Robert HG. Hépatectomie droit réglée. *Presse Med* 1952; 60: 549–51.

3. Ton That Tung, Nguyen Duorg Quang. A new technique for operation on the liver. *Lancet* 1963; i: 192–3.

4. Couinaud C. *Le Foie: Etudes Anatomiques et Chirurgicales.* Paris: Masson, 1957.

5. Bismuth H, Houissan D, Castaing D. Major and minor segmentectomies "réglées" in liver surgery. *World J Surg* 1982; 6: 10–24.

Further reading

Bismuth H, Garden OJ. Regular and extended right and left hepatectomy for cancer. In: Nyhus LM, Baker RJ, eds. *Mastery of Surgery.* 2nd edn. Boston: Little Brown, 1992: 864–72.

Starzl TE, Iwatsuki S, Shaw BW. Left hepatic trisegmentectomy. *Surg Gynecol Obstet* 1982; 155: 21–7.

Special considerations in hepatic resection for malignant disease

O. James Garden BSc, MD, FRCS(Ed), FRCS(Glas)
Senior Lecturer and Honorary Consultant Hepatobiliary Surgeon, University Department of Surgery and Scottish Liver Transplantation Unit, Royal Infirmary, Edinburgh, UK

Henri Bismuth MD, FACS, FRCS(Ed)
Professor of Surgery and Chairman of the Hepatobiliary Centre, Paul Brousse Hospital, Villejuif, France

Principles and justification

Through careful surveillance of 'high-risk' groups of patients by means of improved radiological imaging of the liver and the use of tumour markers, small, often asymptomatic, hepatic lesions are now more frequently detected than formerly. Extensive classical hepatic resections are inappropriate for such small lesions which, when they arise in cirrhotic patients, require the surgeon to preserve as much functioning tissue as possible. The improved anatomical descriptions of the liver have facilitated such segmental liver resections[1-3].

In addition to being able to tailor the type of resection to the individual patient, it has been recognized that morbidity and mortality can be reduced during major and minor hepatic resection by minimizing blood loss and avoiding impairment of the blood supply to the remaining parenchyma. This has led to the development of selective vascular exclusion techniques for use during segmental resection, and of total vascular exclusion of the liver for excision of large tumours involving the hepatic veins[4-6].

Preoperative techniques

A number of preoperative techniques may be employed to minimize the extent of hepatic resection and reduce the risks of postoperative liver failure. In some patients with tumour confined to the liver, systemic chemotherapy may be used to reduce tumour bulk. Hepatic arterial perfusional chemotherapy can be considered in patients in whom there is doubt about the prospects of achieving curative hepatic resection at the time of referral. However, any potential benefit to the patient has to be balanced against the need for an additional laparotomy and the potential risk of hepatic artery thrombosis which would preclude any future attempt at resection.

1a–c One technique which has proved successful in the authors' units has been that of chemoembolization which can be used, not only to reduce tumour bulk, but also to promote hypertrophy of the residual liver. Selective cannulation of the hepatic artery using a transfemoral approach enables instillation of lipiodol and a chemotherapeutic agent such as adriamycin. Although this may produce some mild disturbance of liver function, hepatic pain and fever, further evaluation of the tumour 6–8 weeks later will still demonstrate the embolic material and enables assessment of tumour response. Reduction in tumour size relative to the residual liver may mean that the resection can be less extensive than initially envisaged. *Illustration 1a* is a CT scan of the abdomen showing a diffuse hepatoma in the right posterior sector of the liver. After embolization of the appropriate hepatic artery with lipiodol and adriamycin the appearances at 3 and 6 months are shown in *Illustrations 1b* and *1c*.

Segmental resection

Where a small tumour occupies one or two segments of the liver, resection can be undertaken by either a partial hepatectomy, segmental resection or wedge resection. Segmental resection is anatomically based and is less likely to leave residual tumour, to result in substantial blood loss or to compromise the blood supply to the remaining liver. It also conserves functioning hepatic parenchyma when compared with more extensive resections. Segmental resections should be specifically considered for the following lesions: (1) hepatocellular carcinoma in a cirrhotic liver; (2) centrally situated hepatic metastases; (3) hilar cholangiocarcinoma; and (4) carcinoma of the gallbladder. Intrahepatic calculi and hepatic trauma are non-malignant conditions which may also be dealt with by segmental resection.

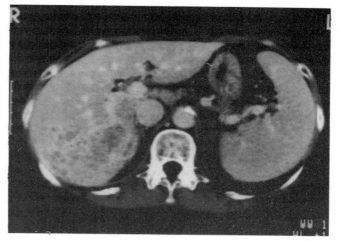

1a

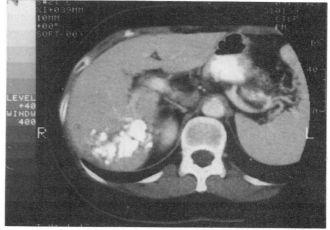

1b

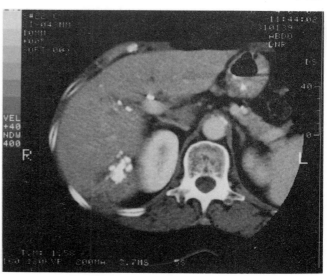

1c

Preoperative

The preoperative and peroperative management of patients undergoing segmental resection is identical to that for patients undergoing major hepatic resection.

Operations

Access to the liver is achieved by an extended right subcostal incision and the degree of mobilization of the liver depends on the procedure to be undertaken. For segmental resection on the right side of the liver total mobilization of the liver is necessary, whereas for anterior lesions involving segment IV complete mobilization can be avoided. Intraoperative ultrasonography is essential to demonstrate the relationship of the lesion to the intrahepatic vessels.

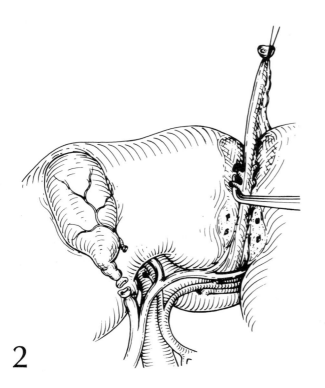

2

Vascular control

Segmental resection in a non-cirrhotic liver can be undertaken without any vascular control and without the risk of excessive bleeding. When necessary, blood loss can be minimized by employing the following techniques: suprahilar vascular exclusion; pedicular or sectoral occlusion; hilar occlusion (Pringle manoeuvre); total vascular exclusion; *in situ ex vivo* resection; *ex situ ex vivo* resection. Both techniques of *ex vivo* resection have been employed for the resection of multiple and complex hepatic tumours. Any apparent advantage is outweighed by the need to reconstitute the vascular attachments of the liver and the bile duct[7] so that *ex vivo* resection is not commonly undertaken.

Suprahilar vascular exclusion

The transverse bisegmental resection of segments IV and V illustrates well the technique of suprahilar vascular control and is normally undertaken for gallbladder carcinoma.

2 The dissection commences with isolation of the cystic duct and artery which are then divided between ligatures. The falciform ligament is incised and the round ligament is held taut by the assistant. Any bridge of liver between segments III and IV is incised by diathermy and then divided using an ultrasonic dissector (Cavitron). This manoeuvre exposes the subsegmental pedicles supplying segment IV. These pedicles may be prominent enough to be secured with a ligature mounted on a Lahey right-angled dissecting forceps. Occasionally, the capsule of the liver has to be incised with diathermy and the Cavitron is then employed to skeletonize the pedicles before ligature and division.

3 As the subsegmental pedicles are secured, a line of demarcation becomes apparent in the anterior portion of segment IV which separates viable from non-viable liver. The dissection is carried down to the undersurface of segment IV at the hilar plate, the left hepatic duct being carefully swept away from the undersurface of segment IV as the dissection is continued into the gallbladder bed.

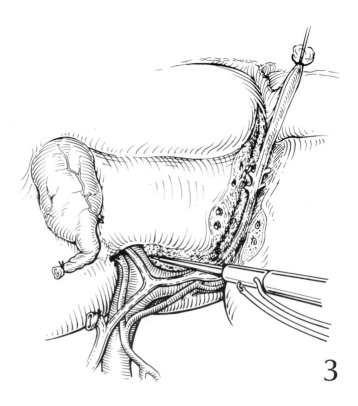

3

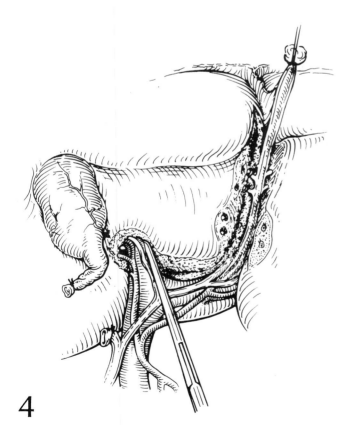

4

4 In this bloodless plane, the anterior sectoral pedicle of the right liver can be skeletonized, thereby allowing the pedicle to segment V to be identified. This pedicle is again secured with ties using Lahey forceps. Once the segmental pedicle has been divided, the line of demarcation between the two segments and the rest of the liver is identified.

5 The liver capsule is incised using diathermy, the line of incision running approximately 0.5 cm from the viable liver. It is preferable to begin this dissection on the free edge of segment IV and then to move transversely to the right of the liver, dividing the terminal portion of the middle hepatic vein between ties. Any small vessels can be divided following diathermy or ligature. When opening up the plane between segments V and VI, care should be taken to avoid damage to the right hepatic vein which should be preserved on the segment IV side. Once the dissection has been carried posteriorly towards the hilar plate, the specimen can be removed and haemostasis secured.

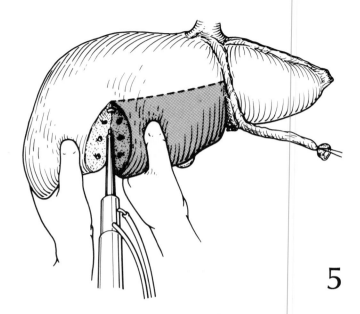

5

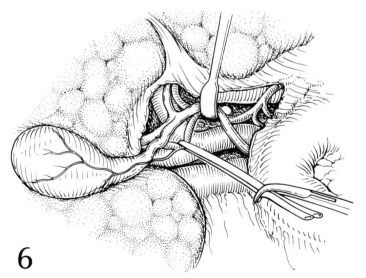

6

Segmental or subsegmental resection with ultrasound-guided suprahilar control

6 Since this resection is generally undertaken for right-sided segmental lesions, the right hemiliver is mobilized from its peritoneal attachments and the right hepatic artery is dissected at the hilus of the liver and secured with a Silastic sling.

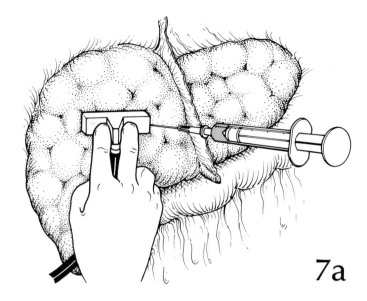

7a

7a, b The portal branch corresponding to the segment to be resected is identified by careful positioning of a 7.5 MHz linear array ultrasound transducer. Once the portal venous supply to the segment has been identified, it is punctured in its longitudinal axis with a 22 gauge Chiba needle. The position in the vein is confirmed by ultrasonography and by aspiration of venous blood on withdrawal of the stillette. A flexible guidewire is passed into the portal vein before the fine gauge needle is withdrawn.

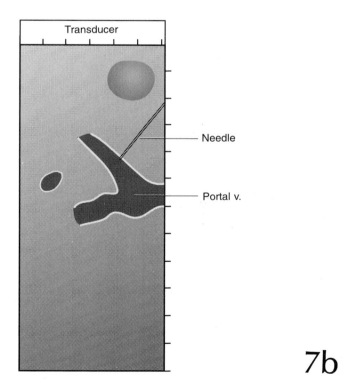

7b

8 A dilator and 5-Fr introducing catheter are passed into the portal venous branch over the guidewire. A 5-Fr balloon catheter is passed through the seal of the introducer catheter before the balloon is inflated with up to 1 ml of isotonic saline and positioned under ultrasound guidance so that it occludes the portal segmental vein. The right hepatic artery is clamped to delineate the segment to be excised, and the segment can be further outlined by injecting methylene blue dye in the side port of the introducing catheter.

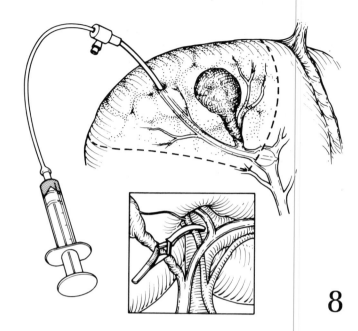

8

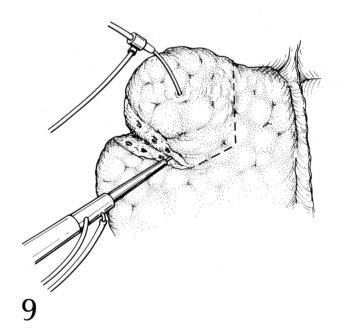

9

9 Resection of the involved segment is undertaken using standard techniques, and more substantial vessels are best ligated with 4/0 silk ties. Once the resection is complete, the right hepatic artery is unclamped and the balloon is deflated before removing it and the introducer catheter from the vessel which is secured by a 4/0 silk suture.

Pedicular or sectoral occlusion

Isolation of the right or left portal pedicles will allow resection of lesions in either the right or left hemiliver. For lesions situated in the right liver, isolation of the anterior or posterior sectoral pedicles may assist in controlling blood loss during segmental resection without compromising the function of the non-resected liver.

10 For lesions involving the right side of the liver, it is preferable to dissect out the right branch of the portal vein and right hepatic artery as for a right hepatectomy, but merely to encircle these vessels with Silastic slings so that clamps can be applied during the segmental resection.

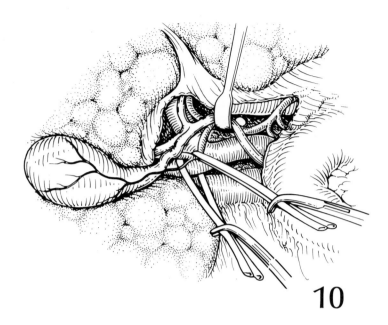

10

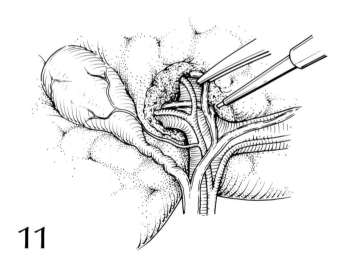

11

11 For lesions situated in segments V and VIII, it may be possible to isolate the anterior sectoral pedicle within the liver substance by incising the capsule of segment IV as it meets the porta hepatis and by extending the plane of dissection laterally into the gallbladder bed. This dissection is greatly facilitated by the Cavitron dissector. There is a variable amount of hepatic parenchyma at this site and the plane of dissection may be identified by intraoperative ultrasonography.

Hilar occlusion

12 During any form of hepatic resection, blood loss may be minimized by mass clamping the porta hepatis. This is usually effected by placing the left index finger through the gastroepiploic foramen and incising the lesser omentum lateral to the left hepatic artery and portal vein. By guiding a right-angled dissector through the lesser omental defect, a Silastic sling or tape can be used to encircle the porta hepatis. A soft occlusion clamp can then be readily applied at the porta hepatis. There are no strict guidelines as to the duration of portal clamping, but it is the authors' practice to apply the clamp for periods of no more than 20 min, releasing the clamp for 5-min periods in order to minimize the risk of compromising liver function.

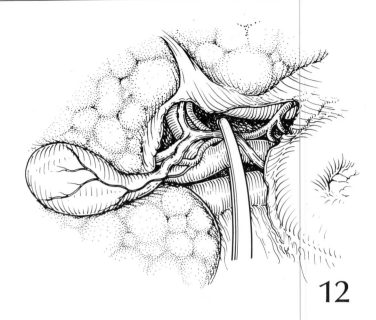

12

Total vascular exclusion

Safe resection of large centrally placed lesions may only be achieved by first establishing control of the vena cava and the hepatic veins.

13 The liver is completely mobilized by dividing the triangular ligaments and by exposing the inferior vena cava on its right side. The caval side of the divided right adrenal vein is sutured to avoid bleeding during manipulation of the liver and clamps. The vein is not divided if the infrahepatic caval clamp can be applied above the adrenal vein. The cava is mobilized above the liver following division of the lesser omentum and clearance of the tissues on the left hand border of the vena cava. The suprahepatic cava is encircled by careful placement of a tape. The infrahepatic cava is similarly mobilized and encircled with a second tape, taking care to avoid damaging any lumbar veins posteriorly.

Vascular exclusion is achieved by applying a vascular clamp to the hepatic pedicle to occlude inflow and the vena cava is then clamped below and above the liver. The circulating blood volume is expanded with crystalloid fluids before clamping; central venous pressures in excess of $12\,\mathrm{cmH_2O}$ are avoided during vascular exclusion so as to prevent excessive hepatic venous bleeding after release of the clamps. An initial trial exclusion is undertaken for a period of up to 5 min to ensure that both the systemic blood pressure and pulmonary wedge venous pressure are maintained. Once the surgeon and the anaesthetist are agreed that the procedure can be tolerated by the patient, the

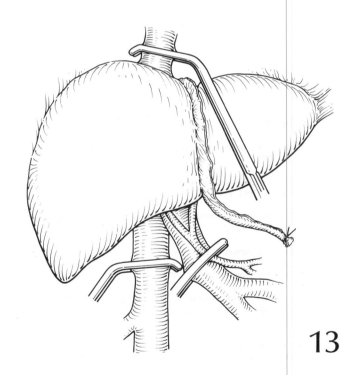

13

clamps are reapplied and the resection undertaken. The techniques previously described for hepatic resection and haemostasis are employed. Small vessels on the resected surface of the liver can be coagulated using argon diathermy and can be sealed with thrombin glue. The glue is allowed to dry before removing the clamps in the reverse order to that in which they were initially placed.

Postoperative care

Selective use of the resectional techniques described will minimize morbidity and mortality. When such surgical procedures are undertaken safely, hepatic dysfunction will be reduced in the postoperative period and hepatic regeneration will be observed within a few weeks.

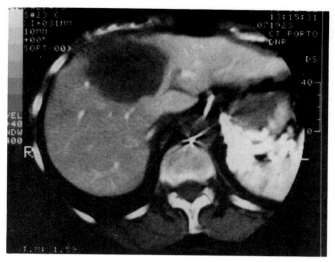

14a

14a, b
A CT scan of the abdomen is shown in *Illustration 14a* with a metastasis from colorectal cancer occupying liver segments IV, V and VII. The CT scan in *Illustration 14b* taken 6 months later shows hypertrophy of the residual liver after excision of the tumour.

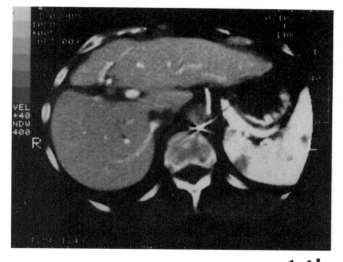

14b

References

1. Couinaud C. *Le Foie: Etude Anatomique et Chirurgicale*. Paris: Masson, 1957.

2. Bismuth H. Surgical anatomy and anatomical surgery of the liver. *World J Surg* 1982; 6: 3–9.

3. Tung TT, Quang ND. A new technique for operating on the liver. *Lancet* 1963; i: 192–3.

4. Shimamura Y, Gunven P, Takenaka Y, Shimizu H, Akimoto H, Shima Y. Selective portal branch occlusion by balloon catheter during liver resection. *Surgery* 1986; 100: 938–41.

5. Castaing D, Garden OJ, Bismuth H. Segmental liver resection using ultrasound-guided selective portal venous occlusion. *Ann Surg* 1989; 210: 20–3.

6. Bismuth H, Castaing D, Garden OJ. Major hepatic resection under total vascular exclusion. *Ann Surg* 1989; 210: 13–19.

7. Pichlmayr R, Grosse H, Hauss J, Gubernatis G, Lamesch P, Bretschneider HJ. Technique and preliminary results of extracorporeal liver surgery (bench procedure) and of surgery on the in situ perfused liver. *Br J Surg* 1990; 77: 21–6.

Further reading

Bismuth H, Castaing D, Garden OJ. Segmental surgery of the liver. In Nyhus LM, ed. *Surgery Annual 1988*. Norwalk: Appleton and Lange, 1988: 291–310.

Illustrations by Angela Christie

Management of hepatic malignancy by hepatic arterial infusion of chemotherapy

Colin S. McArdle MD, FRCS, FRCS(Glas), FRCS(Ed)
Consultant Surgeon, University Department of Surgery, Royal Infirmary, Glasgow, UK

The results of systemic chemotherapy for patients with multiple liver metastases secondary to colorectal cancer are disappointing. For example, single agent 5-fluorouracil has a response rate of approximately 10–15%. Most cytotoxic drugs have a steep dose-response curve, but attempts to increase the response rate by escalating the dose has been limited by unacceptable toxicity. Since colorectal liver metastases of more than 1 cm in diameter receive their blood supply predominantly from the hepatic artery, the intra-arterial route of delivery would appear to be preferable.

Intra-arterial therapy is based on the premise that, if cytotoxic drugs are delivered selectively to a tumour-bearing organ, higher levels of exposure to tumour drug and hence higher response rates can be achieved. In addition, depending on the proportion of drug extracted within that organ, systemic drug levels and hence systemic toxicity may be low.

Early attempts to use the intra-arterial route in patients with colorectal liver metastases were abandoned because of the high incidence of complications such as catheter displacement, sepsis and gastroduodenal haemorrhage. The recent introduction of inert siliconized catheters connected to implantable, refillable subcutaneous ports or pumps has led to renewed interest in intra-arterial chemotherapy.

Anatomy

In patients with classical anatomy the common hepatic artery arises from the coeliac axis and gives off the gastroduodenal branch before dividing into right and left hepatic arteries (*see* page 83). Anatomical variations are common (*Table 1*) and include trifurcation, where the gastroduodenal branch originates less than 2 cm from the bifurcation of the common hepatic artery or where the origin of the left hepatic artery lies proximal to the gastroduodenal branch. Approximately 20% of patients have a dual blood supply. Most commonly, the right hepatic artery arises from the superior mesenteric artery while the left hepatic artery (with its gastroduodenal branch) originates from the coeliac axis. Less frequently, the left hepatic artery arises from the left gastric artery while the right hepatic artery (with its gastroduodenal branch) arises from the coeliac axis. Rarely, the liver has a triple supply from branches of the superior mesenteric artery, coeliac axis and left gastric artery.

Table 1   Frequency (%) of anomalous hepatic arterial anatomy

Normal	65
Abnormal	35
Trifurcation	9
Early origin of left hepatic artery	3
Common origin of coeliac axis and superior mesenteric artery	5
Right hepatic artery originating from superior mesenteric artery	14
Left hepatic artery originating from left gastric artery	4

Preoperative

Before surgery a computed tomographic (CT) scan of the chest and abdomen is performed to exclude extrahepatic disease and to measure the extent of hepatic replacement. Locoregional recurrence is excluded by barium enema, colonoscopy or CT scan of pelvis, as appropriate. Histological confirmation of liver metastases is obtained by ultrasound- or CT-guided fine needle aspiration or Tru-Cut biopsy. Selective coeliac axis and superior mesenteric angiography is advisable to establish the vascular anatomy.

Anaesthesia

Most patients are relatively elderly and careful preoperative anaesthetic assessment is required. Coagulation status should be checked but is seldom abnormal.

Standard antithrombotic measures including subcutaneous heparin and compression stockings are employed. Although blood loss is usually minimal, in patients with greatly enlarged livers the combination of difficult access and increased portal venous pressure may result in increased blood loss. In these patients it is prudent to monitor central venous and intra-arterial pressure throughout surgery. All patients are catheterized to monitor urinary output.

Operation

Depending on the position of previous scars, the abdomen may be opened through an upper midline or right subcostal incision. Formal laparotomy is undertaken to detect locoregional recurrence or extrahepatic disease. If unsuspected local recurrence is present, it may be possible to resect the recurrence and then insert the hepatic artery catheter. The presence of enlarged lymph nodes around the hepatic artery need not preclude insertion of a catheter; biopsy and frozen section may determine whether such nodes are infiltrated with tumour.

1 In most patients the hepatic artery and its gastroduodenal branch are easily palpated. The common hepatic artery is dissected free by incising the overlying peritoneum and, if necessary, by mobilizing the superior aspect of the first part of the duodenum. As the common hepatic and gastroduodenal arteries are identified, sloops are passed around them and, depending on the anatomy, it may also be advisable to pass sloops around the hepatic artery proper and the right and left hepatic arteries. Gentle traction on the sloops facilitates further dissection and identification of other branches, in particular the right gastric artery and the many small branches running posteriorly from the gastroduodenal artery to the duodenum and pancreas. These vessels should be ligated or diathermy applied to avoid unwanted perfusion of the lesser curve of stomach and adjacent organs. To avoid the possibility of chemical cholecystitis, cholecystectomy is performed. A subcutaneous pocket over the right lower ribs is then prepared, the port is secured in position and the arterial catheter passed through the anterior abdominal wall. Depending on the type of arterial catheter used, it may need to be trimmed in length before use.

The gastroduodenal artery is ligated 2–3 cm from its origin. Flow through the common hepatic artery and the hepatic artery proper should be temporarily occluded using bulldog clamps. The gastroduodenal artery is then opened through a longitudinal arteriotomy and the tip of the beaded catheter inserted retrogradely so that its tip lies at the origin of the gastroduodenal artery, thereby gaining access to the hepatic artery without compromising hepatic arterial flow. The use of fine stay sutures to hold the arteriotomy open may facilitate this manoeuvre. The beaded tip of the catheter is held in position by non-absorbable silk or linen ties, the ties being placed immediately above and below the bead. It is important that these ties are tight enough to prevent dislodgement of the catheter but not so tight as to occlude the lumen. The adequacy of liver perfusion can then be checked by injecting methylene blue through the port. After the operation the patency of the catheter is maintained by flushing weekly with heparinized saline.

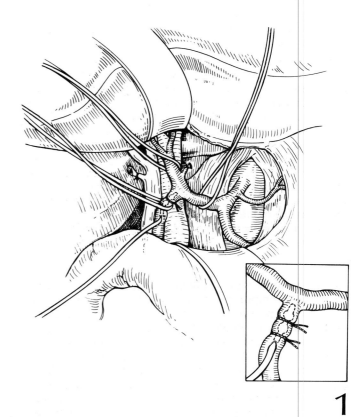

1

If the primary tumour is being resected at the same operation, the hepatic artery catheter is inserted first. The peritoneal cavity is then lavaged with warm saline and the transverse mesocolon clipped to the wound, thus isolating the supracolic compartment and restricting the spread of infection. After the primary tumour has been resected the infracolic compartment is copiously lavaged with warm saline before closure.

2 In patients with a trifurcation, cannulation of the gastroduodenal artery often leads to poor mixing of injectate and uneven distribution in the liver due to streaming. In these patients adequate liver perfusion may be obtained by inserting the catheter retrogradely into the splenic artery. The common hepatic artery is followed back to the coeliac axis and the proximal 2–3 cm of the splenic artery is then mobilized. Additional access can be gained through the lesser sac, if required. The artery is ligated distally and the catheter inserted retrogradely into the splenic artery so that its tip lies at the origin of the artery; the gastroduodenal artery is then ligated. Alternatively, a saphenous vein graft (*see later*) can be anastomosed proximal to the trifurcation to act as a conduit for the catheter.

In patients where the left hepatic artery arises proximal to the gastroduodenal artery, it is usually possible to achieve adequate cross-perfusion via the right hepatic artery having ligated the left hepatic artery.

In patients with a dual blood supply (in whom the branchless right hepatic artery arises from the superior mesenteric artery while the left hepatic artery with its gastroduodenal branch originates from the coeliac axis), the right hepatic artery should be identified as it lies behind the common bile duct in the free edge of the gastrohepatic ligament. A catheter can then be inserted into the gastroduodenal branch of the left hepatic artery. The contribution of the right hepatic artery to liver perfusion can be assessed by temporarily occluding the vessel. In patients with a non-dominant right hepatic artery, in whom adequate perfusion of the right lobe may be obtained by allowing cross-perfusion from the left hepatic artery, the right hepatic artery can then be formally ligated.

3 In patients with a dominant right hepatic artery, where temporary occlusion of the vessel results in inadequate perfusion of the right lobe, adequate perfusion can be achieved by inserting two catheters, one into the gastroduodenal artery to perfuse the left lobe and a second into the right hepatic artery using a saphenous vein graft. A 5–6-cm portion of long saphenous vein is prepared and anastomosed end-to-side to the unbranching right hepatic artery as it lies in the free fold of the gastrohepatic ligament. The catheter is then introduced into the vein graft so that the tip lies at the anastomosis. In this way the saphenous vein graft acts as a conduit for the catheter.

In those patients in whom the left hepatic artery arises from the left gastric artery while the right hepatic artery, with its gastroduodenal branch, arises from the coeliac artery, adequate perfusion can usually be achieved by ligating the non-dominant left hepatic artery (or the left gastric artery) and inserting a catheter into the gastroduodenal branch of the dominant right hepatic artery.

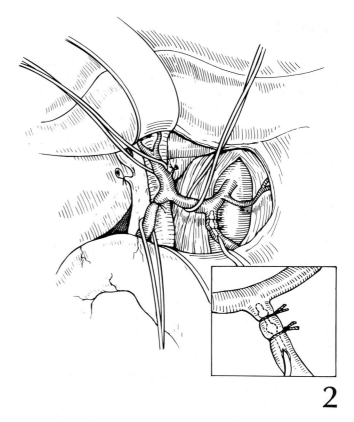

2

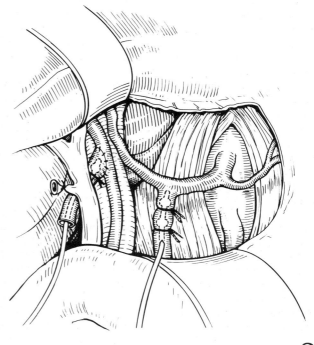

3

Postoperative care

After surgery all patients should receive prophylactic H_2 antagonists to reduce the risk of gastroduodenal ulceration. Catheters should be flushed weekly with heparinized saline.

Complications

If the subcutaneous port becomes infected during the immediate postoperative period, the collection should be drained and packed. Eventually the port will be extruded from the granulating subcutaneous 'pocket'. With care the catheter can still be used for treatment by soaking the extruded port in antiseptic solution for 20 minutes before injection of chemotherapy and simply wrapping it in a dry dressing when not in use. After 3 months the extruded port and exposed segment of the catheter can be excised, leaving the distal end *in situ*. A new port and catheter can be positioned at a fresh site and a double-ended male metal connecting piece used to join the two catheters.

Thrombosis of the catheter is inevitable with time. Suspected thrombosis can be confirmed radiologically by injecting contrast medium via the port. If replacement of the catheter is desirable, angiography should be performed to demonstrate the site of occlusion and confirm that the hepatic artery remains patent.

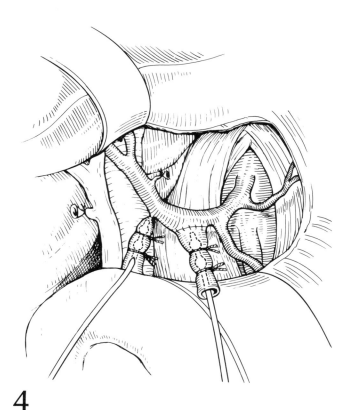

4 A replacement catheter can then be inserted proximal to the blocked catheter using a saphenous vein graft. At laparotomy the common hepatic artery is mobilized proximal to the insertion of the blocked catheter and a segment of vein anastomosed end-to-side to the hepatic artery. The replacement catheter is then inserted into the vein graft so that the tip lies flush with the hepatic artery.

Gastrointestinal bleeding may occur. Endoscopy usually confirms the presence of duodenitis or an area of gastritis in the lesser curve of the antrum. Frank ulceration is seldom present. Further intervention is not normally required and the bleeding usually settles spontaneously. Further bleeding can be prevented by the use of omeprazole.

The ideal chemotherapy regimen for hepatic artery infusion is still to be defined but 5-fluorouracil and floxuridine are among the agents used to date. Depending on the chemotherapy regimen used, systemic side effects including nausea, vomiting, diarrhoea, dehydration and mucositis may occur. Clearly these patients require to be looked after by a dedicated team of clinicians and nurses familiar with the administration and toxic side effects of intra-arterial chemotherapy.

Outcome

Several studies where the results of intra-arterial therapy have been compared with those of systemic therapy have recently been reviewed. Response rates were consistently higher with intra-arterial therapy, although this did not always translate into a survival advantage. This may have been due in part to the small numbers in some studies and the crossover design employed in others. Although these preliminary results are encouraging, further studies are required to determine the optimal chemotherapy regimen. Until then, intra-arterial chemotherapy must be regarded as offering potential rather than proven benefit to patients with liver metastases.

Further reading

Allen-Mersh TG, Earlam S, Fordy C, Abrams K, Houghton J. Quality of life and survival with continuous hepatic artery floxuridine infusion for colorectal liver metastases. *Lancet* 1994; 344: 1255–60.

Kemeny N. Review of regional therapy of liver metastases in colorectal cancer. *Semin Oncol* 1992; 19(Suppl. 3): 155–62.

Rougier P, Laplanche A, Huguier M *et al*. Hepatic arterial infusion of floxuridine in patients with liver metastases from colorectal carcinoma: long term results of a prospective randomised trial. *J Clin Oncol* 1992; 10: 1112–8.

Warren HW, Anderson JH, O'Gorman P *et al*. A phase II study of regional 5-fluorouracil infusion with intravenous folinic acid for colorectal liver metastases. *Br J Cancer* 1994; 70: 677–80.

Illustrations by Gillian Oliver

Liver transplantation

Tariq Ismail MD, FRCS
Senior Registrar in Surgery, The Liver and Hepatobiliary Unit, The Queen Elizabeth Hospital, Edgbaston, Birmingham, UK

Ben-Hur Ferraz-Neto MD
Transplant Fellow, The Liver and Hepatobiliary Unit, The Queen Elizabeth Hospital, Edgbaston, Birmingham, UK

Paul McMaster MCh, FRCS
Consultant Surgeon, The Liver and Hepatobiliary Unit, The Queen Elizabeth Hospital, Edgbaston, Birmingham, UK

History

The first heterotopic liver transplant was performed in a dog by Welch in 1955. Moore and his colleagues at the Peter Brent Brigham Hospital in Boston subsequently performed orthotopic liver transplants in dogs. The first *successful* human liver transplant was performed in 1967 by Starzl in Denver, Colorado for hepatocellular carcinoma in an 18-month-old girl who survived 13 months. In 1968 Calne reported the Cambridge experience of five liver transplants. Today, numerous centres throughout the world perform liver transplantation with over 80% of recipients surviving 1 year.

Principles and justification

Refinements in surgical technique, including non-heparin-requiring extracorporeal venovenous bypass, better organ preservation and the introduction of cyclosporin A, and more recently, FK 506 as immunosuppressants, have contributed to the improvement in results. The technique of liver transplantation is now well established, and recent innovations include segmental grafts, 'split livers' and segmental liver transplants from living-related donors.

Indications

Liver transplantation should be considered in all patients with progressive or end stage liver disease which is unresponsive to medical management. The indications for transplantation in the first 1000 transplants performed in Birmingham are listed in *Table 1*.

Table 1   Indications for liver transplantation

Indication	Number
Primary biliary cirrhosis	266
Other cirrhotics	64
Fulminant hepatic failure	140
Retransplantation	119
Primary sclerosing cholangitis	86
Biliary atresia	74
Metabolic disease	71
Chronic active hepatitis	46
Malignancy	32
Alcoholic liver disease	32
Hepatitis C	23
Hepatitis B	19
Miscellaneous causes	28

Operations

DONOR HEPATECTOMY

Donor preparation

Heart-beating, brain-stem dead individuals without systemic infection or extracranial malignant tumours are potential organ donors. Most liver retrievals are carried out as part of a multiorgan procurement and it is mandatory that the different teams discuss the techniques and sequence of organ retrieval that they wish to adopt. Key features of donor liver procurement include maintenance of the organ's anatomical integrity, recognition of vascular anomalies, and cold preservation.

Incision

1 A long midline incision running from jugular notch to pubic symphysis and including a sternal split provides adequate exposure for all procurement teams. Haemostasis is achieved with electrocautery and bone wax. The falciform ligament is cut between ligatures.

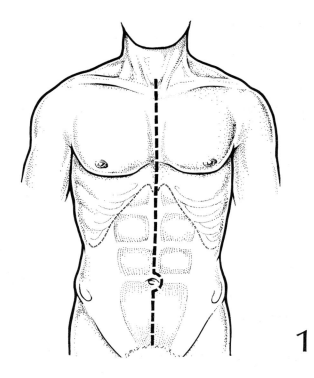

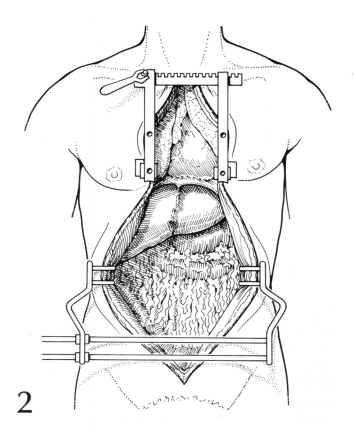

2 Exposure is aided by wide self-retaining sternal and abdominal retractors.

Evaluation and identification of anatomical variants

Once adequate exposure is obtained, the abdominal cavity is examined fully. The liver is checked for its appearance, colour, shape, size and consistency. The portal triad is examined to define variant anatomy. Great care must be taken to identify and deal with the frequent variations in hepatic arterial supply. The normal hepatic artery is located to the left of the bile duct in the hepatoduodenal ligament.

3 The right hepatic artery (or rarely the common hepatic artery) sometimes arises from the superior mesenteric artery and runs posterior to the portal vein into the right lobe of the liver. It can be located by palpation through Winslow's foramen just behind and to the right of the bile duct and can be preserved in continuity with the proximal superior mesenteric artery.

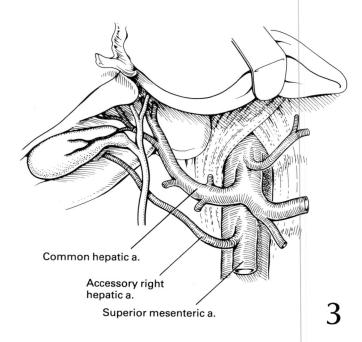

Common hepatic a.

Accessory right hepatic a.

Superior mesenteric a.

3

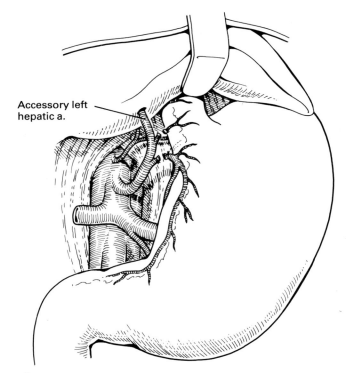

Accessory left hepatic a.

4 The left hepatic artery sometimes originates from the left gastric artery or coeliac artery and runs in the gastrohepatic ligament. Once identified, the branch of the left gastric artery to the lesser curvature of the stomach can be safely ligated and divided.

4

Dissection of retroperitoneum

The right colon, its mesentery and duodenum are mobilized to the left to expose the retroperitoneum. Both common iliac arteries are taped and the inferior mesenteric artery is ligated with silk. The right common iliac artery is mobilized in preparation for cannulation for perfusion. The inferior vena cava is carefully dissected and encircled with umbilical tape just above its bifurcation.

The next step is the dissection of the superior mesenteric vein in the base of the mesentery. The vessel is encircled with silk ties. The common hepatic artery is then taped. The left triangular ligament is sectioned and the lesser omentum divided after excluding an accessory left hepatic artery. Caudal traction maintained on the duodenum allows the common bile duct to be identified at the anterior edge of the hepatoduodenal ligament. It is dissected to the superior margin of the pancreas and transected here with a ligature on the duodenal side. The gallbladder is aspirated of bile and the biliary tree irrigated through it with normal saline until drainage from the cut end of the bile duct is clear. The superior mesenteric artery may be ligated, provided an anomalous right hepatic artery has been excluded and the pancreas is not to be retrieved.

By incising the right crura of the diaphragm, the aorta is exposed. The supracoeliac aorta at the level of the right crus is dissected through the preaortic fascia and surrounded by a tape.

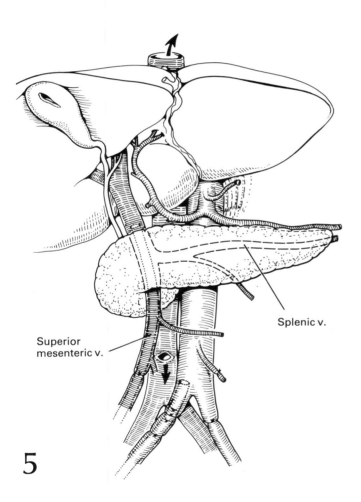

Splenic v.

Superior
mesenteric v.

5

Cold preservation and perfusion

5 The donor liver is heparinized (300 units/kg body weight). A cannula is introduced into the distal aorta via the right common iliac artery and secured. The left common iliac artery is ligated. A cannula is placed into the superior mesenteric vein, positioned in the portal vein just above the pancreas, and secured. The proximal aorta is then either ligated with tape or cross-clamped and the vena cava is cut infrarenally or intrathoracically as agreed with the thoracic surgeons ('vented' or 'bled out') to remove excess volume and prevent hepatic congestion. Simultaneous cold perfusion with preservation fluid via the superior mesenteric vein and aortic cannulae is begun.

Aortic and portal perfusion is achieved *in situ* with 3 litres of Marshall's and 1 litre of University of Wisconsin (UW) solutions, respectively, with gravity pressure ($60-100\,cmH_2O$). Ice slush is placed around the liver to aid surface cooling.

Cold phase dissection

This is performed when the liver is cool and blanched. In sequence, the left gastric and splenic arteries are ligated and divided. The hepatic artery is taken with the coeliac artery and a cuff of aorta. After performing a Kocher's manoeuvre the fingers of the left hand are placed behind the head and body of the pancreas while the left thumb feels the front of the neck to palpate the superior mesenteric vein. This is dissected, displaying the superior mesenteric artery on its left. Careful dissection of the right edge of the superior mesenteric artery will reveal any anomalous right hepatic artery branch.

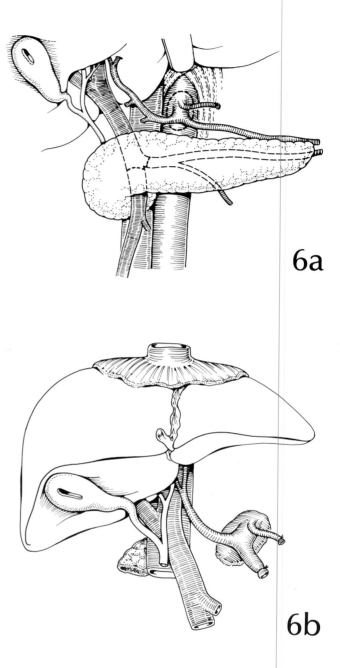

6a

6b

6a, b The aorta is divided at the supracoeliac and infracoeliac level. The superior mesenteric vein and splenic vein are divided after removal of the cannula. The subhepatic suprarenal vena cava is dissected. The right kidney is lowered, the right renal vein skeletonized so that the inferior vena cava can be divided above it, and the right adrenal is divided in half. The diaphragm is cut leaving a wide cuff containing the suprahepatic vena cava. The right and left crura are divided, completely freeing the liver.

The iliac artery and vein are also harvested in case they are required for vascular reconstruction at the recipient operation.

Back table perfusion

The donor liver is taken to the back table, placed in a bowl and given a second flush with UW solution into the hepatic artery, common bile duct (250 ml each) and portal vein (500 ml). The liver is placed in fresh solution (Marshall's or UW) and the bowl is placed in two sterile plastic bags which are vacuumed with suction and placed in an ice box for storage and transport.

Back table preparation of the liver

Graft preparation is carried out at the transplant centre, usually by the same retrieval team. The liver is kept in its preservation fluid and surrounded by ice slush to maintain the temperature at 4°C. The back table work involves preparation for venous and arterial anastomoses and repair of any iatrogenic injuries.

A precise methodical approach in a craniocaudal direction is essential. Excess diaphragm, fat, lymphatic and adrenal tissue are removed and collateral vessels (especially the phrenic and adrenal veins) are carefully ligated. The vena cava can be filled with UW solution to detect any untied collateral veins. The portal vein is then pressure tested and collaterals are ligated. The hepatic artery is skeletonized from its Carrel patch at the coeliac trifurcation, but not proximally as this may devascularize the bile duct.

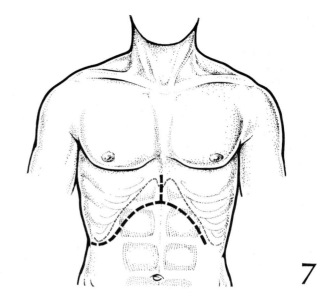

RECIPIENT HEPATECTOMY

Incision

7 A bilateral subcostal incision with an upper midline extension, removing the xiphoid process, usually gives excellent exposure for the recipient operation. Haemostasis of the wound is essential.

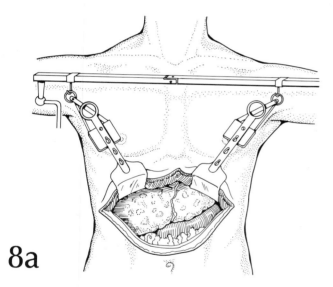

8a

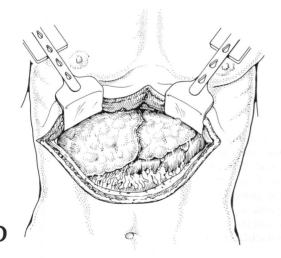

8b

Exposure

8a, b Optimal exposure is achieved by adjustable self-retaining retractors fixed to a Rochard bar.

The falciform ligament is ligated and divided. Extensive vascular adhesions are often present, especially in cirrhotic patients, as a result of preoperative invasive procedures or previous surgery. These require careful ligation. This can be a difficult and dangerous dissection because of venous collaterals in portal hypertension.

9 Dissection is commenced at the level of the cystic duct, freeing all peritoneal reflections. The common bile duct is ligated close to the liver and divided. The hepatic artery is then freed to beyond the gastroduodenal artery, carefully preserving the blood supply to the bile duct. The right gastric artery is usually ligated and divided. Skeletonization of the portal vein now begins, freeing it from periportal lymph nodes (sometimes large, friable and highly vascular) and collaterals. A long section of the vessel is exposed from the hilum to the upper edge of the pancreas.

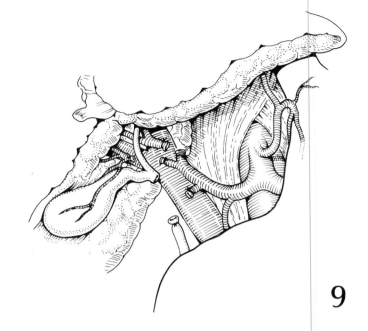

9

Venovenous bypass

Most patients have significant portal hypertension and flows of up to 2 litres are often achieved. In patients without spontaneous portal systemic shunts, use of bypass is advantageous in maintaining cerebral perfusion. If the portal vein is thrombosed, the inferior mesenteric vein can be used to achieve portal decompression. Pump-driven venovenous bypass without systemic heparinization is now used routinely during the anhepatic phase of the recipient operation. This has permitted technical modifications, decreased transfusion and fluid requirements, and reduced cardiopulmonary and renal complications by providing a more haemodynamically stable anhepatic phase.

10 The left axillary vein is explored through a 3–4-cm longitudinal skin incision in the apex of the axilla. The vein is cannulated with a large-bore catheter and tied distally. The authors do not routinely reconstruct the vein after use. The right saphenofemoral junction is next exposed through a 5-cm longitudinal incision in the groin and the long saphenous vein is cannulated with a Gott tube passed into the iliac veins and inferior vena cava. The portal vein is then tied close to the liver, divided and the distal (recipient) end is held open with three haemostats by an assistant while the operator occludes the portal vein with the thumb and index finger. A Gott tube is now inserted for 5–8 cm into the portal vein and then secured. Bypass is established from the saphenofemoral and portal veins with return via the axillary vein.

The authors have also performed portoaxillary bypass only without significant haemodynamic or postoperative sequelae, especially in patients with established portal hypertension.

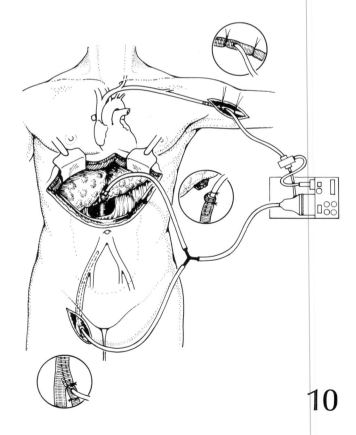

10

Hepatectomy

11 The liver is now skeletonized. The left and right triangular ligaments, the left coronary ligament and the lesser omentum are divided.

The suprahepatic and infrahepatic segments of the vena cava are then encircled with tape. The bare area is separated from the diaphragm and the adrenal gland. The adrenal vein is ligated in continuity and divided. If venovenous bypass is used, the lower vena cava is next trial clamped. Provided haemodynamic stability is maintained this is followed by cross-clamping of the suprahepatic vena cava which is then divided inside the liver leaving as long a segment of recipient cava as is possible. After the infrahepatic cava has been divided the hepatectomy is completed and the specimen removed.

Haemostasis of the retroperitoneum is achieved using electrocautery, argon beam coagulation, suturing and fibrin glue (Tis-Seal). Coagulation status is monitored by conventional tests and thromboelastography during the operation.

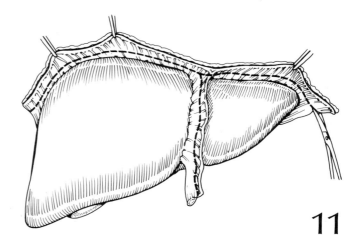

11

IMPLANTATION PHASE

Suprahepatic vena cava

This is the most important vascular anastomosis because, if the available donor and recipient vessels are short, exposure in the presence of the new liver can be difficult and the posterior part of the anastomosis cannot easily be re-exposed if control is required later. If the vessels are too long, kinking and venous outflow obstruction may occur.

12 The donor graft, once in position, can be retracted towards the assistant with his left hand on the right lobe to facilitate exposure. The posterior walls of the vessels are anastomosed by a 3/0 continuous polypropylene (Prolene) suture from within the lumen after placing initial stay sutures in the extremities. The formation of an intraluminal shoulder posteriorly in both donor and recipient vessels, full thickness bites, and an everting over and over anterior row with a single knot complete the anastomosis.

Infrahepatic vena cava

The lower inferior vena cava is anastomosed in a similar fashion, including intraluminal suture of the posterior wall using 4/0 polypropylene. Just before completion of the anterior wall, a cannula is inserted into the donor cava to facilitate outflow of washout fluid on reperfusion. The last stitch is not tied at this stage.

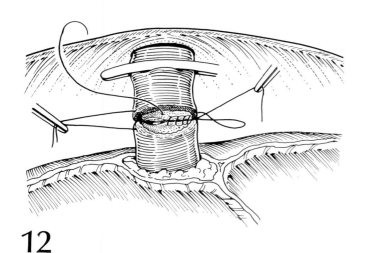

12

Portal vein

The portal limb of the bypass is clamped, the cannula removed and the portal vein checked for the presence of clot. Excess lengths of both host and graft vein are excised to allow approximation without kinking, tension, twisting or narrowing. The continuous intraluminal technique using 5/0 polypropylene is employed.

13 Before completion a cannula is inserted into the donor portal vein and the graft is washed out with 1 litre of 5% dextrose solution at 37°C to rinse out the preservation fluid and other metabolites via the infrahepatic vena cava. The authors have recently used a blood flush from the portal vein which requires transfusion of usually no more than 1 unit of blood.

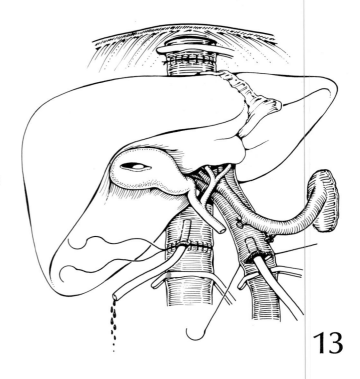

13

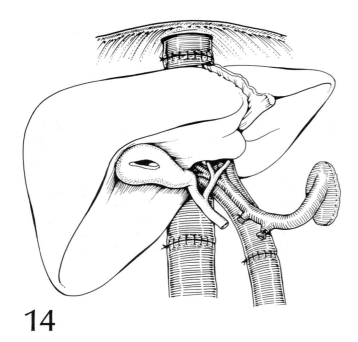

14

14 The portal cannula is removed, the portal vein clamp momentarily released to flush out any clot, and the anastomosis is completed. The knot is tied some distance from the vein. This growth factor technique allows expansion and prevents pursestringing. Hepatic reperfusion may now take place by releasing first the lower, and then the upper caval clamps.

The clamp on the recipient portal vein is removed and, if the anastomosis is intact, the clamp on the donor portal vein is also removed. The portal venous inflow is controlled by digital compression with careful monitoring of haemodynamic parameters. The warm ischaemic time for these three anastomoses should be 30–60 min.

Hypotension and changes in right-sided pressures and ECG are frequently observed but are usually transient, although a defibrillator is always on standby in this critical phase. If portal vein thombosis is suspected in the recipient before the operation, arterioportography is essential to map out venous anatomy. In such cases, continuity can be achieved by a donor iliac conduit to the infrapancreatic superior mesenteric vein. Alternatively, a large collateral vein or left gastric vein may be anastomosed to the donor portal vein.

Hepatic artery

This is the most delicate and the most important phase of the whole transplant procedure. Thrombotic complications nearly always result in retransplantation.

15 The recipient artery is dissected and trimmed back, usually to the junction with the gastroduodenal artery.

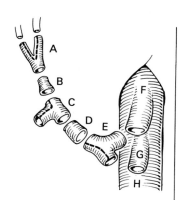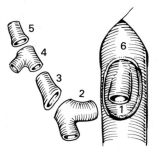

A. Bifurcation of hepatic a.
B. Hepatic artery trunk
C. Bifurcation of gastroduodenal a.
D. Common hepatic a.
E. Bifurcation of splenic a.
F. Coeliac axis
G. Superior mesenteric a.
H. Aorta

1. Aortic patch
2. Coeliac axis stem
3. Patch at splenic a.
4. Common hepatic a. stem
5. Patch at division of gastroduodenal a.
6. Aortic conduit

15

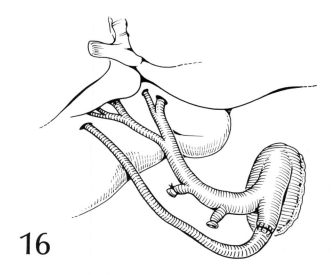

16

16 The donor vessel is anastomosed using continuous 6/0 polypropylene, usually on a patch with the splenic artery, using magnifying loops. If there is an accessory right vessel from the donor superior mesenteric artery a further reconstruction is necessary. The graft right hepatic artery is usually anastomosed to the recipient splenic artery. When a small left hepatic artery arises from the left gastric artery, the graft coeliac axis is used for anastomosis. Papaverine injected into the adventitia of the vessels may be useful to reverse vessel spasm.

Biliary drainage

17 The authors' preferred method of biliary reconstruction is by choledochocholedochostomy, with or without a T tube stent. Cholecystectomy is first performed. A continuous 5/0 polydioxanone sulphate (PDS) suture is used for the duct-to-duct anastomosis. The T tube (if used) is brought out through a small stab incision in the recipient duct. However, significant morbidity is associated with T tubes and many centres have now abandoned their use.

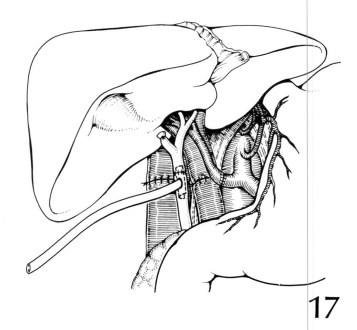

17

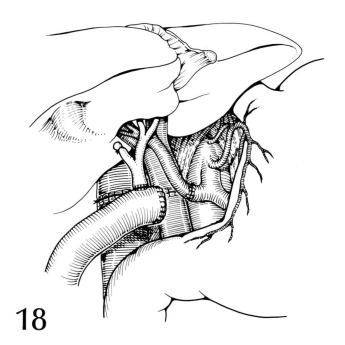

18

18 If a duct-to-duct anastomosis is not possible, as in primary sclerosing cholangitis, biliary atresia, Caroli's syndrome, paediatric recipients and some retransplants, choledochojejunostomy using a Roux limb of jejunum is preferred.

Closure

One abdominal drain is placed below the liver. Primary mass closure with continuous loop nylon with subcuticular 3/0 polypropylene to the skin is performed.

PAEDIATRIC TRANSPLANTATION

The shortage of donor organs has encouraged the development of innovative techniques.

19 Adult cadaveric livers can be reduced in size for transplantation into small infants by resection of one of the major lobes. This segmental liver grafting has provided the foundation for the development of living-related transplantation.

Many children have had previous surgery (e.g. a Kasai procedure) which increases the risk of bleeding when recipient hepatectomy is performed. Venovenous bypass is rarely used in children. If a child has had a previous Kasai portenterostomy the jejunal loop is taken down and preserved.

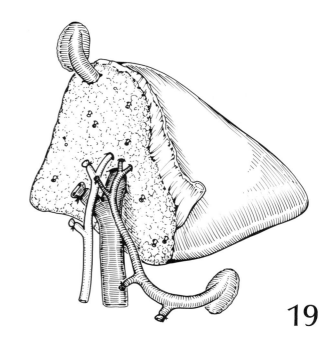

19

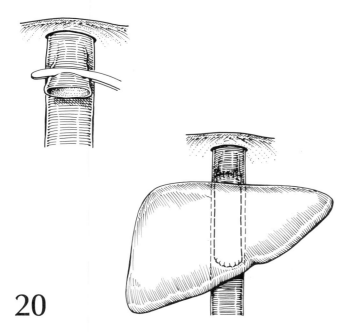

20

20 For orthotopic whole liver transplantation a segment of inferior vena cava can be sacrificed, but when a segmental graft is used the whole vena cava is preserved.

Most paediatric recipients do not have a sufficiently large bile duct or have no bile duct at all, as in biliary atresia, so that a Roux-en-Y choledochojejunostomy is usually performed.

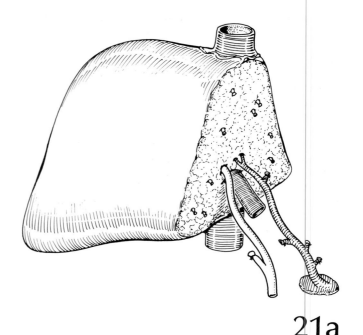

21a

21a, b The left lateral segments II and III (*see page 3*) are commonly used, the left hepatic vein being anastomosed directly to the recipient vena cava. The right hemiliver (segments V, VI, VII and VIII) with the right portal structures and inferior vena cava can be used for a second, usually adult, recipient. Thus, a single liver can be used for two recipients in this 'split liver' procedure. Segment IV is usually removed *ex vivo* and discarded.

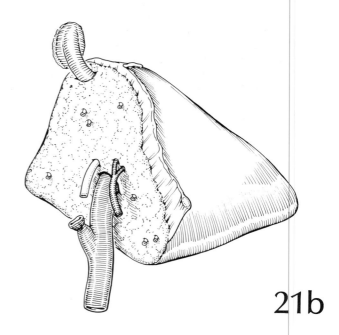

21b

LIVING-RELATED TRANSPLANTATION

Living-related donors are usually parents of the recipient who undergo extensive preparation including volumetric computed tomographic scanning, selective coeliac and mesenteric angiography and hepatic ultrasonography. Potential donors and their families need to be extensively counselled. Major ethical issues remain unresolved, however, and many transplant centres do not perform this procedure.

The principles of the operation are as follows. The donor left lateral hepatectomy (segments II and III) is performed *in vivo*. The recipient hepatectomy is performed but with the vena cava left *in situ* and without using venovenous bypass. The recipient hepatic vein confluence is anastomosed to the donor hepatic vein. An interposition vein graft to the portal vein is used and the hepatic artery is anastomosed to the infrarenal aorta. A Roux-en-Y loop of jejunum is used for biliary drainage.

Postoperative care

The monitoring instituted during surgery is continued in the intensive care unit. As the liver recovers following revascularization, potassium is taken out of the blood by the liver and the serum potassium level may fall. Potassium supplements are given with frequent checking of serum levels. There is danger of overloading the circulation and this may be avoided by monitoring the central venous pressure and pulmonary artery and wedge pressures.

Complications

One of the commonest complications in the early period is continuing haemorrhage which, if not arrested by correction of any coagulopathy, will require re-exploration. Other complications include hepatic artery thrombosis, biliary leaks, bile duct obstruction and sepsis. Acute rejection still occurs in up to 70% of patients, despite the newer immunosuppressive regimens, with a 4% graft loss due to chronic rejection. Late complications include bone disease, renal impairment, malignancy and metabolic sequelae.

Further reading

Bismuth H, Houssin D. Reduced-sized orthotopic liver graft in hepatic transplantation in children. *Surgery* 1984; 95: 367–70.

Broelsch CE, Emond JC, Whitington PF *et al*. Application of reduced-sized liver transplants as split grafts, auxiliary orthotopic grafts, and living related segmental transplants. *Ann Surg* 1990; 212: 368–77.

Calne RY, McMaster P, Bortmann B, Wall WJ, Williams R. Observations on preservation, bile drainage and rejection in 64 human orthotopic liver allografts. *Ann Surg* 1977; 186: 282–90.

Starzl TE, Demetris AJ, Van Thiel D. Liver transplantation (1). *N Engl J Med* 1989; 321: 1014–22.

Starzl TE, Demetris AJ, Van Thiel D. Liver transplantation (2). *N Engl J Med* 1989; 321: 1092–9.

Starzl TE, Porter KA, Putnam CW *et al*. Orthotopic liver transplantation in 93 patients. *Surg Gynecol Obstet* 1976; 142: 487–505.

Orthotopic liver transplantation with caval preservation

Jacques Belghiti MD
Professor of Surgery, Department of Surgery, University Paris VII and Beaujon Hospital, Clichy, France

Roger Noun MD
Assistant of Surgery, Department of Surgery, University Paris VII and Beaujon Hospital, Clichy, France

Principles and justification

Conventional orthotopic liver transplantation involves resection of the retrohepatic vena cava as part of the recipient hepatectomy, and cross-clamping of the portal vein during the anhepatic phase. The retrocaval dissection in the presence of venous collaterals is sometimes difficult, making subsequent haemostasis a problem. Total hepatic vascular exclusion is characterized by significant changes in cardiovascular indices, which include a decrease in renal perfusion pressure and stasis in the splanchnic venous bed, particularly in non-cirrhotic patients. Although venovenous bypass has been proposed in order to reduce these haemodynamic upsets, it is not feasible in children, has associated morbidity, and prolongs the operation. Several technical modifications have been introduced to preserve the recipient vena cava, caval flow and both portal and caval flows. This chapter describes preservation of caval flow during hepatectomy and graft implantation in combination with a temporary portocaval shunt as a means of avoiding haemodynamic variations, preserving renal function and preventing splanchnic stasis. The procedure now offers a viable alternative to the use of venovenous bypass.

The technique of orthotopic liver transplantation with preservation of the inferior vena cava previously reported by others has been modified to allow vena caval patency to be preserved without resort to cross-clamping. This ability to preserve caval blood flow during ligation of the caudate branches and major hepatic veins has evolved from our experience with hepatic resection.

Technically, the most favourable conditions are encountered in fulminant hepatic failure when the liver is atrophic, whereas the least favourable circumstances tend to be in some cirrhotic patients and those with Budd–Chiari syndrome where there is massive enlargement of the retrocaval caudate lobe. The procedure may be contraindicated in patients with liver malignancies if the tumour-free resection margin is jeopardized. From January 1992 to December 1994, this technique was feasible in 95 (98%) of 97 transplants including 57 patients with chronic liver disease, four with Budd–Chiari syndrome, 27 cases of fulminant hepatic failure and seven undergoing retransplantation for chronic rejection. Caval flow was maintained during the anhepatic phase in all except six cirrhotic patients where transient total caval clamping was required for 3–23 min to control substantial venous branches associated with a large caudate lobe.

Operation

Temporary portocaval shunt

1   The recipient operation begins with dissection of the porta hepatis with ligature and transection of both hepatic artery and bile duct. The portal vein is cross-clamped and transected just beyond its bifurcation. After exposure and lateral clamping of the infrahepatic cava, the proximal end of the portal vein is anastomosed end-to-side with the cava using a running 4/0 polypropylene (Prolene) suture.

Completion of this end-to-side portocaval shunt has been technically feasible irrespective of graft size in all of our patients. The additional time taken for dissection of all hilar structures was 5–17 min and did not affect the completion of the portal anastomosis in any patient.

In patients with a previous portosystemic shunt, the shunt must be left intact during the procedure until completion of the graft vascular anastomosis. However, there are technical differences between portocaval and non-portocaval shunts. In patients with non-portocaval shunts the portal vein can be clamped, graft portal perfusion flow being restored at the end of the procedure by ligation of the shunt. Suppression of the shunt is easy in patients with mesocaval shunts while in patients with distal splenorenal shunts (DSRS) dissection around the splenic vein may be difficult.

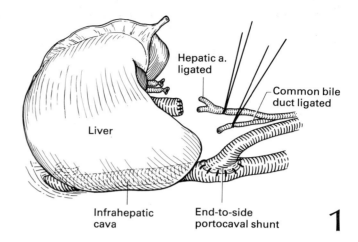

2   In patients with a previous portosystemic shunt the inferior vena cava and portal vein are isolated above and below the shunt. In patients with side-to-side shunts the portal vein is clamped distal to the shunt, so preserving portal flow during the procedure.

However, isolation of the shunt before dissection and its suppression at the end of the procedure can be difficult, especially when a polytetrafluoroethylene (PTFE) graft has been used. In three patients in whom a PTFE graft was used 3–27 months before transplantation dense fibrovascular adhesions developed around the graft which increased technical difficulties and blood loss.

The increased use of liver transplantation raises new issues with regard to the management of bleeding oesophageal varices in patients who are or may become candidates for transplantation. When surgery is being considered, factors influencing the choice of shunts include an estimate of the technical effects of a portosystemic shunt on subsequent liver transplantation. Portosystemic shunting in a transplant candidate has several goals including the need to: (a) assure efficient decompression of portal flow; (b) preserve portal vein patency; (c) minimize technical difficulties during total hepatic resection; and (d) allow easy

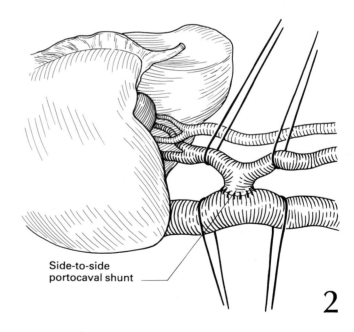

suppression of the shunt to maintain portal perfusion flow to the graft.

According to the literature and the authors' experience, the mesocaval shunt appears to be the shunt of choice in patients who are candidates for liver transplantation.

Hepatectomy

Early hepatic devascularization with transection of the hepatoduodenal ligament facilitates the division of all ligamentous attachments and allows complete mobilization of the liver. The retrohepatic inferior vena cava is exposed by rolling the liver to the left. The recipient liver is dissected from the cava, ligating all caudate venous branches. Complete exposure of the right hepatic vein requires division of a tongue of fibrous tissue (hepatocaval ligament) which normally obscures the right side of the upper part of the retrohepatic cava. During the learning phase of this procedure, it is wise to obtain prior control of the vena cava by passing slings around the infrahepatic suprarenal vena cava and around the inferior vena cava above the liver but just below the diaphragm.

3 The right hepatic vein is then divided, clamped, transected and oversewn using a running 4/0 polypropylene suture.

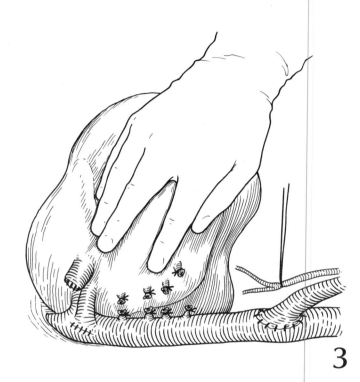

3

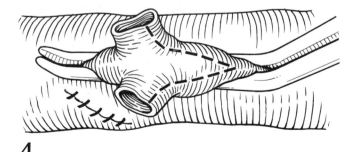

4

4 The middle and left hepatic veins are exposed and a Satinsky side clamp is applied to the caval side without occluding caval flow. The middle and left hepatic veins are transected and, after resection of the caudate lobe, the recipient liver is removed. A single hepatic venous outflow orifice is created from the middle and left hepatic venous trunks, and this can be extended caudally.

Throughout the dissection and after hepatic vein clamping, the inferior vena cava remains patent, thus preserving both portal and caval blood flows.

Graft implantation

5 The donor liver is placed orthotopically and rolled to the right if caval anastomosis is to be performed from the left side of the patient. An end-to-side caval anastomosis is performed between the donor suprahepatic cava and the outflow orifice of the recipient inferior vena cava using a running 4/0 polypropylene suture. While performing this anastomosis the liver is flushed with albumin solution.

In cases of small donor livers with larger recipient vessels, Bismuth and colleagues have described a 'face-à-face' venacavaplasty for matching the size of the donor and recipient vena cava. This technique requires clamping of the vena cava and the use of venovenous bypass. Tzakis in his 'piggy-back procedure' used the three hepatic veins to fashion a single orifice for the outflow anastomosis. The distance between the right hepatic vein and the common trunk of the left and middle hepatic veins usually necessitates caval cross-clamping during implantation of the graft.

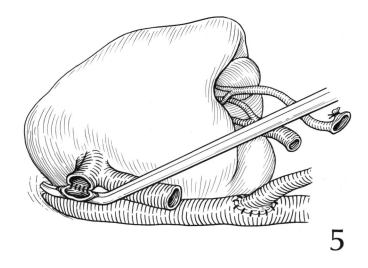

5

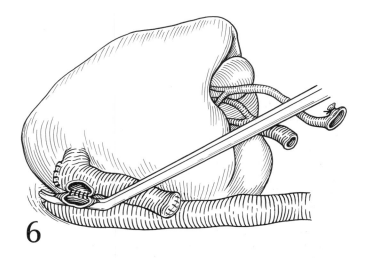

6

6 In order to avoid cross-clamping the cava a side-to-side caval anastomosis was originally used by the authors. However, exposure during implantation of large grafts was often inadequate so this manoeuvre has now been modified to employ an end-to-side anastomosis using only the left and middle hepatic veins. While maintaining continual caval flow, this technique is easier to perform irrespective of graft size. Furthermore, the end-to-side anastomosis allows transjugular hepatic catheterization in the majority of cases.

Revascularization

7 The portocaval anastomosis is taken down and the caval defect is oversewn using a running 4/0 polypropylene suture. An end-to-end portal vein anastomosis is then performed using a running 5/0 polypropylene suture on the posterior side of the anastomosis; the anterior part of the anastomosis is closed by an interrupted suture. The lower end opening of the donor inferior vena cava is left open to allow efflux following liver washout with preservation solution and is subsequently flushed with blood following reperfusion. It is then occluded with a vascular stapling device.

Arterial and biliary reconstructions are similar to those undertaken in conventional orthotopic liver transplantation.

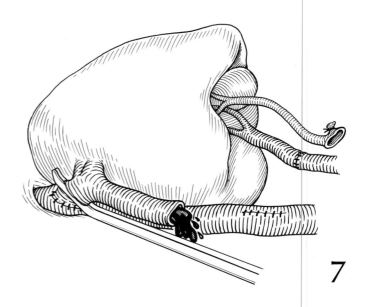

7

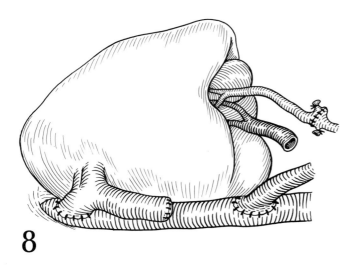

8

8 Alternatively, as portal flow is maintained through the temporary portocaval shunt, the arterial anastomosis can be performed before dismantling the portocaval anastomosis. This does not appear to be detrimental in terms of postreperfusion syndrome, duration of operation and early liver graft function.

Outcome

The preservation of both portal and caval blood flows throughout the procedure maintains haemodynamic stability and renal perfusion pressure. This is particularly important in patients with fulminant hepatic failure in whom intraoperative episodes of intracranial hypertension are the rule and renal failure is frequent. Moreover, this procedure may be of special value in the transplantation of partial livers (split graft, living-related graft, auxiliary graft) as it permits greater versatility than the standard procedure.

Further reading

Belghiti J, Noun R, Sauvanet A. Temporary portocaval anastomosis with preservation of caval flow during orthotopic liver transplantation. *Am J Surg* 1995; 169: 277–9.

Bismuth H, Castaing D, Sherlock DJ. Liver transplantation by "face-à-face" venacavaplasty. *Surgery* 1992; 111: 151–5.

Brems JJ, Hiatt JR, Klein AS, Millis JM, Colonna JA. Effect of a prior portasystemic shunt on subsequent liver transplantation. *Ann Surg* 1989; 209: 51–6.

Lerut J, De Ville De Goyet J, Donataccio M, Reding R, Otte JB. Piggyback transplantation with side-to-side cavocavostomy is an ideal technique for right split liver allograft implantation. *J Am Coll Surg* 1994; 179: 573–6.

Shaw BW, Martin DJ, Marquez JM *et al.* Venous bypass in clinical liver transplantation. *Ann Surg* 1984; 200: 524–34.

Tzakis A, Todo S, Starzl TE. Orthotopic liver transplantation with preservation of the inferior vena cava. *Ann Surg* 1989; 210: 649–52.

Illustrations by Peter Cox

Hepatic transplantation: special issues

C. E. Broelsch MD, PhD, FACS
Professor and Chairman, Chirurgische Klinik, Universitäts Krankenhaus Eppendorf, Hamburg, Germany

X. Rogiers MD
Assistant Professor, Universität Hamburg, Chirurgische Klinik, Hamburg, Germany

The bench procedure

Working at the bench

1 The graft is prepared under sterile conditions on a back table. Care should be taken not to warm up the graft. The operating room should be cool and the bench time should be kept as short as possible. The liver is kept submerged in its conservation medium and cooled by immersing the plastic bag containing the graft in iced water. Fine anastomoses are performed with magnifying loupes, using fine monofilament sutures. In paediatric transplantation, interrupted sutures or resorbable sutures are used.

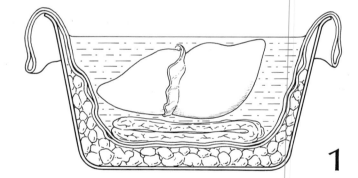

1

Preparing the liver

The bench procedure starts with a close inspection of the graft. The preparation of the liver encompasses the following steps in sequence.

Inferior vena cava

2 Excessive diaphragmatic tissue is first removed. The phrenic veins entering the inferior vena cava (IVC) above the liver are suture ligated. The right adrenal gland, if still present, is removed and the adrenal vein is suture ligated. The IVC is checked for other sites of leakage and the vascular cuffs on both sides are prepared.

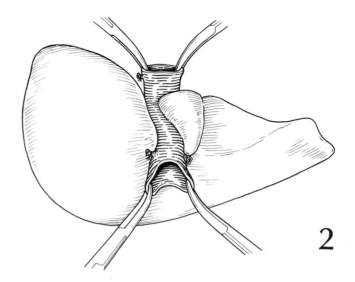

2

Portal vein

The portal vein is freed from the posterior aspect of the hepatoduodenal ligament and is then mobilized up to the level of the portal bifurcation. The vein is checked to ensure that it is watertight and any small branches are suture ligated.

Hepatic artery

The hepatic artery is then progressively freed from the remaining tissue. This dissection is carried out to a point beyond the gastroduodenal artery. The various branches proximal to this point are also suture ligated.

3 Variations in arterial anatomy are dealt with as appropriate.

Bile duct

If cholecystectomy has not been performed, it is undertaken at this stage. The common bile duct itself is left untouched, retaining as much tissue as possible around it. It is advisable to flush the duct with the conservation solution.

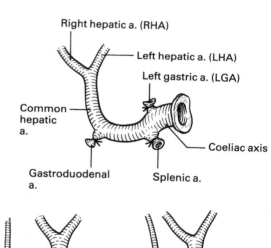

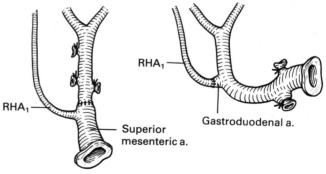

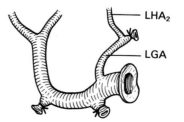

3

Paediatric transplantation

Most children who need liver transplantation weigh less than 10 kg and appropriate donors are rare. This results in long waiting times, high mortality rates on the waiting list (> 15%), and poor condition of recipients at the time of transplantation. To solve this organ shortage, techniques have been developed which make use of larger donors.

Graft reduction

Types of graft and indication

Anatomically the liver can be divided into eight functional segments, each of which has their own portal and arterial inflow (*see* chapter on pp. 1–4). This segmental anatomy is the basis for graft reduction procedures. Venous outflow occurs, mainly through three large hepatic veins; the right and the left hepatic veins drain their respective halves of the liver, while the middle hepatic vein drains the median part of both hemilivers. Anatomical variations in arterial, portal and biliary anatomy are frequent.

4 A variety of reduced grafts allow size differences between donor and recipient to be bridged. The surgeon should compare the sizes of the graft and the need of the recipient before starting the reduction procedure, taking into account factors that determine the amount of space available in the abdomen (notably the size of the recipient's own liver, the amount of ascites and the width of the thoracic cage). In very small infants weighing less than 5 kg the bridgeable size difference is smaller than in larger infants. The relative size of the left lateral segment is particularly variable so that sometimes a larger size difference can be accepted.

On the other hand, the amount of liver transplanted should not be too small. This would lead to congestion of the graft because of the high relative blood flow or even to hepatic failure because of lack of hepatocellular mass. Empirical evidence suggests that a graft weight of 1% of the recipient's body weight is a safe lower limit.

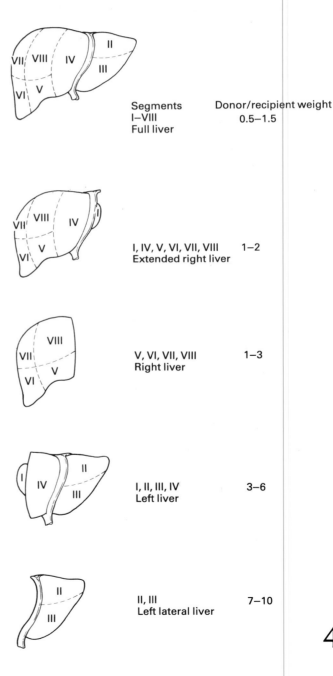

Segments	Donor/recipient weight
I–VIII Full liver	0.5–1.5
I, IV, V, VI, VII, VIII Extended right liver	1–2
V, VI, VII, VIII Right liver	1–3
I, II, III, IV Left liver	3–6
II, III Left lateral liver	7–10

4

Graft preparation

The reduction of a graft is essentially an *ex vivo* hepatectomy. The procedure is illustrated using the left lateral graft as an example.

The graft is inspected and excessive diaphragm is removed. The arterial anatomy is inspected and cholecystectomy is performed.

Preparation of the hepatic vein

5　When preparing a full left or a left lateral graft, the donor cava is removed, leaving only the hepatic veins with a patch. For the right graft the donor vena cava is usually retained. In full right and full left grafts it is best to keep the middle hepatic vein in order to diminish venous congestion and avoid bleeding at the resection surface.

Resection of the caudate lobe

It is generally advisable to resect the caudate lobe since its perfusion may be ambiguous and it may compress the recipient's inferior vena cava.

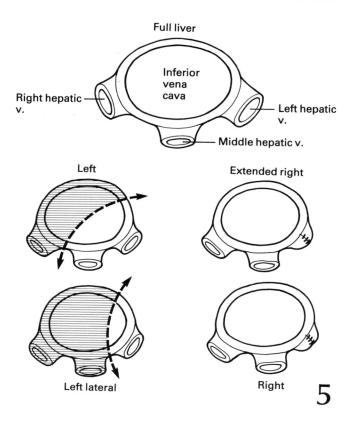

5

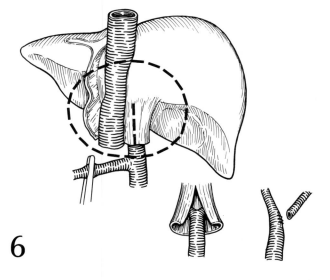

6

Preparation of the hilum

6　The preparation of the hilum starts with the liver turned back to front. The peritoneal sheet covering the back of the portal vein is incised up to the bifurcation. The right or left portal vein is then transected and the defect is oversewn.

7 The graft is then turned over and the hepatic artery
is freed up to the bifurcation, taking care to leave as
much tissue as possible around the bile duct. The
superfluous arterial branch is transected and suture
ligated. The bile duct to the segment that needs to be
removed can either be dissected and taken care of at
this stage, or the bile duct can be dealt with
intrahepatically during transection of the parenchyma.

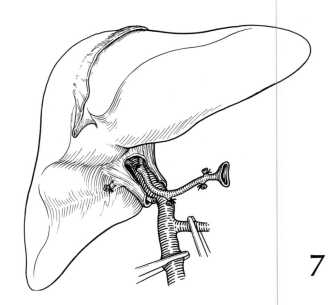

7

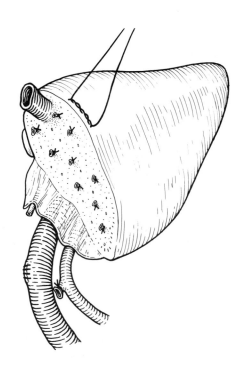

8

Parenchymal transection

8 The parenchymal transection can be performed by
any of the techniques used for hepatic resection
and the transection planes are similar. Blood vessels are
occluded by fine ligatures, suture ligation or clips.
Additionally, horizontal mattress stitches which rely on
the liver capsule for support may be employed. Care has
to be taken not to narrow the hepatic vein or hilar
structures by such sutures. Fibrin glue is used by some
to seal the cut liver surface.

9 The full left and right grafts are prepared using the
same technique. With the right graft, the donor
vena cava is usually conserved.

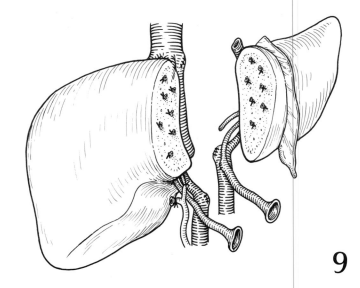

9

Graft implantation

Left lateral graft

10 The recipient liver is removed while conserving the vena cava. After application of a vascular clamp, a large triangular hole is made high on the vena cava and the left hepatic vein of the graft is anastomosed to it, using a triangulation technique with a running resorbable monofilament suture. Great care has to be taken to position the graft correctly in order to prevent kinking of the hepatic vein. The portal vein must be left sufficiently long. The hepatic artery of the graft can be anastomosed to the hepatic or coeliac artery or to the infrarenal aorta.

Full left graft

Implantation of a full left graft is similar to that of a left lateral graft.

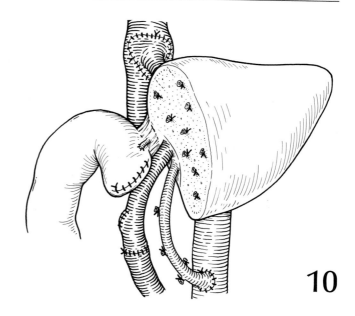

10

Full right graft

The technique of implantation of a right graft depends on whether the donor vena cava was preserved. If the cava is preserved, the technique does not differ from that of an adult liver transplant. If the cava is not preserved, the operation is similar to the left lateral graft or a side-to-side cavocavostomy can be employed.

Perioperative management

After reperfusion, a relatively low central venous pressure should be maintained in order to avoid bleeding from the resection surface. Postoperative haematomas or collections at the resection surface are dealt with by laparotomy to exclude bile leakage and prevent infection.

To prevent vascular thrombosis in small children, the haematocrit is kept below 30 and intravenous heparin (150 units/kg/24 h) is started as soon as haemostasis is complete. Aspirin (5 mg/kg three times/week) is started as soon as oral intake is possible. Regular follow-up by Doppler ultrasonography is performed.

Graft splitting

In split liver transplantation the graft is reduced in such a way that both sides can be used for transplantation.

Indications

Prerequisites for split liver transplantation are (1) a donor previously in excellent health and preferably young; (2) two recipients with size match to the respective parts of the liver; (3) organizational arrangements which would allow both transplants to be performed with an acceptable cold ischaemic time; and (4) vascular and biliary anatomy that is compatible with safe splitting of the liver.

Technique of splitting

The technique of splitting is similar to that of reducing livers. Special attention has to be paid to the vascular and biliary anatomy, as well as to the blood supply of the bile duct.

The actual splitting procedure can be performed either *ex situ* on the back table, or *in situ* in the heart-beating cadaveric donor.

Ex situ splitting

11 The bench procedure starts in the usual fashion and follows the same steps as for graft reduction. However, a choice has to made regarding the side on which the vessel is going to be cut short. For the portal vein, the decision as to which branch to cut depends on the anatomy and on any portal vein problems which may be anticipated in the recipients.

After freeing the hepatic artery bifurcation, the left branch is followed up to its entry into the left lateral lobe in order to make sure that there is no second branch to the right liver. Usually the artery with the larger calibre is divided. If need be, this short artery can be extended with an interposition graft using iliac artery from the same donor. Dissection along the right hepatic artery should be avoided since this can affect the blood supply of the bile duct.

The left hepatic vein is cut at its entry into the inferior vena cava, either with or without a cuff. If a cuff of vena cava wall is taken, the defect has to be reconstructed by sewing in a vein patch. Alternatively, a piggy-back implantation on to the preserved recipient vena cava can be performed. The vena cava and right and middle hepatic veins remain with the right liver.

The authors usually divide the left hepatic duct at the end of the parenchymal dissection. This is performed blindly, without dissection of the bifurcation and at a distance from it to avoid devascularizing the bile duct. This carries a risk of having two bile ducts for the left graft. Some groups determine the site of division of the vessels by performing angiography and cholangiography on the back table. Others dissect the bifurcation of the bile duct.

Split-liver transplantation has not been employed as much as might have been expected. Reasons for this are apprehension about the results and potential complications with the right graft, and the organizational difficulties associated with the procedure. One-year patient survival rates range from 60% to 78%, while graft survival ranges from 52% to 69%. Recently, the results may have improved further. Most surgeons agree that special informed consent is needed and that patients in very poor condition should not be considered for this type of approach.

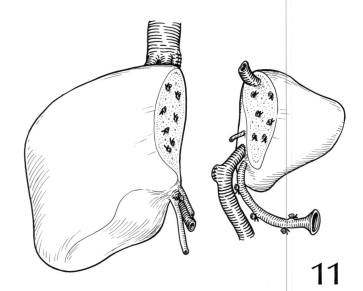

11

In situ splitting

12 *In situ* splitting of the liver in the cadaveric organ donor was developed by the authors to decrease the risk for the recipient of the right liver, allowing haemostasis and observation of the perfusion of the grafts, and decreasing the cold ischaemic times (*Table 1*). The operation is the same as the living donor liver procurement (*see below*) followed by normal procurement of the right liver. It results in a right graft containing segments I, IV, V, VI, VII and VIII and a left lateral graft (segments II and III). The technique requires an experienced donor surgery team.

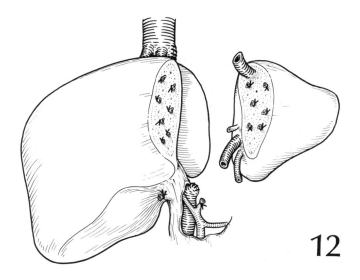

12

Table 1   Results of split-liver transplants

	Classical split-liver transplant	In situ split-liver transplant
Site of splitting	Back table	Heart-beating donor
Site of haemostasis	Recipient	Donor
Procurement time	Short	Long
Bench time	Long	Short
Right graft segments	V, VI, VII, VIII	(I), (IV), V, VI, VII, VIII
Left graft segments	II, III	II, III
Discarded segments	IV	(None)

Living-related donor

Donor operation

The decision-making process in living-related liver transplantation requires that informed consent is obtained on two separate occasions (*Figure 1*).

Preoperative

The preoperative evaluation includes a thorough medical examination with emphasis on cardiovascular risk factors, and a psychological evaluation to confirm mental stability and freedom of choice. A computed tomographic scan with volumetry and angiography are performed to confirm the suitability of the potential graft. In parents of children with Allagille's disease an endoscopic retrograde cholangiogram is performed to confirm normal size of the bile ducts.

Preoperatively, 2–3 units of packed red cells should have been self-donated. Intraoperatively, a cell-saver is used. Thrombosis prophylaxis includes low-dose low molecular weight heparin subcutaneously started preoperatively, elastic stockings, and mobilization up until the time of surgery.

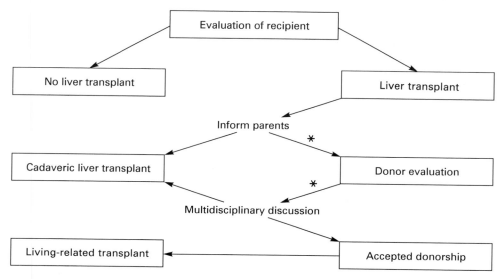

Figure 1 Decision-making process in living-related liver transplantation. *Informed consent required.

Operation

13 A transverse incision is made, encompassing the width of both rectus muscles, with a median extension to the xiphoid process. Both costal margins are retracted upwards using a Rochard retractor.

The abdomen is explored to exclude any abnormalities. The falciform, left triangular and gastrohepatic ligaments are transected in order to mobilize the left lateral lobe fully. The left hepatic artery and portal vein are carefully dissected free down to the bifurcation from their main stem. If possible, a branch from the artery or the portal vein to segment IV is saved. Small portal branches to the caudate lobe are suture ligated and divided.

Dissection is carried to the right side of the round ligament. Portal branches to segment IV are suture ligated and cut so that the ligament is progressively rolled to the left, and a free view on the hilar plate and the portal bifurcation is finally obtained. At the end of this dissection, some blue discoloration of the tip of segment IV may be apparent.

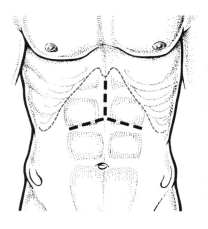

13

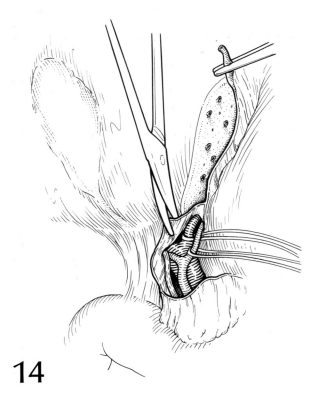

14

14 The hilar plate, containing the bile duct(s) to segments II and III, can now be divided. This should be done with vascular scissors or a knife in order to avoid devascularization of the edges. In some 30% of cases, two separate bile ducts are found for segments II and III. The donor side of the duct(s) which will remain is oversewn with a 5/0 resorbable monofilament suture.

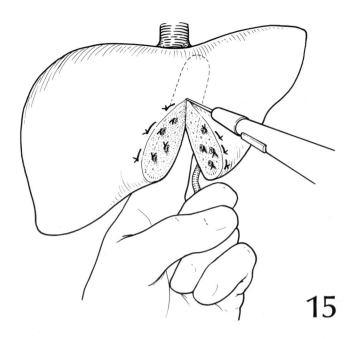

15 Parenchymal transection is performed along the line of the falciform ligament. The operator's finger, put through above the portal bifurcation and resting on the caudate lobe, can help with orientation.

Any of the traditional liver resection techniques may be used but vascular exclusion is not performed. As the transection progresses, haemostasis is obtained on both sides. Finally, the left lateral lobe is only attached to the rest of the donor liver by its vessels.

The artery, portal vein and hepatic vein of the segment are clamped and cut sequentially. The segment is handed over immediately to the back table where it is flushed with University of Wisconsin solution through the portal vein and the hepatic artery. The bile duct(s) are flushed clean with the same solution. If needed, vascular interposition grafts can be sewn onto the artery and/or the portal vein. Fresh saphenous vein from the donor or cryopreserved vein can be used for this purpose.

The vascular stumps in the donor are oversewn and haemostasis is checked. The abdomen is closed, leaving one Penrose drain close to the cut section of the liver.

Perioperative care
Much attention is paid to prophylaxis against thromboembolic disease. This complication has been responsible for the only death after living liver donation and for most of the few deaths after kidney donation thus far. Subcutaneous mini-dose low molecular weight heparin is commenced preoperatively and continued throughout the postoperative course. The patient is kept mobile up to the moment of the operation and mobilization is restarted on the first postoperative day.

Outcome
More than 300 living-related liver procurements have been performed worldwide up to the end of 1994. The procedure has earned an important place in the treatment of children with end-stage liver disease. To date there has been one death after living-related liver donation (due to massive pulmonary embolism). Complications have been very limited and similar to those of elective minor liver resections. After operation, liver regeneration has been adequate. The procured organ has generally been of excellent quality and primary non-function has not been described.

Recipient operation

The recipient operation is similar to the implantation of a left lateral lobe graft from a cadaveric donor. Care must be taken while handling the graft, since it is much softer than a cadaveric graft.

The biliary anastomosis has been the Achilles' heel of the procedure. Care must be taken to ensure that the bile duct(s) is well vascularized and that no segmental duct is missed. In one-third of cases two bile ducts will need to anastomosed. The anastomosis should be performed by a rested surgeon using magnifying loupes. The suture material used is usually a 7/0 slowly resorbable monofilament suture.

Results

More than 350 living-related liver transplants have been performed worldwide with excellent results (*Table 2*). In the authors' centre it allowed mortality on the waiting list to be reduced to 5.2% on the cadaveric list and to zero on the living-related waiting lists.

Table 2   Results of living-related liver transplants

Principal author	No. of patients	One-year patient survival (%)	One-year graft survival (%)
Broelsch (1991)	29	82	75
Emond (1993)	18	94	83
Tanaka (1993)	33	82	—

Further reading

Broelsch CE, Whitington PF, Emond JC *et al*. Liver transplantation in children from living related donors. Surgical techniques and results. *Ann Surg* 1991; 214: 428–39.

De Hemptinne B, Salizzoni M, Yandza TC *et al*. Indication, technique and results of liver graft volume reduction before orthotopic transplantation in children. *Transplant Proc* 1987; 19: 3549–51.

Emond JC, Whitington PF, Thistlethwaite JR *et al*. Transplantation of two patients with one liver: analysis of a preliminary experience with "split liver" grafting. *Ann Surg* 1990; 212: 14–22.

Rogiers X, Malago M, Habib N *et al*. *In-situ* splitting of the liver in the heart beating cadaveric donor for transplantation in two recipients. *Transplantation* 1995; 59: 1081–3.

Tanaka K, Uemoto S, Tokunaga Y *et al*. Surgical techniques and innovations in living related liver transplantation. *Ann Surg* 1993; 217: 82–91.

Liver cysts: non-parasitic

Henry A. Pitt MD
Professor and Vice Chairman, Department of Surgery, The Johns Hopkins Medical Institutions, Baltimore, Maryland, USA

Cystic lesions of the liver are commonly encountered by modern imaging techniques or at laparotomy. Asymptomatic, simple liver cysts account for the vast majority of these lesions. However, a variety of other cystic lesions must be considered in the differential diagnosis. Cystic lesions of the liver have been classified into four broad categories: (1) congenital, (2) neoplastic, (3) traumatic and (4) inflammatory[1].

Inflammatory cysts include pyogenic and amoebic liver abscesses which are discussed in the chapter on pp. 110–121, and echinococcal cysts which are the subject of the chapter on pp. 101–109. Traumatic cysts result from injury to the liver, with formation of a subcapsular haematoma or disruption of an intrahepatic bile duct, and represent less than 1% of all liver cysts[2]. These lesions may resolve, form a cyst without an epithelial lining or become a pyogenic abscess. The indications and options for treating these lesions are similar to congenital cysts or liver abscesses. Neoplastic liver cysts may be primary or metastatic. Hepatocellular carcinoma may outgrow its blood supply and cavitate, but the solid portion of the tumour is usually still apparent. Cystadenocarcinomas of the pancreas or ovary may spread to the liver giving rise to cystic liver metastases. Cystadenomas and cystadenocarcinomas may also develop in the liver. These rare neoplasms comprise less than 5% of hepatic cysts[2], and their management will be included in this chapter. Congenital cysts are the most common cystic lesions in the liver and include simple cysts and polycystic liver disease. They will be the primary focus of this chapter.

History

Congenital liver cysts arise from abnormal development of the intrahepatic bile ducts. In 1906 Moschowitz postulated that aberrant ducts formed during embryogenesis while Von Meyenberg later proposed that excessively developed intralobular bile ducts become dilated with time[2]. More recent work in mice suggests a defect in the production of the basement membrane of the bile ducts, while another theory proposes that cystic dilatation of biliary microhamartomas results in polycystic liver disease[2]. Cystadenomas, and the very rare cystadenocarcinomas, are also thought to arise from the biliary ductal epithelium. These lesions are usually multiloculated and, histologically, cystadenomas often contain a densely cellular ovarian stroma as well as a mucin-producing columnar epithelium. In comparison, simple cysts as well as those in polycystic liver disease are lined by a cuboidal epithelium.

Principles and justification

The indications for and type of treatment vary considerably for simple cysts, polycystic liver disease and neoplastic cysts. Small, asymptomatic, simple cysts pose no risk to health and should be observed. Moderate sized, asymptomatic solitary cysts (usually less than 10 cm in diameter) that are detected by imaging may also be followed. If the carcinoembryonic antigen (CEA) level is normal, the echinococcal titre is negative, and serial ultrasonographic examinations show no change in size over 12 months, no further follow-up is necessary. Moderate sized, asymptomatic cysts that are encountered at laparotomy or laparoscopy may be aspirated. If the fluid is clear, has no bacteria on Gram's stain and culture, and cytological examination is negative, no further treatment is required. If a portion of the cyst wall can be easily excised and examined histologically, the presence of a flat, cuboidal epithelium confirms the presence of a simple cyst.

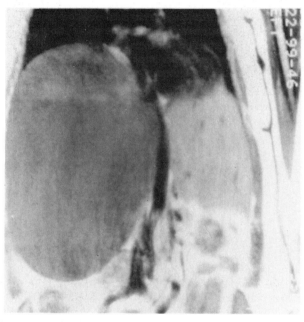

MRI scan of a massive cyst.

1

1 Large simple cysts (usually more than 10 cm in diameter) often cause symptoms and require therapy. Symptoms usually develop insidiously as the cyst expands and compresses adjacent organs. A dull aching pain is frequently a problem, and displacement of the stomach or duodenum may result in nausea, vomiting and, ultimately, weight loss. Respiratory compromise may be another indication for treatment. Haemorrhage is an unusual complication which is usually heralded by acute abdominal pain. Secondary infection is also unusual if the cyst has not been manipulated. Biliary obstruction rarely occurs, but compression of intrahepatic ducts may result in enough stasis for stones to form. If small stones leave the intrahepatic ducts, cholangitis or gallstone pancreatitis may occur. Compression of the intrahepatic vena cava by a massive cyst may also cause clots to form with resulting pulmonary emboli or peripheral oedema.

2 Some patients may have multiple simple cysts. However, patients with polycystic liver disease have innumerable cysts distributed throughout the liver and, occasionally, also in the pancreas or spleen. Despite massive replacement of the liver by cysts, polycystic liver disease is often asymptomatic and rarely causes biliary obstruction or liver failure. However, the majority of patients with polycystic liver disease also have autosomal dominant polycystic kidney disease. Progressive renal failure and the need for dialysis and kidney transplantation are usually more pressing problems than the liver cysts. However, since end stage renal disease can be treated effectively, progressive hepatomegaly can cause the same symptoms as those that occur with large simple cysts and are an indication for surgery. Only rarely would hepatic insufficiency be an indication for liver transplantation.

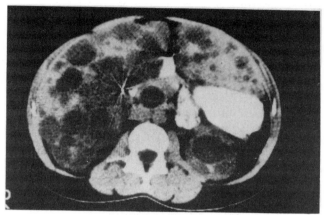

Computed tomographic scan showing polycystic disease.

2

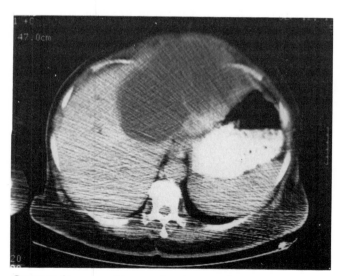

Computed tomographic scan showing cystadenoma.

3

3 Differentiation of simple cysts, cystadenomas and cystadenocarcinomas may not be possible without histological examination of the cyst. Symptoms are identical and cyst size is not helpful[3]. Simple cysts are usually circular or oval, lack septae and have uniformly thin walls The presence of septae or any nodularity or irregular thickening of the cyst wall is a clue that the lesion may be a cystic neoplasm. Simple cysts usually have clear fluid. Cystic neoplasms are more likely to have bilious or chocolate-coloured fluid, but the character of the fluid is not sufficiently characteristic to be diagnostic[3]. Similarly, neither fluid analysis for CEA nor cytological examination have been accurate enough to make appropriate clinical decisions regarding treatment.

Preoperative

In addition to a complete history and physical examination, liver function tests, serum amylase and CEA levels, and coagulation studies should be performed. However, these studies are almost always normal. If the history or presentation suggest an inflammatory process, amoebic or echinococcal titres may be indicated. The diagnostic accuracy of ultrasonography, computed tomographic (CT) scanning and magnetic resonance imaging (MRI) are similar. Ultrasonography is preferred for following asymptomatic lesions because of cost and lack of radiation exposure. However, CT scanning provides a broader view of the entire liver, and newer spiral techniques provide the vascular anatomy that was formerly best visualized by MRI. In addition, CT scanning is excellent for detecting thin septae, daughter hydatid cysts or fine calcification that may be present in echinococcal cysts or cystic neoplasms.

Percutaneous needle aspiration, with or without the introduction of sclerosing agents, has been proposed as a treatment option. However, secondary infection and a high recurrence rate are problems with this mode of therapy. The introduction of sclerosing agents into the biliary tree may also result in long-term problems with sclerosing cholangitis. In addition, the accuracy of fluid analysis for differential diagnosis is low. Moreover, the differentiation between simple cysts, premalignant cystadenomas and cystadenocarcinomas requires histological examination of the entire cyst wall. Thus, cyst aspiration is usually not indicated before surgery. If a cystic neoplasm is suspected, endoscopic retrograde cholangiography may be helpful in defining the biliary communication. Angiography may also be indicated if hepatic resection is contemplated. However, preoperative cholangiography and angiography are usually not necessary if ultrasonography or CT scanning suggest a simple cyst. For antibiotic prophylaxis, a single dose or 24 h of perioperative treatment with a first generation cephalosporin will usually be adequate.

Anaesthesia

In most instances general endotracheal anaesthesia will be appropriate for surgery in patients with liver cysts. This principle applies regardless of whether a laparoscopic or an open approach is undertaken. A high epidural anaesthetic may also be feasible. However, a large cyst may already be causing respiratory compromise and, if a laparoscopic technique is employed, the pneumoperitoneum may further compromise the respiratory system. In this situation general endotracheal anaesthesia would usually be the safest alternative.

Operation

The operation and the approach – whether laparoscopic or open – should be based on the anatomy of the cyst and the suspected and eventual pathology. For example, most anterior simple cysts can be approached and partially excised with a laparoscopic technique. On the other hand, the ability to manage patients with polycystic liver disease adequately through a laparoscopic approach is limited. These patients will usually require a combination of resection of major cystic areas as well as excision of the common wall between the cysts (fenestration). If the lesion is a cystadenoma, complete excision of the cyst wall is required. This goal may be achieved either through enucleation or hepatic resection. Proper management of a cystadenocarcinoma is formal hepatic resection. However, if metastases are encountered, partial excision may provide palliation of pressure symptoms.

Incision

4a–c The choice of incision is also based on the anatomy of the cyst and suspected pathology. If a laparoscopic approach is undertaken, four ports similar to those employed for laparoscopic cholecystectomy will usually be adequate. However, the use of an 11-mm trocar for one of the lateral ports will facilitate removal of cyst tissue If an open approach is undertaken for a simple cyst, a standard right subcostal or midline incision may be used depending upon the position of the cyst and the anatomy of the costal margins. If a major hepatic resection is required, either an extended right subcostal or a long midline incision will be appropriate for lesions on the right or left, respectively.

Exploration

Regardless of the approach or the liver pathology, a thorough exploration of the abdomen is indicated. A search for peritoneal metastases is particularly appropriate if a cystadenoma or a cystadenocarcinoma is suspected. The number, size and location of the liver cysts should be assessed. However, with modern imaging techniques this information is usually known before surgery is undertaken. If cyst enucleation is contemplated in the case of a cystadenoma, or if resection is indicated, intraoperative ultrasonography may be helpful to search for other lesions and to determine the relationship of the lesion to major vascular structures.

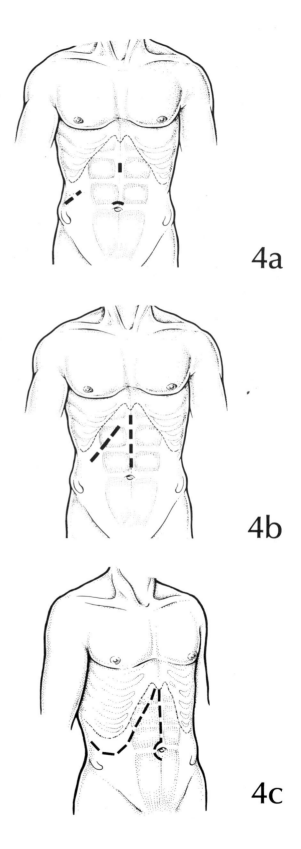

Aspiration

5 The first step in determining the nature of the cyst is to aspirate its contents Aspiration can be performed safely with either an open or a laparoscopic approach. The presence of bile or secondary infection may change the operative plan. Fluid should be sent for Gram's stain, culture and cytological examination. Cytological examination will not be helpful in making operative decisions. However, some neoplastic cysts have large areas where the epithelium is denuded. Thus, a positive cytological result may establish the diagnosis if partial cyst excision is inappropriately performed. If the slightest suspicion exists that echinococcal cyst disease is present, open exploration with fastidious packing of the adjacent area with laparotomy pads soaked in hypertonic saline should be performed before aspiration. In this setting, pathological examination of the fluid for scolices may also be indicated.

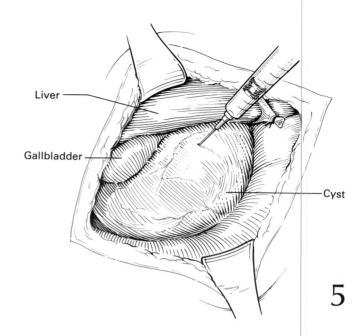

5

Biopsy

6a–c The next step is to biopsy a portion of the cyst wall. Again, biopsy can be performed easily with both the laparoscopic and open techniques. Cautery is appropriate regardless of the approach, as a moderate sized portion of cyst should be excised to increase the likelihood of establishing the correct diagnosis. Once the cyst is opened, residual fluid should be suctioned from the most dependent portions. The inner lining of the cyst should then be observed to look for any unusual areas. Further biopsy of suspicious lesions should be undertaken to be sure that a cystic neoplasm is not being missed because of a sampling error.

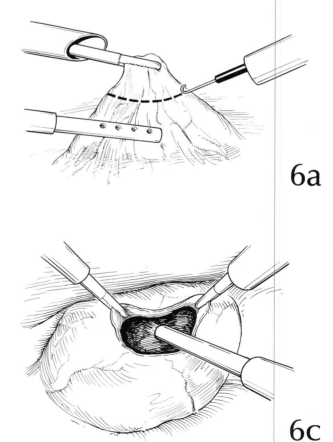

6a

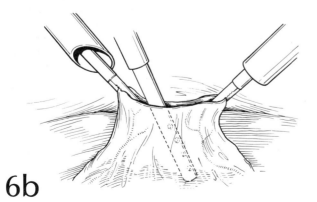

6b

6c

Partial resection

7 If no intracystic lesions or bile are found, the superficial cyst wall is excised with cautery. Less than 1 cm of the rim of the cyst is left attached to the liver. Vascular and biliary radicles should be clipped or oversewn as encountered. This additional cyst wall is also sent for frozen section to be sure that a cystic neoplasm is not being overlooked. For a simple cyst, complete excision of the cyst wall is not necessary as long as the remaining wall is in wide contact with the peritoneal cavity. Postoperative closed suction drainage is usually not necessary as serous secretions will be absorbed by the peritoneum. In patients with polycystic disease the septa should be avoided as bile ducts often traverse them. However, multiple adjacent cysts may be placed in communication with the peritoneal cavity by excising the common wall between cysts (fenestration)[2,4]. If a cystic neoplasm is encountered, partial resection is not appropriate except as palliation of a metastatic cystadenocarcinoma.

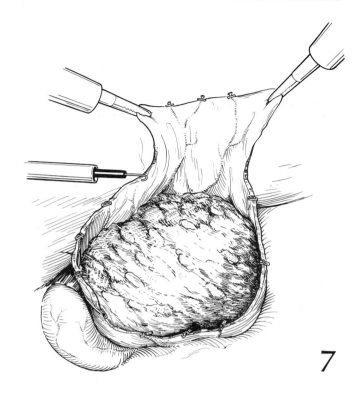

7

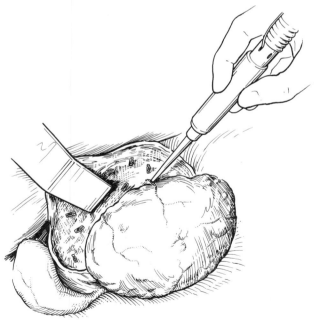

8

Enucleation

8 Complete removal of the cyst wall is not necessary for a simple cyst as long as the remaining wall is in wide contact with the peritoneal cavity. Cyst enucleation is also not appropriate for patients with polycystic liver disease nor is it adequate therapy for a cystadenocarcinoma. However, enucleation is an excellent option for patients with a cystadenoma[5]. In these patients a plane can often be established between the cyst wall and the adjacent liver parenchyma. An ultrasonic dissector may facilitate this dissection. Ligation of feeding blood vessels and identification and ligation of an attached bile duct will also be required. Closed suction drainage may also be indicated if bile leakage is a concern.

Hepatic resection

The techniques of formal liver resection have been adequately described in the chapters on pp. 30–45 and 46–55. Liver resection is not necessary for simple cysts. In patients with polycystic liver disease, non-anatomical resections should be individualized on the basis of the anatomy of the cystic disease and the patient's symptoms. In some patients with a cystadenoma, hepatic resection may be simpler than enucleation. In patients with cystadenocarcinoma of the liver, formal hepatic resection is the procedure of choice. As with other hepatic malignancies, an adequate margin between the line of resection and the tumour is important to prevent local recurrence.

Postoperative care

Even with a major hepatic resection, return of gastrointestinal function is usually prompt. With partial resection or enucleation no liver parenchyma is removed so liver insufficiency is not a concern. Similarly, in patients with polycystic liver disease, very little parenchyma is removed even when a formal liver resection is performed. When major hepatic resection is required, the remaining liver is usually not cirrhotic in these patients so that liver failure is rarely a problem. If a closed suction drain has been placed because of concerns about a bile leak, the drain should be left in place until bile flow has been stimulated by food intake. The drain can then be safely removed if no bile is observed. Considerable serous drainage may follow resection in patients with polycystic liver disease. In this setting, however, the drain may be removed promptly if the drainage is not bile-stained because the peritoneum should absorb this excess fluid.

Outcome

The results of partial resection of simple cysts are excellent[2,5,6]. Cyst recurrence is only likely if most of the cyst wall was intrahepatic and loculation by adjacent structures allows the cyst to reform. Whether the recurrence rate will be higher with laparoscopic partial resection of simple cysts, because of a less adequate procedure, has yet to be determined. However, initial reports of laparoscopic management of patients with polycystic liver disease have been disappointing. On the other hand, the results of combined liver resection and cyst fenestration for polycystic liver disease have been excellent with almost all patients having prompt as well as sustained relief of preoperative symptoms[2,4].

Partial resection or marsupialization of a cystadenoma will result in recurrence and the subsequent need for resection[2,3]. However, if the entire cystadenoma is removed by enucleation, recurrence is not a problem[5,6]. The results of surgery for cystadenocarcinomas of the liver are similar to those for other primary hepatic malignancies. If metastatic disease is encountered, median survival is less than 1 year. If resection is possible, approximately 25% of patients will survive 5 years[2].

References

1. Doty JE, Pitt HA. Cystic lesions of the liver and biliary tree. In: Moody FG, ed. *Surgical Treatment of Digestive Disease.* Chicago: Year Book Medical Publishers, 1986: 334–51.

2. Que FG, Gores GJ, Welch TJ, Nagorney DM. Noninflammatory hepatic cysts. In: Pitt HA, Carr-Locke DL, Ferrucci JT, eds. *Hepatobiliary and Pancreatic Disease.* Boston: Little, Brown: 1995, 71–80.

3. Shermack MA, Pitt HA, Sitzmann JV, Hruban RH, Cameron JL. Symptomatic noninflammatory hepatic cysts: can cyst fluid or size predict pathology? *Proceedings of the International Hepato-Pancreato-Biliary Association,* 1994: 87.

4. Turnage RH, Eckhauser FE, Krol JA *et al.* Therapeutic dilemmas in patients with symptomatic polycystic liver disease. *Am Surg* 1988; 54: 365–72.

5. Sanchez H, Gagner M, Rossi RL *et al.* Surgical management of nonparasitic cystic liver disease. *Am J Surg* 1991; 161: 113–9.

6. Henne-Bruns D, Klomp HJ, Kremer B. Non-parasitic liver cysts and polycystic liver disease: results of surgical treatment. *Hepato-gastroenterology* 1993; 40: 1–5.

Liver cysts: hydatid disease

Henry A. Pitt MD

Professor and Vice Chairman, Department of Surgery, The Johns Hopkins Medical Institutions, Baltimore, Maryland, USA

Hydatid cysts of the liver are one of the inflammatory processes that can result in cystic hepatic lesions. The other processes are hepatic abscesses, including pyogenic and amoebic abscesses, which are discussed in the next chapter.

Hepatic hydatidosis can be caused by one of two organisms, *Echinococcus granulosus* or *Echinococcus multilocularis*. *Echinococcus granulosus* is endemic in several areas of the world where sheep, the intermediate host, and sheep dogs, the primary host, are commonly found. Endemic areas include southern Europe, the Middle East, portions of South America, Australia and New Zealand[1,2]. *Echinococcus multilocularis* occurs in arctic regions of Canada and Scandinavia where it is usually harboured by foxes while the intermediate host is often a rodent such as the vole[1].

History

Echinococcus granulosus causes well circumscribed cysts with an inner layer (endocyst) which produces internal daughter cysts. The compressed liver parenchyma around the cyst and the associated inflammatory process form an ectocyst. These layers may become calcified and difficult to separate. In the past a number of surgical procedures were designed to excise the endocyst without resecting any liver parenchyma. However, in recent years, as surgery of the liver has become safer, many experienced groups have been performing more liver resections and fewer local cyst excisions. *Echinococcus multilocularis* causes a much more infiltrative process which, until recently, has not been thought to be amenable to surgery. However, a few recent reports claim that hepatic resection may benefit selected patients with this form of hydatid liver disease[1].

Principles and justification

As the majority of surgery for hydatid disease of the liver is performed for *Echinococcus granulosus*, the remainder of this discussion will focus on this form of the disease.

The most common presenting symptom is pain[1-3]. However, these cysts may rupture into the biliary tree, through the diaphragm into the chest or into the peritoneum or adjacent abdominal organs. To avoid these complications, surgery is usually recommended for patients with symptomatic cysts and also for moderate-sized asymptomatic cysts[1-4]. Patients with small, asymptomatic, centrally located cysts may be observed. Antihelminthic therapy with agents such as mebendazole or albendazole may be tried in these patients with minimal disease. However, evidence that these agents can eradicate the disease is lacking, and hepatic toxicity is a problem[1-3].

The timing and type of surgery to be performed will depend upon the presentation as well as the number and position of the cysts. If a dull, aching pain is the only symptom, surgery can be performed electively. However, if the patient presents with cholangitis due to rupture into the biliary tree or with a productive cough due to rupture through the diaphragm into the bronchial tree, surgery should be performed with moderate urgency as soon as the evaluation is complete. In the rare instance where a cyst ruptures into the peritoneal cavity and the patient presents with peritoneal signs, surgery may need to be performed as an emergency without a definitive diagnosis.

Preoperative

A history of exposure to sheep or sheep dogs should be sought but may not be forthcoming. A history of living in, having immigrated from, or frequently travelled to an endemic region should also raise the suspicion that a hepatic cyst is echinococcal. Physical examination is usually normal, but hepatomegaly or a large, non-tender cyst, especially in the left lobe, may be palpable. Liver function tests and amylase levels are usually normal but may be raised if a cyst ruptures into the biliary tree causing cholangitis and/or pancreatitis. Examination of sputum for scolices will establish the diagnosis if the patient has a productive cough due to a bronchial communication. Confirmation that a liver cyst is hydatid can also be achieved by performing serological tests. Several serological tests are available that are highly accurate and provide information in a few days[1–3].

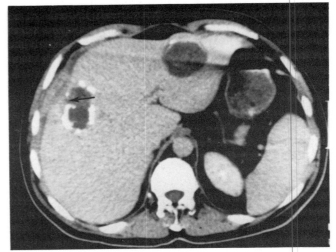

1a

1a,b Ultrasonography, computed tomographic (CT) scanning and magnetic resonance imaging (MRI) can all detect hydatid liver disease with similar accuracy[1–3]. As with simple cysts, ultrasonography is most appropriate if the cyst is being followed. However, CT scanning gives a better picture of the entire liver and therefore provides the surgeon with more information to plan an appropriate operation. CT scanning can also demonstrate rupture through the diaphragm (*Illustration 1a*, arrow), fine calcifications (*Illustration 1a*, left), small cysts (*Illustration 1b*, left) as well as daughter cysts (*Illustration 1b*, right). However, it is not accurate in predicting communication with the biliary tree.

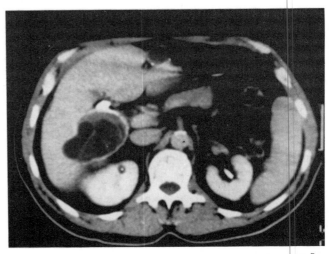

1b

2 If the patient presents with cholangitis or pancreatitis, cholangiography should be performed preoperatively. Transhepatic cholangiography may be dangerous because of the presence of intrahepatic cysts that may be ruptured, so endoscopic retrograde cholangiopancreatography (ERCP) is the procedure of choice[1–3]. Endoscopic sphincterotomy may be indicated if daughter cysts remain in the bile duct. However, the sphincter may be quite patulous if cyst contents have recently passed into the duodenum. Whether ERCP should also be performed routinely before elective surgery is debatable. However, having the information that a cyst communicates with the biliary tree before commencing surgery can be quite helpful.

If a major hepatic resection is contemplated, angiography may also provide useful information. Most authorities believe that percutaneous aspiration is contraindicated. Some recent reports suggest that percutaneous drainage with injection of sclerosing agents can be performed safely in carefully selected patients[5, 6]. However, the number of reported patients is small and concerns remain about anaphylactic reactions if cyst contents are spilled, as well as potentially high recurrence rates which, to date, have not been reported. Surgery therefore remains the treatment of choice for most patients with hepatic hydatid disease.

For antibiotic prophylaxis for elective surgery, a single dose or 24 h of perioperative treatment with a first generation cephalosporin will usually suffice. If the patient presents with cholangitis, a longer course of antibiotics more specific for common biliary organisms is appropriate. Whether antihelminthic drugs should also be given to patients with cholangitis or for perioperative prophylaxis has not been proven. However, if an analogy to prophylactic antibiotics can be drawn, a short course of perioperative mebendazole or albendazole may be appropriate.

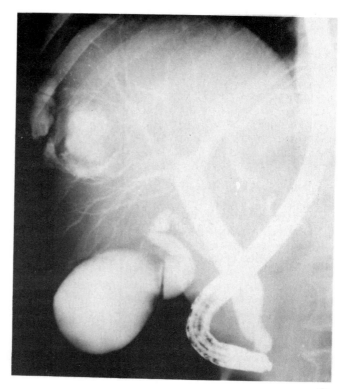

2

Anaesthesia

General endotracheal anaesthesia is indicated for patients undergoing surgery for hepatic hydatid disease. Most of these operations will be performed as open procedures but, rarely, a small superficial cyst may be approached laparoscopically. However, concerns about spillage of cyst contents limit the applicability of laparoscopy for these patients. Even with open surgery, the possibility of an anaphylactic reaction should be anticipated by the anaesthetist. Ready availability of adrenaline and steroids should be adequate to manage most allergic reactions.

Operation

3 The operation should be based on the individual patient's presentation as well as the size and location of the cysts. In the patient whose CT scans and ERCP are shown in *Illustrations 1* and *2*, four hydatid cysts were present – two on the left and two on the right. A calcified cyst in segment II communicated with, but had not ruptured into, the biliary tree. A second small cyst was present on the edge of segment III. A third, heavily calcified cyst occupied portions of segments V and VI near the gallbladder. The fourth calcified cyst near the junction of segments VII and VIII had ruptured through the diaphragm into the bronchial tree. As a result, the patient had presented with a productive cough and preoperative diagnosis had been established by identification of scolices in the sputum.

Incision and exploration

A variety of incisions may be appropriate depending on the number, size and location of the cysts, as well as the anatomy of the costal margins. A right subcostal incision, an extended right subcostal incision, a bilateral subcostal incision or a midline incision may all provide adequate exposure in individual patients. As with all laparotomies, complete exploration of the abdomen should be performed before dealing with the primary pathology. If a complete abdominal and pelvic CT scan has been performed preoperatively, the likelihood of finding additional hydatid cysts is low. Nevertheless, the minimal time spent doing a complete exploration will occasionally yield unexpected pathology.

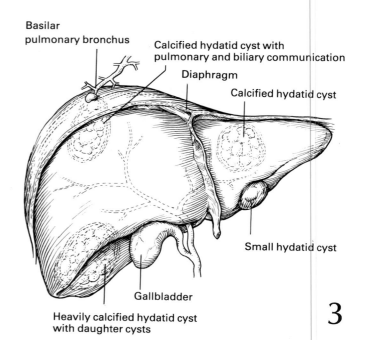

Basilar pulmonary bronchus

Calcified hydatid cyst with pulmonary and biliary communication

Diaphragm

Calcified hydatid cyst

Small hydatid cyst

Gallbladder

Heavily calcified hydatid cyst with daughter cysts

3

Cyst excision

4a–c The calcified cyst in segment II was completely excised without removal of adjacent liver parenchyma (pericystectomy). With multiple daughter cysts the pressure within hydatid cysts is usually quite high so injection of scolicidal agents, such as 20% hypertonic saline, is unlikely to be very effective. Similarly, aspiration of cyst contents, even with a large bore needle, is usually not very rewarding. Moreover, injection of a scolicidal agent such as formaldehyde can cause sclerosing cholangitis if it gains access to the biliary tree. In the case illustrated, the area was therefore packed with laparotomy pads soaked with hypertonic saline before approaching the cyst so that its contents would not spill into the peritoneal cavity. The cyst was opened, and daughter cysts were evacuated to avoid accidental spillage. With some cysts, however, this step is not necessary. A plane was then established between the calcified wall and the adjacent liver resulting in complete excision of the cyst.

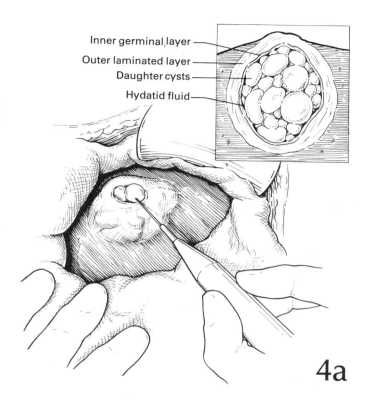

Inner germinal layer
Outer laminated layer
Daughter cysts
Hydatid fluid

4a

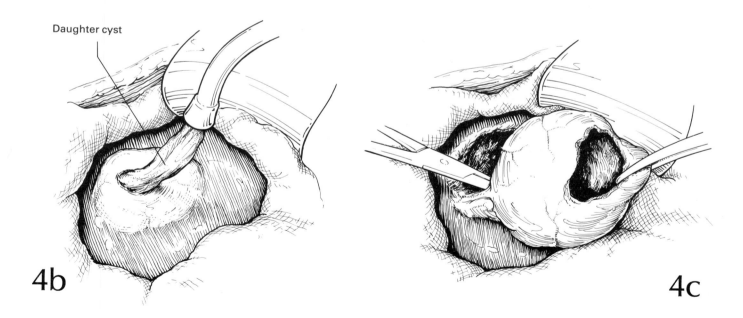

Daughter cyst

4b

4c

Biliary communication

5 Once the cyst was removed from segment II, the cavity was irrigated briefly with hypertonic saline and a biliary communication was easily identified. The bile duct was then oversewn, and a closed suction drain was placed into the cavity (inset). In this instance the cavity could also be obliterated by large, chromic liver sutures. Since this patient had no history of cholangitis, normal liver function tests and amylase levels and an otherwise unremarkable ERCP, no further biliary procedures were performed.

In patients who present with cholangitis or pancreatitis due to rupture of cyst contents into the biliary tree, bile duct exploration is usually indicated. This exploration should be performed in a similar fashion as described for bile duct stones in the chapter on pp. 337–350. Some authorities debate as to whether the gallbladder should be removed in these patients. However, the function of the sphincter of Oddi may be altered after passage of cyst contents. As a result, normal filling and emptying of the gallbladder may also be impaired which may result in subsequent gallstone formation and/or cholecystitis. Cholecystectomy is therefore usually advisable if the common duct needs to be explored for hydatid disease.

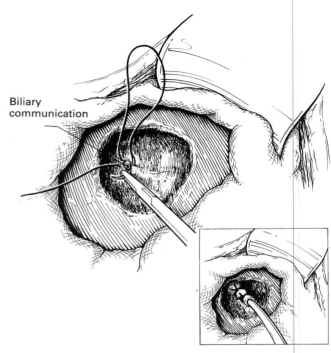

Biliary communication

5

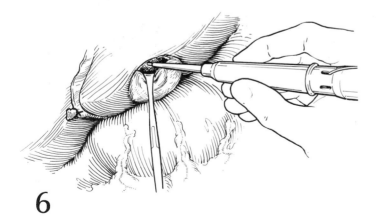

6

Wedge resection

6 In the case illustrated, the small superficial cyst on the edge of segment III was easily excised with a small amount of adjacent hepatic parenchyma using the ultrasonic dissector. Alternatively, chromic sutures could be placed in the adjacent liver, and cautery could be used to perform a bloodless local wedge resection. The very superficial excision that was performed for this cyst was unlikely to result in a bile leak and did not therefore require drainage.

Omental packing

7a–c The heavily calcified cyst adjacent to the gallbladder could not be easily separated from the adjacent liver parenchyma, nor was wedge resection feasible because of concerns about disruption of the blood supply to and bile ducts from segment VI. After careful packing with hypertonic saline-soaked laparotomy pads, the cyst was therefore widely unroofed and daughter cysts were removed. Fastidious dissection of the endocyst containing the germinal layer was also performed to prevent recurrence. Adjacent omentum was then packed into the residual cavity as a further measure to prevent subsequent problems.

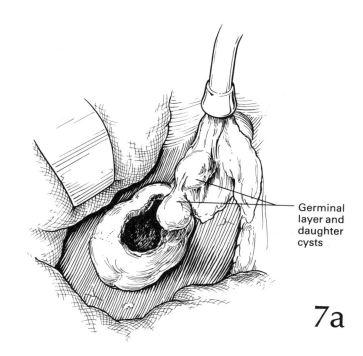

Germinal layer and daughter cysts

7a

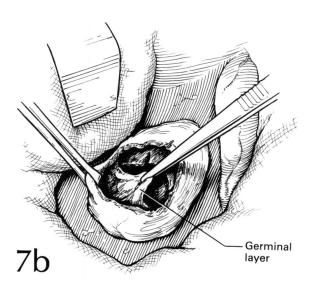

Germinal layer

7b

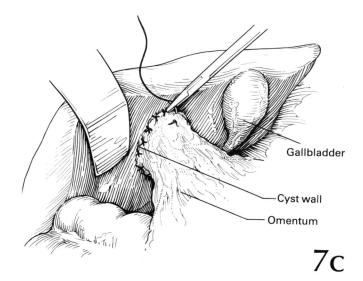

Gallbladder

Cyst wall

Omentum

7c

Diaphragmatic rupture

The fourth cyst near the dome of the right lobe of the liver had ruptured through the diaphragm and also communicated with the biliary tree. The CT scan had demonstrated minimal disease above the diaphragm so the entire procedure was performed from the abdomen. Even with moderate disease in the chest originating from a hepatic hydatid cyst, resection and reclosure of a small portion of the diaphragm may allow adequate exposure from below. However, if extensive cyst disease is present in the chest, a thoracotomy may also be required to adequately remove all of the hydatid elements.

8a–d In the patient presented, inflammatory adhesions between the dome of the liver and the diaphragm were initially dissected to reveal a fistulous communication between the cyst and the bronchus (*Illustration 8a*). This cyst was also heavily calcified, and wedge resection would not have been safe because of its proximity to the right hepatic vein. The cyst was therefore unroofed, daughter cysts were removed, and the germinal layer was carefully excised. The fistulous opening through the diaphragm was closed with sutures and a closed suction drain was placed into the cavity because of the biliary communication and the risk of a bile leak.

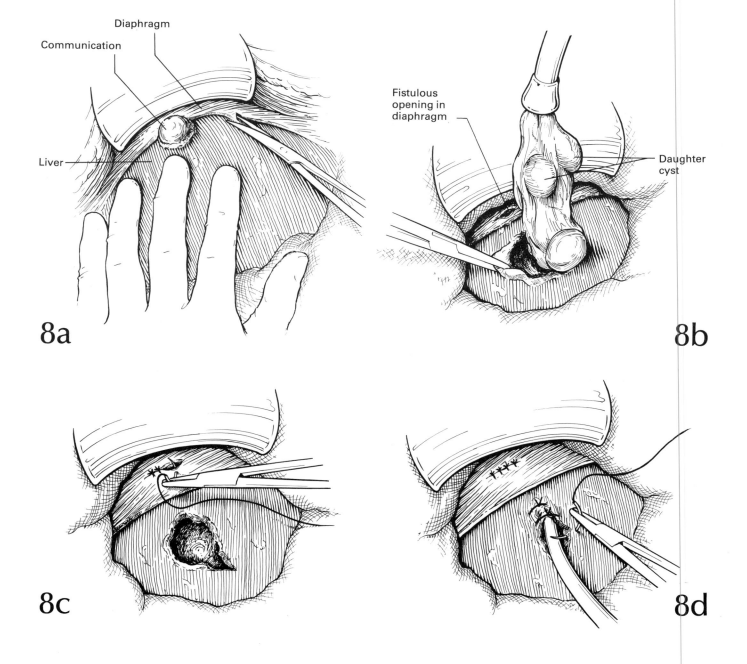

8a

8b

8c

8d

Hepatic resection

As previously mentioned, a trend toward more formal segmental and lobar hepatic resections for hepatic hydatid disease has evolved in recent years. The techniques for these liver resections are described in detail in the chapters on pp. 30–45 and 46–55. In performing these operations for echinococcal cysts, care should be taken not to rupture the cyst during the dissection. However, unlike surgery for hepatic malignancies, only a minimal margin is required on the outer wall of the cyst to prevent recurrence.

Postoperative care

As with other hepatic surgery, gastrointestinal function usually returns relatively rapidly. The majority of patients with hepatic hydatid disease have otherwise normal liver parenchyma so hepatic insufficiency is rarely a problem, even when major hepatic resection is performed. Any drains that have been placed because of concerns about a bile leak should be left in until bile flow has been stimulated by food intake. If a bile leak occurs, the drain should be kept in place until bile drainage ceases. If leakage persists for more than 10–14 days, a sinogram should be performed through the drain. If a cavity persists, the drain should not be moved. However, if no cavity is present, the drain should be pulled back slightly or replaced by a shorter, smaller diameter drain until the sinus tract closes. The drain can be safely removed when the bile leakage has stopped.

Outcome

The morbidity and mortality of surgery for hepatic hydatid disease should be low[1–4]. The most common complication is bile leakage which can usually be managed without difficulty as described above. Some recent data suggest that this complication is somewhat diminished by omental packing. With local cyst excision, even with biliary communication or diaphragmatic rupture, the mortality rate should be as low as 1–2%, and for major hepatic resection for hydatid disease it should not be much higher. The fact that these patients rarely have underlying cirrhosis makes these procedures somewhat safer than hepatic resection for hepatocellular carcinoma.

Reliable data on the long-term outcome of these patients are difficult to obtain. If the cysts do recur, this process may take many years to evolve. As a result, follow-up for 10 years or more is required to determine the eventual outcome of surgery. However, some recent data suggest that recurrence rates are lower with hepatic resection than with local cyst excision. Of course, these improved long-term results must be weighed against the slightly increased morbidity and mortality associated with major hepatic resection.

References

1. Liddle C, Little JM. Hydatid disease. In: Pitt HA, Carr-Locke DL, Ferrucci JT, eds. *Hepatobiliary and Pancreatic Disease.* Boston: Little, Brown, 1995: 91–100.

2. Langer B. Hepatic echinococcosis. In: Cameron JL, ed. *Current Surgical Therapy.* 5th edn. St Louis: Mosby-Year Book, 1995: 270–3.

3. Pitt HA, Korzelius J, Tompkins RK. Management of hepatic echinococcosis in Southern California. *Am J Surg* 1986; 152: 110–5.

4. Moreno-Gonzalez E, Selas PR, Martinez B, García IG, Carazo FP, Pascual MH. Results of surgical treatment of hepatic hydatidosis: current therapeutic modifications. *World J Surg* 1991; 15: 254–63.

5. Giorgio A, Tarantino L, Francica G *et al.* Unilocular hydatid liver cysts: treatment with US-guided double percutaneous operation and alcohol injection. *Radiology* 1992; 184: 705–10.

6. Khuroo MS, Dar MY, Yattoo GN *et al.* Percutaneous drainage versus albendazole therapy in hepatic hydatidosis: a prospective randomized study. *Gastroenterology* 1993; 104: 1452–9.

Liver abscess

I. S. Benjamin BSc, MD, FRCS
Professor, Academic Department of Surgery, King's College Hospital, London, UK

History

The first description of liver abscess is generally attributed to Bright of Guy's Hospital and was published in 1836. One of the earliest modern series was that of Ochsner et al. (1938)[1] who reported a series of 47 pyogenic abscesses of the liver. This was said to represent an incidence of about 1% of post-mortem examinations, and 0.008% of hospitalized patients. The peak age incidence was in the third and fourth decades, a different spectrum from the present situation in which the peak is in the sixth to eighth decades of life. In the pre-antibiotic era, open drainage was the only management option, but as long ago as 1900, percutaneous drainage of liver abscesses was described by Laurent using a specially designed long trocar and cannula.

Principles

The principles of management of hepatic abscesses do not differ fundamentally from the principles of abscess management elsewhere in the body, nor from the general principles governing surgery of the liver. Broadly, the presence of the abscess is established initially on clinical grounds and subsequently on imaging supported by generalized evidence of infection (such as leucocytosis) and, as a general rule, pus within a closed cavity must be released. The causative organism should be established whenever possible, either from blood culture or from direct aspiration of the abscess contents. Finally, the predisposing cause should be identified and, if necessary, eradicated. According to the general principles of liver surgery, the abscess can be localized within the hepatic segmental anatomy and an appropriate method of drainage selected which will cause least damage to normal liver tissue. If the underlying cause of the abscess is thought to be neoplastic, then consideration should be given to radical resection if possible, and if due to biliary disease then free drainage of as much of the intrahepatic biliary tree as possible should be secured by appropriate means. Other general principles of liver surgery such as attention to coagulation and support of impaired hepatocyte function should also form a part of the general management.

Aetiology

Liver abscesses are generally classified according to the nature of the infecting organism i.e. pyogenic, specific bacterial infection (such as tuberculosis), amoebic, parasitic and fungal. Both amoebic abscesses and hydatid cysts may contain only the primary infecting organism or parasite, or may be secondarily infected with pyogenic organisms. Pyogenic abscesses per primum are generally also subdivided according to the underlying cause. The most common varieties are taken into account in the classification shown in Table 1.

The frequency of these various causes displays distinct geographical variations. Pyogenic abscesses are by far the most common type of abscess in Western series, whereas in Eastern countries and in much of the Third World a liver abscess may be assumed to be of amoebic origin until proven otherwise.

Pyogenic abscess

The source of infection may be classified as in *Table 1*. In earlier series infection within the gastrointestinal tract was the commonest cause of pyogenic liver abscess, and most frequently appendicitis was responsible. The decreasing frequency of severe untreated appendicitis probably accounts for much of the shift in age spectrum from the third to the fifth decade with the passage of time. Complicated diverticular disease is now more common than appendicitis as a portal source. Umbilical sepsis remains common in Third World countries, particularly where it is the custom to dress the umbilical cord with infected materials. Portal blood is usually sterile, but chronic sepsis anywhere within the gastrointestinal tract may produce transient episodes of portal bacteraemia. This may be enhanced by obstructive jaundice, and there is also evidence that translocation of bacteria across the mucosa of the gastrointestinal tract is enhanced by starvation and by associated alterations in gastrointestinal microbial flora[2]. Sepsis associated with diverticular disease and thrombosed haemorrhoids may also be sources of portal pyaemia. Liver abscesses are rare in association with Crohn's disease, despite the bacteraemia which may occur in that condition. Benhidjeb *et al.*[3] reported a case of Crohn's disease which presented initially with a hepatic abscess. Pyogenic abscesses of gastrointestinal tract origin are frequently multiple.

Organisms of biliary origin now give rise to almost one-third of all pyogenic liver abscesses, usually as part of a syndrome of cholangitis and biliary obstruction. Garrison and Polk[4] reported that 22% of pyogenic hepatic abscesses arose from sepsis within the portal venous drainage region, compared with 32% of biliary origin. Cholangitis due to choledocholithiasis (or rarely other foreign bodies within the biliary tract), benign or malignant biliary strictures, congenital disorders of the biliary tree and primary sclerosing cholangitis may all be sources of such infection. Direct spread from acute cholecystitis or empyema of the gallbladder may also be included in this category.

1 Patients with chronic incomplete biliary tract obstruction, such as those with primary sclerosing cholangitis, recurrent biliary strictures after previous surgical repair, or occluded biliary stents are particularly prone to forming multiple small intrahepatic abscesses, initially in communication with the peripheral biliary radicals. The endoscopic retrograde cholangiopancreatogram shown is of a woman with a malignant bile duct stricture and an abscess can be seen in communication with a right sectoral hepatic duct.

Table 1   Aetiology of liver abscess

Pyogenic
  Biliary tract origin
    'Ascending' cholangitis
    Stent occlusion
    Primary sclerosing cholangitis
  Portal origin
    Appendicitis
    Diverticular disease
    Inflammatory bowel disease
    Umbilical sepsis
  Traumatic
    Iatrogenic (e.g., biliary surgery, liver biopsy, post-embolization)
    Penetrating injuries
    Blunt liver trauma
  Neoplastic
    Degeneration
    Post-embolization
  Infected cysts
    Simple
    Choledochal
    Parasitic
  Contiguous spread
    Gallbladder
    Gastrointestinal perforation
  Metastatic from systemic sepsis (especially in immunocompromised hosts)
  'Cryptogenic'

Specific bacterial infections
  Tuberculosis

Fungal

Parasitic
  Amoebic
  Hydatid
  Clonorchis sinensis
  Ascaris lumbricoides

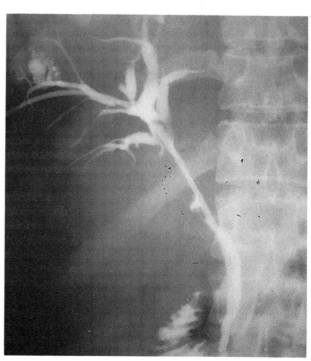

1

The symptoms of pyogenic abscess may be difficult to distinguish from those of the underlying suppurative cholangitis and, indeed, the principles of management may be similar, with the primary objective of securing good biliary drainage.

Asiatic pyogenic cholangitis is a separate category in which there is gross dilatation of the intrahepatic ductal system in association with intrahepatic stone formation, multiple strictures, and invasive sepsis which may partially destroy one or more segments of liver. This syndrome is frequently associated with parasitic infestation of the biliary tract. Such abscesses may not respond to drainage and may require partial liver resection for their eradication.

Chronic pancreatitis is said to produce biliary tract obstruction in about 15% of cases, but liver abscesses in this condition remain uncommon[5]. The combination of long-standing biliary obstruction and sepsis with impaired hepatic blood supply may be a potent cause of liver abscess; the author has seen one such patient in whom an indolent *Streptococcus milleri* liver abscess occurred following an otherwise uncomplicated pancreatoduodenectomy for chronic pancreatitis.

Haematogenous abscesses arising from systemic infection are much more common in immunocompromised patients. They constitute about 9% of all liver abscesses, and drug abusers, patients with leukaemia, diabetes or HIV infection, and those with other systemic infections such as subacute bacterial endocarditis may be at particular risk.

Iatrogenic causes (other than those associated with benign biliary strictures) are responsible for an increasing number of cases. Liver infection may follow percutaneous biopsy, percutaneous transhepatic cholangiography, or biliary stenting, when the stents become occluded (*Illustration 1*). Cases have also been reported following ethanol injection for hepatocellular carcinoma[6]. Embolization of large liver tumours may also result in a liver abscess, occasionally with gas-forming organisms.

Trauma (other than iatrogenic injury) is responsible for about 6% of pyogenic abscesses and this includes blunt injuries causing subcapsular haematomas which subsequently become infected. Contiguous spread from subhepatic, pleural or perinephric sepsis gave rise to the liver abscess in about 10% of patients in the series reported by Garrison and Polk[4].

The number of pyogenic abscesses described as 'cryptogenic' has diminished with improved investigation. In the series reported by Ochsner *et al.*[1] cryptogenic abscesses constituted 55–60% of the total, while in the series of Garrison and Polk[4] no cause could be found in only 15% of cases.

Amoebic abscess

This is caused by the organism *Entamoeba histolytica* which, while not indigenous to most Western countries, is found much more commonly with the increase of foreign travel. It has become indigenous in some immigrant populations such as the Hispanic population in the south and west of the United States. This may be particularly important because the organism may have a long latent period, occasionally up to 20 years. While amoebic abscesses classically contain the primary infecting organism, secondary infection with pyogenic organisms may also occur and can follow intervention.

Fungal abscess

These abscesses are found primarily in immunocompromised patients and may have a characteristic radiological appearance[7].

Tuberculous abscess

This form of abscess is extremely rare. Multiple small abscesses may be present in miliary tuberculosis or a single large granuloma (tuberculoma) can develop in the absence of any evidence of systemic tuberculosis. Organisms are rarely isolated from the lesion and treatment with antituberculous drugs may have to be empirical. The author has seen one case in which liver resection was required for a left-sided tuberculoma, the differential diagnosis being that of necrosis and superinfection within a primary liver tumour.

Parasitic disease

Hydatid disease
Although the diagnosis of hydatid disease of the liver is usually readily made on scanning, supported by positive serology, there may be confusion with other forms of liver abscess, especially if there is secondary infection. Bacterial infection may follow previous surgical treatment or may be spontaneous. Infection within simple cysts or hydatid cysts constituted 4% of all cases of pyogenic hepatic abscess in the series of Garrison and Polk[4].

Other parasites
Rare in Western medical practice, infestation of the biliary tree with *Ascaris lumbricoides* or with *Clonorchis sinensis* is extremely common in Asia, Africa and Central and South America. The biliary tract becomes secondarily infected, resulting in suppurative cholangitis, following which nests of worms within the liver parenchyma may cause pyogenic cholangitic liver abscesses. Chronic suppurative cholangitis (pyogenic Asiatic cholangitis) is a common sequel of infestation with *Clonorchis sinensis*.

Microbiology of pyogenic liver abscesses

In early reports, 38% of abscesses were reported to be sterile on culture[1] but this would now be uncommon. Bowers et al.[8] in a series of 34 patients reported a single organism in 15, polymicrobial growth in 11, and no positive culture in seven (material for culture was not obtained from one patient). The organisms found are usually of enteric origin. *Escherichia coli* and other organisms predominated in the 38 abscesses analysed by Barnes et al.[9] (*Table 2*). Staphylococcal infection was more common in earlier series but has now diminished in importance.

Anaerobic species are more commonly identified in recent times, the commonest being *Bacteroides fragilis*. More sensitive methods such as estimation of volatile and non-volatile fatty acids by gas liquid chromatography in the pus from abscesses allowed demonstration of the presence of anaerobic or microaerophilic bacteria in 14% of cases in one series[10]. However, *Streptococcus milleri* has also often been reported[11].

Lactobacilli have been found in an abscess following ethanol injection for hepatocellular carcinoma, and *Listeria* and *Yersinia* have also been reported. The responsible mycobacterium is only rarely cultured in cases of tuberculous infection[12], although infection with tubercle bacilli has been reported in association with HIV infection[13].

Pathology

Pyogenic liver abscesses are multiple in 50% of cases. There is a predilection for the right lobe rather than the left. Abscesses are frequently related to the portal venous radicals or to biliary radicals, in which case they may be bile-stained. The wall of the abscess may display characteristic features according to the infecting organism, but the common finding is of inflammatory infiltration of the surrounding liver. This may wall off the abscess so that in most cases it loses its communication with the biliary tree. The purulent contents may be foul smelling and contain gas, and the smell may be suggestive of a mixed aerobic/anaerobic infection.

Ameobic abscesses frequently reach a large size but are usually solitary. While 75% are on the right, those on the left side may be prone to intrapericardial rupture. The content of amoebic abscesses has the characteristic 'anchovy sauce' appearance and contains few pus cells but a great deal of debris.

Presentation and diagnosis

The presentation is characteristically one of pyrexia of unknown origin[14]. The classic constellation of signs includes sweating, anorexia, malaise, vomiting and weight loss, often associated with pain in the upper abdomen. Although swinging fever is described as classical, an analysis of clinical features in 58 cases revealed this feature in only 25% of cases[15]. Ameobic abscesses may have an insidious onset with hepatomegaly, abdominal pain and fever; diarrhoea occurs in less than 20% of patients. Evidence of atelectasis or pleural effusion may be found in any case of hepatic abscess, with occasional pain referred to the shoulder tips, but this is a non-specific finding. Haemobilia has been reported in one child secondary to liver abscess, treated by selective arterial embolization[16]. Khan et al.[17] reported obstructive jaundice secondary to an amoebic liver abscess.

Choice of treatment

There are essentially three forms of treatment: antibiotic therapy without any invasive treatment, radiological aspiration or drainage, and open surgical drainage.

Long courses of high dose antibiotics may be used in some patients with multiple small hepatic abscesses when the underlying cause is unknown or has been eradicated but, in general, drainage is also necessary. While open drainage used to be the standard treatment for all liver abscesses, in recent years it has been overtaken by percutaneous drainage techniques on the grounds of equal efficacy and greater safety. The changing practice over the last decade or two has paralleled the increased use of percutaneous drainage for other intra-abdominal collections. During the years 1979–1988 the author encountered 36 such collections in a specialist hepatobiliary unit; prior to 1984, surgical drainage was the norm. Following the adoption of percutaneous drainage methods for intra-abdominal collections there was a significant fall in overall mortality from serious postoperative sepsis[18]. Others have also reported the increasing use of percutaneous drainage[19,20].

Table 2 Pathogenic aerobic organisms in 38 cases of liver abscess. Data from Barnes et al.[9].

Organism	n
Escherichia coli	16
Klebsiella pneumoniae	6
Streptococcus sp.	6
Enterococcus	4
Proteus sp.	4
Enterobacteriaceae	3
Other Gram-negative rods (*Pseudomonas aeruginosa* 1)	3
Staphylococcus aureus	1

Table 3 Retrospective comparison of surgical *versus* percutaneous tube drainage. Data from Bertel *et al.*[21].

	Surgical	Percutaneous
Number of patients	23	16*
Morbidity (%)	48	69
Hospital stay (days)	26	46

* Three required surgery.

The issue does not readily lend itself to controlled trial because of the differing circumstances surrounding liver abscesses in individual patients. A retrospective study of patients treated at the Mayo Clinic from 1977 to 1984[21] suggested that non-surgical drainage has significant disadvantages (*Table 3*). However, much of the morbidity in this series was associated with dislodged catheters and several patients undergoing percutaneous drainage required surgery because of inadequate aspiration of viscous abscess contents.

2a–f It has been the author's recent experience that it is rarely necessary to abandon percutaneous drainage because of viscous contents and frequent tube changes, regular flushing, and even breaking down of the walls between loculi by manipulating the catheter allows continued effective use of drainage techniques. A sequence of CT scans in a patient with a pyogenic abscess of unknown aetiology treated by percutaneous drainage is shown. *Illustration 2c* shows a contrast study performed after insertion of the catheter and reveals the complex abscess contents. The catheter was used to break down loculi within the cavity, and drainage and antibiotics continued for several weeks was followed by complete resolution without recurrence.

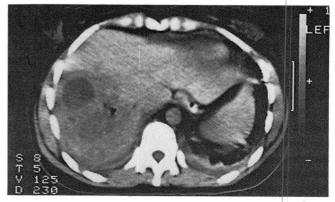

2a

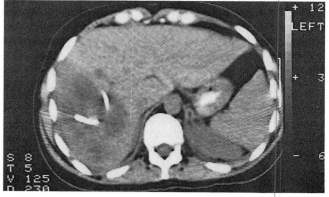

2b

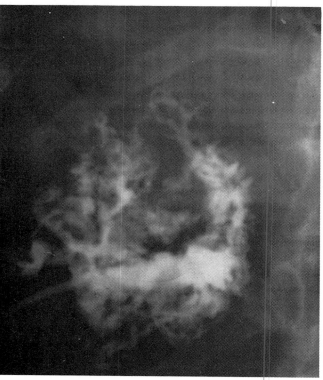

2c

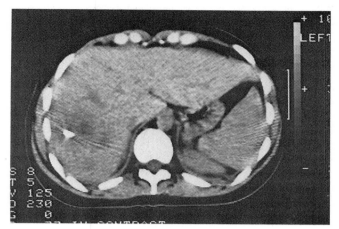

2d

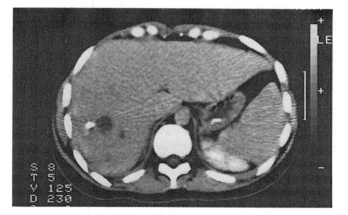

2e

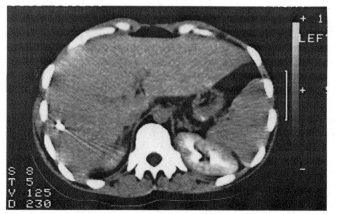

2f

Failure of drainage may, however, still result from technical factors or multiple abscesses. In such cases a combination of external drainage with prolonged systemic antibiotics is indicated. Attar *et al.*[22] used CT-guided drainage in 15 patients with abscesses of 5–1000 ml in volume, including some with multiple abscesses; only one patient required surgical drainage because of a true failure to respond. Enormous abscesses with a thick wall are unlikely to collapse completely, and may leave the problem of a residual cavity. It may be that such patients should be selected for surgical drainage.

For amoebic abscesses the issue of whether to aspirate or not remains controversial. De La Rey Nel *et al.*[23] prospectively randomized 80 patients to undergo aspiration or non-aspiration along with metronidazole treatment. This series, pursued over a period of 1 year in Durban, South Africa, suggested that aspiration did influence the course and outcome of treatment and the authors suggested a number of criteria for selection.

It should be emphasized again that it is important to consider the possibility of hydatid disease when considering aspiration, since percutaneous puncture of hydatid cysts with intraperitoneal leakage may both disseminate the disease and produce a potentially fatal anaphylactic reaction. Increasing experience suggests that percutaneous aspiration and instillation of alcohol or other scolicidal agent may be safe[24], but the author would still urge caution.

Preoperative

Clinical

Liver abscess should be considered in any case of pyrexia of unknown origin, especially in the presence of known biliary disease or when there has been biliary surgery, intervention or trauma. General examination is aimed at eliciting signs of systemic sepsis and multi-organ failure. Careful assessment of renal and hepatic function is undertaken, particularly in patients with associated jaundice. It is important to consider causes of immune deficiency in patients with otherwise unexplained liver abscesses. The abdomen is examined with a view to identifying localizing signs in the liver or elsewhere, with particular reference to other pathology within the gastrointestinal tract.

Haematological investigation is vital. Haemoglobin levels may fall precipitously in the presence of hepatic abscess (often in association with haemolysis and a raised ESR) and a neutrophil leucocytosis is typical of pyogenic abscess. Coagulation should be checked as a preliminary to surgical or radiological intervention. Biochemical testing usually shows an increased serum alkaline phosphatase concentration even in the absence of biliary obstruction. Aspartate aminotransferase (AST) levels may remain normal except in advanced disease. The albumin levels may fall precipitously in the presence of continuing liver sepsis, and this may also be predictive of a poor outcome. Where relevant, serological tests such as the ELISA test should be performed for amoebic or hydatid disease. IgG ELISA is a sensitive and specific test for invasive amoebiasis in comparison with evidence of previous exposure[25].

The importance of microbiology has already been mentioned. Blood cultures must be performed, though these are frequently negative. The question of aspiration of suspected abscesses is controversial because, although valuable for microbiological diagnosis of pyogenic abscesses, it may be unnecessary or unhelpful in amoebiasis and many would regard it as positively contraindicated in hydatid disease.

Imaging

The imaging results in 100 liver abscesses from two different geographical areas have been reviewed recently[26] and showed a preponderance, respectively, of amoebic and pyogenic or fungal abscesses. Plain abdominal radiography may give useful indicators such as elevation of the diaphragm, associated pleural effusion or consolidation of the underlying lung. Chest radiography may suggest extension of the infective process into the lung tissue or the formation of a bronchopleural fistula. An air/fluid level may be seen in some cases. However, ultrasonography has become the investigation of first choice and has, to a large extent, displaced colloidal liver scans in this role. Overall, ultrasonography will reach a correct diagnosis in 93% of cases[9]. Computed tomographic (CT) scanning may offer some increase in diagnostic accuracy as lesions as small as 2 cm can be identified. Because the pus in some abscesses is very thick, distinction between a solid lesion and an abscess is not always straightforward. In the case of multiple abscesses, other forms of diffuse parenchymal liver disease such as fatty infiltration, cirrhosis and multiple metastases have to be considered. Nevertheless, with CT scanning the diagnostic accuracy should approach 100%. Labelled white cell scanning or gallium scanning may be of complementary value. The value of magnetic resonance imaging (MRI) relative to CT scanning has yet to be established.

It should not be forgotten that the majority of liver abscesses are now of biliary origin, so that imaging of the biliary tract (usually by ERCP but occasionally by PTC) may form a critical part of the evaluation of liver abscesses.

Operations

OPEN SURGICAL DRAINAGE

It is important to appreciate the surgical anatomy of the liver (*see* chapter on pp. 1–4). The most important surgical implication for patients with liver abscesses is the relationship between cavities and the major vessels, particularly the hepatic veins. An expanding liver abscess will push segmental vessels aside, so that the wall of an abscess cavity may be partially formed by displaced and compressed major vessels and biliary radicals. In the case of large abscesses (those usually treated surgically) the use of intraoperative ultrasonography may help to define these margins. If there is any suspicion of underlying malignancy then multiple biopsies should be performed. If this is strongly suspected and the general condition of the patient and anatomy of the lesion allows, immediate resection with a clearance margin should be considered.

Incision

3 The usual approach is transperitoneal, and a long right subcostal incision is recommended. This can be extended well across the midline to the left side and into the right flank if extensive mobilization of the liver is required. The disadvantage of this incision is the inaccessibility of the lower abdomen to palpation, particularly if a source of sepsis in the colon is considered likely. Nevertheless, a full laparotomy is indicated as far as is possible. The alternative retroperitoneal approach is no longer recommended. Although this minimizes the risk of peritoneal contamination, it is impossible to assess or to deal with other pathology, and careful packing and antibiotic therapy will avoid generalized peritonitis in any event.

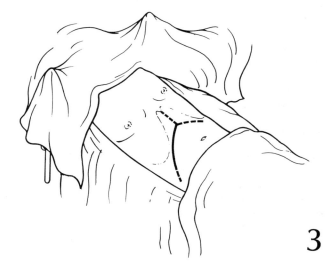

3

Localization of the abscess

4a,b The abscess can usually be localized by inspection and palpation. If the liver is greatly enlarged it may initially prove difficult to mobilize the right lobe of the liver, or even to insert a hand between the liver and the costal margin. Vigorous retraction of the costal margin using a fixed retractor system is recommended (*Illustration 4a*) but, in the case of a large abscess with risk of rupture, an initial aspiration using a trocar and cannula may be valuable (*Illustration 4b*). A large-bore needle may help to identify the site of an abscess, and samples are immediately taken for aerobic and anaerobic culture. Intraoperative ultrasonography is helpful in defining the extent of the abscess and its relationship to the major vessels and ducts.

A decision must also be taken on how to deal with any other abdominal pathology that is found. There is no absolute contraindication to resection of diverticular disease, for example, in combination with drainage of a liver abscess, but the general principles guiding multiple operative procedures at one laparotomy should be observed. The chief aim of the procedure is to deal with the liver abscess, and other pathology may be better dealt with through a different incision at a different time.

Once the site of the abscess has been identified, packs are used to wall off the rest of the abdominal cavity. Hydatid disease is considered in the chapter on pp. 101–109, but if it is thought to be a possibility then packs soaked in an appropriate scolicidal agent such as aqueous povidone-iodine (Betadine) should be used.

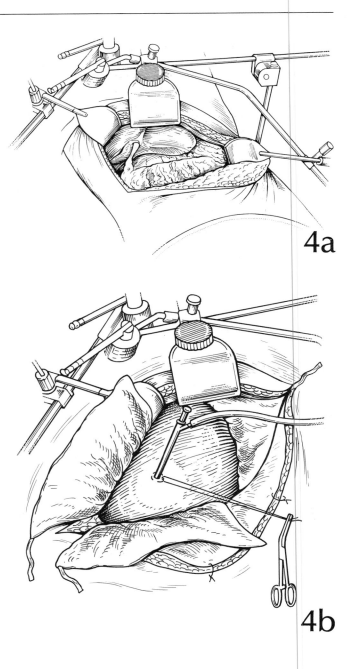

4a

4b

Aspiration of abscess

5 Following trocar aspiration an incision is made over the most superficial part of the abscess. If the liver parenchyma is thick at this level the incision can be made with the diathermy point. A large bore sucker is inserted into the cavity and the contents fully aspirated. A finger can then be inserted to assess the extent of the cavity and to help break down any internal loculi.

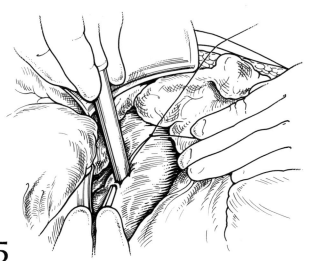

5

6a,b Although the simplest procedure is then to insert some form of large-bore drainage tube, deroofing is more likely to speed the resolution of large cavities. Deroofing is performed using the diathermy point, but care must be taken not to enter deeply into the liver parenchyma, since this may be the site of compressed segmental vesels and bile ducts which should not be disrupted. There is almost invariably some bleeding from the cut edges of the liver, and this is controlled by suturing small individual vessels (paying particular attention to small bile radicals which should be sutured separately) and then, if necessary, by controlling the cut rim of the deroofed cavity with a continuous locking mattress suture.

At the conclusion of this procedure it should be possible to inspect the lining of the cavity. The cavity should be carefully washed out and then packed for a few minutes to check for haemostasis and for bile leaks. Any small leaking bile radicals should be evident on removal of the packs and are carefully closed with a fine suture. If in doubt, radiological screening after injection of contrast medium into the biliary tree (via the gallbladder or bile duct) may reveal leaks. Injections of saline or diluted methylene blue dye may be used as a simpler alternative. In practice, it is less common to use these techniques for pyogenic abscess than for hydatid disease.

Consideration is now given to the type of tube drainage. Simple tube drains of the largest size available may be adequate and should be brought out through a separate stab wound. Suction drains become blocked and are usually unhelpful. Sump drains, particularly those of the irrigating variety, may be helpful for large cavities. The drains should be placed so that they exit in a dependent position and they must be securely fixed to the abdominal wall. Finally, if a flap of omentum is easily raised and can be laid into the cavity, this may also be helpful.

The abdominal cavity is finally washed out thoroughly with saline and closed in the usual fashion.

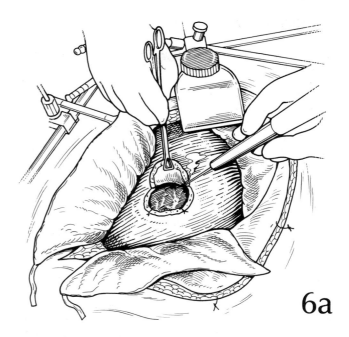

6a

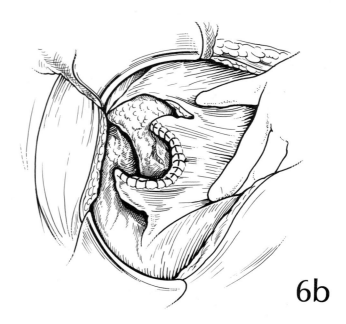

6b

LAPAROSCOPIC DRAINAGE

Cappuccino *et al.*[27] described the use of laparoscopy to guide and place intrahepatic and perihepatic drains in a patient in whom CT-guided drainage had failed to produce resolution. Robles *et al.*[28] described the technique in a patient with amoebic abscess. Extensive experience of these techniques has not yet been reported in the literature, and any advantages over percutaneous drainage with laparotomy in selected cases are as yet uncertain.

Postoperative care

Following open surgery a closed system of drainage is preferred to avoid ascending infection by exogenous organisms. If irrigation is to be used, a dilute antiseptic solution (such as aqueous povidone-iodine) is acceptable. A rate of 1 litre/24 h is usually adequate. The presence of drains is helpful since, in addition to postoperative ultrasonography, contrast medium can be instilled to determine whether the cavity is closing. Any postoperative bile leakage can be managed conservatively since the tube effectively functions as a controlled external biliary fistula. This drainage normally ceases spontaneously but, if not, a combination of ERCP and contrast tubography will identify the site and nature of the leak and determine whether any further action is needed. The tubes are removed when they have ceased to drain any significant amount of fluid and when the cavity is seen to be closing down around the tubes and a track is well established.

Antibiotics are usually continued for several weeks and follow-up antibiotics for a longer period are often used in the case of multiple abscesses. The choice of antibiotics, initially blind, can now be directed according to the microbiology and sensitivities determined on the operative samples.

Outcome

Until 1968 a mortality rate of 80–90% was regularly reported for liver abscesses, but overall mortality is now less than 10%. Factors which will determine outcome are age, multiplicity of lesions, associated biliary disease and malignancy. Adverse prognostic features include a raised serum AST level, low serum albumin level, persistently high white cell count and other complicating pathology. If a liver abscess fails to respond to treatment (whether conservative, percutaneous, or surgical) one should suspect continued obstruction to the biliary tree, a foreign body, or underlying malignancy.

References

1. Ochsner A, De Bakey M, Murray S. Pyogenic abscess of the liver. An analysis of 47 cases with review of the literature. *Am J Surg* 1938; 40: 292–319.

2. Ding JW, Andersson R, Soltesz V, Willen R, Bengmark S. Obstructive jaundice impairs reticuloendothelial function and promotes bacterial translocation in the rat. *J Surg Res* 1994; 57: 238–45.

3. Benhidjeb T, Ridwelski K, Wolff H, Gellert K, Luning M, Perschy J. Lover abscess as a first manifestation of Crohn's disease. *Dig Surg* 1992; 9: 288–92.

4. Garrison RN, Polk HC. Liver abscess and subphrenic abscess. In: Blumgart LH, ed. *Surgery of the Liver and Biliary Tract*. Edinburgh: Churchill Livingstone, 1994: 1091–102.

5. Reddy KR, Jeffers L, Livingstone AS, Gluck CA, Schiff ER. Pyogenic liver abscess complicating common bile duct stenosis secondary to chronic calcific pancreatitis. A rare presentation. *Gastroenterology* 1984; 86: 953–7.

6. Okada S, Aoki K, Okazaki N *et al.* Liver abscess after percutaneous ethanol injection (PEI) therapy for hepatocellular carcinoma. A case report. *Hepatogastroenterology* 1993; 40: 496–8.

7. Pastakia B, Shawker TH, Thaler M, O'Leary T, Pizzo PA. Hepatosplenic candidiasis: wheels within wheels. *Radiology* 1988; 166: 417–21.

8. Bowers ED, Robison DJ, Doberneck RC. Pyogenic liver abscess. *World J Surg* 1990; 14: 128–32.

9. Barnes PF, DeCock KM, Reynolds TN, Ralls PW. A comparison of amebic and pyogenic abscess of the liver. *Medicine* 1987; 66: 472–83.

10. Gupta U, Sharma MP. Etiology of liver abscess with special reference to anaerobic bacteria. *Indian J Med Res* 1990; 91: 21–3.

11. De Mestier P, Gujez C, Chakkour K, Khayat M, Chevalier T. Liver abscess caused by *Streptococcus milleri*. *Gastroenterol Clin Biol* 1992; 16: 1007–8.

12. Goh KL, Pathmanathan R, Chang KW, Wong NW. Tuberculous liver abscess. *J Trop Med Hyg* 1987; 90: 255–7.

13. Weinberg JJ, Cohen P, Malhotra R. Primary tuberculous liver abscess associated with the human immunodeficiency virus. *Tubercle* 1988; 69: 145–7.

14. Cohen JL, Martin FM, Rossi RL, Schoetz DJ Jr. Liver abscess. The need for complete gastrointestinal evaluation. *Arch Surg* 1989; 124: 561–4.

15. Ahmed L, el-Rooby A, Kassem MI, Salama ZA, Strickland GT. Ultrasonography in the diagnosis and management of 52 patients with amebic liver abscess in Cairo. *Rev Infect Dis* 1990; 12: 330–7.

16. Khalil A, Chadha V, Mandapati R *et al.* Hemobilia in a child with liver abscess. *J Pediatr Gastroenterol Nutr* 1995; 12: 136–8.

17. Khan JA, Jafri SMW, Khan MA. Obstructive jaundice: an unusual presentation of amebic liver abscess. *J Trop Med Hyg* 1990; 93: 194–6.

18. Pace RF, Blenkharn JI, Edwards WJ, Orloff M, Blumgart LH, Benjamin IS. Intra-abdominal sepsis after hepatic resection. *Ann Surg* 1989; 209: 302–6.

19. Falk KA, Angeras UJ, Friman VZ, Gamklou GR, Lukes PJ. Pyogenic liver abscesses: have changes in management improved the outcome? *Acta Chir Scand* 1987; 153: 661–4.

20. Farges O, Leese T, Bismuth H. Pyogenic liver abscess: an improvement in prognosis. *Br J Surg* 1988; 75: 862–5.

21. Bertel CK, Van Heerden JA, Sheedy PF. Treatment of pyogenic hepatic abscesses: surgical vs percutaneous drainage. *Arch Surg* 1986; 121: 554–8.

22. Attar B, Levendoglu H, Cuasay NS. CT-guided percutaneous aspiration and catheter drainage of pyogenic liver abscesses. *Am J Gastroenterol* 1986; 81: 550–5.

23. De La Rey Nel J, Simjee AE, Patel A. Indications for aspiration of amoebic liver abscess. *S Afr Med J* 1989; 75: 373–6.

24. Bastid C, Azar C, Doyer M, Sahel J. Percutaneous treatment of hydatid cysts under sonographic guidance. *Dig Dis Sci* 1994; 39: 1576–80.

25. Sathar MA, Simjee AE, De La Rey Nel J, Bredenkamp BLF, Gathiram V, Jackson TFHG. Evaluation of an enzyme-linked immunosorbent assay in the serodiagnosis of amoebic liver abscess. *S Afr Med J* 1988; 74: 625–8.

26. Barreda R, Ros PR. Diagnostic imaging of liver abscess. *Crit Rev Diagn Imaging* 1991; 33: 29–58.

27. Cappuccino H, Campanile F, Knecht J. Laparoscopy-guided drainage of hepatic abscess. *Surg Laparosc Endosc* 1994; 4: 234–7.

28. Robles PJ, Lara JG, Lancaster B. Drainage of hepatic amebic abscess successfully treated by laparoscopy. *J Laparoendosc Surg* 1994; 4: 451–4.

Liver trauma

O. James Garden BSc, MD, FRCS(Ed), FRCS(Glas)
Senior Lecturer and Honorary Consultant Hepatobiliary Surgeon, University Department of Surgery and Scottish Liver Transplantation Unit, Royal Infirmary, Edinburgh, UK

History

The earliest hepatic surgery was almost exclusively concerned with trauma. By the turn of the century, the principles of managing hepatic trauma were well established, it being recognized that minor wounds could stop bleeding spontaneously or be dealt with successfully by a variety of suture techniques, and that more significant haemorrhage might require to be controlled by packing or hepatic resection[1–3]. In 1908 Pringle also described the use of gauze packing to achieve temporary haemostasis, but this publication was more notable for its advancement of the concept of temporary occlusion of the portal triad as a means of controlling hepatic haemorrhage and division of the ligamentous attachments to gain access to posteriorly situated liver injuries[4].

The Second World War witnessed a change in the management of liver injuries, but experience in subsequent conflicts and in civilian practice has provided a better definition of the role of exploratory laparotomy, packing, abdominal drainage and hepatic resection[5,6]. Since 1980 refinements in imaging have hearalded an era of conservative management of hepatic trauma in selected patients, while at the same time an aggressive approach to the management of caval and hepatic venous injuries has gained popularity[7,8]. Major liver injuries, often in association with multiple organ trauma, are difficult to manage and are associated with high morbidity and mortality rates. This type of injury is relatively uncommon in civilian practice in the UK compared with the USA, and most surgeons consequently have only a limited experience.

Principles and justification

In the management of liver trauma, the nature of the injury and the extent of associated injuries play a major part in determining outcome. Simple penetrating injuries caused by stab wounds or low energy missiles result in minimal tissue devitalization and are associated with relatively minor haemorrhage unless a major vascular structure is traversed. Blunt injuries or gunshot wounds, on the other hand, more commonly disrupt the hepatic parenchyma extensively and result in massive haemorrhage. Deceleration injuries may tear or avulse the right hepatic vein as the posterior sector of the liver is detached from the right triangular ligament. The middle hepatic vein is more often injured within the liver parenchyma as a consequence of anterior-posterior compression of the liver against the vertical column.

Diagnosis

Injury to the liver will normally be suspected from the mechanism of injury and the clinical presentation. The hypovolaemic patient with abdominal signs requires urgent aggressive resuscitation and immediate laparotomy may become an integral part of the resuscitation process. The use of thoracotomy prior to laparotomy is controversial, but if an associated chest injury is present, thoracotomy may take precedence in order to achieve intrathoracic haemostasis and permit clamping of the aorta above the diaphragm. In the absence of a cardiac or thoracic injury, aortic compression below the diaphragm is as effective while resuscitative measures are continued.

1a–c In the resuscitated and haemodynamically stable patient, peritoneal lavage may be helpful in detecting significant intra-abdominal injury. The presence of freely aspirated blood from the peritoneal cavity may signify hepatic injury. Evaluation of liver trauma by ultrasonography, computed tomographic (CT) scanning and arteriography may also be considered after the initial phase of acute injury. Subcapsular haematoma without intraperitoneal bleeding may be identified and, with minor stab wounds to the liver, laparoscopy may be performed in order to defer or avoid exploratory laparotomy. Operation, however, is generally necessary to exclude associated injuries of other organs and to permit drainage of the liver wound.

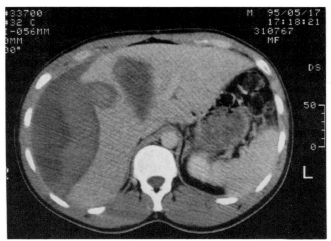

1a

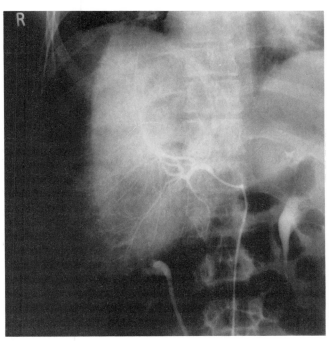

1b

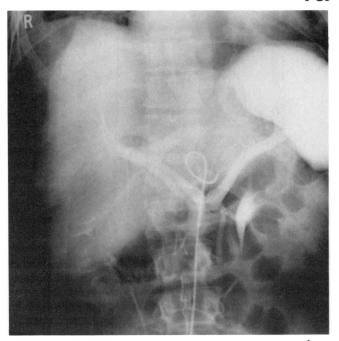

1c

The classification given in *Table 1* may be of value in assessing the amount of tissue disruption and haemorrhage and in planning operative management. Grade I and II injuries are by far the most common in surgical practice in the UK. Grade III injuries can be controlled by temporary clamping of the porta hepatis and grade IV injuries carry the highest mortality.

Table 1   Grading of liver injury

Grade	Injury
I	Capsular tear. Minor bleeding that stops spontaneously or after a few simple sutures. Parenchyma not damaged.
II	Parenchymal damage. Local haemostasis possible by careful suturing.
III	Parenchymal damage. Major haemorrhage from intrahepatic arteries and/or veins threatening life and producing shock.
IV	Grade III injury with a tear of the inferior vena cava or major hepatic vessels.

Preoperative

For patients with severe injuries, aggressive management will follow the principles of initial care of all trauma patients. Endotracheal intubation is utilized and blood volume replacement is initiated with warm Ringer's lactate solution via a large-bore upper extremity or central vein catheter. Large volumes of blood, frozen plasma and platelets will be necessary and a broad-spectrum cephalosporin is administered. If initial fluid replacement exceeds 50 ml/kg, type-specific blood is commenced with the use of O negative blood being reserved for the agonal patient. All blood is given through warming devices and filters. If the patient's blood pressure cannot be maintained above 60 mmHg a left lateral thoracotomy is made in the fifth intercostal space and the descending aorta above the diaphragm is occluded until haemorrhage from the liver has been controlled at laparotomy.

Operations

PRIMARY REFERRAL

Incision

2 An upper midline incision extending from the xiphoid process to below the umbilicus is generally recommended, although others prefer a right subcostal incision with thoracic extension when necessary. The upper midline incision is the most rapid and bloodless and allows thorough exploration for other injuries. For major hepatic injuries it can be extended by median sternotomy or by lateral extension beneath the right subcostal margin; this is preferred by the author to avoid unnecessary thoracic exploration.

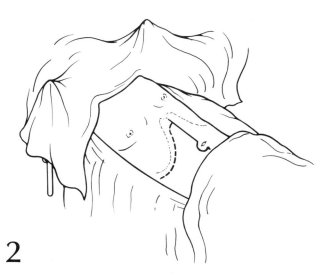

2

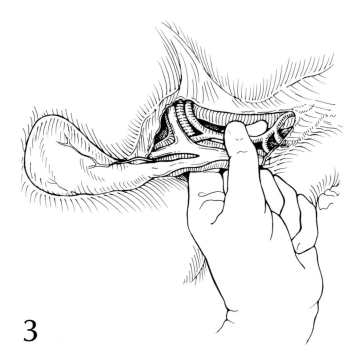

3 Blood and blood clots are rapidly evacuated as the peritoneal cavity is opened and the surgeon grasps the porta hepatis of the liver between finger and thumb, while applying gentle but firm pressure on the liver wound. In this way, temporary control of bleeding will allow careful inspection of the wound and the rest of the abdominal cavity.

3

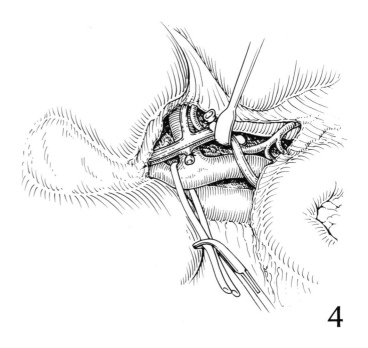

4 The porta hepatis can be secured by a sling or tape and this will facilitate subsequent placement of a soft occlusion clamp. The clamp can be applied intermittently for periods of up to 20 minutes. Initial control of active bleeding permits replacement of blood volume, stabilization of blood pressure and a more deliberate assessment of the patient's status. In certain cases involving localized injury to one lobe of the liver, it may be possible to isolate the right branch of the portal vein and the right hepatic artery in such a way that control of the vessels to one side of the liver will minimize the risk of liver failure whilst control of bleeding points is undertaken.

Specific procedures

Type I and II injuries

Superficial capsular lacerations will generally have stopped bleeding by the time the abdomen is opened and should not be manipulated for fear of precipitating further haemorrhage. Continued pressure with a swab or the application of a haemostatic agent will be useful if there is minor persistent ooze of blood. Haemostasis may be achieved by the use of diathermy coagulation. Drainage is unnecessary if the tear is limited to the capsule.

5 Non-bleeding superficial parenchymal lacerations such as those resulting from stab wounds and small calibre gunshot wounds do not need to be sutured unless they are situated in the periphery of the liver and can be confirmed as non-penetrating wounds. A 20 gauge soft silicone rubber drain is placed at the site of the wound and brought out laterally through a separate stab incision and is left in place as long as bile or fresh blood continues to drain.

Subcapsular haematomas most frequently occur over the dome of the right lobe of the liver and, if encountered at laparotomy for abdominal trauma, it is the author's practice not to disturb the lesion. The increasing use of diagnostic scans in patients with abdominal trauma has made it less likely that such lesions are diagnosed by laparotomy. The abdomen should be explored and definitive treatment undertaken if the liver size is increasing on abdominal examination, an enlarging defect is shown on scanning, or there is an increase in symptomatology. At operation, blood and clot have to be removed while temporary control of haemorrhage is established by portal clamping. Bleeding is controlled by direct suture ligation of bleeding points and postoperative drainage is established.

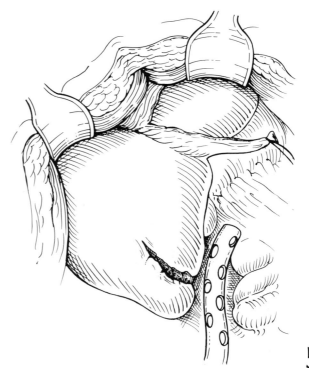

Type III injury

6 Once blood and clots have been removed from the operating field the liver is compressed by a pack held in the hands of the assistant. Bleeding is controlled by temporary portal clamping for up to 20 minutes. This enables the laceration to be gently explored while bleeding points are suture ligated with 3/0 and 4/0 polypropylene (Prolene). Deep large chromic catgut sutures should not be used because the use of such sutures in secondarily referred patients does not always control haemorrhage, may promote necrosis of the liver, and may injure major bile ducts or vessels. Devitalized liver tissue is best debrided with the Cavitron or with a Kelly clamp, preserving as much of the viable surrounding liver tissue as possible. Entry and exit sites of penetrating wounds are not sutured since this may produce uncontrolled bleeding within the liver substance, resulting in the development of major intrahepatic haematomas and hepatic disruption.

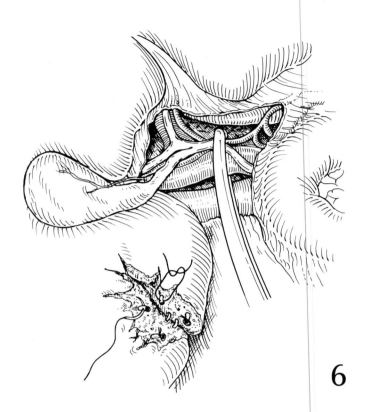

6

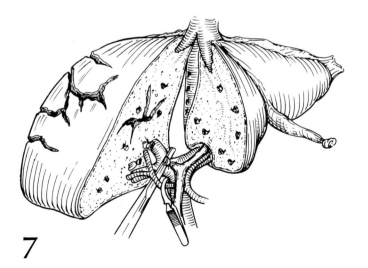

7

7 Hepatic lacerations requiring segmental or classical hepatic resection are rare, but resection is more often indicated for extensive injuries involving the right lobe of the liver. Although atypical resection and debridement of an acute injury can be undertaken, formal hepatic resection along anatomical lines ensures a clean transection through the liver, and the vessels and ducts can be secured with haemostatic clips or by suture ligation. Although some have advocated the insertion of a T tube into the biliary tree, the author does not use this for injuries not involving the extrahepatic biliary tree. The abdomen is drained in the same way as for elective hepatic resections.

Type IV injury

In severe liver injury the continuation of haemorrhage despite clamping of the porta hepatis is strongly suggestive of an injury to the major hepatic vein, trunks or the retrohepatic vena cava. With such injuries, adequate access must be ensured. Several approaches have been used in an attempt to control this form of haemorrhage but no one of these has met with consistent success.

8 The injured retrohepatic inferior vena cava is isolated by freeing the liver from its peritoneal attachments and encircling the suprahepatic and infrahepatic vena cava. Intermittent portal clamping may reduce blood loss, but in the hypovolaemic patient it may be necessary to clamp the abdominal aorta temporarily above the coeliac trunk. Exposure of the injured vessels, either from above the liver or by resection of the right hemiliver, may then be undertaken and any bleeding points can be controlled by suture ligation. However, such extensive manoeuvres all produce significant additional blood loss and most centres report uniform failure.

Other attempts at maintaining venous return to the heart have included creation of an atriocaval shunt by insertion of a balloon tip catheter through an opening in the inferior vena cava up into the atrium, and establishing the patient on venovenous bypass as for a liver transplant. Although the latter approach has been favoured by the author, his success with the technique has been no greater than that reported in the literature.

9 In centres not familiar with the management of major trauma, patients with such injuries have an improved chance of survival if their bleeding is controlled by temporary insertion of abdominal packs. Insertion of such packs may be particularly judicious in hypovolaemic patients with major liver injury, established coagulopathy and failing cardiorespiratory function. Folded packs should be inserted above and below the liver to compress the injury. Packs should not be placed within the liver injury since this may further disrupt the wound. A temporary closure of the abdominal incision is undertaken. The author does not recommend the use of abdominal drains in such cases and prefers to re-explore the abdomen 2 days later to remove the packs, rather than to have them accessible through an open wound.

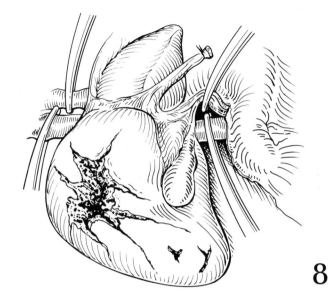

8

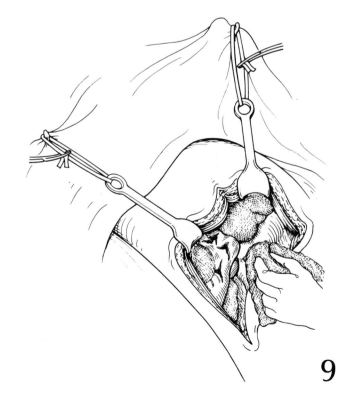

9

SECONDARY REFERRAL

Early referral

Patients may require to be transferred from non-specialist centres for further management. Such patients would normally be transferred following insertion of abdominal packs, with the patient haemodynamically stable. Following further stabilization with adequate resuscitation and administration of coagulation factors, the packs can be removed and the injury dealt with on its merits employing the principles of management described above.

Late referral

Patients in this group are generally referred because they develop specific complications such as sepsis, jaundice or a biliary fistula. Intra-abdominal sepsis may develop due to the presence of devitalized liver tissue. Such patients require CT scanning to determine the extent of the injury and devitalization of the liver. Once the patient is resuscitated, early surgical intervention may be necessary to enable debridement and provide adequate intra-abdominal drainage. The late development of intra-abdominal sepsis following liver injury may be managed adequately by percutaneous drainage of well defined collections, but control of sepsis is extremely difficult while necrotic liver is present.

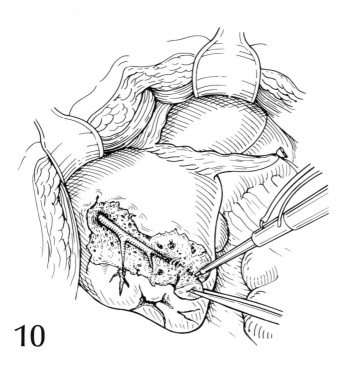

10

10 Detached fragments of liver and blood clot may lie free within the peritoneal cavity. Such fragments may have a tenuous attachment to the liver and therefore may be readily removed. The author prefers to use the Cavitron to debride the injury and it may be unnecessary to undertake a formal hepatic resection. Dissection is undertaken along anatomical planes avoiding damage to vessels. Any divided segmental pedicles can be secured by suture ligation with 4/0 or 5/0 polypropylene. Care must be taken not to tear branches of the hepatic veins as they course between the sectors of the liver to the vena cava.

Jaundice is common following liver trauma and may be associated with the presence of sepsis. If ductal injury is suspected and ultrasonography does not exclude the possibility of mechanical obstruction, ERCP may be necessary to demonstrate the anatomy of the biliary tree. In the unlikely event of injury to the extrahepatic biliary system, temporary drainage of the biliary tree may be achieved by endoscopic insertion of a biliary stent.

Postoperative care

The systemic hypotension often seen from such extensive injuries and loss of blood may produce impaired hepatocellular function as well as diminished function of other organs. Coagulopathy occurs in over 50% of patients and an aggressive prophylactic regimen, consisting of the administration of platelets and fresh frozen plasma, may reduce blood transfusion requirements and assist in arresting haemorrhage. Monitoring should be undertaken in an intensive care unit as ventilatory support may be required. Renal dysfunction is common and haemofiltration may be necessary.

Complications

Intra-abdominal sepsis following major hepatic injury may declare itself as the discharge of tissue, pus or bile through the wound or abdominal drain. In the absence of biliary obstruction, the fistula will resolve if sepsis is controlled. If the drainage of bile persists, a tubogram through the fistula tract or an endoscopic retrograde cholangiogram will determine if there is obstruction of the biliary tree. Liver function is assessed immediately after the operation by estimation of blood glucose and lactate levels and a coagulation screen. These tests may be repeated frequently to monitor hepatic function. Because of the significant risk of respiratory complications, physiotherapy, incentive spirometry and early ambulation are employed routinely. Upper gastro-intestinal haemorrhage is not uncommon and patients should be managed prophylactically with an H_2 receptor antagonist such as cimetidine. Postoperative jaundice reaches a peak at about 10 days after surgical intervention, although it may persist for some weeks with severe injury. Serum bilirubin and other tests reflecting liver damage return slowly to normal over the next 2–3 months.

References

1. Beck C. Surgery of the liver. *JAMA* 1902; 38: 1063–8.

2. Schroder WE. The progress of liver hemostasis – reports of cases. *Surg Gynecol Obstet* 1906; ii: 52–61.

3. Burckhardt H. Beitrag zur Behandlung der Leberverlezungen. *Zentralbl Chir* 1887; 14: 88–99.

4. Pringle JH. Notes on the arrest of hepatic haemorrhage due to trauma. *Ann Surg* 1908; 48: 541–9.

5. Madding GF, Lawrence KB, Kennedy PA. Forward surgery of the severely injured. *Second Auxiliary Group 1*, 1942–1945, 307.

6. Trunkey KK, Shires GT, McClelland R. Management of liver trauma in 811 consecutive patients. *Ann Surg* 1974; 179: 722–8.

7. Feliciano DV, Mattox KL, Jorden GL, Burch JM, Bitondo CG, Cruse PA. Management of 1000 consecutive cases of hepatic trauma (1979–1984). *Ann Surg* 1986; 204: 438–45.

8. John TG, Greig JD, Johnston AJ, Garden OJ. Liver trauma: a 10-year experience. *Br J Surg* 1992; 79: 1352–6.

Budd–Chiari syndrome

Jacques Belghiti MD
Professor of Surgery, Department of Surgery, University Paris VII and Beaujon Hospital, Clichy, France

Jean Pierre Benhamou MD
Professor of Medicine, Department of Hepatology, University Paris VII and Beaujon Hospital, Clichy, France

Roger Noun MD
Assistant of Surgery, Department of Surgery, University Paris VII and Beaujon Hospital, Clichy, France

Dominique Valla MD
Professor of Medicine, Department of Hepatology, University Paris VII and Beaujon Hospital, Clichy, France

Principles and justification

The Budd–Chiari syndrome is a disorder caused by a blockage of the hepatic venous outflow located at the major hepatic veins and/or at the portion of the inferior vena cava (IVC) situated between the ostia of the hepatic veins and the right atrium. The clinical presentation depends on the number of involved hepatic veins, the degree of obstruction and the rapidity of thrombosis.

Physiopathological and histopathological consequences of hepatic venous outflow blockage

The obstruction of a single main hepatic vein is clinically silent. When occlusion of the different hepatic veins is asynchronous, atrophy of the formerly affected liver segments may coexist with congestive enlargement of more recently affected segments. In approximately half of the cases of occlusion of the hepatic veins, a hypertrophic caudate lobe is found[1]. Hypertrophy of the caudate lobe is caused by the anatomy of its outflow tract and can result in compression of the IVC. Impairment of venous drainage has two consequences: raised sinusoidal pressure and liver cell ischaemia. Raised sinusoidal pressure results in portal hypertension and enhances the filtration through the liver capsule of a high protein ascites. Massive production of ascitic fluid can induce hypovolaemia and functional renal failure. The consequences of ischaemia are liver failure and parenchymal cell atrophy. Within a few weeks, centrilobular fibrosis develops. In late stages of the disease, established cirrhosis is evident.

Causes and manifestations of the Budd–Chiari syndrome

The causes of hepatic venous outflow blockage can be classified into four groups according to the mechanism of obstruction: (1) primary lesions of the main hepatic veins; (2) tumorous invasion of the main hepatic veins or IVC; (3) compression by space-occupying lesions; and (4) primary lesions of the IVC[2]. The term 'veno-occlusive disease' should be restricted to the well defined lesion affecting intrahepatic venules and will not be used in this chapter. Primary lesions of the main hepatic veins account for most cases of blockage of the hepatic venous outflow in western countries, in contrast to membranous occlusion of the IVC which represents the main cause in the Orient. The proportion of idopathic cases is now less than 10% given that a systematic search for an associated thrombogenic condition (paroxysmal nocturnal haemoglobinuria or primary myeloproliferative disorder) is performed.

The main clinical manifestations of hepatic vein occlusion in a series of 50 patients admitted to Hôpital Beaujon are shown in *Table 1*. Patients can be ascribed to one of three clinical variants (*Table 2*) depending on the number of involved hepatic veins, the degree of obstruction and the rapidity of thrombosis.

Table 1 Clinical manifestations of hepatic venous outflow blockage due to primary lesions of the hepatic veins in a series of 50 patients admitted to Hôpital Beaujon

Signs and symptoms	Prevalence (%)
Ascites	96
Liver enlargement	90
Abdominal pain	80
Splenomegaly	64
Oedema	46
Jaundice	44
Fever	40
Hepatic encephalopathy	22
Gastrointestinal bleeding	14

Diagnosis

The diagnosis of hepatic venous outflow blockage should be suspected whenever ascites and liver enlargement are present, especially in patients with an already recognized thrombogenic condition. In the majority of cases, ultrasonography provides evidence of obstruction of the hepatic outflow (echogenic material in the lumen, stenosis with upstream dilatation, hyperechogenic cord replacing the veins, intrahepatic venous collaterals) and changes in liver morphology with the characteristic enlargement of segment I. Inferior vena cavography must be performed whenever patency cannot be clearly demonstrated by non-invasive imaging procedures, coupled with pressure measurement. Tumours invading or compressing the hepatic veins are well delineated by computed tomographic scanning. Magnetic resonance imaging might be better than ultrasonography and computed tomographic scanning for studying the IVC. In patients in whom the non-invasive imaging procedures fail to establish the diagnosis, liver biopsy early in the course of the disease can yield classical features. Rarely, opacification of the hepatic vein is needed. The patency of the portal vein and superior mesenteric vein can be evaluated by ultrasonography and knowledge of patency is essential when making therapeutic decisions.

Treatment

Non-specific measures

Non-specific measures include the prevention of other venous thromboses and the treatment of ascites. Prevention of extension of venous thrombosis is justified in patients with primary lesions of the hepatic veins and IVC when a thrombogenic condition is present. Full-blown primary myeloproliferative disorders must be treated urgently. Control of ascites is usually achieved with diuretics. When diuretics are not sufficient, paracentesis with infusion of serum albumin is indicated. Peritoneovenous shunting should only be performed when ascites is resistant to medical therapy and portosystemic shunting is not feasible. However, obstruction of the valve and thrombosis of the recipient vein are common due to the protein-rich ascitic fluid and to the frequently associated thrombogenic condition.

Restoration of hepatic blood outflow

This essential aspect of treatment aims to correct sinusoidal and portal venous hypertension, thereby controlling ascites and preventing gastrointestinal bleeding. Another goal is to reduce hepatic ischaemia and prevent disease progression. The indications for the currently available procedures mainly depend on the patency of the IVC and portal vein.

Table 2 Classification of clinical forms of the Budd–Chiari syndrome

Form	Incidence	Main symptom	Raised transaminases	Prothrombin time
Fulminant failure	Rare	Fulminant liver	Massive	< 20%
Acute and subacute jaundice	25%	Ascites +++	Moderate	< 40%
Chronic malnutrition	75%	Ascites +	Slight or none	> 40%

Operations

PATENT PORTAL VEIN AND PATENT IVC

Transformation of the portal vein into an outflow tract is the rationale for portosystemic shunting. In cases of high IVC pressure without thrombosis, some authors have suggested that a shunt with the superior vena caval system should be performed. The authors advise against this approach and believe that a standard shunt using IVC can be used in most of these cases. Shunts using the right atrium or innominate vein are associated with a higher postoperative thrombosis rate, probably because of the long prosthetic graft. The most important determinant of patency is the gradient pressure between portal vein and IVC before shunting; a portal shunt using the IVC can be performed despite high IVC pressure if a significant gradient exists between the portal vein and IVC and no (or minimal) residual gradient persists after shunt opening. Following portal decompression, the hypertrophied caudate lobe gradually reduces in size with progressive relief of IVC compression, thus improving the shunt flow. The higher incidence of shunt thrombosis observed in patients with extensive fibrosis or cirrhosis could be due, in part, to a persistent retrohepatic caval compression and to a low flow rate.

From our experience and from the literature it appears that: (a) both side-to-side portacaval and mesocaval shunts have given the best results; (b) in-hospital mortality ranges from 0 to 30%; (c) shunt thrombosis occurs in less than 10% of patients and is usually an early complication; (d) massive ascites may develop if extensive fibrosis or cirrhosis is present; and (e) most patients have no ascites at 1 year follow-up[1-4].

Side-to-side portacaval shunt

This type of shunt is the first to be considered in almost every patient with a patent portal vein as it seems to be associated with the lowest rate of thrombosis[5]. The procedure may be compromised in cases with caudate lobe hypertrophy that widens the distance between the portal vein and IVC. The procedure begins with an extensive circumferential mobilization of the infrahepatic vena cava in order to facilitate its displacement towards the portal vein. In Budd–Chiari syndrome, the approach to the IVC is rendered difficult by the presence of a developed collateral and lymphatic circulation in the peritoneum over its anterior surface. Once collaterals have been dealt with, attention is directed to mobilization of the portal vein. The hepatoduodenal ligament in the Budd–Chiari syndrome is usually stretched by liver enlargement and is overlaid by a thickened peritoneum.

The portal vein should be approached from the right posterolateral aspect to obviate the need to dissect the common bile duct and to minimize bleeding from collaterals. Ligation before division of the engorged lymphatic trunks in this area is mandatory. When its anterior wall is exposed, a vein retractor is inserted to retract the common bile duct medially. Care must be taken to avoid inadvertent injury to a right hepatic branch arising from the superior mesenteric artery. The portal vein is isolated, encircled with an umbilical tape, and isolated upwards to its bifurcation in the hilum and downwards behind the pancreas after division of the pancreatic tributary that enters the posterolateral aspect of the vein. Before making the anastomosis, pressures in the IVC and portal vein are measured by direct puncture as the gradient across the two veins is essential for shunt patency.

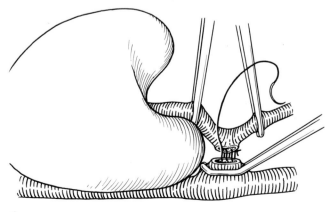

1

1 After it is established that the two vessels can be approximated without excessive tension, a Satinsky clamp is applied to the anterior wall of the IVC in a direction parallel to the portal vein. In some cases the pressure in the IVC is so high that it is necessary to isolate the vein between two clamps to avoid slippage of a partially occlusive clamp. The portal vein is occluded between two vascular clamps. An ellipse is removed from both the medial aspect of the IVC and posterior aspect of the portal vein. The portal vein is anastomosed side-to-side with the IVC with a minimum anastomotic length of 1.5 cm using a running polypropylene (Prolene) 5/0 suture.

Before completion of the anastomosis, the clamps on the portal vein are temporarily released to flush out any clots and the anastomosis is irrigated with heparinized solution. The Satinsky clamp is first released to allow expansion of the anastomosis and the suture is tied. This is followed by removal of the clamps from the portal vein. The patency of the shunt is then demonstrated by showing reversed portal flow on intraoperative Doppler ultrasound and a minimal gradient between both sides of the shunt. If difficulty is found in approximating the two vessels as a result of an enlarged caudate lobe, a mesocaval shunt may be used, as resection of the caudate lobe to allow apposition of the two vessels is hazardous.

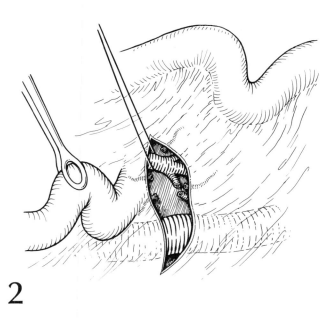

2

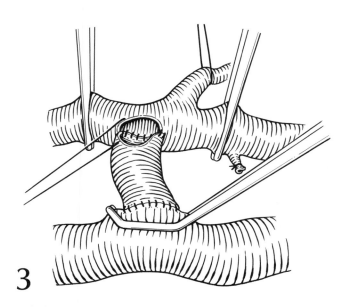

3

Mesocaval interposition shunt

When hepatic enlargement and/or a huge caudate lobe precludes a side-to-side portacaval shunt, a mesocaval interposition shunt is indicated. This was originally described using a jugular venous graft and later using a prosthetic graft. The authors prefer to use a short jugular venous H graft, although when the vein is not suitable a prosthesis can be used. The widest part of the superior mesenteric vein below the pancreas can be identified by intraoperative ultrasonography and is dissected free. Extensive dissection of the vein is tedious and harmful in the presence of lymphatic engorgement.

2 When isolating the mesenteric vein, the peritoneal leaf and all the lymphatic channels must be secured. The first colic vein that enters the right lateral aspect of the mesenteric vein must be divided to obtain sufficient length. The mesentery of the ascending colon is incised and the anterior wall of the IVC only is exposed to avoid bleeding from retroperitoneal collaterals. A Satinsky clamp is applied to the anterior surface of the IVC and an ellipse is removed from its medial aspect.

3 An anastomosis between the graft and the IVC is first effected with a running 4/0 polypropylene suture. The graft is then anastomosed to the side of the superior mesenteric vein after its isolation between two clamps using a posterior running 5/0 polypropylene suture.

Interrupted sutures are used for the anterior layer to allow expansion of the anastomosis. Care is taken to choose the level of the anastomosis to the mesenteric vein so as to avoid compression or kinking of the graft by the third part of the duodenum. Usually a conduit of 4–6 cm in length is required. As described above, pressure measurements are taken both before and after opening of the shunt.

Liver transplantation

Liver transplantation is an alternative to portacaval and mesocaval shunt[6]. However, it requires lifelong medication and increased susceptibility to infections. Since portacaval and mesocaval shunting have achieved good results in patients without severe liver lesions, liver transplantation should probably be reserved for patients with cirrhosis. Preservation of the vena cava in this setting is not recommended because of the marked caudate lobe hypertrophy and the developed collateral channels. Permanent anticoagulation is necessary after transplantation as the disease may recur in the new liver.

PATENT PORTAL VEIN AND OCCLUDED IVC

Portosystemic shunts with the right atrium or superior vena cava must be reserved for the rare cases in which associated IVC thrombosis has been clearly demonstrated by cavography or magnetic resonance imaging. This form of the Budd–Chiari syndrome is managed either by creating an anastomosis between the portal system and the superior vena caval system, or by an anastomosis between the portal system and the IVC associated with IVC decompression.

Mesoatrial shunt

The widest level of the superior mesenteric vein is identified by intraoperative ultrasonography through a midline incision and is dissected free in the root of the mesentery. In a modification of the standard technique, a synchronous median sternotomy is carried out and the pericardium is opened. The graft used is an externally supported expanded polytetrafluoroethylene (PTFE) graft which is sutured end-to-side to the superior mesenteric vein with a continuous 5/0 polypropylene suture.

4 The graft is then tunnelled under the transverse colon and over the left liver lobe, and is passed into the mediastinum through a subxiphoid incision in the diaphragm.

The lateral wall of the right atrium is cross-clamped just below the auricule and anastomosed to the graft using a continuous 5/0 polypropylene suture. After pressure measurements, the pericardium is left open and the wounds are closed.

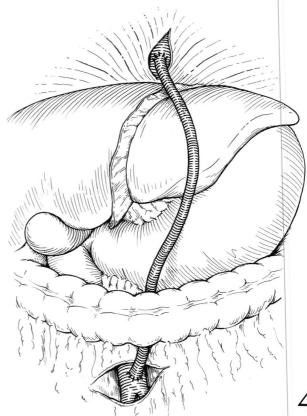

4

5 Alternatively, the graft can be anastomosed to the innominate vein to avoid opening the pericardium with its ensuing risk of tamponade. The risk of thrombosis with these techniques ranges from 0 to 40%[2].

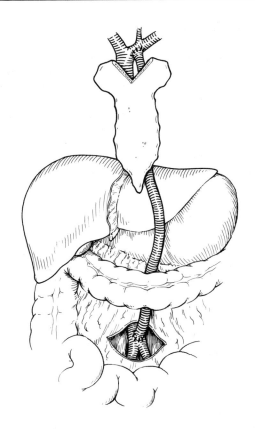

5

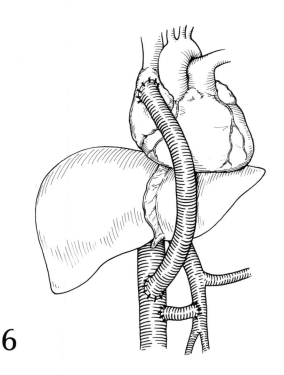

6

6 In order to improve the rather low blood flow in a long prosthetic graft, a variant of this procedure combines a side-to-side portacaval shunt and a cavo-atrial shunt with a large externally supported expanded graft, thus decompressing both the vena cava and the portal system[5].

Recently, balloon dilatation followed by expandable stent placement have been proposed for patients with vena caval obstruction or for selected patients with severe caval stenosis. Such treatment may eliminate the need for a mesoatrial shunt and facilitate portacaval decompression[7].

In patients with membranous occlusion of the IVC, transcardiac surgical membranotomy or percutaneous transluminal angioplasty can be performed. These procedures are justified only when the area of caval obstruction is short and thin and located at or above the level of the hepatic venous orifices. Through a midline incision associated with a median sternotomy, supported by total heart-lung bypass, a longitudinal incision is made in the thoracic IVC. The narrow channel is enlarged by excision of the causative fibrous tissue and the hole in the IVC is closed in a transverse fashion. Transluminal angioplasty may be followed by massive pulmonary embolism, as there is often a thrombus under the membrane, and should be reserved for recurrent stenosis.

OCCLUDED PORTAL VEIN

When the portal vein is extensively thrombosed, neither portosystemic shunting nor liver transplantation can be performed. Several therapeutic procedures have been proposed in this situation, but the experience with each of them is limited and a clear evaluation is impossible.

Thrombolytic therapy has achieved uncertain results[2] and should be used early, but only when recent thrombosis can be clearly documented. When thrombolytic therapy is used, no invasive diagnostic procedure should be performed.

Percutaneous transluminal angioplasty

Percutaneous transluminal or surgical angioplasty has been attempted in patients with a short stenosis of the hepatic veins. Although immediate relief of obstruction is obtained in some reported cases, recurrence is common.

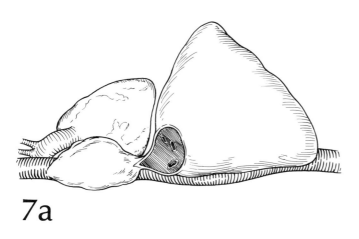

7a

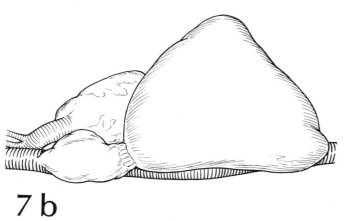

7b

Senning's procedure

Dorsocranial liver resection with direct hepatoatrial anastomosis or Senning's procedure was proposed on the basis of the observation that hepatic veins are usually occluded in their terminal portion. It can be considered in Budd–Chiari syndrome with extensive portal thrombosis, since it is the only effective treatment for liver decompression. Senning's procedure improves liver outflow by partial liver resection, including resection of the confluence of the occluded hepatic veins, thus creating direct communications between hepatic venules and the right atrium. Through a midline incision associated with a median sternotomy the pericardium is opened. Under a total heart-lung bypass or a venous bypass between the infrarenal IVC and the axillary vein, the infrahepatic IVC, portal triad and lower part of the right atrium are clamped.

7a, b The suprahepatic IVC is opened by a longitudinal 5 cm incision extending from the cranial part of the liver to the lower part of the right atrium. A wedge resection of the dorsocranial part of the liver, including the confluence of the occluded hepatic veins, is performed until a prompt decrease in liver size is observed[8]. The incised right atrium is then sutured to the liver capsule around the resection area.

Postoperative care

Early management after shunting procedures includes monitoring of liver and renal function, correction of fluid and electrolyte imbalance, treatment of ascites, evaluation of shunt patency by Doppler ultrasound and systemic anticoagulation. Continuous infusion of heparin, adjusted to maintain the partial thromboplastin time at twice normal, is converted on the seventh postoperative day to heparin calcium (Calciparine) given subcutaneously for 6 weeks, after which oral anticoagulants are used indefinitely.

Long-term management focuses on treatment of the concurrent haematological disorder and regular assessment of liver status and shunt patency. An adequately decompressed liver should avoid progression of the liver disease if appropriate patients were selected for shunting.

References

1. Panis Y, Belghiti J, Valla D, Benhamou JP, Fékété F. Portosystemic shunt in Budd–Chiari syndrome: long-term survival and factors affecting shunt patency in 25 patients in western countries. *Surgery* 1994; 115: 276–81.

2. MacIntyre N, Benhamou JP, Bircher J, Rizetto M, Rodes J, eds. *Oxford Textbook of Clinical Hepatology*. Oxford: Oxford University Press, 1991.

3. Cameron J, Herlong HF, Sanfey H, Boitnott J, Kaufman SL, Gott VL. The Budd–Chiari syndrome: treatment by mesenteric-systemic venous shunts. *Ann Surg* 1983; 198: 335–46.

4. Bismuth H, Sherlock DJ. Portasystemic shunting versus liver transplantation for the Budd–Chiari syndrome. *Ann Surg* 1991; 214: 581–9.

5. Orloff MJ. Budd–Chiari syndrome and veno-occlusive disease. In: Blumgart LH, eds. *Surgery of the Liver and Biliary Tract*. Edinburgh: Churchill Livingstone, 1988: 1425–53.

6. Campbell DA, Rolles K, Jamieson N, O'Grady J, Wight D, Williams R. Hepatic transplantation with perioperative and long-term anticoagulation as treatment for Budd–Chiari syndrome. *Surg Gynecol Obstet* 1988; 166: 511–18.

7. Kohli V, Pande GK, Dev V, Reddy KS, Kaul U, Nundy S. Management of hepatic venous outflow obstruction. *Lancet* 1993; 342: 718–22.

8. Sauvanet A, Panis Y, Valla D, Vilgrain V, Belghiti J. Budd–Chiari syndrome with extensive portal thrombosis: treatment with Senning's procedure. *Hepatogastroenterology* 1994; 41: 174–6.

Surgery in the cirrhotic liver

Jacques Belghiti MD
Professor of Surgery, Department of Surgery, University Paris VII and Beaujon Hospital, Clichy, France

Roger Noun MD
Assistant of Surgery, Department of Surgery, University Paris VII and Beaujon Hospital, Clichy, France

Principles and justification

Hepatocellular carcinoma is the most common primary malignant liver tumour. Cirrhosis, particularly when associated with hepatitis B or C, is the main factor associated with the development of hepatocellular carcinoma. The severity of the postoperative course after surgical resection in patients with a cirrhotic liver depends on the following factors: (a) stage of cirrhosis and general condition of the patient; (b) intraoperative haemorrhage due to portal hypertension and difficulties in obtaining haemostasis; (c) extent of resection; (d) ability of the cirrhotic parenchyma to regenerate after resection; (e) electrolyte imbalance largely due to the presence of postoperative ascites; and (f) sepsis. All of these factors may contribute to the disappointing early experience with surgical resection of hepatocellular carcinoma in non-selected cirrhotic patients, especially in western countries[1]. The therapeutic strategy for dealing with hepatocellular carcinoma has now significantly changed with an increase in the resectability rate, a decrease in postoperative mortality and improved survival rates[2]. These changes reflect early detection of hepatocellular carcinoma, careful selection of candidates and technical advances in liver surgery.

Although alcohol injection, transcatheter arterial embolization and liver transplantation have greatly extended the range of options available for the treatment of hepatocellular carcinoma complicating cirrhosis, hepatic resection remains the treatment of choice[3]. The two aims of hepatic resection are apparently in opposition: one is to resect the maximum amount of malignant tissue with effective clearance, and the other is to leave enough non-tumorous hepatic tissue to prevent postoperative liver failure. It is now possible to achieve both objectives with an acceptable operative risk by means of careful patient selection, technical advances such as ultrasound and vascular occlusion techniques, and adequate perioperative care. The key to a successful outcome is careful patient selection so that alternative methods of management can be used for those at high risk.

Preoperative

The preoperative evaluation of the cirrhotic patient undergoing surgical resection focuses on the patient, the liver and the tumour.

Evaluation of the patient

Careful preoperative assessment and optimization of the patient's status will reduce operative risk. The nutritional status is evaluated and malnutrition corrected. Adequate renal, pulmonary and cardiac function are mandatory to withstand the enhanced postoperative hyperdynamic state. Varices are evaluated and the presence of risk factors for bleeding warrants preoperative sclerotherapy. Fluid and electrolyte imbalance and coagulation disorders must be corrected. Patients with ascites are poor candidates for laparotomy and alternatives should be explored.

Evaluation of the liver functional reserve

The risk of postoperative liver failure depends upon the quantity and quality of the remaining parenchyma. It is now possible to use ultrasound and a three-dimensional scanner to measure precisely the volume of the parenchyma that would remain after an oncologically acceptable resection. However, it is difficult to estimate the probable functional capacity of the remaining cirrhotic liver. The system of classification used to evaluate functional reserve is that of Child-Pugh, and class A patients have significantly lower operative mortality and incidence of postoperative liver failure than combined class B and C patients[4,5]. Thus, a Child-Pugh C classification indicates that the patient most probably will not survive surgery, while a Child-Pugh B classification indicates that only limited resection can be considered. Liver resection is indicated in Child-Pugh A patients, but there are diverging opinions as to whether major surgery is indicated in this category. Indeed, although the Child-Pugh system provides a baseline, it does not take into account the residual functional reserve, the ability of the remaining liver to regenerate, and the ability of the patient to survive surgery. For this reason some surgeons plan the extent of the resection on the results of specific dynamic tests such as indiocyanine green (ICG) and bromosulphophthalein retention tests. Other factors suggesting active liver pathology have a detrimental effect on operative risk, and acute alcoholic hepatitis as well as viral chronic hepatitis must be investigated. The presence of a high preoperative level of transaminases, indicating the presence of active hepatitis, means that surgery should be postponed.

Assessment of the tumour

Hepatic resection is considered if the tumour is solitary and there is no associated thrombosis of the portal trunk. Preoperative investigations include ultrasonography, coeliac and superior mesenteric arteriography, and computed tomographic (CT) scanning. The arteriographic contrast medium should contain a lipid, and this investigation is followed by a CT scan 3 weeks later. The lipid substance is taken up by the tumour cells, increasing the diagnostic sensitivity of the test and enabling the detection of pathology which is otherwise invisible. Concomitant embolization of the arterial branch supplying the tumour may result in a decrease in tumour size[3].

Anaesthesia

The anaesthetist should be informed of the severity of the underlying liver disease and plan anaesthetic requirements accordingly. Intravascular volume is maintained by colloid or fresh frozen plasma rather than crystalloid. Cardiovascular indices are monitored by the placement of a Swan-Ganz catheter and a radial arterial line. A Foley catheter is required to monitor urine output. Continuous monitoring of oxygen saturation is helpful, as are frequent electrolyte measurements and coagulative profiles. Blood and blood products should be available, but with technical advances are often not required. Prophylactic antibiotics and histamine H_2 blockers should be given.

Operation

Position of patient

The position of the patient is important and can make the difference between an easy and difficult operation. The patient should be positioned supine with the right arm extended along the body. The rib margin is positioned over a rolled blanket to facilitate exposure of the liver. The hips are taped in the supine position to allow rotation of the table to either side.

Incision

1   The choice of incision is influenced by several goals. It is important to give a good access to all parts of the liver, to use an incision which can be extended in any situation, and to prevent leakage of ascitic fluid from the incision. The procedures are usually performed through either a bilateral subcostal incision (with or without upper midline extension), or through an upper midline incision which is extended to the right at the level of the umbilicus and then taken to the mid axillary line. The latter incision is indicated for surgery of the right lobe and provides particularly good access to the area around the junction between the inferior vena cava and the right hepatic vein.

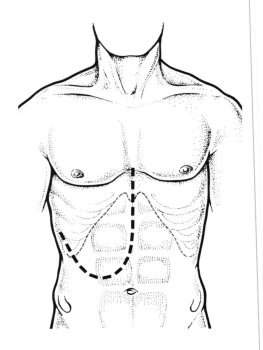

1

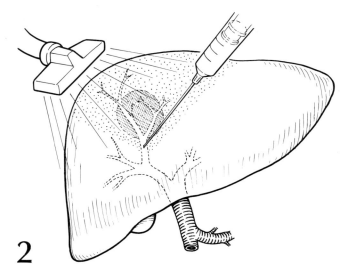

2

Extent of resection

2   The tumour appears to spread by invasion of the portal blood supply and then disseminates by embolization from that main portal branch. It is therefore possible to define an area at risk of secondary deposits by identifying the portal blood supply to the tumour, and so define the extent of the area to be resected. A satisfactory approach to exclude potential spread of the tumour would be to excise the entire area supplied by the identified portal branch leaving a margin of 1 cm around the actual tumour.

Intraoperative tumour staging

Abdominal exploration

Abdominal exploration may detect intrahepatic or extrahepatic spread. Needle biopsy is helpful in the evaluation of a suspect nodule, but it is often difficult to distinguish on frozen section between a cancerous nodule and a nodule of regeneration. Satellite nodules can be resected at the time of operation if this does not involve massive resection of the liver. Abdominal exploration reveals hilar node involvement which precludes further hepatic resection in 5% of patients with otherwise operable tumours.

Intraoperative ultrasonography

This method of assessment is essential to the practice of surgery in patients with a cirrhotic liver and the surgeon may be surprised by the presence of invisible and non-palpable tumour. Intraoperative ultrasonography localizes the tumour accurately and determines its relationship to vascular structures. It may detect tumour thrombus or occult intrahepatic lesions (which are not apparent on preoperative radiological examination or on palpation) that would influence the surgical procedure intended.

The technique is also useful to guide peroperative biopsies, allow transportal methylene blue staining, permit selective portal clamping by intraportal balloon catheter and provide guidance during parenchymal transection (*see below*).

Vascular occlusion

In patients with cirrhosis, operative blood loss is a major decisive factor in determining short-term prognosis. The cirrhotic parenchyma appears to tolerate liver ischaemia, within certain limits, better than it withstands the consequences of bleeding and transfusions.

Continuous vascular occlusion can be used in all cirrhotic patients for 30 minutes. Prolonged intermittent clamping for periods of up to 90 minutes also appears to be tolerated in cirrhotic patients[6].

No particular method of vascular occlusion appears superior, but total hepatic vascular exclusion seems to be poorly tolerated in this patient population. Hemiliver exclusion with preservation of blood flow to the other hemiliver seems a very attractive approach which has minimal haemodynamic consequences. There is no definitive preference between continuous and intermittent clamping (periods of 10 min clamped and 5 min unclamped), although intermittent clamping naturally leads to a greater blood loss during surgery.

Margin of safety and choice of resection

The tumour must be excised with a margin of 1 cm of non-affected parenchyma. This margin appears to be sufficient as recurrence of the tumour occurs in 80% of cases at a distance from the resected zone. As hepatocellular carcinoma usually involves cirrhotic livers, major resections (resection of more than three segments) should only be considered in patients with Child-Pugh A tumours involving more than one segment.

In all other cases resection must be limited in order to spare the non-cancerous parenchyma as much as possible. However, anatomical resections are indicated as hepatocellular carcinoma infiltrates the portal venous branches and intrahepatic metastases may develop even if the tumour appears to be very small. The portal unit to be resected is accurately delineated after dye injection or occlusion of the portal branch supplying the tumour by means of intraoperative ultrasonography. The branch can be occluded by an intraportal balloon catheter or by transparenchymal application of clips to the vessel. This technique of occlusion spares the remaining parenchyma from ischaemia, permits prolonged occlusion, and is truly curative in that it deals with the possibility of metastatic spread due to venous emboli.

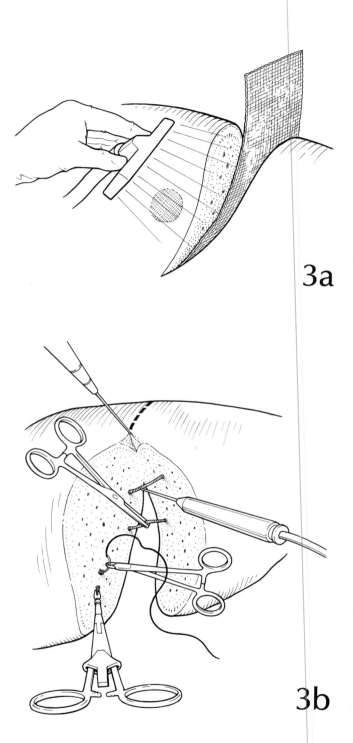

3a

3b

Parenchymal transection

3a, b   Liver transection in cirrhotic patients does not differ markedly from that used in non-cirrhotic patients. The tumour is localized by intraoperative ultrasonography and the portal unit to be resected is accurately delineated by dye injection into the portal branch of the segment containing the tumour. The incision is then traced on Glisson's capsule with electrocautery and the parenchymal transection is guided by ultrasound. The appropriate safety margin is estimated by determining the interrelationship between the tumour and a Mersilene mesh introduced into the cut section, and all the vascular and biliary radicles are ligated at the transection margin. Because the cirrhotic liver is hard to cut, the ultrasound dissector is less suitable for parenchymal transection than other classical methods.

Treatment of the raw surface

4 After the specimen is removed, the clamps are released and the cut surface is packed for 5 min. The gauze packs are placed over a plastic drape which is laid against the raw surface. This non-adherent material prevents the gauze packs from sticking to the exposed parenchyma, so causing bleeding at the time of their removal. Bleeding vessels must be secured with fine polypropylene (Prolene) 5/0 sutures. Biliary leakage is controlled by injecting methylene blue through the cystic duct. Ultimate sealing of the raw surface by fibrin glue is warranted as infected collections, usually attributable to oozing, bile leakage and fluid accumulation, are poorly tolerated in cirrhotic patients. Moreover, the presence of ascites may preclude the natural sealing of the cut surface by neighbouring organs and omentum.

Drainage

After liver resection in the cirrhotic patient there is a considerable risk of developing ascites. In this setting, a one-way suction drain prevents parietal and pulmonary complications while avoiding the risk of infection ascending the drain. Drains must be withdrawn early in the absence of ascites or bile leakage. Alternatively, elective paracentesis may be indicated to minimize the risk of infection from routine drain insertion.

Postoperative ascites is prevented by reducing the administration of sodium-containing intravenous fluids and by using diuretics if there is adequate renal function. Intravascular volume expanders are used if the patient is hypotensive, oliguric, or has a rising serum creatinine. Volume expansion is best achieved by albumin or fresh frozen plasma. One week of prophylactic antibiotics is used to avoid infection of the ascitic fluid.

Postoperative care

Most cirrhotic patients require a short stay in the intensive care unit. The primary goals are to: (a) establish an adequate cardiopulmonary status; (b) correct fluid and electrolyte imbalance; (c) monitor liver and renal function; and (d) diagnose and treat infection promptly. Bleeding from the liver margin is monitored by drain outputs, haemodynamic parameters, and serial haemoglobin assays. Fluid balance and renal function are monitored by weighing the patient daily, recording input/output fluid levels, serum and urine electrolyte concentrations and serum creatinine level.

Hepatic function is monitored by serial biochemical tests. The prothrombin time and clotting factor V levels are the most useful indicators of liver function.

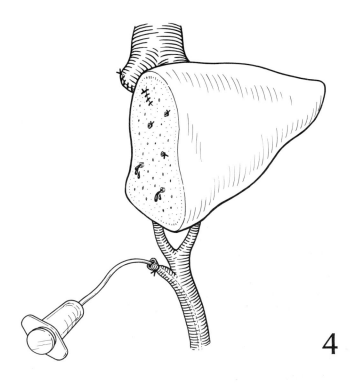

4

Progressive increase in alkaline phosphatase and gamma GT levels are indicators of active regeneration. A high index of suspicion of infection is important if there is any unexplained deterioration, as fever and leucocytosis may be absent. The possibility of infected ascites must always be considered. Perihepatic fluid collections are treated by percutaneous aspiration/drainage and appropriate antibiotic therapy.

References

1. MacIntosh EL, Minuk GY. Hepatic resection in patients with cirrhosis and hepatocellular carcinoma. *Surg Gynecol Obstet* 1992; 174: 245–54.

2. Nagasue N, Kohno H, Chang YC *et al.* Liver resection for hepatocellular carcinoma: results of 229 consecutive patients during 11 years. *Ann Surg* 1993; 217: 375–84.

3. Farmer DG, Rosove MH, Shaked A, Busuttil RW. Current treatment modalities for hepatocellular carcinoma. *Ann Surg* 1994; 219: 236–47.

4. Nagao T, Inoue S, Goto S *et al.* Hepatic resection for hepatocellular carcinoma: clinical features and long-term prognosis. *Ann Surg* 1987; 205: 33–40.

5. Franco D, Capussoti L, Smadja C *et al.* Resection of hepatocellular carcinomas: results in 72 European patients with cirrhosis. *Gastroenterology* 1990; 98: 733–8.

6. Elias D, Desruennes E, Lasser P. Prolonged intermittent clamping of the portal triad during hepatectomy. *Br J Surg* 1991; 78: 42–4.

Surgery for biliary atresia

Edward R. Howard MS, FRCS, FRCS(Ed)
Consultant Hepatobiliary and Paediatric Surgeon, King's College Hospital, London, UK

History

Atresia of the extrahepatic bile ducts is the end result of a variable inflammatory process of unknown aetiology which occurs before birth and which, if untreated, leads to death from cirrhotic liver failure within 2 years. The incidence is between 0.8 and 1.0 per 10 000 births. Extrahepatic anomalies are associated with biliary atresia in approximately 20% of cases and the most common association (known as the polysplenia syndrome) comprises polysplenia, situs inversus and a preduodenal portal vein[1]. Abnormalities of the heart, kidneys and inferior vena cava may also occur.

The patency of a proximal segment of the hepatic or common hepatic ducts is preserved in 10–15% of patients and bile may be aspirated from the duct during surgery. These rare variants were originally called 'correctable' cases because they could be treated with conventional biliary–enteric anastomoses such as hepaticojejunostomy.

Most cases, however, show obliteration of the extrahepatic bile ducts up to the capsule of the liver in the porta hepatis. Segments of the distal bile duct may remain patent, although without communication with the hepatic ducts, and in some cases injection of contrast material into the gallbladder may show free flow to the duodenum without filling of the proximal ducts. Occlusion of the proximal bile ducts was once believed to be surgically 'non-correctable' and the problems of treatment are reflected in reports of only 52 surgical successes between 1927 and 1970[2].

A new operation for biliary atresia was suggested by Kasai[3], who observed that excision of the obliterated bile duct remnants in the porta hepatis could result in bile drainage in a proportion of the patients with 'non-correctable' atresia. This operation is now known as portoenterostomy.

Classification

1 The historical division of biliary atresia into 'correctable' and 'non-correctable' types depending on the presence or absence of a residual segment of bile-containing proximal bile duct has been superseded by a classification which describes three major types of atresia. The Japanese Society of Paediatric Surgeons[4] has subdivided these main types to include details of the structure of the gallbladder and the distal bile ducts. These details have been omitted from the illustration as they have no influence on the results of surgical treatment.

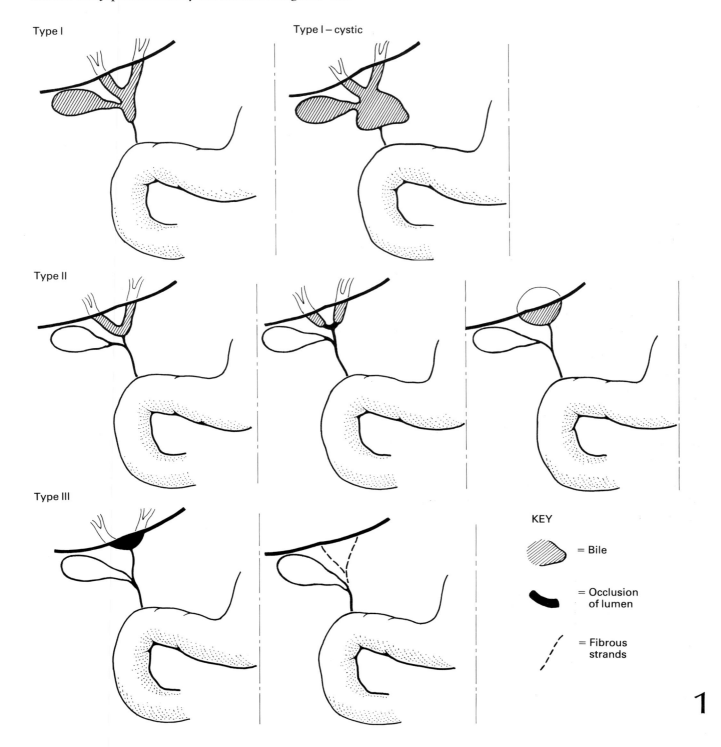

Type I

Type I – cystic

Type II

Type III

KEY

= Bile

= Occlusion of lumen

= Fibrous strands

1

Diagnosis

The differential diagnosis of prolonged jaundice in neonates and infants includes giant cell hepatitis, intrahepatic bile duct hypoplasia, choledochal cyst, spontaneous perforation of the bile ducts and inspissated bile syndrome. Infection, metabolic abnormalities and α_1-antitrypsin deficiency may be detected as causes of neonatal hepatitis by appropriate screening tests, but the aetiology is unknown in 70% of patients with intrahepatic cholestasis. These patients must be separated immediately from patients with surgical causes of jaundice.

Choledochal cysts, bile duct perforation and cases of obstruction from inspissated bile can be confidently diagnosed with ultrasonography and hepatobiliary scintigraphy using technetium-labelled iminodiacetic acid compounds. Liver function tests are of little value in differential diagnosis of atresia, but percutaneous liver biopsy is diagnostic in most cases. However, liver biopsies from patients with α_1-antitrypsin deficiency may be confused with atresia and it is essential to rule out this condition by α_1-antitrypsin phenotyping.

Other investigations useful for confirming the diagnosis of biliary atresia include laparoscopy combined with gallbladder cholangiography, endoscopic retrograde cholangiography and duodenal intubation (for the identification of bile). Unfortunately no single test is diagnostic in all cases, but two or more tests in combination usually differentiate biliary atresia from other causes of prolonged jaundice. Accurate preoperative diagnosis is imperative as the findings at laparotomy may be difficult to interpret or frankly misleading. It may be particularly difficult, for example, to identify small, proximal bile ducts in cases of biliary hypoplasia and the patency of such ducts may be difficult to determine even using operative cholangiography.

Preoperative

Vitamin K (phytomenadione, 1.0 mg/day) is administered intramuscularly for at least 4 days before surgery. Blood is cross-matched and oral neomycin (50 mg/kg/day) given, in six divided doses, for 24 h preoperatively. An adequate intravenous line is set up and a nasogastric tube inserted.

Antibiotics (cephalosporins) are given intravenously after induction of anaesthesia and should be continued for at least 5 days after surgery.

Operations

PORTOENTEROSTOMY

Originally the surgical management of suspected cases of biliary atresia was separated into two stages. The 'diagnostic' stage consisted of making a short transverse incision in the right hypochondrium, followed by operative cholangiography and liver biopsy. This was followed by definitive surgery a few days later. The author prefers to make the diagnosis using the techniques described above and to restrict surgery to only one procedure.

2 Tissue excised from the porta hepatis during portoenterostomy shows epithelium-lined ductules which may measure up to 300 μm in diameter. Partial destruction and desquamation of the epithelium has occurred and the ductules are surrounded by fibrous tissue, which contains inflammatory cells.

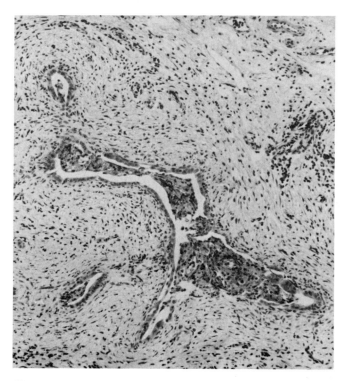

Haematoxylin and eosin, ×16. Courtesy of Dr M. Driver

2

3 Large ductules are often absent but serial sectioning has shown that even small channels may communicate with intrahepatic ducts. Biliary drainage is achieved in the portoenterostomy operation by transecting these ductules and anastomosing a Roux-en-Y loop of jejunum to the edges of the area of excision in the porta hepatis. This operation is most effective in patients under 6 weeks of age[5].

Position of patient

The patient is placed supine on a thermostatically controlled heated operating table with facilities for intraoperative cholangiography.

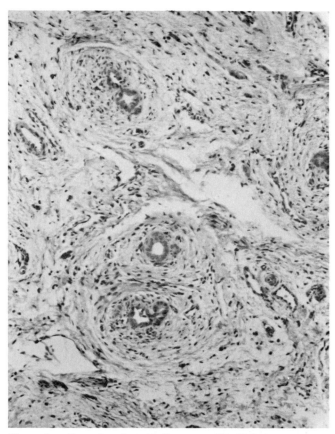

Haematoxylin and eosin, ×13. Courtesy of Dr M. Driver

3

Incision

4 A bilateral subcostal incision, dividing the right and left rectus muscles, exposes the inferior margin of the liver. The appearance of the liver, and the presence or absence of ascites and portal hypertension, are noted. Associated anatomical anomalies (such as polysplenia, asplenia, malrotation or preduodenal portal vein) will be encountered in 15–20% of patients.

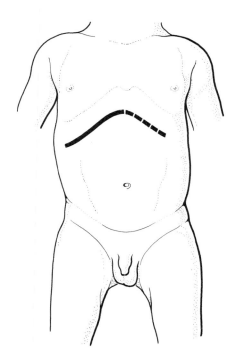

4

Cholangiography

5 Operative cholangiography via a gallbladder catheter is indicated either if the diagnosis remains in doubt following the preoperative investigations or if bile is detected upon aspiration of the gallbladder. The presence of bile within the gallbladder is an absolute indication for radiographic studies of the biliary tract.

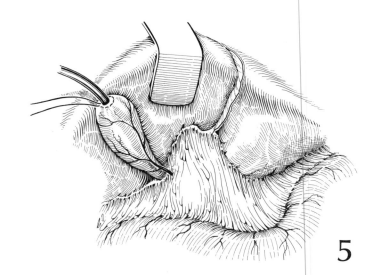

5

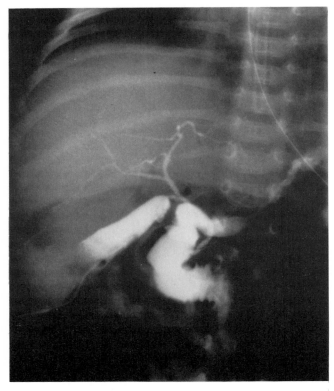

6

6 The demonstration of a patent common bile duct and a communication with intrahepatic ducts excludes a diagnosis of biliary atresia and terminates the operation.

...

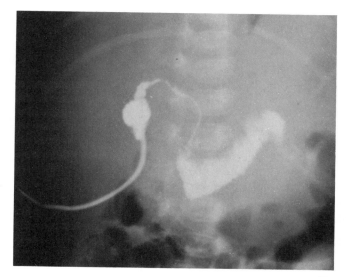

7

7 In 20–25% of patients with biliary atresia the cystic and distal common bile ducts are patent and the duodenum will be opacified by injecting contrast material into the gallbladder. However, it is impossible to visualize the atretic proximal ducts even after occluding the supraduodenal portion of the bile duct with a soft clamp.

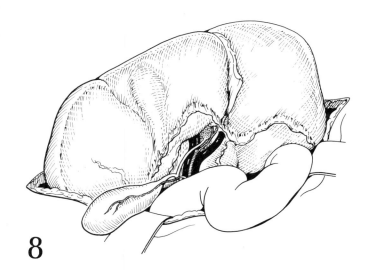

8

Mobilization of the liver

8 For accurate dissection in this operation it is imperative that the porta hepatis is clearly visualized. This is achieved by dividing the falciform and left and right triangular ligaments and completely mobilizing the liver. It is possible to evert the liver into the wound to expose the porta hepatis.

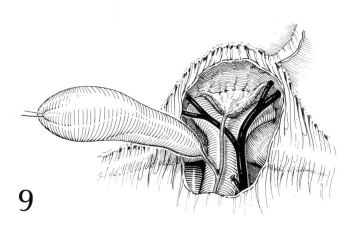

9

Mobilization of gallbladder and bile ducts

9 The remainder of the operation is more easily performed under magnification. The cystic artery, which is often enlarged, is ligated and divided and the gallbladder dissected from its bed. Care must be taken not to mistake the right hepatic artery for the cystic artery. The mobilized gallbladder is used as a guide to the fibrous remnant of the common bile duct, which may be partially obscured by thickened peritoneum and enlarged lymph nodes.

Dissection and exposure of porta hepatis

10 The lower end of the common bile duct is divided between ligatures at the upper border of the duodenum and the upper portion, with the gallbladder attached, is dissected upwards above the bifurcation of the portal vein. The portal vein and the hepatic arteries are exposed along their whole course until they disappear within the liver substance.

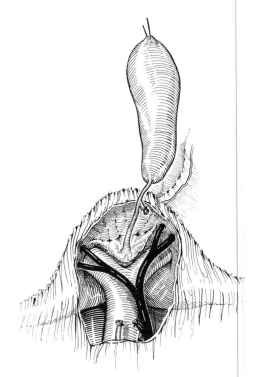

10

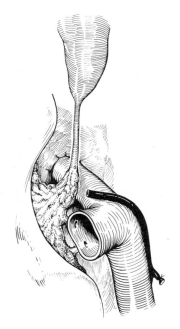

11

11 Clear identification and mobilization of the bifurcation of the portal vein is essential and may necessitate ligation and division of small venous radicles to the caudate lobe of the liver. Enlarged lymphatics should be ligated meticulously to prevent postoperative ascites caused by leakage of lymphatic fluid.

Excision of bile duct remnants

12a, b The remnant of the bile duct and the gallbladder are removed after transecting the fibrous tissue in the porta hepatis. The plane of transection is flush with, and outside, the liver capsule or 'portal plate'. All residual tissue is removed within the area bounded by the right and left branches of the portal vein and the accompanying hepatic arteries. The transection can be performed very accurately using angled scissors designed specifically for this stage of the operation[5].

Inferiorly the transection should extend behind the posterior surface of the portal vein. Bleeding points are controlled with direct pressure: diathermy could damage the small biliary ductules on the undersurface of the liver and should not be used.

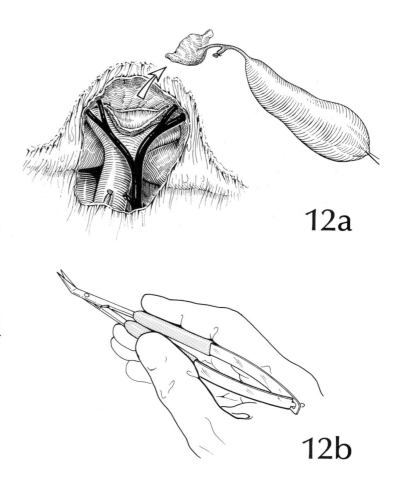

12a

12b

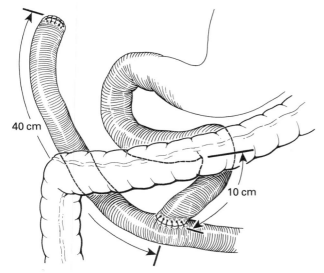

13

40 cm

10 cm

Preparation and anastomosis of Roux-en-Y loop

13 A 40-cm Roux-en-Y loop is prepared by transecting the jejunum approximately 10 cm distal to the duodenojejunal flexure. The distal end is oversewn and passed in a retrocolic position to the hilum of the liver. Continuity of the small bowel is established with an end-to-side enteroenterostomy.

14a, b

An anastomosis is fashioned between the edge of the transected area in the porta hepatis and the side of the Roux loop using sutures of 5/0 polydioxanone. The anastomosis is achieved by inserting the whole of the posterior row of sutures before tying them. The jejunal loop is then 'railroaded' into position and the sutures are tied in series. An anterior row of sutures completes the anastomosis. A small drain is placed down to the porta hepatis and a needle biopsy of the right lobe of the liver taken before closing the abdomen.

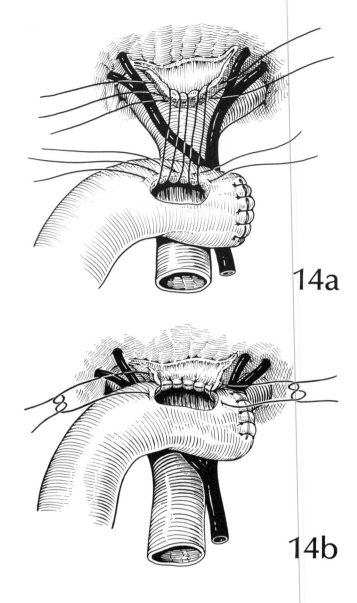

14a

14b

CHOLECYSTPORTOENTEROSTOMY

15

Presence of a patent gallbladder and distal common bile duct, demonstrated by operative cholangiography, may allow a more natural conduit for bile drainage to be constructed following anastomosis of the gallbladder to the transected tissue of the porta hepatis. This procedure may reduce the incidence of ascending cholangitis after operation but may be complicated by bile duct obstruction and leakage from kinking.

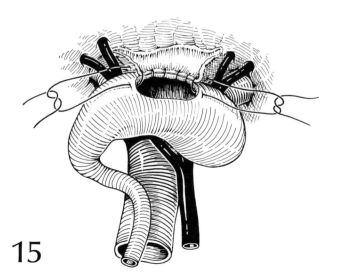

15

HEPATICOJEJUNOSTOMY

16 The rare finding of a large remnant of common hepatic duct may allow the construction of a hepaticojejunostomy as an end-to-side anastomosis between the bulbous end of the common hepatic duct and the side of the Roux loop.

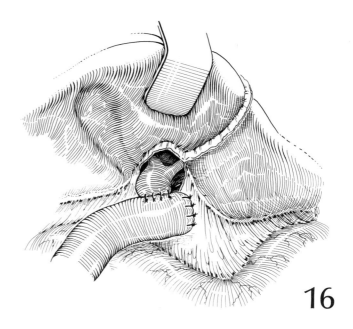

16

CUTANEOUS ENTEROSTOMY

Attempts to prevent attacks of ascending bacterial cholangitis following portoenterostomy have included fashioning cutaneous stomas and constructing a variety of 'valves' in the Roux loop conduit. However, there is no evidence that the incidence of cholangitis is lessened by these procedures, which do cause additional complications. For example, enterostomies tend to develop stomal varices and to haemorrhage repeatedly. Enterostomies also complicate liver transplantation, if it becomes necessary at a later date, and they are now generally avoided.

Postoperative care

Nasogastric drainage is continued until bowel activity returns and intravenous antibiotics (cephalosporins) administered for 5 days after surgery. An oral cephalosporin is then substituted for a further 3 weeks as prophylaxis against ascending bacterial cholangitis. The onset of any unexplained pyrexia, particularly if accompanied by a rise in serum bilirubin levels, suggests an ascending bacterial cholangitis, the cause of which must be identified with blood and liver biopsy cultures. Common organisms include *Escherichia coli, Proteus* spp. and *Klebsiella*.

The onset of effective bile drainage and an improvement in liver function tests are difficult to predict after portoenterostomy and may not occur for 2–3 weeks after surgery. Histological analysis of the tissue excised from the porta hepatis may aid prognosis, and early satisfactory bile flow may be expected if ductules with diameters greater than 150 μm are identified.

Phenobarbitone and cholestyramine are prescribed to encourage bile flow and vitamins D and K given routinely. At the time of discharge from hospital the parents and the referring physicians are given full information on the signs and hazards of any future episodes of cholangitis and the necessity for urgent treatment with intravenous antibiotics.

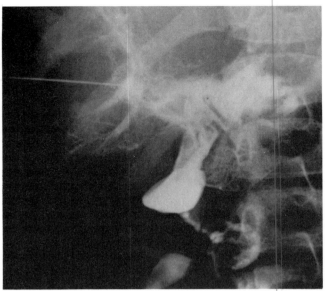

17 A Roux loop will occasionally become obstructed by adhesions and this requires urgent surgical correction. Children who present with an episode of jaundice following a long trouble-free period should therefore be investigated with percutaneous cholangiography.

17

Outcome

Since the portoenterostomy operation was introduced more than 30 years ago, refinements in surgical technique and earlier referral for surgery have caused a steady improvement in the results. Children operated before 6 weeks of age have a much better chance of establishing effective bile drainage than older children. Bile drainage is achieved in more than 90% of patients under 6 weeks, but the success rate falls to less than 35% in infants over 12 weeks of age.

Although most patients continue to show some abnormalities in liver function after portoenterostomy, survival to adulthood is possible. Long-term complications include recurrent cholangitis, hepatic fibrosis, cirrhosis and portal hypertension. Injection sclerotherapy is the treatment of choice for haemorrhage from oesophageal varices.

Current surgical techniques have increased the 10-year survival of patients with biliary atresia to more than 60%. Liver transplantation is reserved for those patients who either completely fail to respond to portoenterostomy or who develop liver failure at a later stage.

References

1. Davenport M, Savage M, Mowat AP, Howard ER. Biliary atresia splenic malformation syndrome: an aetiological and prognostic subgroup. *Surgery* 1993; 113: 662–8.

2. Bill AH. Biliary atresia – introduction. *World J Surg* 1978; 2: 557–9.

3. Kasai M, Kimura S, Asakura Y, Suzuki H, Taira Y, Ohashi E. Surgical treatment of biliary atresia. *J Pediatr Surg* 1968; 3: 665–75.

4. Hays DM, Kimura K. *Biliary Atresia: The Japanese Experience*. Cambridge, Massachusetts: Harvard University Press, 1980: 52–6.

5. Howard ER. Biliary atresia: aetiology, management and complications. In: *Surgery of Liver Disease in Children*. Oxford: Butterworth-Heinemann, 1991: 39–59.

Illustrations by Angela Christie

Oesophageal varices: pathophysiology and management of the acute bleed

Alan G. Johnson MChir, FRCS
Professor of Surgery, Department of Surgical and Anaesthetic Sciences, Royal Hallamshire Hospital, Sheffield, UK

Principles

Oesophageal and gastric varices are complications of an underlying disease and therefore any direct treatment of them does not deal with the cause and can sometimes make the liver disease worse. Varices are collaterals which open as a result of venous obstruction (whether in the liver or a thrombosed portal or splenic vein) and perform a useful function. They are only clinically important where they impinge on a mucosal surface and then bleed. Oesophageal varices, while looking terrifying when seen down an endoscope, are only a small part of the widespread bed of collaterals. The questions that have puzzled clinicians and researchers alike are why many varices do *not* bleed, and why some bleed at a particular time when they have been present for years. It is extremely rare for an intra-abdominal varix to bleed spontaneously into the peritoneal cavity.

Applied anatomy

1 The gastro-oesophageal junction is also the junction between the portal and azygos venous systems. Below the diaphragm, the major veins that drain the region are the left gastric vein (with its constant tributary the 'cardiac vein' from the upper part of the fundus of the stomach) which drains to the portal vein, and the short gastric veins which drain to the splenic vein. In some patients there is a 'polar gastric vein' which drains from the posterior wall of the gastric fundus to the middle section of the splenic vein.

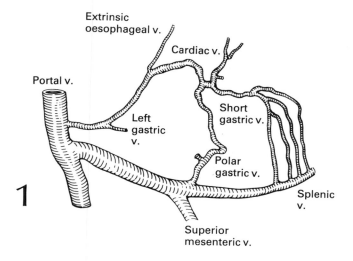

Extrinsic oesophageal v.
Cardiac v.
Portal v.
Short gastric v.
Left gastric v.
Polar gastric v.
Splenic v.
Superior mesenteric v.

1

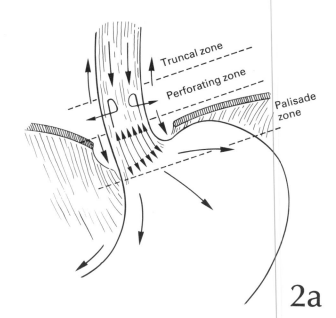

2a

2a,b There are three zones in the lower oesophagus with different venous patterns. From below upwards they are: (1) the palisade zone, (2) the perforating zone and (3) the truncal zone. Most of the perforators which run to the outside of the oesophagus are found in the 'perforating zone'. In patients with portal hypertension they become grossly dilated as can be demonstrated in radio-opaque anatomical casts (*Illustration 2b*). There are no perforating veins in the 'palisade zone' which is surrounded by the lower oesophageal sphincter. The 'truncal zone' lies proximal to the perforating zone and contains large longitudinal venous trunks which run within the folds; it extends upwards from about 5 cm above the gastro-oesophageal junction for some 8 or 10 cm. As bleeding from oesophageal varices nearly always occurs in the lower 5 cm, it comes from the palisade or lower perforating zone.

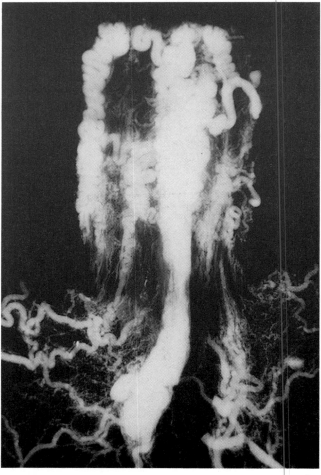

2b

3a,b There are also three groups of veins at different depths in the oesophageal wall and a large perioesophageal plexus. They are (1) the intraepithelial channels, (2) the superficial venous plexus and (3) the deep intrinsic veins which drain into the perioesophageal plexus ('adventitial' veins). Linking the subepithelial and submucosal plexus with the perioesophageal plexus (but only in the perforating zone) are perforating veins which may be as important in the pathogenesis of oesophageal varices as the perforating veins in the calf and ankle are in the varicose veins of the leg. Sclerotherapy usually leaves the perioesophageal adventitial plexus intact and so leaves a good collateral channel. The apparently single trunk seen on endoscopy may therefore be more than one vein and, in the lower oesophagus, the veins lie superficial to the muscularis mucosa and so are less well protected and are more likely to bleed.

As in the leg, sclerotherapy may be most effective when it thromboses the veins just opposite a perforating vein. It has the advantage over devascularization/transection procedures that it leaves the perioesophageal plexus intact to act as an effective collateral circulation.

'Pull through' pressure studies of the normal oesophagus show a 3-cm high pressure zone in the lower oesophagus with the respiratory reversal point (the boundary between the abdominal and the thoracic cavities – from the positive pressure in the inspiration to negative pressure on inspiration) at about 1.5 cm.

The following anatomical facts are relevant to the pathophysiology and the mechanical and pharmacological control of bleeding from varices: (1) the veins in the lower 5 cm of the oesophagus run more superficially beneath the mucosa; (2) there is a constant area of perforating vein about 3 cm above the gastro-oesophageal junction; (3) the lower oesophagus lies at the junction between the thoracic and abdominal cavities; and (4) flow in the perforators is reversed towards the mucosa rather than out to the perioesophageal area. During tamponade the gastric balloon is inflated in the stomach and then drawn up with gentle traction against the undersurface of the diaphragm. The finding that the Linton tube (which does not have an oesophageal balloon) is fairly effective in preventing *oesophageal* bleeding suggests that it acts by compressing intramural and perforating veins at the lower oesophageal junction against the diaphragm, thus reducing flow. It would be unlikely to be effective in patients with a large hiatus hernia.

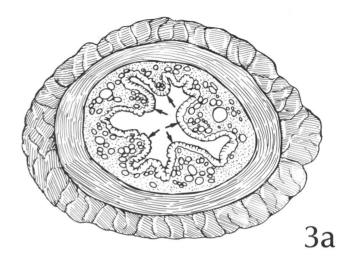

3a

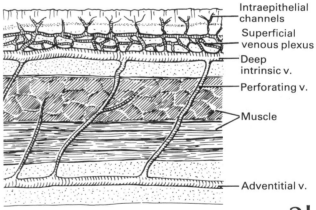

Intraepithelial channels
Superficial venous plexus
Deep intrinsic v.
Perforating v.
Muscle
Adventitial v.

3b

Applied physiology

Normally the flow in the lower oesophageal veins is downwards to the stomach or outwards from the mucosa to the perforating venous plexus and then upwards into the azygos vein. Inspiration increases flow by producing a negative pressure in the chest, drawing blood up from the abdomen. The flow through the upper stomach is normally downwards to join the gastric vein and portal venous system. When flow in the portal vein is obstructed by cirrhosis or thombosis, the connecting veins dilate and collateral flow from the portal system to the azygos system increases. Flow in the portal vein continues towards the liver in many cases (hepatopedal), especially in the earlier stages of cirrhosis, but later it becomes hepatofugal. It is possible that this change is one of the key factors in initiating variceal bleeding. However, flow in the submucosal variceal vessels, which are those likely to bleed, is more variable. Studies with miniature endoscopic Doppler probes suggest that flow *into* the varices in portal hypertension may take place through the dilated perforators just as flow in varicose veins of the leg comes from the perforators deep in the calf. If flow back down to the stomach is also obstructed, the pressure within the subepithelial vessels is considerable.

Flow in the upper gastric vessels in some patients is upwards across the junction but in others the direction of flow is still downwards. This explains how an injection in the lower oesophagus can thrombose a type I gastric varix. When a patient inspires, upward flow is increased but flow into the varices through the perforators is also increased. The Valsalva manoeuvre slows or stops flow up the varices but, interestingly, does not increase the pressure gradient across the variceal wall because both the intravariceal and the intraoesophageal pressures rise to about the same degree. This makes it unlikely that pressure changes induced by the Valsalva manoeuvre initiate bleeding and further evidence comes from the observation that varices very rarely bleed in the second stage of labour when Valsalva manoeuvres are frequent and marked. The 'Muller' manoeuvre produced by *inspiration* against a closed or partly closed glottis is far more likely to produce a sudden rise in pressure, and may occur during coughing, retching or exercise. It is the negative pressure of inspiration which suddenly distends the varices when there is a fall in intraoesophageal and intrathoracic pressure.

The physiology is different in the relatively rare situation when oesophageal varices develop above a sliding hiatus hernia where all the lower oesophagus and part of the stomach is in the chest.

Reflux oesophagitis rarely accompanies varices, partly because the varices may produce an effective seal in the lower oesophagus by virtue of their size. Erosive factors are not therefore the normal cause of variceal bleeding. Similarly, trauma by fish bones or 'rough' food is very unusual. While we still do not understand what initiates bleeding in a particular patient, we do know that larger varices under higher pressures are more likely to bleed than small, low pressure varices, and that when the vessel wall and mucosa are very thin, a sudden change in local pressure could well initiate a bleed, especially if it follows a general rise in portal pressure such as occurs with acute alcoholic hepatitis after a heavy drinking bout.

The lower oesophageal sphincter responds to peptide hormones and to drugs. Gastrin contracts the sphincter whereas cholecystokinin relaxes it. Therefore, a different balance of hormones could also lead to changes in the local pressure in the veins. Some drugs contract the sphincter and have been used in treatment (*see below*).

Management of the acute bleed

As with any emergency, attention to airway, breathing and circulation are the first priorities. Colloids and blood are given as soon as they are available. Intravenous normal saline should be avoided as the sodium is retained in cirrhotic patients and ascites can be made worse.

NON-OPERATIVE MANAGEMENT OF VARICEAL BLEEDING

Whatever the definitive treatment of bleeding oesophageal varices may be (see chapters on pp. 163–173 and 174–182), initial control of bleeding is essential. Rapid transport to a unit with expertise is vital but this may be some distance away. During transfer, tamponade is effective but needs the presence of experienced personnel or it can be disastrous. A Sengstanken tube inflated in the right lower lobe bronchus in a patient with a bleeding duodenal ulcer does nothing for that patient's chances of survival! Just because a patient is known to have cirrhosis and portal hypertension, it must *not* be assumed that he is necessarily bleeding from varices. In the present state of knowledge, the best emergency treatment while transporting the patient, in the absence of local experience with tamponade, is an intravenous infusion of the somatostatin analogue octreotide (50 μg bolus followed by 50 μg/h).

Ideally, the diagnosis of variceal bleeding (as opposed to peptic ulcer bleeding) should have been confirmed. The mechanism of action of octreotide has not been fully explained but some controlled trials have found it to be effective. As an alternative, metoclopramide 10 mg intravenously is effective in the short term and acts by constricting the lower oesophageal sphincter and so tamponading the varices.

Vasopressin has also been used but is contraindicated in older patients with heart disease because it constricts the coronary arteries as well as the visceral arteries supplying the gut. Attempts to overcome this complication have been made by the use of its analogue, glypressin, or by giving glyceryl trinitrate at the same time.

BALLOON TAMPONADE

The principle of tamponade is to compress the varices with a balloon within the oesophagus and upper stomach. It is a very effective way of controlling bleeding but is not a definitive form of treatment and there should be no surprise if a patient rebleeds when the balloons are deflated. Further measures are required as soon as possible after control has been obtained. However, tamponade is only effective if the balloon is in the right position and at the right pressure for the right indication. The single-balloon Linton tube is not as effective as the two-balloon Sengstaken–Blakemore type of tube for the control of oesophageal varices. Most Sengstaken tubes have an oesophageal balloon that is far too long and which nearly reaches the upper oesophageal sphincter. Whichever tube is used, there must be an oesophageal suction channel so that swallowed saliva can be aspirated to prevent it accumulating and spilling over into the lungs causing aspiration pneumonia.

Once the tube is fixed in position, it must not be left inflated for more than 24 h, preferably 12 h, because pressure necrosis can occur. A very restless patient such as an alcoholic with delirium tremens may occasionally try to pull out the inflated balloon causing oesophageal rupture. This is one of the very few situations where heavy sedation and tracheal intubation is required during the treatment of bleeding varices.

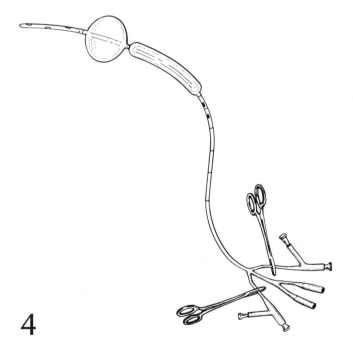

4

Insertion of the Sengstaken tube

4 It is important to check that the balloons inflate with air and stay inflated satisfactorily without leaks (it is not uncommon for a tube to have been on the shelf for several years before use and for the rubber to have perished).

The gastric balloon will take 300–400 ml and the oesophageal balloon should be inflated until it is evenly distended but not distorted (usually about 100–120 ml). The pressure in both balloons is measured and recorded and both balloons are then emptied completely and the connecting tubes clamped for ease of intubation.

5 A well lubricated flexible guidewire is passed down the gastric aspiration channel to the closed end (making sure it does not emerge through a side opening). If there is time, the patient's throat may be sprayed with lignocaine, or it may have already been sprayed for the recent gastroscopy.

The well lubricated tube is inserted through the mouth into the stomach and passed well beyond the 40 cm mark from the incisor teeth. The gastric balloon is filled with 100 ml of air initially and then pulled back gently to ensure that it is in the stomach and impacts below the lower oesophageal sphincter at 35–43 cm from the teeth depending on the size of patient.

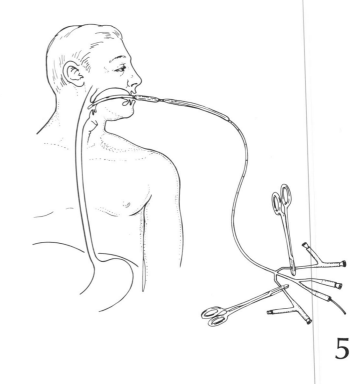

5

6 The guidewire is withdrawn and the gastric balloon inflated to its full 300–400 ml. The pressure is measured and should be the same or only slightly higher than before it was inserted at the test inflation. The patient should not experience any pain.

With gentle traction on the tube, the oesophageal balloon is *slowly* inflated with a volume of air, a little less than that used at the test inflation. If there is severe pain the inflation should be stopped. The pressure is measured and should be 20–25 mmHg *higher* than the test pressure because of the squeeze of the oesophageal wall. If it is not higher, a further 5 ml of air is introduced and the pressure remeasured. If it is considerably higher than the appropriate level, 5 ml increments of air are withdrawn until the right pressure is achieved.

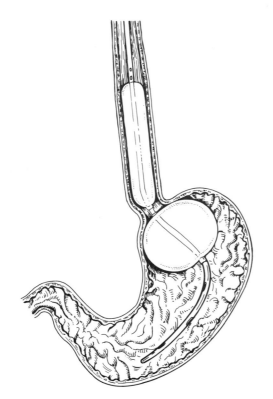

6

7 Once the tube is at the right pressure and in the right position it is fixed in order to stop it being drawn down into the stomach. A split tennis ball at the mouth is effective and does not cause pressure sores on the lips or cheeks. The length of tube inserted when there is gentle traction is noted and recorded using the incisor teeth as the reference point.

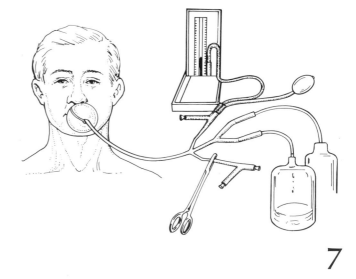

7

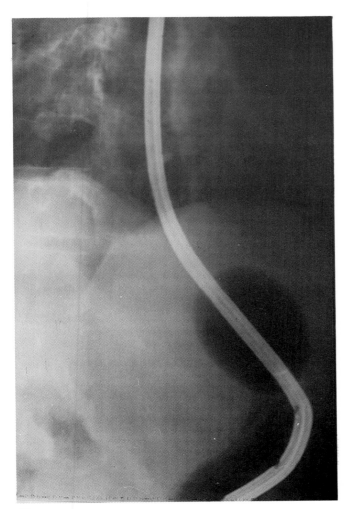

8

8 Each time the patient's pulse and blood pressure are measured, the balloon pressures are checked, as is the position of the tube at the teeth. If there is any doubt, its position may be checked by radiography.

The oesophageal suction channel is attached to continuous low pressure suction and the gastric aspiration channel is put on free drainage and hand-aspirated from time to time. The absence of any fresh blood in the oesophageal or the gastric aspiration channel is confirmation that the bleeding has been controlled.

Sedation and opiates should be avoided if possible or given in small doses because of their slow metabolism by the diseased liver. The patient is encouraged to take good breaths and to be as mobile as possible to avoid bronchial pneumonia.

Definitive treatment

Plans are now made for definitive treatment (e.g. sclerotherapy or transection/devascularization). If this treatment is likely to be delayed for some reason, the *oesophageal* tube may be deflated and the traction lessened but the *gastric* balloon is kept inflated. In the event of a further bleed, the tube can quickly be pulled back into position and the oesophageal balloon reinflated. If sclerotherapy is to be undertaken within 12 h, which is the ideal, the balloons are kept inflated until the last minute to give the best possible view and the least chance of rebleeding. The aspiration ports are aspirated by hand and then the balloons are emptied completely and the inflation channels are clamped to minimize trauma during withdrawal of the tube.

Other measures

Patients in whom a major bleed has occurred rapidly develop portosystemic encephalopathy. A lactulose enema is very effective and lactulose can also be given down the gastric aspiration channel of the Sengstaken tube. Spironolactone is needed to treat or prevent ascites.

PROPHYLACTIC TREATMENT

There is no evidence that prophylactic portacaval shunt or prophylactic sclerotherapy improve survival in patients with varices which have not bled. There have been a number of well conducted randomized controlled trials of sclerotherapy and most show no benefit, although some show benefit in subgroups such as alcoholics. Prophylactic devascularization is commonly performed in some countries but its value has not been confirmed by prospective controlled trials. Beta blockers reduce rebleeding in the long term, but side effects from a dose that is sufficient to reduce portal pressure

make it unacceptable to many patients, and treatment is difficult to justify if the patient has never bled and may, indeed, never bleed. If prophylactic treatment is being considered, it should be given to selected patients with a high risk of bleeding such as those with large varices with a high wedged hepatic venous pressure and the endoscopic signs of 'cherry red' varices or 'haematocystic spots' on their surface (*Table 1*).

Acknowledgement

Illustration 2b is reproduced from *Oxford Textbook of Clinical Hepatology*, Vol 1, by André Vianne published by Oxford University Press, 1991.

Table 1   Endoscopic classification of oesophageal varices

Red wale markings*	**Diffuse redness***
Absent	Absent
Mild	Present
Moderate	
Severe	
Size*	**Haematocystic spots***
Small	**(resembling blood blisters**
Medium	**>4 mm in diameter)**
Large	Absent
	Present
Cherry red spots* (about	**Colour of varices**
2 mm in diameter)	White
Absent	Blue
Mild	
Moderate	
Severe	
Location*	**Oesophagitis**
Inferior	Absent
Median	Present
Superior	

* Significant predictive value for bleeding.
Adapted from *N Engl J Med* 1988; 319: 986.

Injection sclerotherapy of oesophageal varices

J. E. J. Krige FRCS, FCS(SA)
Associate Professor, Department of Surgery, University of Cape Town, South Africa

John Terblanche ChM, FRCS, FCS(SA)
Professor and Head, Department of Surgery and Co-Director, MRC Liver Research Centre, University of Cape Town, South Africa

Techniques

The three techniques of injection sclerotherapy are intravariceal, paravariceal and the combination of both intravariceal and paravariceal methods.

Intravariceal technique

Injection of sclerosant directly into the varix to induce variceal thrombosis is the most widely used technique. The injections are localized to the lower 5 cm of the oesophagus. The authors use 5% ethanolamine oleate.

Paravariceal technique

Sclerosant is injected into the submucosa adjacent to a varix, as described by Wodak[1] and Paquet[2]. The most widely used sclerosant is polidocanol (0.5% or 1% concentration). The sclerosant is administered as 30–40 separate injections (0.5–1 ml each) in a helical fashion, commencing at the gastro-oesophageal junction and extending approximately one-third of the way up the oesophagus. The aim is to produce oedema to compress the varix during acute bleeding and subsequently to provoke tissue reaction, fibrosis and thickening of the mucosa over the varices to prevent bleeding. This technique will not be described further.

Combined technique

The combination of intravariceal and paravariceal injections is used in Cape Town for the emergency management of actively bleeding varices, and in the elective management of large varices to prevent needle-puncture bleeding[3]. The authors use 5% ethanolamine oleate although other agents have been used successfully by other groups. A small volume (1 ml) of sclerosant is injected paravariceally to partially compress the varix, followed by an intravariceal injection of a larger volume (up to 5 ml) to thrombose the varix. As with the intravariceal injection technique, the injections are restricted to the lower 5 cm of the oesophagus.

Equipment

Endoscopes

1 Either single- or twin-channel endoscopes are suitable for injection sclerotherapy. The single-channel endoscope should have a large channel so that suction is not reduced after the injector has been inserted. The twin-channel endoscope is useful for acute bleeding because one channel allows unimpeded suction during injection. Either end- or oblique-viewing endoscopes are effective for injection sclerotherapy. For general purposes an end-viewing instrument is more versatile, enabling both diagnostic and therapeutic functions to be performed. The advantages of an oblique-viewing endoscope are better visualization of the greater and lesser curves of the stomach and the built-in forceps elevator which is helpful in aiming the injector, particularly when small varices are being injected electively.

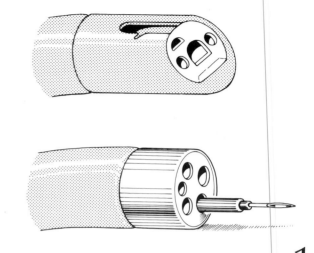

1

Injectors

Several types of sclerotherapy injectors with retractable needles are commercially available (*Illustration 1*). The flexible metal injectors are robust and reusable, but the narrower internal calibre and greater resistance during injection restricts the volume of sclerosant administered per unit time compared with the disposable injectors. Injectors are equipped with either 23 or 25 gauge needles. The larger needle is preferred as it facilitates injection of viscous sclerosant solutions and is not associated with any greater risk of bleeding after withdrawal of the needle.

Sclerosants

Several different sclerosant agents have been successfully used. The Cape Town group uses 5% ethanolamine oleate for both the intravariceal and the combined injection technique[3]. The most widely used alternative solutions are sodium tetradecyl sulphate (1%) and sodium morrhuate (2%) while polidocanol (0.5% or 1%) is used almost exclusively by proponents of paravariceal sclerotherapy[4].

Procedures

ELECTIVE SCLEROTHERAPY

Preparation of patient

The procedure is explained to the patient and signed consent obtained. Two assistants, including a qualified nurse trained in endoscopy techniques, should be present throughout the procedure. One assistant provides suction of the patient's mouth to avoid aspiration, ensures that the bite guard is not dislodged and comforts the patient. The other assistant advances and retracts the injector needle and administers the sclerosant under the direction of the endoscopist. The posterior tongue and pharynx are sprayed with a local anaesthetic (10% xylocaine). A small butterfly needle is inserted into a superficial hand vein and remains in place for the duration of the procedure. The appropriate analgesia and sedation are administered intravenously according to the medical status of the patient. The desired sedation is achieved by injecting small incremental doses, being cautious to avoid oversedation in the aged and in those with liver compromise. The authors' preference is 2.5 mg midazolam and 25 mg pethidine.

Before passing the endoscope the fully connected instrument should be checked for satisfactory function of the light source and lens, focus and tip deflection controls, air, suction and water channels. The assistants should be familiar with the technique and equipment. Commands such as 'advance needle' and 'retract needle' should be rehearsed before injection. The endoscopist indicates the volume to be injected and the assistant acknowledges that the desired volume has been injected. It is important that the assistant should comment when more resistance than expected is encountered during injection, because the varix may be thrombosed or the needle incorrectly positioned.

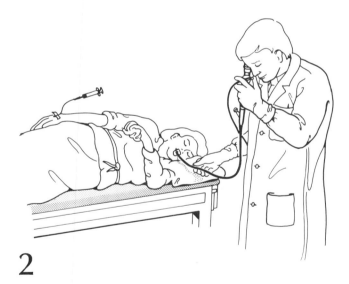

2

Position of patient

2 The patient is placed in the left lateral decubitus position at the top of the bed with the head on a pillow and the neck slightly flexed. The distal endoscope tube is lubricated with a water-soluble medical-grade lubricant, dentures are removed and a comfortable mouthpiece (bite guard) is used in patients with teeth to protect the endoscope.

Endoscopy

3   Passage of the fibreoptic endoscope is initiated by guiding the gently flexed tip over the tongue and then extending the tip in the upper pharynx. The opening of the cricopharynx is identified and negotiated with gentle pressure coinciding with a swallow. The instrument is passed under direct vision, keeping the oesophageal lumen in full view by controlling the tip. Intermittent insufflation of air is used to maintain sufficient distension of the lumen for visibility. Constant or excessive air insufflation should be avoided. Mucus and fluid are removed through the suction channel and the lens cleared with a jet of water when necessary. After passing the cricopharynx, the entire oesophagus is examined for oesophageal varices. The extent, number and size are noted for documentation. Unless varices are bleeding, panendoscopy is first performed to exclude other lesions before commencing injection of varices.

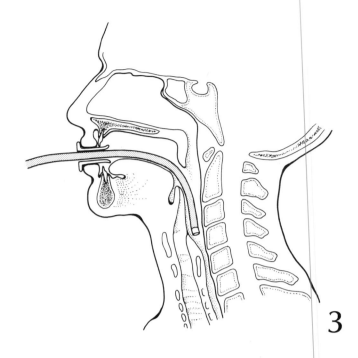

3

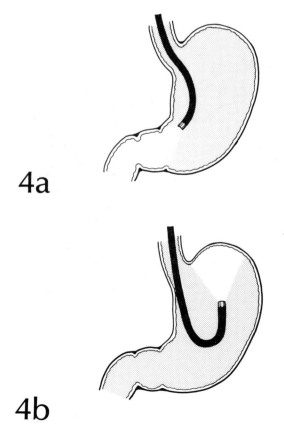

4a

4b

4a, b   When the stomach is reached, the tip is passed distally under vision, insufflating only enough air to display the channel ahead. The pylorus is centred in the field of view and air is insufflated to distend the distal stomach and relax the pylorus; as this occurs the tip is gently advanced into the duodenal bulb. The proximal duodenum is carefully evaluated. Thereafter, the endoscope is withdrawn into the stomach and the cardia, gastric fundus and upper portion of the lesser curve are viewed by reversing the tip in the moderately distended body of the stomach. If gastric varices or evidence of portal hypertensive gastropathy are present they are noted and documented.

5   On completion of panendoscopy the endoscope is partially withdrawn and positioned above the gastro-oesophageal junction, and the varices in the lower 5 cm of the oesophagus are injected.

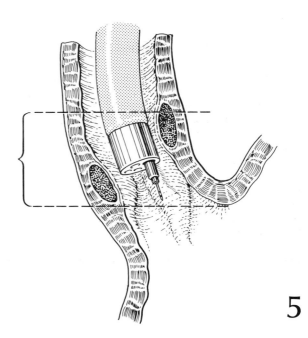

5

Injection technique

6   The endoscope tip is manoeuvred into position and the target varix identified. The endoscopist passes the injector through the channel into the field of view and the tip is positioned 2 cm beyond the end of the endoscope. Care should be taken to avoid inadvertent puncture of the plastic injector sheath and damage to the endoscope channel by the needle when advancing the injector. The injector should not be passed through the channel with the endoscope tip in a position of acute flexion. The needle should remain in the retracted position until the tip of the injector has passed through the endoscope and is visible to the endoscopist. All movements and manipulation of the injector are performed *only* by the endoscopist. A practice aiming pass with the needle retracted is useful to determine the direction of the advancing needle.

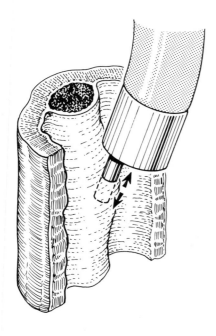

6

7 The assistant is instructed to advance the needle and a small volume of solution is discarded into the oesophageal lumen in order to fill the injector. The endoscopist inserts the needle directly into the centre and most prominent part of the varix by advancing the injector a further 5 mm: the length of the visible needle and the angle of insertion determine the depth of puncture. If the needle is well placed and appears intravariceal, the assistant is instructed to inject 1 ml of sclerosant. If this is achieved without resistance the assistant injects further sclerosant. With further injection of sclerosant the varix will be seen to distend above and below the injection site and become paler. This is the indication to stop the injection. A total volume of no more than 5 ml is usually required for a large varix: smaller varices require proportionately less sclerosant. On completing injection of the first varix, the remaining varices are injected. After a previous series of injections, varices will be smaller and less sclerosant is injected. During subsequent endoscopy, varices may be thrombosed and appear firm and cord-like. If increased resistance to insertion of the needle and injection of sclerosant with leakage around the needle is noted, confirming obliteration of the variceal channel, no further injection should be undertaken.

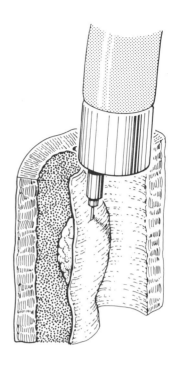

7

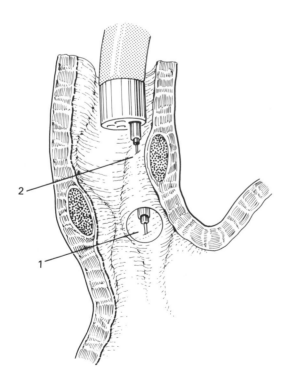

8

8 A second series of injections is performed at a higher level for large varices (site 2). The fibrescope is withdrawn 2–3 cm and the varices injected (usually 2–3 ml of sclerosant is sufficient). As the varices become smaller after several previous injections, they are injected only at the lower site (site 1).

9 Accurate placement of the needle is critical in obtaining effective delivery of sclerosant and avoiding complications which may follow incorrect injection. A tangential flat angle of insertion as shown in *Illustration 7* is preferable to avoid deep injection: a less acute angle with a perpendicular approach may transfix the varix and penetrate the oesophageal wall, resulting in an intramuscular injection. In this situation increased resistance to injection will be noted by the assistant and no blanching or distension of the varix will occur. The injector and needle should be withdrawn and a further injection performed after accurate placement of the needle.

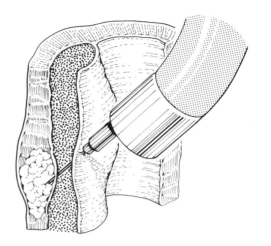

9

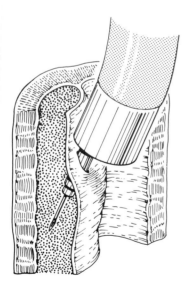

10

10 The needle should not be left protruding while selecting a further varix for injection because inadvertent laceration of a varix with accompanying bleeding may occur, especially with coughing or peristalsis. Needle insertion and variceal puncture requires a delicate wrist action by the endoscopist while manipulating the injector. This provides a limited controlled forward momentum of about 5 mm.

Injection by attempting to spear the varix or forceful jabbing of the varix with the needle may result in deep insertion and cannulation of the varix with entry of both needle and the hub of the catheter sheath and resultant bleeding from the varix on extraction.

EMERGENCY SCLEROTHERAPY

Initial measures

Urgent intravenous fluid resuscitation is started. The authors' group uses pharmacological therapy in patients with suspected variceal bleeding, although the efficacy remains controversial[4]. Vasopressin, its synthetic analogue terlipressin, and somatostatin have been used to lower portal pressure[4]. The most commonly used agent is vasopressin, which should be administered as a continuous intravenous infusion. Combination of glyceryl trinitrate with vasopressin reduces the side effects caused by vasopressin alone and potentiates the portal haemodynamic effects. The glyceryl trinitrate can be administered intravenously, sublingually, or transdermally. A combination of continuous intravenous vasopressin (0.4 units/min) and sublingual glyceryl trinitrate (one tablet every half hour for up to 6 hours) was used[4], but currently the authors, like others, have converted to using a continuous infusion of somatostatin or octreotide.

Endoscopy

Urgent endoscopy is essential. The patient is positioned as for elective sclerotherapy as shown in *Illustration 2*. One-third of patients with suspected variceal bleeding do not, in fact, have varices. Patients shown to have varices on endoscopy fall into one of three groups although the differentiation may be difficult during active bleeding: (1) those with actively bleeding varices; (2) those whose varices have stopped bleeding; (3) those who have varices but are bleeding from another lesion. At endoscopy, variceal bleeding that has stopped is diagnosed if adherent blood clots are noted on a varix, or when varices are present in a patient with upper gastrointestinal bleeding in whom panendoscopy demonstrates no other cause of bleeding.

Emergency endoscopy should be performed in the endoscopy unit where all the necessary equipment is available. Many units have a fully equipped emergency endoscopy trolley and if necessary this can be taken into the operating room or to the intensive care unit. It is imperative that full resuscitative facilities are available together with skilled staff experienced in dealing with emergencies. Two endoscopy assistants should be present throughout. Adequate monitoring is necessary during the procedure. Emergency endoscopy should not commence until satisfactory venous access and central venous pressure measurement are established and volume replacement and resuscitation procedures with blood transfusions are initiated to correct hypovolaemia. If bleeding is extensive, endotracheal intubation is essential before endoscopy to protect the airway and avoid aspiration.

Intravariceal injection

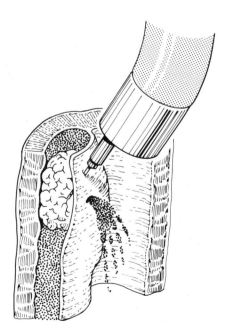

11 Active variceal bleeding with a jet of blood or rapid oozing is immediately dealt with by controlling the bleed with intravariceal sclerotherapy. Urgent control of bleeding with accurate placement of the needle and sclerosant should be performed without delay while there is adequate visibility. No attempt should be made to inject distal to the active bleeding site or to insert the needle into the bleeding point, because this may enlarge the hole and aggravate bleeding with extravasation and loss of sclerosant. A technique similar to elective intravariceal sclerotherapy is used with needle insertion proximal to the bleeding site. A total volume of 5 ml of sclerosant is usually sufficient. Distension and blanching of the varix indicate that the needle is in the correct position and that the appropriate volume of sclerosant has been injected. After the bleeding has been controlled, the other variceal channels are sclerosed. A second series of injections is usually performed at a higher level, as depicted in *Illustration 8*. Panendoscopy is undertaken on completion of sclerotherapy to exclude other lesions.

Combined paravariceal and intravariceal injection

12a–c The authors' group prefers this technique to control active variceal bleeding. The needle is inserted in a paravariceal position and sclerosant injected proximal to the bleeding point to compress the bleeding site by raising a weal (*Illustration 12a*). Sufficient sclerosant is injected to control the bleeding (*Illustration 12b*). If this does not completely control the acute bleeding, the paravariceal injection is repeated alongside the bleeding point. The procedure is completed by injecting the varix intravariceally (*Illustration 12c*). The volume injected paravariceally should not be more than 1 ml at each site to avoid ulceration of mucosa. The remaining variceal channels are then sclerosed. Panendoscopy is performed on completion of sclerotherapy to exclude other lesions.

If variceal bleeding is profuse, vigorous lavage through the endoscope channel and elevation of the head of the table to 30° may improve visibility and allow identification of the bleeding site. No blind attempts at injection should be used. The procedure is usually performed with the patient on his/her side as depicted in *Illustration 2*. With profuse bleeding the patient requires endotracheal intubation. The procedure may be facilitated by placing the patient on his/her back on the bed (or operating table) and adjusting the headpiece to an angle of 45°. If immediate sclerotherapy cannot be performed because of lack of expertise or inadequate visibility, bleeding should first be controlled by balloon tube tamponade before the patient is subjected to further sclerotherapy[4].

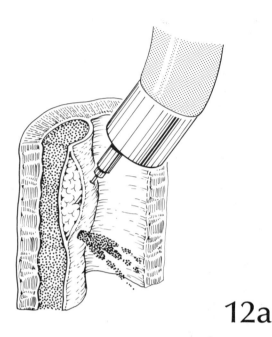

12a

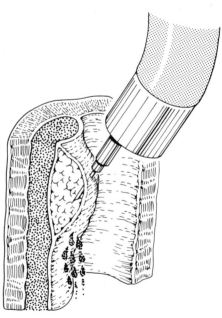

12b

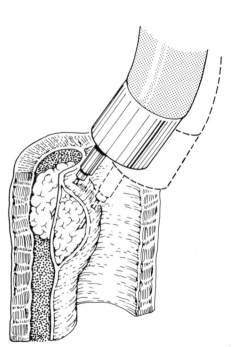

12c

Balloon tube tamponade

13 The four-lumen balloon tube (Minnesota tube) is effective in temporarily controlling variceal bleeding and gaining time for resuscitation and management planning[3,4]. Before inserting the balloon tube in stuporous or comatose patients, the airway should be protected by an endotracheal tube to prevent aspiration. A new tube should always be used and the inflated gastric and oesophageal balloons tested underwater to confirm a complete air seal. The deflated lubricated tube is passed through a bite guard via the mouth after adequate topical pharyngeal anaesthesia. Passage via the nose should not be used because of potential pressure necrosis of the nasal cartilage. The left index finger in the mouth facilitates initial passage of the tube by guiding the tip of the tube over the posterior tongue, through the cricopharynx and prevents coiling of the tube in the pharynx. If difficulty is encountered negotiating the cricopharynx, especially when an endotracheal tube is in place, a McGills forcep and laryngoscope are used to pass the tube under direct vision. The tube is inserted almost fully and the epigastrium auscultated to confirm that the gastric balloon is in the stomach by instilling air with a 50-ml syringe into the aspirating lumen. The gastric balloon is inflated with 50-ml increments of air to 200 ml. If the patient shows signs of discomfort, inflation *must* stop as the gastric balloon may be in the lower oesophagus and the position should be rechecked. When fully inflated, the tube is pulled back until the balloon engages the gastro-oesophageal junction and abuts on the cardia. A partially split tennis ball, secured over the tube, maintains firm traction against the bite guard and ensures constant compression on the cardia by the gastric balloon.

The oesophageal balloon is inflated only if bleeding continues after traction on the gastric balloon. The oesophageal balloon pressure should not exceed 40 mmHg or be maintained for more than 14 h. Thereafter, preferably within 6–12 h, sclerotherapy should be undertaken to achieve more lasting control because of the high rate of recurrence of bleeding (60%) after removal of the tube. If bleeding persists or recurs after the tube has been placed, the tube should be checked and, if found to be correctly situated, a further diagnostic endoscopy should be performed. A bleeding source that has been missed during the initial endoscopy may be the cause of continued bleeding. Because of associated dangers, a balloon tube should be used only when required to control endoscopically confirmed variceal bleeding[5,6].

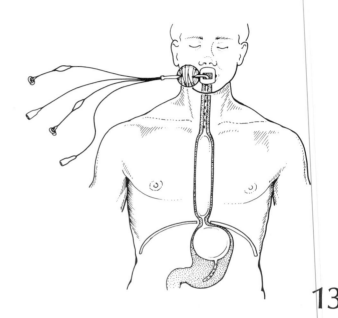

13

Postoperative care

Elective sclerotherapy

After elective outpatient sclerotherapy, patients are observed in the endoscopy suite recovery room for an hour before discharge. Bleeding following elective sclerotherapy is rare. Retrosternal discomfort is treated with antacids. After admission for acute variceal bleeding, the first two injection sclerotherapy sessions are performed in hospital. Further injection treatments are performed on an outpatient basis.

Injection sclerotherapy is repeated at weekly intervals until the varices have been eradicated. The first subsequent assessment is performed at 3 months and then repeated 6-monthly or yearly for life[7]. Any recurrent variceal channels noted during repeat endoscopy require a further course of injection sclerotherapy. If ulceration extending over more than one-quarter of the circumference of the oesophagus is present at the site of previous sclerotherapy, further injections are deferred for 2 weeks to allow the ulceration to heal. Minor ulceration or slough is usually ignored.

Emergency sclerotherapy

The patient is returned to an intensive care unit for 24 h after injection. Unless the patient is stuporous or comatose, oral fluids are allowed for the first 24 h and thereafter a regular diet is recommended. Prophylactic antibiotics are not administered routinely in uncomplicated cases. Hepatic encephalopathy and ascites are treated with standard therapy. Mild retrosternal discomfort and low-grade pyrexia may occur for 24 h after injection. If either is excessive or if the patient has dysphagia, a Gastrografin contrast swallow is obtained to exclude an injection site leak[6].

No further bleeding will occur in 70% of patients. If bleeding does recur, vasopressin or somatostatin is commenced and the patient re-endoscoped. Recurrent bleeding from oesophageal varices is treated by repeat injection similar to the initial procedures. If bleeding is massive and satisfactory control is not achieved by sclerotherapy, a balloon tube is placed for acute control and followed by sclerotherapy within 6–12 h. Bleeding from oesophageal ulceration or slough is treated conservatively with oral sucralfate. In the unusual event of persistent bleeding from injection ulceration, intravenous somatostatin is administered.

In patients who have continued acute variceal bleeding after two emergency sclerotherapy injection sessions during a single hospital admission, we recommend that bleeding be temporarily controlled with balloon tube tamponade followed by a surgical procedure[4,6,8]. Unfortunately, it is not possible to predict during initial evaluation and variceal injection which patients will not ultimately respond to sclerotherapy.

Outcome

Elective sclerotherapy

In the Cape Town 10-year prospective study evaluating the long-term management of patients after oesophageal variceal bleeding[7], oesophageal varices were eradicated in 123 of 140 patients. A median number of five injections were required to eradicate the oesophageal varices which remained eradicated for a mean of 19 months. Varices recurred in 37 patients after a mean of 15 months and were easily re-eradicated by further injection sclerotherapy. Recurrent variceal bleeding was unusual after the varices had been eradicated and occurred in only 13 of the 123 patients.

Acute variceal injection

The success rate of a single injection treatment is 70%[4,6]. The 30% of patients who have further bleeding after initial injection of sclerosant should have a second injection performed; in this group the success rate is more than 90%[4,6].

References

1. Wodak E. Akute gastrointestinale Blutung; Resultate der endoskopischen Sklerosierung von Osophagusvarizen. *Schweiz Med Wochenschr* 1979; 109: 591–4.

2. Paquet K-J, Oberhammer E. Sclerotherapy of bleeding oesophageal varices by means of endoscopy. *Endoscopy* 1978; 10: 7–12.

3. Terblanche J, Krige JE, Bornman PC. Endoscopic sclerotherapy. *Surg Clin North Am* 1990; 70: 341–59.

4. Terblanche J, Burroughs AK, Hobbs KE. Controversies in the management of bleeding oesophageal varices. *N Engl J Med* 1989; 320: 1393–8, 1469–75.

5. Burnett DA, Rikkers LF. Nonoperative emergency treatment of variceal haemorrhage. *Surg Clin North Am* 1990; 70: 291–306.

6. Kahn D, Bornman PC, Terblanche J. A 10-year prospective evaluation of balloon tube tamponade and emergency injection sclerotherapy for actively bleeding esophageal varices. *HPB Surg* 1989; 1: 207–19.

7. Terblanche J, Kahn D, Bornman PC. Long-term injection sclerotherapy treatment for oesophageal varices: a 10 year prospective evaluation. *Ann Surg* 1989; 210: 725–31.

8. Bornman PC, Terblanche J, Kahn D, Jonker MA, Kirsch RE. Limitations of multiple injection sclerotherapy sessions for acute variceal bleeding. *S Afr Med J* 1986; 70: 34–6.

Oesophageal varices: oesophageal transection and devascularization procedures

George W. Johnston MCh, FRCS
Honorary Professor, Queen's University Belfast, and Consultant Surgeon, Royal Victoria Hospital, Belfast, UK

History

Since Boerema and Crile first described direct ligation of oesophageal varices by a transthoracic approach there have been many modifications of the method. Japanese surgeons, disillusioned by the results of shunt surgery, employed transthoracic paraoesophageal devascularization and oesophageal transection combined with an abdominal component consisting of splenectomy and devascularization of the upper stomach together with vagotomy and pyloroplasty[1]. This extensive operation has never gained popularity in the West, and even in Japan thoracotomy is now included less frequently. The advent of mechanical staplers has renewed interest in the transection–devascularization procedures.

Principles and justification

Portal hypertension in itself does not require treatment and there is, as yet, insufficient evidence to support prophylactic therapy for oesophageal varices which have not bled. When varices do bleed the clinician is presented with a life-threatening situation, not only because of haemorrhage but because of the risk of liver failure in cirrhotic patients with limited liver reserve. Where efficient emergency sclerotherapy is available only a small proportion of patients require urgent surgery, either in the form of a portal systemic shunt or a devascularization–transection procedure. Burroughs and colleagues consider that if two attempts at sclerotherapy fail to control acute bleeding, one should proceed to emergency transection[2]. Where sclerotherapy is unavailable, emergency transection–devascularization is a viable alternative. Even if the initial bleeding episode is controlled by acute sclerotherapy, consideration has to be given to the prevention of recurrent bleeding whether by chronic injections, portal systemic shunt, or some form of oesophageal transection–devascularization procedure. Perhaps transection–devascularization is the preferred option in countries where compliance with a chronic injection programme is poor or where the risk of encephalopathy after the shunt procedure is high. A recent three-centre controlled trial demonstrated similar survival following either transection or repeated sclerotherapy[3].

Preoperative

Emergency oesophageal transection carries a high rate of mortality in these seriously ill patients and should be avoided in most patients with Child's grade C disease. Even in the elective situation the operation should probably be confined to those with Child's grade A and B disease. All patients should have documented varices which have bled. Where doubt exists about the source of bleeding, ultrasonographic examination is useful to assess splenic size when the organ is not palpable or percussible (one cannot have bleeding varices without splenomegaly). The aetiology of the liver disease should be established where possible by liver function tests, serological, immunological and histological examination. Coagulation studies are essential and replacement therapy should be employed where indicated. One dose of an intravenous cephalosporin is indicated at the time of surgery because of the necessary gastrotomy in these immunocompromised patients.

Anaesthesia

Halothane is probably best avoided for medicolegal rather than good scientific reasons. The volume distribution of most non-depolarizing muscle relaxants is increased, thereby giving rise to relative resistance but a longer duration of action. Obviously good hydration with adequate diuresis is desirable to reduce the risk of the hepatorenal syndrome, but overloading should be avoided in those patients with a high risk of postoperative ascites. Care is required with postoperative analgesia because of the impaired detoxication rate of the liver.

Operations

CONTROL OF OESOPHAGEAL VARICES USING A CIRCULAR STAPLER

Position of patient and incision

The patient is placed supine on the operating table and a midline epigastric incision used in most patients. Where splenectomy is considered necessary because of hypersplenism a left subcostal incision gives better exposure. Exploration of the abdomen is carried out to confirm the diagnosis and exclude other disease. In portal hypertension the spleen is always enlarged and can be damaged by careless retraction. The hard, cirrhotic liver can also cause difficulties of access to the lower oesophagus.

Exposure of the left gastric pedicle

1 The most important route transmitting the high portal pressure to the oesophageal varices is the left gastric or coronary vein. This vessel requires ligation and can be approached either through the gastrohepatic omentum or via a window in the gastrocolic omentum. The latter route gives excellent access to the lesser sac and also to the splenic artery, should one wish to carry out a splenic artery ligation for hypersplenism in patients where the spleen is not being removed.

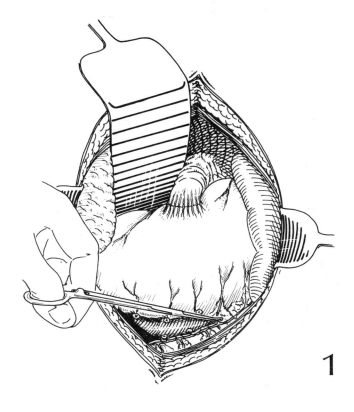

Ligation of the left gastric pedicle

2 The mobilized stomach is retracted upwards and adhesions in the lesser sac are divided until the left gastric pedicle is reached at the upper border of the pancreas. Even in portal hypertension these adhesions are generally not very vascular and diathermy is sufficient to control bleeding. The pedicle of the left gastric vessels is cleared sufficiently to allow vision of the main left gastric vein. It is not necessary to dissect out the individual vein, as this can give rise to unnecessary bleeding. The group of vessels present in the pedicle can be ligated in continuity using a non-absorbable suture placed by fine right-angled forceps. A number of ligatures should be applied. The largest size of metal ligaclip should also be used as it provides a useful marker in later radiology.

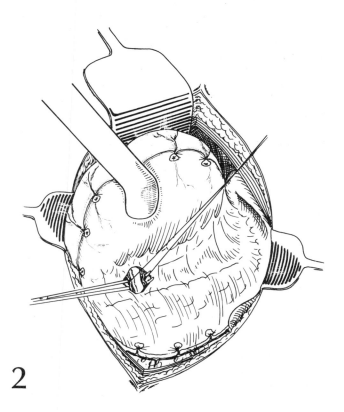

Mobilization of the oesophagus

3 Attention is now turned to the region of the gastro-oesophageal junction. In portal hypertension the peritoneum on the front of the oesophagus generally contains multiple spidery venules. In spite of this extra vasculature it is usually possible to visualize the 'white line' underneath the peritoneum marking the position of the phreno-oesophageal ligament. A transverse incision is made in the peritoneum at this level, bleeding from the small peritoneal vessels being controlled by diathermy. When the phreno-oesophageal ligament has been exposed it is brushed upwards with a small gauze dissector. This exposes the oesophagus and the large perioesophageal collateral veins which lie deep to the peritoneum. The lateral and posterior aspects of the lower oesophagus are mobilized under direct vision using gauze dissection, bringing into view the large collateral channels which run with the posterior vagus nerve. This mobilization should not be done blindly, particularly if there is perioesophagitis as a result of previous injection sclerotherapy or secondary to previous reflux oesophagitis.

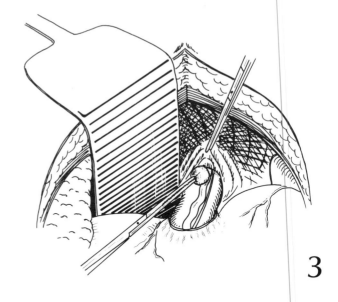

3

4

Devascularization of the lower oesophagus

4 There are usually one or two large collateral channels which run with the anterior vagus and a number of even larger vessels with the posterior vagus. It is usually possible to free these vessels from the vagal nerves which are then protected in Silastic slings. At this stage it is useful to place a rubber catheter sling around the oesophagus, excluding the vagal nerves. The anterior collateral veins are divided between ligatures. With the fingers of the right hand positioned behind the oesophagus the posterior veins are displaced forwards to facilitate their separation from the posterior vagus and subsequent division. It is permissible to sacrifice one of the vagi, usually the anterior, if there is significant difficulty in separating it from the venae comitantes. Some operators consider that these portoazygos collaterals should be preserved. In any case, it is essential to free the oesophagus from these large extrinsic vessels for a distance of about 6–8 cm.

Division of perforating veins

5 Perforating branches passing directly into the oesophagus from the venae comitantes require individual ligation or diathermy coagulation. Usually there are only one or two perforating branches on the front of the oesophagus but three or four such veins usually penetrate the oesophagus from the posterior vessels. It is often stated that dissection around the hiatus carries a high risk of serious haemorrhage in patients with portal hypertension but this is rarely the case. However, mobilization of the oesophagus can be more difficult in patients with perioesophagitis.

The extent of devascularization of the upper stomach depends on whether or not it is considered necessary to undertake a splenectomy. In Western society hypersplenism is not a major problem and splenectomy is indicated in a minority of patients only. If the spleen is not being removed, perhaps it is wiser not to divide the short gastric vessels since one can easily encounter troublesome bleeding, particularly if these vessels are very short.

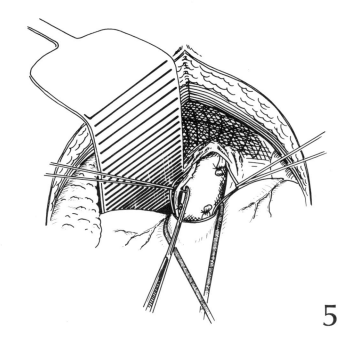

5

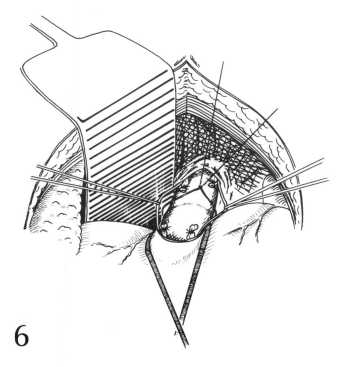

6

Placement of encircling ligature

6 A 0 linen or silk ligature is passed around the now cleared oesophagus and loosely tied. It is important to place this ligature in position before the insertion of the stapling device; with the rigid gun in position it is technically more difficult and increases the risk of damage to the oesophageal wall. Again it is important to ensure that both vagal nerves lie outside the encircling ligature.

Insertion of stapling gun

7 A small gastrotomy is made in a relatively avascular part of the anterior wall of the stomach and an obturator sizer is passed into the oesophagus to determine the largest size of gun head that can be slipped into the oesophagus without risk of damage. The correct size of EEA stapler (usually no. 28 or 31) or ILS stapler (usually 29 or 32) is selected. The closed gun is advanced via the gastrotomy into the lower oesophagus, making sure that neither the encircling ligature nor the sling around the oesophagus impede the passage of the gun up the lumen.

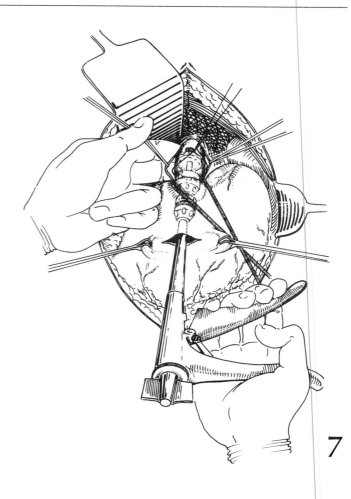

7

Technique of transection

8 When the gun has been advanced into the oesophagus for 5–6 cm, a 3-cm gap is opened up in the head and the instrument is drawn back down the oesophagus until the lowest part of the gap lies immediately above the gastro-oesophageal junction. Light traction is applied to the oesophageal sling while the assistant carefully maintains the gun in the correct position. The encircling ligature is tightened around the stem of the gun into the gap between the anvil-carrying nose cone and the staple-carrying cartridge immediately above the cardia. It is important to remove the rubber sling from around the oesophagus at this point before the head of the gun is tightened, otherwise one risks entrapment of the sling, thereby interfering with stapling. The head of the gun is closed and the trigger pulled to complete the anastomosis.

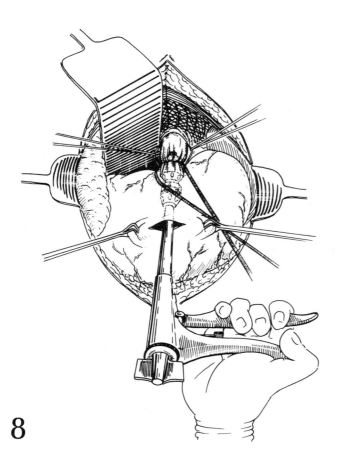

8

Confirmation of a satisfactory transection

9 The head of the gun is opened and the instrument drawn through the newly completed anastomosis. A complete 'doughnut' indicates a satisfactory transection. A finger is gently introduced through the gastrotomy to confirm a satisfactory suture line and to direct a nasogastric tube into the stomach for postoperative decompression. The gastrotomy wound is closed in two layers. Since a vagotomy has not been carried out, a gastric drainage procedure is not required. The abdomen is closed without drainage.

Modifications of circular stapler technique

Simple transection

In a patient with acute bleeding the operating time can be reduced by doing a simple transection alone without any devascularization. However, the risk of rebleeding may be greater although there is no controlled trial to prove this.

Addition of splenectomy

In Western society hypersplenism is rarely a significant problem. In areas where schistosomiasis is prevalent, however, massive splenomegaly is often present and splenectomy should therefore be considered almost as a routine. Splenic artery ligation alone can be useful in non-schistosomiasis patients in helping to lower portal pressure, at least on a temporary basis.

Addition of vagotomy and drainage

Although this is part of the Sugiura operation, there is no logical justification for the procedure as a routine. If there is a concomitant peptic ulcer, however, the gastrotomy for the introduction of the gun should be made in the most dependent part of the stomach and this opening subsequently used for a gastrojejunostomy in conjunction with vagotomy.

Transection of the mucosa only

Since full thickness oesophageal transection removes a portion of the lower oesophageal sphincter, Hirashima and colleagues[4] advocate mucosal transection only,

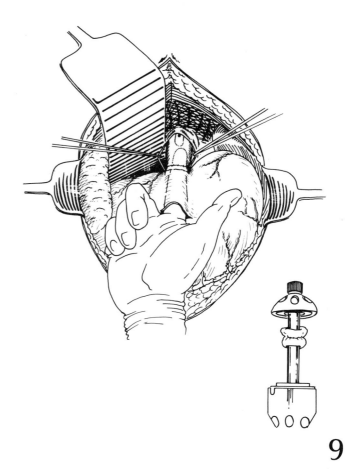

9

leaving the muscle intact. A longitudinal incision is made in the muscle layer of the distal oesophagus and a mucosal cuff isolated circumferentially using scissor dissection. A ligature is placed around the mucosa inside the oesophageal muscular tube. When the stapling gun is inserted only the mucosal flange is resected, leaving the muscular mechanism intact. The oesophageal muscle coat is then sutured over the mucosal staple line.

Addition of an antireflux procedure

Vankemmel advocates a cardioplasty using a linear stapler to provide a valvular flange in the fundus[5]. He claims that this 'gastro-oesophageal dam' minimizes gastro-oesophageal reflux. Some advocate the use of a Nissen fundoplication. This is technically easy if the spleen has been removed or the short gastric vessels divided, but is somewhat more difficult if the fundus has not been mobilized, since one cannot safely pull down on the recently sutured oesophagus.

CONTROL OF GASTRO-OESOPHAGEAL VARICES USING A LINEAR STAPLER

Transabdominal subcardiac linear stapling for oesophageal varices

Although the technique of managing bleeding varices using linear staplers is described in the literature supplied by the manufacturers of stapling instruments, very few procedures have been reported and there is little evidence of the long-term effectiveness of the technique. Subcardiac linear stapling does not attack the site of bleeding in 90–95% of patients, i.e. the lower 3–5 cm of the oesophagus, and thus late rebleeding rates are high. The technique, however, has merit in a few well defined situations in patients with acutely bleeding varices:

1. Where there is a fixed hiatus hernia which causes difficulty in mobilization of the oesophagus.
2. Where the oesophagus is likely to be friable in a patient bleeding within a few days of recent sclerotherapy, particularly if there have been a number of episodes of sclerotherapy.
3. Where there is gross perioesophagitis related to previous repeated sclerotherapy, making mobilization of the oesophagus dangerous.

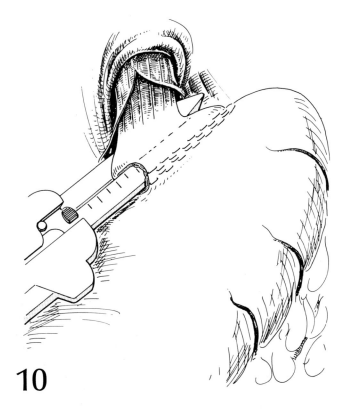

10 The stomach is exposed and the region of the gastro-oesophageal junction identified. A small gastrotomy is made on the lesser curvature of the stomach, 2 cm below the cardia, and the bleeding from the edges of the wound controlled. An SGIA 50 stapler, which contains no blade, is used. One limb is inserted inside the stomach via the gastrotomy and advanced to the top of the fundus. The second limb is placed on the anterior gastric wall on the serosal aspect and the gun closed and fired. Four lines of staples are inserted into the anterior gastric wall. The identical procedure is carried out on the posterior gastric wall and the gastrotomy closed. Nasogastric aspiration is advisable for a few days.

10

Cardiofundectomy for gastric varices

Although gastric varices account for well under 10% of all cases of variceal bleeding, they are a particularly difficult problem. Sclerotherapy is technically difficult and often ineffectual. Direct suturing gives temporary control but rebleeding is common. Even portal systemic shunts do not always stop bleeding from gastric varices. Yu and colleagues have described an oblique cardio-fundectomy for the control of bleeding gastric varices[6].

11 Initially the oesophagus and upper stomach are devascularized and Yu and colleagues also advise splenectomy. This gives easy access for the TA90 stapler, applied obliquely across the fundus of the stomach from halfway down the greater curvature to within about 2 cm of the gastro-oesophageal junction. The gun is fired and the redundant fundic area with its tortuous varices excised and the gun removed. It is wise to add a continuous seromuscular suture of 2/0 polyglactin (Vicryl) to ensure complete haemostasis. Nasogastric aspiration is advised for a few days.

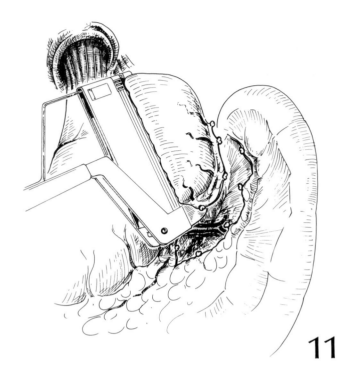

11

Postoperative care

Following transection, nasogastric aspiration continues for 24–48 h after surgery and oral fluids are withheld until the 5th postoperative day. There is no indication for radiological studies before starting oral fluids. In some patients increasing ascites may be a problem postoperatively and the cautious use of diuretics is required. On returning to solid food the patients are warned that they may experience some temporary dysphagia. With modern staplers only about 5% require later oesophageal dilatation.

Outcome

Since January 1976 the author has performed 139 stapled oesophageal transections with devasculariza-tion. Only 29 were done as emergencies, the remainder being performed electively, often during the same hospital admission but usually within a few weeks of the onset of bleeding. In addition to oesophageal tran-section and subdiaphragmatic devascularization, 26 patients had splenectomy and 13 had splenic artery ligation because of hypersplenism. There were 22 operative deaths in the series, 10 of these occurring in patients with Child's grade C disease. There were eight deaths in the 29 patients undergoing emergency transection, giving an emergency mortality rate of 28%

compared with a 13% mortality rate for the 110 patients undergoing an elective procedure. No patient de-veloped a suture line leak. However, two patients did have oesophageal leaks; both occurred about 2 cm above the anastomosis and were thought to be related to intraoperative dilatation before transection. One of these patients died from mediastinitis and the other survived following simple suture. Fifteen patients in the series required oesophageal dilatation because of stricture formation. Of the 117 patients who survived to leave hospital, 46 have had recurrent haemorrhage in a follow-up period extending from 3 months to 19 years. Often recurrent haemorrhage was of a minor nature and only seven of the 46 patients died as a result of bleeding. Where recurrent varices were identified as the cause, post-transection sclerotherapy was used in 30 of the patients. The overall 5-year, 10-year and 15-year cumulative survival rates for the whole series were 49%, 32% and 28%, respectively. Forty-seven patients remain alive at the time of review and the majority are well and free of jaundice, ascites or encephalopathy.

References

1. Sugiura M, Futagawa S. A new technique for treating oesophageal varices. *J Thorac Cardiovasc Surg* 1973; 66: 677–85.

2. Burroughs AK, Hamilton G, Phillips A, Mezzanotte G, McIntyre N, Hobbs KEF. A comparison of sclerotherapy with staple transection of the esophagus for the emergency control of bleeding from esophageal varices. *N Engl J Med* 1989; 321: 857–62.

3. Triger DR, Johnson AG, Brazier JE *et al*. A prospective trial of endoscopic devascularization and oesophageal transection and gastric devascularization in the long term management of bleeding oesophageal varices. *Gut* 1992; 33: 1553–8.

4. Hirashima T, Hara T, Benitani A, Juan I-K, Sato H. A new stapling technique in esophageal mucosal transection. *Jpn J Surg* 1982; 12: 160–2.

5. Vankemmel MH. Highly selective portal decompression for bleeding esophageal varices. *Int Surg* 1985; 70: 125–8.

6. Yu T-J, Cheng K-K, Lai S-T *et al*. A new operation for the management of gastric varix bleeding. *Chinese Med J (Taipei)* 1989; 43: 49–56.

Illustrations by Angela Christie

Gastric varices

A. G. Johnson MChir, FRCS
Professor of Surgery, Department of Surgical and Anaesthetic Sciences, Royal Hallamshire Hospital, Sheffield, UK

Incidence

Gastric varices are a far less frequent cause of bleeding in patients with portal hypertension than oesophageal varices. They account for less than 5% of initial bleeds but form a higher proportion of bleeding episodes in patients on a long-term sclerotherapy programme for oesophageal varices. This may not be a result of the sclerotherapy itself, but rather a sign of the progression of the portal hypertension. However, when gastric varices do bleed, bleeding may be very severe and difficult to control.

Recognition

Gastric varices may be missed at endoscopy as they do not follow the rugal folds and, unless very large, do not produce the characteristic blue appearance of oesophageal varices which lie beneath the squamous mucosa of the oesophagus. Sometimes it appears that the brisk spurt of blood is coming from a normal gastric mucosa.

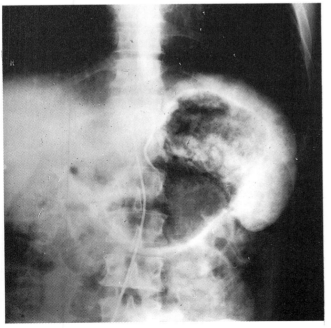

1

1 Portography does not help to distinguish between perigastric varices and those that lie just beneath the mucosa. It can, however, identify type III varices (*see below*).

When a patient is bleeding or has just bled, it is very important to discover whether the haemorrhage is emanating from an oesophageal or gastric varix because the treatment may be different.

Classification

2 Gastric varices can be classified into three types.

Type I: these are lesser curve gastric varices which connect with oesophageal varices across the squamocolumnar junction. They are the most common type and over 50% disappear when the oesophageal varices are successfully injected.

Type II: these are fundal varices and are usually associated with oesophageal varices which converge around the cardia. They have a high risk of bleeding, and bleeding is associated with a high mortality.

Type III: these are isolated gastric varices, unconnected to the oesophagus or cardia, and may develop in the body or even in the antrum of the stomach. They are usually due to segmental portal hypertension from splenic vein thrombosis, often following pancreatitis. The gastric varices are collaterals which enable blood to bypass the blocked vein and so pass from the spleen to the portal vein. Type III varices may be further subdivided into type IIIa varices which are limited to the fundus of the stomach and have the same high risk of bleeding as type II varices, and type IIIb varices which are in the body or antrum and rarely bleed. Other classifications recognize the same subtypes but subdivide them in a different way; classification is important because these different groups of varices have different natural histories and need different treatments.

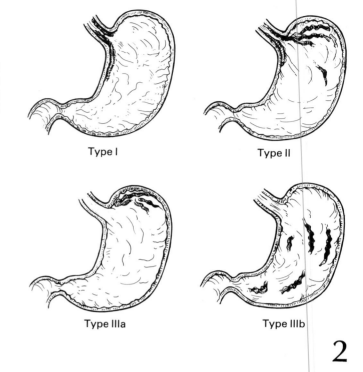

Type I   Type II

Type IIIa   Type IIIb

2

Endoscopic appearance

Varices can also be classified by their form and colour. The form may be tortuous, nodular or tumorous, and the colour white or red, with or without focal red spots. Nodular varices with red spots, especially if they are anterior to the cardia or on the greater curve, have the highest chance of bleeding.

Diagnosis

It is important to distinguish type III varices due to splenic vein thrombosis from other varices because the definitive treatment is different. Doppler ultrasonography or the portal venous phase of a coeliac axis arteriogram can be used to make the diagnosis. Direct splenic puncture, although now less commonly performed, is safe if the needle track is obliterated when the needle is withdrawn.

Treatment

Sclerotherapy

3 Injection sclerotherapy is the treatment of choice for type I (lesser curve) varices but is difficult to perform for types II and III varices where the risk of rebleeding is greater. For fundal varices the gastroscope must be retroverted, which makes the manipulation of the injection needle difficult. The best technique is to protrude the needle from the retroverted endoscope and then pull the whole gastroscope back towards the fundus. Superficial mucosal injections can produce gastric ulceration overlying a non-thrombosed varix and can be catastrophic. One technique is to use paravasal injections initially to reduce the bleeding, and then to employ an intravariceal bleeding injection immediately thereafter. Attempts to inject bucrylate glue have met with limited success and leakage of glue may seriously damage the gastroscope.

A Sengstaken-Blakemore tube is effective for type I varices and, possibly, type II gastric varices, but not for type III varices because pressure cannot be exerted effectively against varices in the body or the fundus of the stomach.

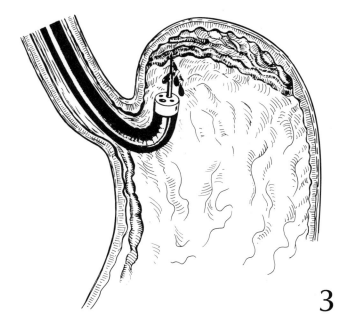

3

Surgery

If sclerotherapy does not succeed immediately for type II or III gastric varices, early surgery should be considered unless there are serious contraindications.

Type II varices

Type II varices can be treated by some form of portacaval shunt or by upper gastric devascularization with or without gastric transection (the oesophageal varices may already have been sclerosed). Whichever operation is chosen, direct suture of the bleeding varices from within the stomach is also necessary to control bleeding.

4 A deep continuous locking synthetic absorbable suture may be used along the length of the varices. The suture must pass beneath the varix, not just through it. Indeed, the suture may pass through the full thickness of the gastric wall and care must be taken not to injure the spleen when inserting a suture in the fundus (unless devascularization has already been performed).

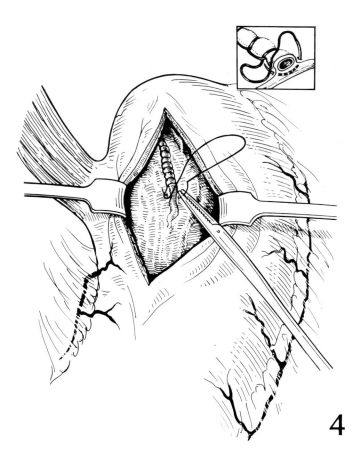

4

Type III varices

As these are usually segmental and not part of a general portal hypertension, the approach is different. Splenectomy with intragastric under-running of the bleeding vein is usually completely successful for type IIIa varices. Type IIIb varices in the antrum may be part of a generalized portal hypertension in which the oesophageal varices have been sclerosed, or it is sometimes related to splenic vein thrombosis. Antral varices may be treated expectantly in the first instance and then by resection or direct ligation, according to the situation.

Portal hypertensive gastropathy may coexist with any form of gastric varices and it is most important that this is recognized. If gastropathy is the cause of bleeding, then the approach is pharmacological with a somato-statin analogue (e.g. octreotide) initially, and beta-adrenergic blockade in the long term. Shunting is occasionally necessary but devascularization does not always stop the bleeding from gastropathy.

In summary, gastric varices are a rare and serious source of haemorrhage and must be identified and classified accurately. Because they can develop once oesophageal varices have been sclerosed, it must not be assumed when patients rebleed that they are rebleeding from the oesophagus; gastric varices must always be considered and treated effectively if present.

Further reading

Hashizume M, Kitano S, Yamaga H, Koyanagi N, Sugimachi K. Endoscopic classification of gastric varices. *Gastrointest Endosc* 1990; 36: 276–80.

Hosking SW, Johnson AG. Gastric varices: a proposed classification leading to management. *Br J Surg* 1990; 75: 195–6.

Sarin SK, Lahoti D, Saxena SP, Murthy NS, Makwana UK. Prevalence, classification and natural history of gastric varices: a long term follow-up study in 568 portal hypertension patients. *Hepatology* 1992; 16: 1343–9.

Illustrations by Angela Christie and University of California

Shunt surgery: total and partial portacaval anastomosis

R. Shields MD, DSc, PRCS(Ed), FRCS (Eng), FACS, FRCPS, FCS(SA), FCSHK
Professor of Surgery, University of Liverpool, and Honorary Consultant Surgeon, Royal Liverpool University Hospital, Liverpool, UK

Principles and justification

Portal hypertension and its main clinical manifestation – bleeding oesophageal varices – are usually the result of an obstruction to the portal blood flow, frequently within the liver, but occasionally at an extrahepatic site. When bleeding from oesophagogastric varices is not controlled or recurs, a definitive treatment is decompression of the portal system by shunt operation between the portal and systemic circulations.

Indications

By far the most common indication for a portacaval anastomosis is bleeding from oesophagogastric varices caused by intrahepatic obstructive disease, usually cirrhosis. There are three circumstances in which a portacaval anastomosis should be considered for patients with oesophagogastric varices and liver disease.

Elective portacaval shunt

Elective portacaval shunt is indicated in patients who have bled from oesophageal varices and in whom the bleeding has stopped, either spontaneously or as a result of therapeutic intervention (e.g. endoscopic sclerotherapy). These patients are put into a programme of treatment such as maintenance sclerotherapy to obliterate the varices, but if this or other treatments such as oesophageal transection fail, and is followed by recurrent bleeding, portasystemic anastomosis should be considered.

Careful selection of patients for elective operation is required. Patients must have moderate to good liver function, and surgery is contraindicated in those with persistent jaundice, intractable ascites, repeated bouts of spontaneous encephalopathy and poor nutrition. Grossly disturbed coagulation which is unresponsive to treatment and a history of alcoholism are also contraindications.

Emergency portacaval shunt

An emergency portacaval shunt may be required in those whose bleeding from oesophageal varices cannot be controlled by simpler measures. After resuscitation, initial attempts at controlling bleeding include balloon tamponade, the use of vasoactive drugs and endoscopic sclerotherapy. If these treatments are not successful, surgical intervention is required and usually takes the form of oesophageal transection. If bleeding continues, decompression of the portal circulation is required. The results in patients in this group are generally not good, partly because they usually have severe liver disease with all its complications, and partly because the patient has been ravaged by continuing bleeding and futile attempts at its control.

Persistent bleeding from gastric varices is not readily controlled by sclerotherapy or ligation of the varices, and a portosystemic shunt is indicated in such cases.

Prophylactic portacaval shunt

This was advocated in the past to prevent bleeding in patients with oesophageal varices which had not yet bled. However, four well conducted controlled trials have shown that prophylactic surgery is of no value to these patients. Although a successful shunt means that bleeding is uncommon, liver failure and other complications of liver disease supervene. Prophylactic surgery is therefore not indicated.

Preoperative

It is assumed that a diagnosis of oesophageal varices has been made, usually by endoscopy but occasionally by radiology. It is then necessary to establish (1) whether the patient has liver disease and, if so, to assess its severity; (2) that the varices are at the site of bleeding and that the bleeding is not caused by a co-existent disease such as a duodenal or gastric ulcer; (3) that the portal vein and the inferior vena cava are patent and therefore suitable for anastomosis.

A detailed history and physical examination are required. Blood should be withdrawn for typing and cross-matching, and for haematological and biochemical investigations aimed particularly at determining the degree of liver damage. Special investigations include hepatic vein catheterization to determine wedged hepatic vein pressure, free hepatic vein pressure and inferior vena cava pressure. Wedged hepatic vein pressure can reflect portal pressure in most forms of cirrhosis and therefore establishes the diagnosis of portal hypertension. Superior mesenteric angiography is helpful in defining the portal vein and its collateral connections, and confirming the patency of the portal vein and the presence of varices. Alternatively, direct percutaneous injection of contrast medium into the spleen to provide direct visualization of the portal venous system can be carried out. Percutaneous splenoportography carries a risk of damage to the spleen and should not be performed unless abnormalities in coagulation have been corrected. Patency of the portal vein can be determined by ultrasonography and this is usually preferable.

The patient should be restored to as good a condition as possible for a major operation. Blood loss should be vigorously replaced using, if possible, blood which is less than 12 hours old. Thrombocytopenia should be corrected by infusion of platelets and fresh frozen plasma is given to correct other coagulation abnormalities.

Hepatic encephalopathy is a common sequel to shunt procedures and an attempt should be made to prevent it by eliminating all nitrogen from the gastrointestinal tract and destroying ammonia-forming bacteria. Thus, blood should be removed from the stomach by lavage through a nasogastric tube, magnesium sulphate and neomycin should be given into the stomach, and the colon should be repeatedly and thoroughly cleansed with enemas containing neomycin.

To support the failing liver, glucose solutions should be given parenterally together with therapeutic doses of vitamins K, B and C. Any abnormality in electrolytes should be corrected, particularly hypokalaemia and metabolic alkalosis.

It is important that vital functions are monitored frequently. Urine output should be measured hourly by means of an indwelling catheter. Central venous pressure should be measured and haematocrit monitored. These patients require admission to the intensive care unit because of the possibility of complications in patients who are so ill.

Choice of portasystemic shunt

The portasystemic shunts most commonly used are:

1. End-to-side total portacaval shunt in which the cut end of the portal vein is anastomosed to the inferior vena cava and blood from the intestine is diverted around the liver. This is an effective form of shunt, but is followed by encephalopathy in 20% of patients. Partial shunting, which preserves a flow of blood to the liver while decompressing the splanchnic circulation, is claimed to be effective in preventing bleeding and reducing the risk of encephalopathy.
2. Side-to-side portacaval shunt is rarely performed and does not carry any special advantage, as well as being more difficult to perform.
3. Interposition mesocaval shunt (*see later*).
4. Selective distal splenorenal shunt (Warren shunt) (*see later*).

Operations

DIRECT TOTAL PORTACAVAL SHUNT

Position of patient

1 The patient is placed on the operating table with the right side elevated to an angle of 30° to the table. The costal margin is at the level of the break of the table and the right arm is suspended from a screeen with towels. The left arm is extended on an arm board.

Monitoring and sampling devices shown include a nasogastric tube, left radial artery catheter for recording of blood pressure, large-bore intravenous catheter inserted into the left arm for blood transfusion, intravenous catheter inserted into the right arm for continuous recording of central venous pressure, blood pressure cuff on the right arm for determination of arterial blood pressure, ECG leads, Foley catheter in position for monitoring of urine output and ground plate for electrocautery.

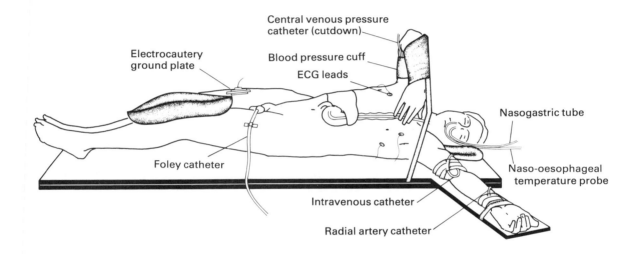

Central venous pressure
catheter (cutdown)

Electrocautery
ground plate

Blood pressure cuff

ECG leads

Nasogastric tube

Foley catheter

Naso-oesophageal
temperature probe

Intravenous catheter

Radial artery catheter

1

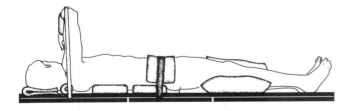

2

2 The elevation of the right side of the body can be maintained with sand bags. The patient's position is secured by a large strap which passes across the iliac crest and a pillow is positioned between the lower extremities.

3 The head-down position is adopted before 'breaking' the table.

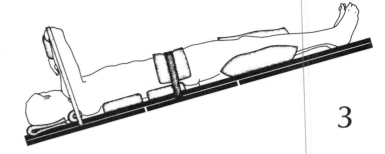

3

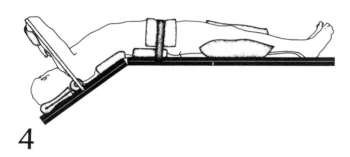

4

4 The table is broken at the level of the costal margin
   to widen the space between the right costal margin
and the right iliac crest.

5 The table is then broken at the level of the knees.

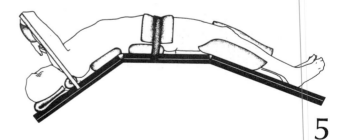

5

Incision

6 A large right subcostal incision is made extending from the xiphoid process into the flank, two finger breadths below the costal margin. The layers under the skin are incised with electrocautery to divide the rectus abdominis, external oblique and the transversus abdominis muscles and the medial 4–5 cm of the latissimus dorsi.

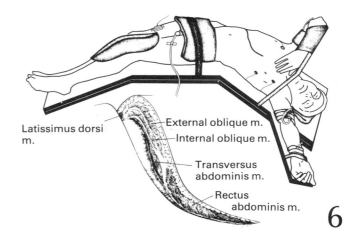

Latissimus dorsi m.

External oblique m.

Internal oblique m.

Transversus abdominis m.

Rectus abdominis m.

6

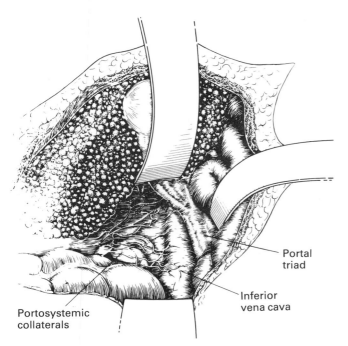

Portal triad

Inferior vena cava

Portosystemic collaterals

7

Exposure of operative field

7 The operative field is exposed by retraction of the viscera by three retractors positioned at right angles. The inferior retractor retracts the hepatic flexure of the colon, the medial displaces the duodenum reflected to the patient's left, and the superior retractor retracts the liver and gallbladder towards the head.

Incision of the posterior peritoneum

8 The posterior peritoneum overlying the inferior vena cava is incised with electrocautery as an extended Kocher manoeuvre along the right side of the descending second part of the duodenum. The many collateral blood vessels in this greatly thickened peritoneum should be obliterated by electrocautery.

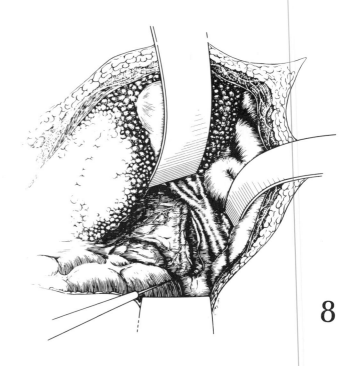

8

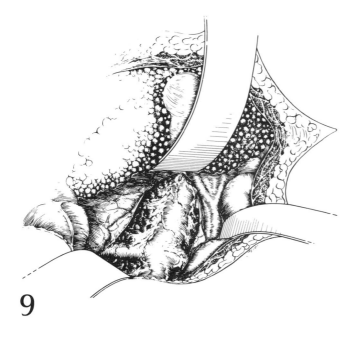

9

Exposure of the inferior vena cava

9 The inferior vena cava is exposed as it lies behind the duodenum by reflecting the descending duodenum and the head of the pancreas to the left. The right kidney and the hepatic flexure of the colon are retracted towards the feet. The anterior surface of the inferior vena cava is then cleared of all adventitia.

Isolation of the inferior vena cava

For end-to-side anastomosis it is not necessary to free the inferior vena cava around its entire circumference.

Exposure of portal vein

10 The portal vein is located in the posterolateral aspect of the portal triad and is approached from behind. The tissue on this aspect of the portal triad contains lymph nodes and lymphatics and can be divided by blunt and sharp dissection. When the surface of the portal vein is exposed, a small retractor is inserted to retract the bile duct medially.

Pressures in the portal vein must be measured before and after the portacaval anastomosis. One of two methods may be employed, both using a saline (spinal) manometer. A small jejunal vein in the mesentery may be dissected and a saline-filled fine plastic catheter inserted until its tip lies in the main superior mesenteric trunk. Alternatively, the portal vein can be punctured directly by a fine needle attached by tubing to the manometer.

The zero point of reference is the inferior vena cava. Significant portal hypertension is indicated by a pressure of 150 mm saline or more.

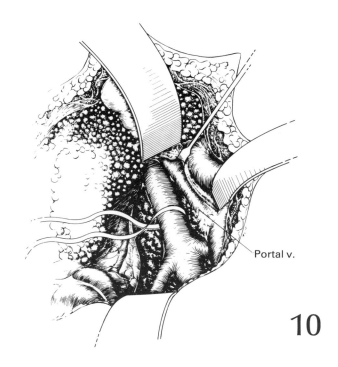

Portal v.

10

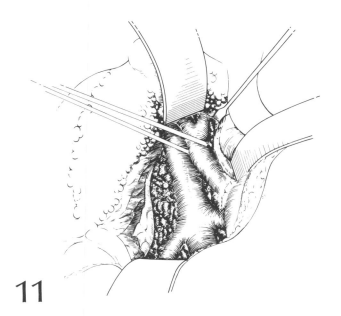

11

Mobilization of the portal vein

11 The portal vein is mobilized circumferentially at its mid point and an umbilical tape is passed around it. It is then mobilized up to its bifurcation in the liver hilum. Several tributaries on the medial aspect are ligated in continuity and divided.

The umbilical tape is used to pull the portal vein out of its bed. The portal vein is cleared to the point where it disappears behind the pancreas and its two major tributaries, the superior mesenteric vein and splenic vein, are identified. Good mobilization of the portal vein is essential to perform end-to-side anastomosis without kinking.

12 A Satinsky clamp is placed obliquely on the anteromedial wall of the inferior vena cava so that it will receive the end of the portal vein at an angle of 45°. A 2-cm long strip of the inferior vena cava is excised and a retraction suture is placed on the lateral wall. The portal vein is doubly ligated at the hilum and an angled vascular clamp is placed across the portal vein near the pancreas. The portal vein is divided obliquely just below the site of ligation.

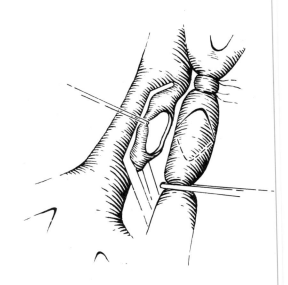

12

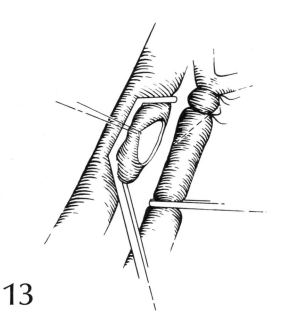

13

13 The portal vein is transected at an angle so that the anterior wall is longer than the posterior wall at the transected end. After transection and before starting the anastomosis, the clamp on the portal vein is released to flush out any clots. This manoeuvre is repeated just before the final sutures are placed in the anterior row of the anastomosis.

14 The end-to-side anastomosis is performed with a continuous over and over 4/0 vascular suture in the posterior row and a second layer of vascular sutures in the anterior row. The portal vein should not be kinked, but should describe a smooth curve as it descends towards the inferior vena cava. Twisting and kinking of the portal vein are the most common causes of a poorly functioning anastomosis.

After completion of the anastomosis the pressure in the portal vein is measured. It should be at the same level as, or only slightly higher than, the pressure in the inferior vena cava. If there has been no appreciable fall in the portal vein pressure, the surgeon must look for and correct any kinking of the portal vein. If pressure remains unreduced, the anastomosis must be taken down and refashioned. Failure to do so will lead to catastrophic bleeding from varices postoperatively.

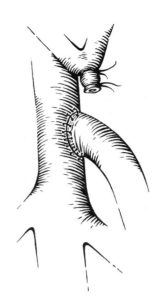

14

Liver biopsy

A wedged liver biopsy specimen is always obtained to confirm the underlying liver disease.

Closure of the wound

The peritoneum is closed with a continuous locking suture of chromic catgut and the muscles are closed with interrupted monofilament nylon. The subcutaneous tissues are closed with interrupted sutures of 3/0 plain catgut and the skin edges are approximated with clips. No drains are used.

Important technical notes

1. A subcostal incision should be used rather than a thoracoabdominal incision, which may cause ascitic fluid to enter the pleural cavity producing intractable pleural effusion.
2. Electrocautery reduces operating time and the amount of blood loss.
3. Bleeding and oozing from many of the collateral vessels is curtailed as soon as the portacaval anastomosis is completed and the portal hypertension reduced. It is not necessary to control each of the bleeding collaterals with ligatures because this prolongs the operation and increases blood loss.

PARTIAL PORTACAVAL SHUNT

Although total end-to-side portacaval shunt produces satisfactory decompression of the portal circulation, the loss of perfusion of the liver by mesenteric blood is considered to be a major factor leading to the increased incidence of postoperative encephalopathy and deterioration in liver function, and a partial portacaval shunt is therefore preferred. The indications and the method of preoperative preparation are as described for an end-to-side portacaval shunt.

Position of patient

The position of the patient on the table is as described for an end-to-side portacaval shunt.

15 A generous right subcostal incision is made. The umbilical vein is divided, as well as the falciform ligament. The falciform ligament is divided to prevent tearing from the costal traction.

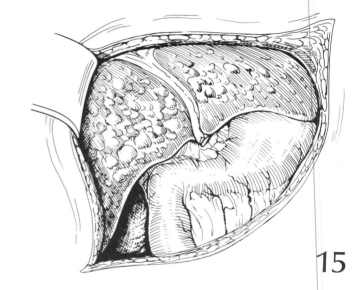

15

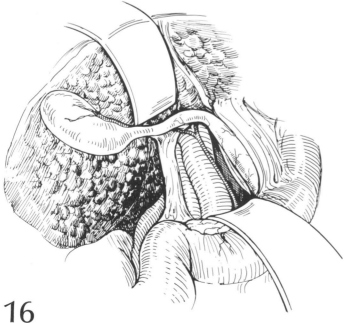

16

16 The retractors are put in position as described for an end-to-side portacaval shunt, and an incision is made in the posterolateral surface of the hepatoduodenal ligament. A long segment of the surface of the portal vein is exposed by gentle dissection. Although not strictly necessary, it is advisable to mobilize the portal vein circumferentially.

17 The vena cava is exposed by mobilizing the duodenum medially. If difficulty is encountered in finding the vena cava in obese subjects, the caudate lobe of the liver is a good landmark because it overlies the vena cava. The adventitial tissues overlying the vena cava should be divided and removed. The anterior, lateral and medial surfaces of the vena cava are exposed from the region of the right renal vein to the caudate lobe of the liver. The vena cava does not need to be circumferentially mobilized, but there must be sufficient mobilization so that a deep Satinsky clamp can be applied.

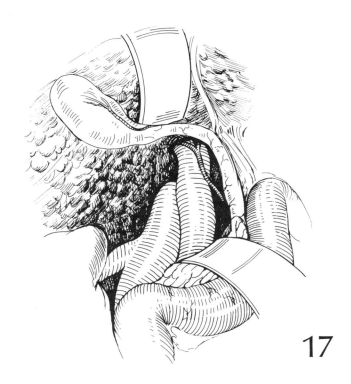

17

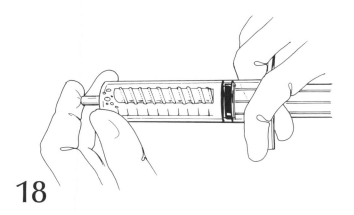

18

18 A segment of 8 mm or 10 mm ringed polytetrafluoroethylene (PTFE) graft is cut to a length estimated to be needed for anastomosis (usually 3–5 cm). A ringed graft is essential because unsupported grafts kink or can be compressed by adjacent viscera or by long-term external fibrosis. The graft is placed in a 20-ml syringe filled with heparin (1000 mg/ml). With the outlet occluded by the finger, the plunger is compressed and released several times until air bubbles cease to emanate from the surface of the graft. Sarfeh and Rypins[1], who pioneered this technique, believe that this is an important manoeuvre to reduce the risk of perioperative graft thrombosis caused by the interaction between blood and air.

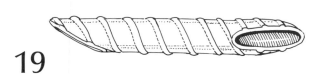

19

19 Bevels are cut on the graft end at 90° to each other, to conform with the angles of anastomosis to the portal vein and inferior vena cava. Large bevels are essential because of platelet deposition at the suture lines.

20 A Satinsky clamp is applied deeply on the inferior vena cava, occluding it partly, and a generous venotomy is made to conform with the length of the bevelled end of the graft.

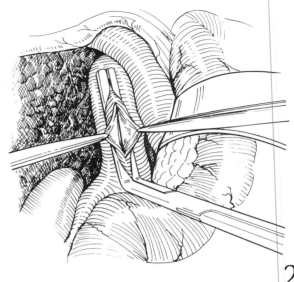

20

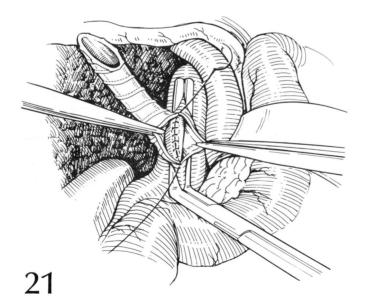

21

21 An everting, continuous, horizontal mattress suture of 5/0 polypropylene (Prolene) is used to prevent inversion and avoid compromise of the width of the anastomosis.

22 The anastomosis between the graft and the inferior vena cava is completed.

The anastomosis with the portal vein is performed by placing a Satinsky clamp deep on the lateral aspect of the portal vein. It does not matter whether this clamp completely or partially occludes the vein.

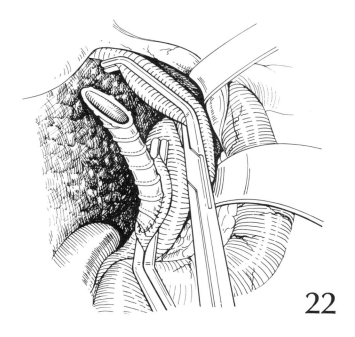

22

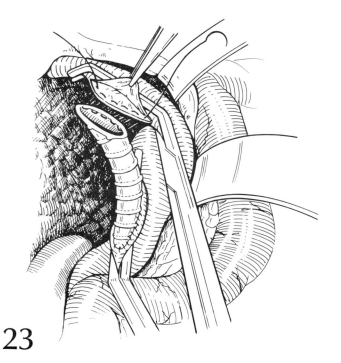

23

23 A posterior row of everting horizontal mattress sutures is inserted using an open technique and, after all sutures have been inserted, the graft is brought into apposition with the portal vein by pulling on both ends of the sutures.

An anterior row of everting sutures completes the anastomosis. Before completing the anastomosis, heparinized saline is forcefully injected into the graft lumen to remove debris and clot.

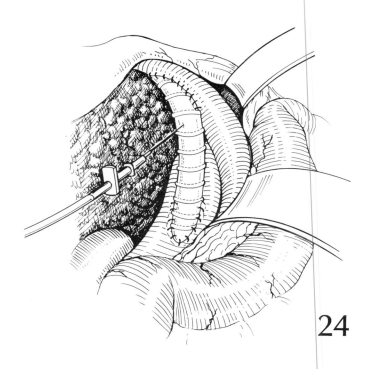

24 The clamp on the vena cava is removed and the suture lines are inspected for any bleeding. Usually an ooze ceases spontaneously within a minute or so, but a definite opening of the anastomosis can be closed by a single suture carefully placed.

A saline manometer is used to measure the portal pressure by inserting a 19-gauge needle into the central portion of the graft. There should be a fall in pressure of at least 10–15 cm of saline. If this is not achieved the graft must be carefully inspected. If there is no fall in graft pressure, a Fogarty balloon catheter should be passed through a small (1 mm) incision in the graft to test the suture lines with the balloon inflated.

If there is any suspicion concerning the inadequacy of the anastomosis, it should be taken down and re-fashioned. To leave the patient with an unreduced portal pressure will only lead to severe haemorrhage in the early postoperative period.

The operation is completed by ligating, in continuity, the left gastric vascular axis by approaching through the gastrohepatic ligament which is incised in its avascular portion. The left gastric vessels are identified and ligated in continuity. The gastroepiploic vessels can also be ligated in continuity with vascular clips.

24

Closure of the wound

This is the same as for a direct end-to-side portacaval shunt.

Postoperative care

Patients should be admitted to an intensive care unit with equipment and staff compentent to manage the complicated problems associated with hepatic disease.

Careful monitoring of the vital signs and parameters, such as central venous pressure, urine output, blood gases, fluid balance, body weight and abdominal girth, are essential. Liver function, blood coagulation and renal function should be serially measured.

Sarfeh and Rypins[1] advise that portography is carried out 5 days after insertion of a partial shunt, the shunt being cannulated via the transfemoral vein. They advise embolization of unligated collaterals and the lysis of any perioperative graft thrombosis, by directly infusing low-dose streptokinase into the portal vein below the anastomosis after graft dilatation by means of a balloon. However, the author has not found it necessary to employ these techniques.

References

1. Sarfeh IJ, Rypins EB. Partial shunting for portal hypertension: surgical technique. *Contemp Surg* 1988; 32: 11–16.

Shunt surgery: distal splenorenal shunt

J. Michael Henderson FRCS(Ed), FACS
Chairman, Department of General Surgery, The Cleveland Clinic Foundation, Cleveland, Ohio, USA

History

The distal splenorenal shunt (DSRS) was developed by Warren, Zeppa and Foman in Miami in the early 1960s. Conceptually, it brought together Warren's experience with portosystemic shunts which gave good control of variceal bleeding, and Zeppa's experience of devascularization procedures which resulted in maintenance of portal perfusion and liver function. These surgeons reasoned that selective decompression of the spleen and gastro-oesophageal junction would control variceal bleeding, and that maintenance of portal hypertension in the superior mesenteric and portal veins would maintain portal flow to the cirrhotic liver. This operation was initially shown to be feasible in dogs, and the first report of its use in man was presented in 1966. Since that time the DSRS has been extensively used worldwide, and has been subjected to intensive clinical, haemodynamic and metabolic study.

Principles and justification

1 The distal splenorenal shunt is illustrated schematically. It must be emphasized that it is not a portosystemic shunt, and that the principle is one of selective decompression of gastro-oesophageal varices with maintenance of portal hypertension and portal flow to the liver. The varices are decompressed through the short gastric veins, spleen and splenic vein by anastomosing the splenic vein to the left renal vein. Disconnection of the splenic vein from the superior mesenteric vein, ligation of the left and right gastric veins, interruption of veins running along the transverse mesocolon to the splenic hilus, and ligation of the inferior mesenteric vein comprise the second component of this operation. This 'disconnection' separates the high pressure superior mesenteric/portal system from the low pressure, shunted splenic system.

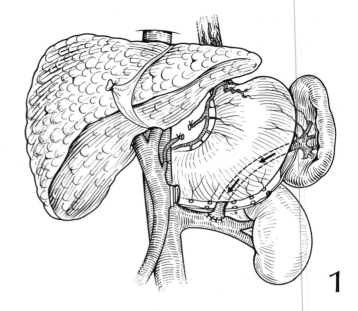

1

Indications

The indication for this operation is the need to control bleeding gastro-oesophageal varices in patients with preserved hepatic function. The majority of patients undergoing the DSRS will have failed to respond to endoscopic sclerotherapy. In some patients with good liver function, DSRS may be considered as a primary form of therapy if: (1) they have very large varices with severe 'risk' factors; (2) they have poor access to medical care and sclerotherapy; or (3) they have gastric varices or portal hypertensive gastropathy. Candidates for DSRS are usually in Child's class A or B, and ideally have no ascites or ascites that is easily controlled. Although used primarily as an elective procedure, DSRS can be performed in urgent cases if evaluation has shown that it is the best option for the patient.

Contraindications

The contraindications for DSRS are thrombosis or absence of the splenic vein, e.g. in patients who have previously undergone splenectomy. An anomaly of the left renal vein may increase the technical difficulty, and the 4% of patients who have a retroaortic left renal vein may have to be dealt with by the alternative operation of distal splenocaval shunt. Ascites that is intractable or difficult to control is a contraindication to the DSRS. Patients with poor liver function (Child's class C) should rarely be considered for DSRS.

The alternative operations which may be considered in this group of patients are liver transplantation, total portosystemic shunts, partial portosystemic shunts, or devascularization procedures. Child's class C patients with variceal bleeding should be considered for liver transplantation. Total portosystemic shunts divert all portal flow away from the liver sinusoids and accelerate hepatic failure in the majority of patients. Partial portosystemic shunts (8 mm diameter) reduce portal hypertension to approximately 12 mmHg, maintain some portal flow to the liver in 80% of patients and do not accelerate liver failure; they may be indicated in some Child's A and B patients with variceal bleeding. Devascularization procedures have a high risk of further bleeding (40% at 5 years) but do maintain good portal flow and liver function. The choice of operation must be made based on full evaluation of patients. DSRS is a good option in carefully selected patients.

Preoperative

Preoperative evaluation

Evaluation for DSRS is similar to that undertaken in any patient who has experienced variceal bleeding, and is completed when the patient has been stabilized after their acute bleed. The two components of this assessment are, firstly, the nature of the liver disease and its severity and, secondly, the technically feasible options.

The aetiology of the portal hypertension is determined from the history, physical examination, laboratory test results and, if necessary, by liver biopsy. The majority of patients have cirrhosis of some type as the cause of their portal hypertension. However, it is important to identify the small percentage of patients with prehepatic causes of portal hypertension, because their normal liver means that they have an excellent prognosis if their bleeding can be controlled permanently. In the context of DSRS, the essential component of this phase of preoperative assessment is to be sure that there is adequate liver function, and preferably that there is no active liver disease before proceeding with the operation.

Upper gastrointestinal endoscopy should be undertaken on all patients once they are stabilized to confirm that they are bleeding from portal hypertension and to exclude other significant upper gastrointestinal pathology. It is then important to assess the vessels which could be used for the shunt. Imaging of the portal, splenic and left renal veins requires angiography. While ultrasonography provides an adequate image of the portal vein, it is not adequate for defining the other vessels. Selective splenic and superior mesenteric arteriography followed through the venous phase will image the splenic, superior mesenteric and portal veins. Patency, position and vessel size are assessed and, in addition, the main collaterals running to the varices can usually be visualized. These collaterals are important; for example, the left gastric vein is encountered at the time of operation and must be ligated. Occasionally, inadequate images are achieved with this technique and a splenoportogram may be needed to be certain of the status of the splenic vein.

The left renal vein is imaged by direct catheterization and venography. In 20% of the population there is some anomaly of this vessel; 4% have a true retroaortic left renal vein which is placed low and cannot be used for DSRS, while 16% have a circumaortic left renal vein in which the anterior limb is superior and in the normal left renal vein position while the posterior limb is retroaortic. In most of these patients the anterior limb is large enough to use for DSRS. In individuals without anomalies it is helpful to define the caudad/cephalad separation of the left renal vein and splenic vein at this time. This is achieved by completing the study of the left renal vein before arteriography and leaving the catheter in the left renal vein while the splenic vein is visualized.

Preoperative preparation

Preoperative preparation aims to optimize the patient's condition and thus minimize postoperative complications. The greatest postoperative threat after DSRS is ascites, and this can be minimized by careful fluid and electrolyte management and appropriate use of diuretics before, during and after surgery. Many patients with variceal bleeding develop some ascites during fluid resuscitation. If this can be eliminated by diuresis, it can also be managed after DSRS. Restriction of dietary sodium intake to 2 g/day and minimizing the amount of sodium given intravenously is important. Spironolactone should be used to reduce renal tubular sodium reabsorption and urine electrolyte output can be monitored. The key to fluid management in DSRS is 'to run the patient dry'.

Anaesthesia

DSRS is performed under general anaesthesia with endotracheal intubation and muscle relaxation. The specific agents must be chosen and used with a knowledge of the patient's underlying liver disease and appropriate dose adjustments made. The greatest challenge to the anaesthetist is in perioperative fluid management, as any excess intravenous fluid (particularly when given as crystalloid) will result in ascites in the postoperative period. Central venous pressure should be maintained in the range 4–6 mmHg if possible. A perioperative urine output of 20–30 ml/h is adequate. Blood and blood products should be available. Platelets do not need to be given solely to correct a low platelet count, but may be required if there is bleeding.

Operation

Position of the patient and incision

The patient is placed supine with 15–20° of hyperextension to open the space between the costal margin and the iliac crest. The table is also rotated slightly to the right to increase the prominence of the left subcostal space.

2a, b A bilateral subcostal incision is used which is more extensive on the left but which is extended to the right to cross the right rectus muscle. Exposure is greatly improved if a fixed retractor system is employed with firm upward retraction on the left costal margin and in the midline superiorly.

The abdomen is fully explored and any ascitic fluid is removed and sent for bacteriological culture. The liver is inspected and biopsied. The area of dissection for the distal splenorenal shunt is approached through the lesser sac to expose the pancreas and dissect on its posterior surface.

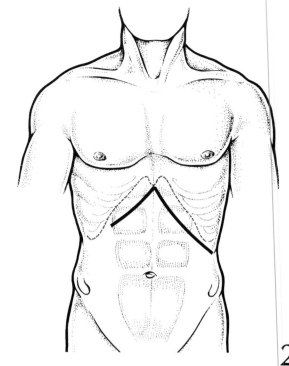

2a

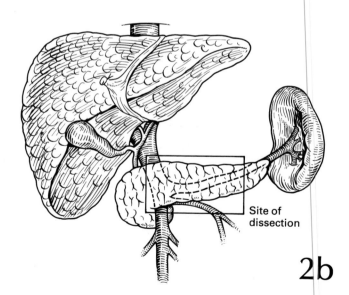

Site of dissection

2b

Access to the pancreas and vessels

3 The lesser sac is opened by dividing the gastrocolic omentum widely from pylorus to short gastric vessels. There are frequently adhesions between the transverse mesocolon and the back wall of the stomach which need to be taken down in order to avoid entering large varices running in the transverse mesocolon. The splenic flexure of the colon should be taken down from the lower pole of the spleen to open the lesser sac widely and expose the pancreas fully. This move also interrupts potential collaterals which run from the high pressure portal vein to the splenic hilus along the mesocolon.

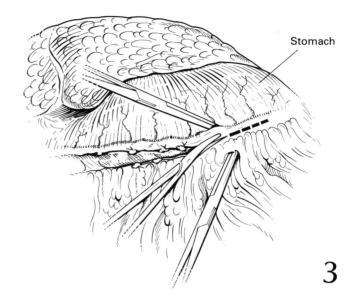

Stomach

3

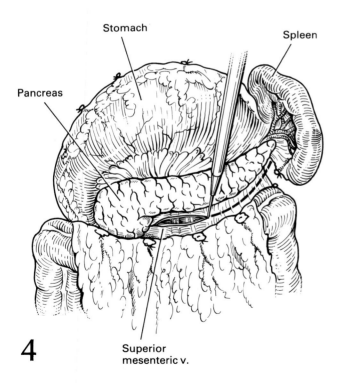

Stomach

Spleen

Pancreas

Superior mesenteric v.

4

Mobilization of the pancreas

4 The stomach is retracted upwards using a fixed retractor. The retroperitoneum along the inferior border of the pancreas is widely opened; this plane is most easily identified over the fourth part of the duodenum. The goal at this stage is to rotate the pancreas upwards from the superior mesenteric vessels on the right to the tail on the left. This allows full exposure of the splenic vein for subsequent dissection.

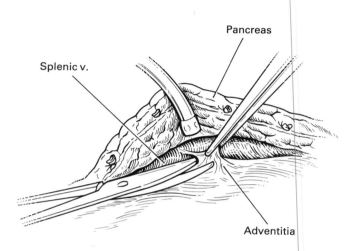

5a

Exposure of the splenic vein

$5a, b$ The inferior mesenteric vein is identified and ligated. Initially the splenic vein should be exposed along its inferior and posterior aspect, with the plane of dissection being right on the splenic vein with division of the overlying adventitia. This plane is relatively safe as few tributaries enter on this side. The more of the vein that can be exposed along its inferior border, the safer the subsequent dissection.

The junction of the splenic vein, superior mesenteric and portal vein should be identified. Again, the posterior plane is a safe plane of dissection and should be developed so that any bleeding can be controlled with finger compression of the vein and pancreas. It is only once this control can be achieved that the plane in front of the three veins can be opened safely.

At this point it is helpful to identify the left renal vein to determine how much of the splenic vein needs to be dissected out of the pancreas.

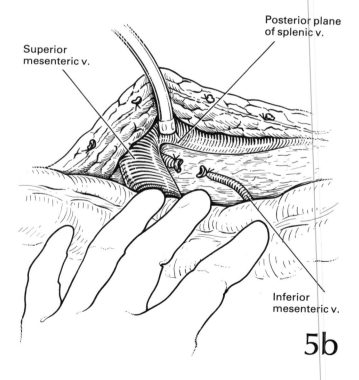

5b

Dissection of the left renal vein

6 This dissection is aided by the preoperative anatomical knowledge obtained at venography. The aorta and superior mesenteric artery can be palpated behind the splenic and superior mesenteric veins. The retroperitoneum is opened in this angle and blunt dissection will identify the left renal vein which has then to be mobilized sufficiently to allow it to come up into a side-biting clamp for subsequent anastomosis. Mobilization is achieved by dividing the left adrenal vein as it enters the left renal vein. The gonadal vein is left intact as it can serve as an outflow from this renal vein.

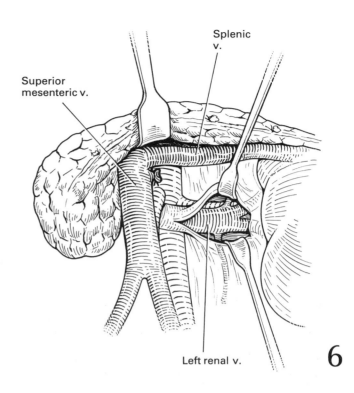

Splenic v.

Superior mesenteric v.

Left renal v.

6

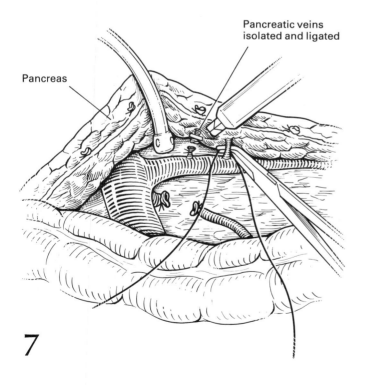

Pancreatic veins isolated and ligated

Pancreas

7

Dissection of the splenic vein from the pancreas

7 The key to this dissection is accurate identification, isolation and ligation of the small tributaries which run from the pancreas into the splenic vein. This is achieved by a delicate dissection of these tributaries using a blunt clamp to dissect tissue at right angles to the splenic vein. To minimize the risk of tearing these small vessels they must be dissected along the line in which they enter the splenic vein. Once isolated they are ligated on the splenic vein side and a vascular clip is placed on the pancreas side. These vessels are serially identified along the upper margin of the splenic vein until enough vein has been freed to allow the splenic vein to come down to the left renal vein without kinking or tension. Preoperative identification of the left gastric vein is helpful as it may come off either the splenic or the portal vein close to their junction. The vein can be a large exceedingly thin walled vessel and it is ligated carefully at its origin.

Ligation and trimming of the splenic vein

8 Once the splenic vein has been sufficiently dissected it is ligated and clamped at the point where it joins the superior mesenteric vein. A 0 silk tie is placed on the splenic vein and a large ligaclip is placed behind this tie just before the junction of the superior mesenteric and portal veins. This has proved to be the best method for dealing with the splenic vein stump and incurs the lowest risk of thrombus formation in the portal vein. The clamp on the splenic vein is moved back close to the pancreatic tissue, and the vein is brought down to the left renal vein trimmed to an appropriate length. This usually requires some excision of the splenic vein. The anastomosis to the renal vein is almost always placed just anterior to the ligated stump of the adrenal vein.

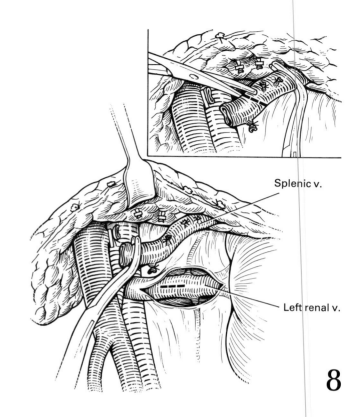

Splenic v.

Left renal v.

8

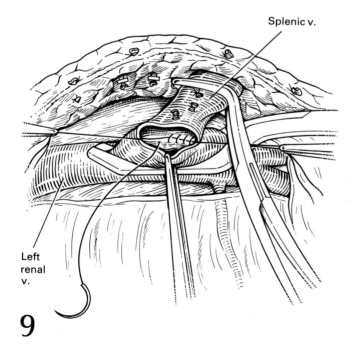

Splenic v.

Left renal v.

9

Anastomosis

9 The anastomosis must be made without tension on the two veins, and requires an assistant on the left side to pull up on the renal vein clamp to keep tension off the anastomosis as it is sewn. Stay sutures of 5/0 Tevdek are placed at each end of the anastomosis. The needle is brought to the inside and the posterior wall sewn on the inside. The needle is again brought out to anchor to the stay suture at the right end.

10 The anterior layer of the anastomosis is fashioned with interrupted 5/0 silk sutures. Interrupting the anterior layer of sutures is important in avoiding a purse-string effect. The renal vein clamp is opened initially and, providing there is no significant bleeding, the splenic clamp is rapidly removed. Flows can be measured in this anastomosis and should be approximately 1 ml/min per ml volume of the spleen.

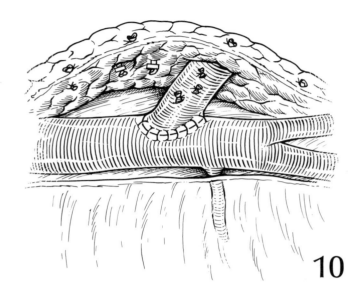

10

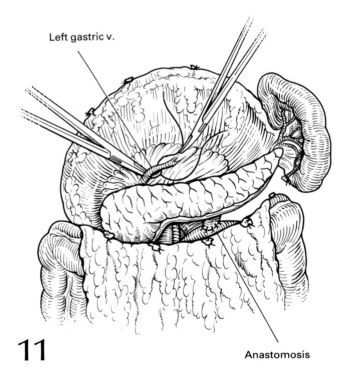

Left gastric v.

11

Anastomosis

Disconnection

11 The superior mesenteric vein and portal system are next disconnected from the shunt. This is achieved by lifting the stomach upwards and identifying the left gastric vein at the upper margin of the pancreas. The vein is carefully dissected and divided at this point along with its main feeding vessels which run from the lesser curve. If the left gastric vein has not been identified flowing into the splenic vein during dissection of the splenic vein, the pancreas should be lifted off the portal vein to identify the left gastric vein behind the pancreas. A clip should be placed in continuity across this vessel.

The supraduodenal right gastric vein, if of identifiable size, is also ligated in continuity.

DSRS with entire splenopancreatic disconnection

12 In patients with alcoholic cirrhosis, total dissection of the splenic vein from the pancreas may help to maintain long-term portal flow. This dissection is more time consuming and tedious but does prevent the formation of large siphoning collaterals which run through the pancreas from the portal vein to the splenic vein when the latter is left attached to the tail of the pancreas.

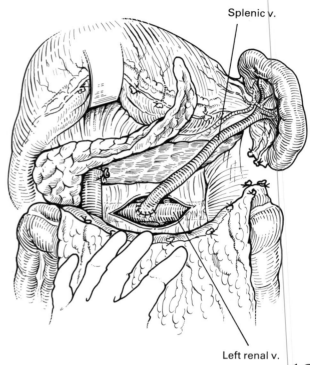

Splenic v.

Left renal v.

12

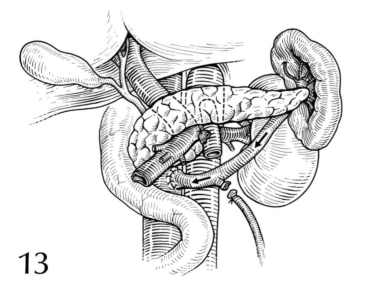

13

Distal splenocaval shunt

13 In patients with an anomalous left renal vein, particularly when it is retroaortic, a splenocaval anastomosis can be used. The exposure and dissection of the splenic vein is identical to that previously described. The inferior vena cava is reached by taking down the ligament of Treitz, displacing the duodenum caudad, and dissecting between the superior mesenteric artery and the aorta to reach the inferior vena cava. With a large spleen and a tortuous splenic vein, the splenic vein will reach the vena cava without an interposition graft.

Postoperative care

The patient is managed for 24–48 h in the intensive care unit. As emphasized previously, it is important to 'run the patient dry' to lessen the risk of ascites. Maintaining a CVP of 3–4 mmHg is adequate, infusion of salt-containing solutions is minimized, and a urine output of 20–30 ml/h is sufficient. The ideal is to maintain a pulse rate below 100 beats/min and a systolic blood pressure of 100–110 mmHg.

Perioperative antibiotics are given but not continued in the postoperative period. A nasogastric tube is left in place for 24 h. The Foley catheter is usually removed at 48 h.

The patient is normally transferred to routine ward care 24 h after the operation. Diet is slowly advanced from clear liquids to a regular diet over the next 2–3 days. Strict dietary restriction to a daily intake of 2 g sodium and 30 g fat is maintained for 6–8 weeks. The fat restriction lessens the risk of chylous ascites (which can occur following division of lymphatics following dissection around the left renal vein) from approximately 30% to < 10%. Patients are started on spironolactone 50–100 mg per day on the second postoperative day. Urine sodium and potassium output are monitored to confirm that the dose of diuretic is adequate. A urine sodium:potassium ratio greater than unity is the target. Paracentesis is occasionally indicated to document the nature of the ascitic fluid and for therapeutic purposes. A peritoneovenous shunt is rarely required.

On the seventh postoperative day a catheter is placed through the groin and up the vena cava, to enter the left renal vein and the anastomosis. Venography is performed and pressures in the splenic vein, left renal vein and the inferior vena cava are measured. There should be no pressure gradient across the anastomosis but there may be a gradient from the left renal vein to the inferior vena cava. Patency of the shunt at this time results in long-term patency in most patients as late thrombosis is unusual. Early thrombosis is dealt with by reoperation.

Patients are usually discharged home 7–10 days after the operation.

Outcome

In large collected series of patients undergoing DSRS the thrombosis rate is 5% or less with control of bleeding in more than 90% of patients. The risk of rebleeding is greatest in the first 4–6 weeks before the short gastric and left renal veins have fully accommodated to flow in the shunt.

In patients with excellent hepatocellular function, 1-year and 5-year survival rates of more than 90% and 70%, respectively, have been achieved in recent series. Prospects are particularly good for patients with schistosomiasis, and good risk patients with cirrhosis, stable disease and good hepatocellular reserve.

Encephalopathy is unusual after DSRS. Four prospective randomized clinical trials which have compared DSRS with sclerotherapy have found a similar rate of encephalopathy. Although cirrhotic patients can develop encephalopathy, DSRS does not accelerate this.

Further reading

Henderson JM. Nontransplant liver surgery. In: Quigley EMM, Sorrell MF, eds, *The Gastrointestinal Surgical Patient – Preoperative and Postoperative Care*. Baltimore: Williams and Wilkins, 1994: 469–89.

Henderson JM, Warren WD, Millikan WJ, Galloway JR, Kawasaki S, Kutner MH. Distal splenorenal shunt with splenopancreatic disconnection: a four year assessment. *Ann Surg* 1989; 210: 332–41.

Henderson JM, Gilmore GT, Hooks MA *et al*. Selective shunt in the management of variceal bleeding in the era of liver transplantation. *Ann Surg* 1992; 216: 248–55.

Jin G, Rikkers LF. Selective variceal decompression: current status. *HPB Surg* 1991; 5: 1–15.

Warren WD, Zeppa R, Foman JS. Selective transplenic decompression of gastroesophageal varices by distal splenorenal shunt. *Ann Surg* 1967; 166: 437–55.

Shunt surgery: mesocaval shunt

R. Shields MD, DSc, PRCS(Ed), FRCS(Eng), FACS, FRCPS, FCS(SA), FCSHK
Professor of Surgery, University of Liverpool, and Honorary Consultant Surgeon, Royal Liverpool University Hospital, Liverpool, UK

Principles and justification

Mesocaval shunts reached the zenith of their popularity for the treatment of portal hypertension in the 1970s because of the high rate of postoperative encephalopathy experienced with end-to-side portacaval shunts. The most popular of these shunts is the interposition mesocaval shunt which will be described here. Variants include the Clatworthy shunt which has been used in children when the portal vein is unusable because of thrombosis; this variant entails anastomosis of the transected inferior vena cava to the superior mesenteric vein and will not be discussed further.

However, time has shown that the operation does not, in fact, enjoy the advantage of lower rates of encephalopathy and liver failure. Indeed, a late problem is thrombosis within the wide-bore shunt, leading to recurrence of portal hypertension and variceal bleeding.

Indications

The shunt may be performed in emergency or semi-emergency circumstances if medical measures and other surgical methods, e.g. oesophageal transection, have failed. The relative speed and ease of its performance make its use particularly attractive in an emergency.

Mesocaval shunts are now rarely used in elective circumstances because other procedures are more successful, e.g. oesophageal transection, distal spleno-renal shunt, hepatic transplantation, transjugular portal-systemic shunt. However, the operation can be performed when other treatments have failed, or are difficult or impossible to perform because of (a) thrombosis of the portal vein or splenic vein with maintained patency of the superior mesenteric vein, (b) a large caudate lobe overlying the inferior vena cava, (c) obesity, and (d) the Budd–Chiari syndrome.

Contraindications

The use of mesocaval shunts is contraindicated in patients in whom occlusion of the superior mesenteric vein is demonstrated radiologically, in those with severe impairment of the hepatic functional reserve (the operation should not be carried out in patients in Child's group C), and in patients who have oesophageal varices and portal hypertension but have not yet bled.

Preoperative

Preoperative evaluation

The patient should be evaluated as described in the chapter on pp. 155–162.

Preoperative preparation

Attempts should be made, as far as possible, to restore blood-clotting mechanisms, haemoglobin and plasma protein levels to normal. Adequate amounts of fresh blood should be available for transfusion.

Operation

Incision

1 The abdomen is opened through a long midline incision. A transverse incision can be used with advantage in the grossly obese patient. Usually there are only a few collaterals in the midline and these can be divided with ease. Large vascular adhesions between the abdominal viscera and the parietes should be carefully identified, ligated and cut. The sponging aside of adhesions, easily possible in most other abdominal operations, should be avoided because of troublesome haemorrhage from small veins.

The abdominal viscera are carefully examined and particular search is made for other sources of gastro-intestinal haemorrhage (especially gastric ulcer and duodenal ulcer) and the presence of a hepatoma (particular search should be made around the posterior surface of the liver) which may occur in 5–10% of patients with longstanding cirrhosis.

At operation the portal pressure can be determined by inserting a fine polyethylene catheter into a mesenteric vein and threading it into the portal vein. Pressure can be measured directly employing a central venous catheter set or, if available, a strain gauge manometer. The zero reference of the venous manometer is adjusted to the level of the right atrium and

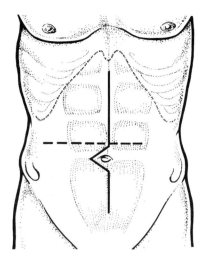

1

mean portal pressure is recorded. Operative venous angiography can be performed if the previous films have been unsatisfactory.

Pressure in the inferior vena cava should also be measured by inserting a fine needle into the vein at the site selected for the shunt. Thrombosis or occlusion of the inferior vena cava is occasionally encountered, in which case a satisfactory fall in portal pressure after shunting would not be obtained.

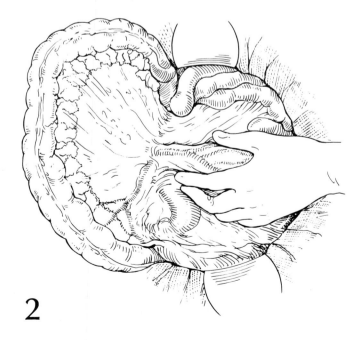

2

2 The transverse colon is lifted out of the wound and reflected to the head end of the patient to put the transverse mesocolon on stretch.

The small intestine is packed into the left lower part of the abdominal cavity and the surgeon places tension on the mesentery of the small bowel by retracting it inferiorly with the right hand. The root of the small intestinal mesentery is therefore displayed and pulsations can be felt in the superior mesenteric artery as it runs across the third part of the duodenum.

3 At the junction of the base of the transverse mesocolon and the base of the small intestinal mesentery an incision is made in the posterior peritoneum over the superior mesenteric vessels, which can usually be palpated.

The third part of the duodenum can often be seen shining through the mesentery in thin subjects. This will not be the case in obese patients and dissection will have to be made through the fat-encased mesentery. A vein of reasonable size, but smaller than the superior mesenteric vein, may be encountered running obliquely from above left to the right lower quadrant. This is not the superior mesenteric vein but the ileocolic vein and should not be dissected further. The surgeon should move further to the patient's left, where the superior mesenteric vein can be identified because it is larger and runs in the sagittal plane.

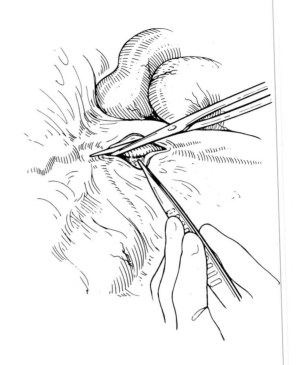

3

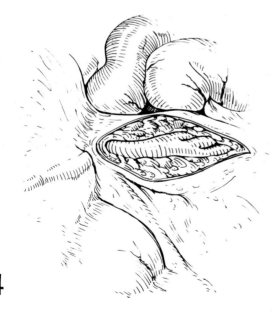

4

4 The mesenteric vein is then cleared cranially and caudally by a process of sharp and blunt dissection. Fine, non-pointed scissors should be used along with non-toothed dissecting forceps. The small but troublesome venous collaterals should be coagulated with diathermy.

5 The superior mesenteric vein is traced caudally until its tributaries are encountered. Of the two major tributaries, one may lie behind the other and may not be immediately apparent; it is therefore liable to damage with clumsy attempts to pass a tape around them. Preferably the two or three tributaries of the mesenteric vein are separately dissected, identified and a tape put around each.

The superior mesenteric vein is then traced cranially over the uncinate process until it passes behind the neck of the pancreas. A well marked fibrous tunnel is evident and this may be elevated, but care should be taken not to damage the small, fragile but broad-based veins which enter the superior mesenteric vein from the pancreas. No attempt should be made to ligate these because troublesome haemorrhage may result.

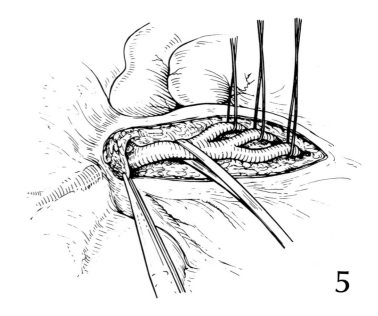

5

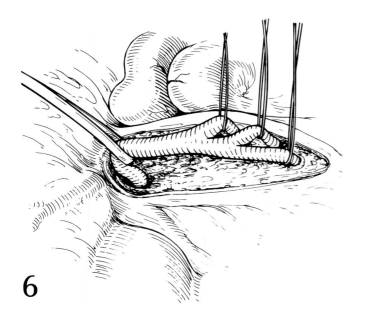

6

6 A tape should then be passed around the cranial part of the superior mesenteric vein and the rest of the vein mobilized.

At any point along its length, the superior mesenteric vein may be joined by small venous tributaries which should not be clamped. Each one should be ligated separately and then divided between ligatures. At least 3 cm of superior mesenteric vein or more, including its main tributaries if necessary, should be displayed so that there is sufficient vein available for anastomosis.

7 The posterior peritoneum at the base of the
transverse mesocolon is then opened further on the
lateral side of the superior mesenteric vein, and the
third part of the duodenum and its junction with the
second part identified. The duodenum is then carefully
mobilized, several vascular adhesions requiring separate
ligation. The retroperitoneal space inferior to the
duodenum is entered.

This direct approach to the inferior vena cava is
preferable to mobilizing the right colon and
approaching the inferior vena cava on its lateral side
because of the large venous collaterals traversing the
retroperitoneal space and the lateral peritoneal gutter.

The duodenum is mobilized as it passes posterior to
the superior mesenteric vessels. The third and fourth
portions of the duodenum are then mobilized completely by incising the ligament of Treitz so that the
duodenum can be lifted cranially out of the operating
field. In this way, postoperative compression of the
duodenum by the graft or impingement on the graft
lumen by the duodenum is avoided.

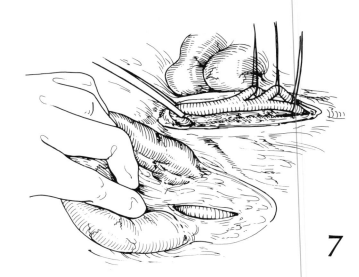

7

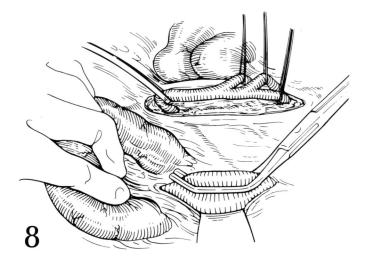

8

8 The anterior surface of the inferior vena cava is
identified and dissected free for a distance of about
5 cm on its anterior, lateral and medial surfaces. It is not
necessary to mobilize the inferior vena cava completely,
and the lumbar vessels need not be ligated.

The caval anastomosis is performed first because it
lies in the depths of the wound. A Satinsky partially
occluding vascular clamp is placed on the anterior
surface of the vena cava and sufficient vena cava is
drawn through the clamp to allow a satisfactory
anastomosis.

9 Using vascular scissors, a small window is then cut on the anterior surface of the inferior vena cava.

The average synthetic graft is about 20–22 mm in diameter, depending on the length of superior mesenteric vein available for anastomosis. The minimum diameter that should be used is 18 mm. Hitherto, knitted Dacron (polyester fibre) has been used, but occasional technical difficulty has been encountered in anastomosing a rigid graft end-to-side with a flimsy, friable superior mesenteric vein. Goretex (expanded polytetrafluoroethylene) is a more pleasant material with which to work, but there is a high rate of graft thrombosis and the use of this graft material in this site is now deprecated. Some surgeons have used autologous vein, e.g. jugular or iliac vein, instead of synthetic material.

In anastomosing the graft to the inferior vena cava, a simple running stitch of 4/0 synthetic vascular suture is employed.

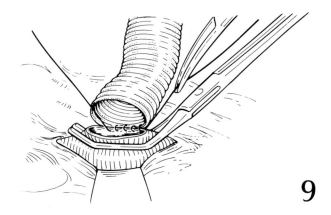

9

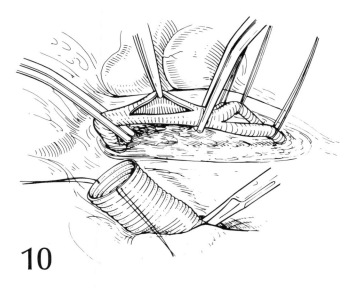

10

10 The graft is then trimmed to adequate length, usually between 4 and 7 cm, avoiding too long a graft which might kink after the viscera have been replaced in the abdomen, or too short a graft which might be under tension and whose sutures may tear out of the delicate wall of the superior mesenteric vein.

A 20–30° clockwise twist is imparted to the graft before starting the anastomosis to the superior mesenteric vein because the normal course of the superior mesenteric vein relative to the inferior vena cava is 20–30° counterclockwise when the viscera are restored to the normal position.

A longitudinal incision is made in the superior mesenteric vein after proximal and distal occlusion with small angled vascular clamps. Partial occlusion clamps should be avoided.

11 Stay sutures are applied between the graft and the superior mesenteric vein. The posterior surface of the vein is anastomosed first and, of necessity, this suturing is done within the lumen of the graft.

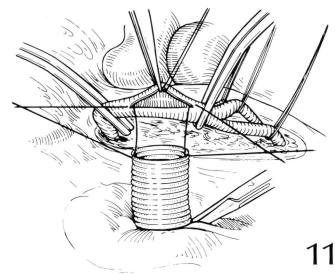

11

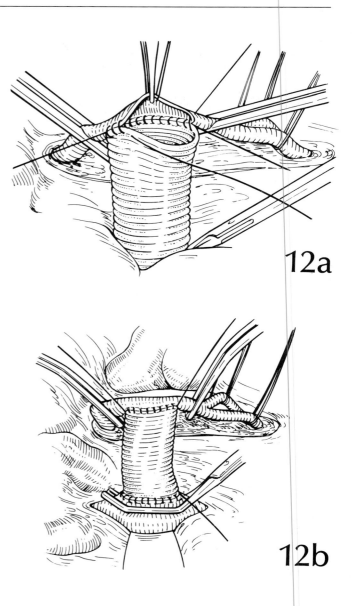

12a, b The anterior part of the anastomosis is then completed. The caval clamp is removed and the anastomosis rechecked for leakage. This should be performed carefully, using interrupted fine vascular sutures. The clamps in the superior mesenteric vein are then removed. With a successful anastomosis the graft fills out and a vascular flow can be easily palpated by the surgeon's fingers.

Pressure measurements can now be obtained from the superior mesenteric vein and the inferior vena cava at the level of the anastomosis. The pressure in the superior mesenteric or portal vein after release of the clamps should drop to approximately 40–60% of the preshunt pressures. It should be emphasized that the residual pressure in the superior mesenteric vein after this type of shunt is considerably higher than that after a standard end-to-side portacaval shunt, probably because of the higher caval pressure at the level of the anastomosis.

If there is any doubt about the patency of the shunt, angiography should be carried out through the fine catheter inserted into the mesenteric vein. If the anastomosis is faulty, usually because of kinking or obstruction of the superior mesenteric–graft junction, it should be taken down and refashioned. It is not justified to stop the operation at this stage until the patency of the graft and of the anastomosis is confirmed, otherwise the portal hypertension remains unrelieved and further bleeding will take place after the operation. It should be remembered that if, for one reason or another, the superior mesenteric vein is, in the course of manipulation, damaged, it can be safely ligated without risk of intestinal infarction. Another form of major shunt should be established at another site.

Closure

The viscera should be replaced and the abdomen closed in the usual fashion. Non-absorbable sutures should be inserted in the linea alba. Drains are not required.

Postoperative care

Transient ascites and hyperbilirubinaemia are usual after operation. The ascites usually responds to sodium restriction and the infusion of salt-poor albumin, 50 g every 12 h during the first 48 h after operation. Careful monitoring of the serum electrolytes is necessary, particular attention being paid to the potassium level and the arterial pH of the blood. Hypokalaemic alkalosis should be avoided because encephalopathy may be precipitated. Potassium-containing solution may have to be infused up to a daily dose of 80–120 mmol potassium. The risk of transient encephalopathy can be reduced by the postoperative administration of neomycin.

Shunt surgery: transjugular intrahepatic portosystemic stent shunt (TIPSS)

Doris N. Redhead DMRD, FRCR
Consultant Radiologist, Department of Radiology, Edinburgh Royal Infirmary, Edinburgh, UK

History

In 1969 Josef Rosch conceived the notion of a non-operative portosystemic shunt using a transjugular approach to the liver[1]. During transjugular cholangiographic studies inadvertent puncture of the portal venous system had been observed. In his experimental studies Rosch used a balloon catheter to dilate the tract through the liver parenchyma between hepatic and portal veins. Colapinto et al. employed this technique in humans[2] but, although these workers were able to create portosystemic shunts and to lower portal pressure, the benefit was short-lived due to premature shunt occlusion. In 1989 Palmaz employed metallic stents to support the tract and was able to achieve long-term patency. These experimental studies stimulated the application of the transjugular intrahepatic portosystemic stent shunt (TIPSS) technique in patients with portal hypertension and variceal haemorrhage. A clinical trial was then performed by Richter and Palmaz[3]. Refinements were later made to the original method to facilitate the procedure and improvements in equipment over the last few years have allowed the technique to be performed with great success and safety. It is estimated that more than 10 000 TIPSS procedures have been performed worldwide and the procedure now has an established place in the management of patients with portal hypertension[4]. The role of TIPSS in the management of variceal haemorrhage in the author's current practice is illustrated in *Figure 1*.

Principles and justification

Indications

TIPSS can be used to control acute bleeding and prevent recurrent bleeding from oesophageal, gastric and ectopic varices, and from portal gastropathy. The technique can also be used to treat intractable ascites, hypersplenism associated with portal hypertension, Budd–Chiari syndrome and hepatorenal syndrome. It can also be used in patients awaiting liver transplantation and when closure of a surgical portosystemic shunt is contemplated.

Contraindications

Absolute contraindications are cardiac failure, severe liver dysfunction and polycystic liver disease. Relative contraindications are hepatic neoplasia and partial portal vein occlusion.

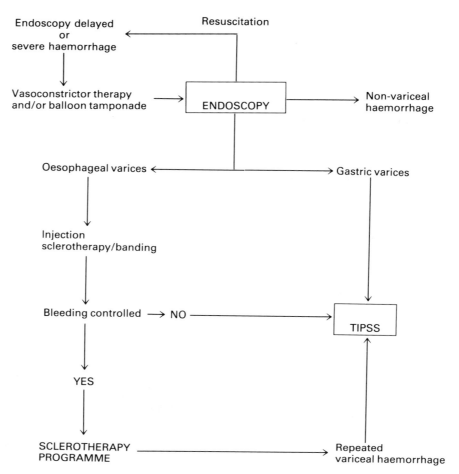

Figure 1   Role of TIPSS in the management of suspected variceal haemorrhage

Preoperative

Preparation of the patient

Prior to TIPSS insertion a full clinical examination is undertaken, with full haematological assessment, coagulation screen, determination of serum urea and electrolyte levels and biochemical assessment of hepatic and renal function. Prothrombin time should be brought to within 5 s of control values, platelet count should exceed 30 000/mm³, and grouped blood must be available. Paracentesis may be advisable if there is gross ascites and fluid intake is restricted for 6–8 h before the procedure. Indirect portography is performed to assess patency and flow pattern in the portal vein.

Sedation and analgesia

The majority of TIPSS procedures are performed using local anaesthesia. Sedation, usually in the form of midazolam, is administered intravenously immediately prior to the procedure. Pethidine is given when appropriate. Oxygen is administered continuously and monitoring is carried out using pulse oximetry. Most patients tolerate this regimen well. In patients with poor hepatic reserve, eliminating the added risk of general anaesthesia is desirable. In the emergency situation, however, where the patient is actively bleeding and restless, a general anaesthetic may be preferable.

Cirrhotic patients are susceptible to infection so cefotaxime and clavulanic acid + amoxycillin (Augmentin) are given 1 h before the procedure and for 48 h thereafter.

Operation

Jugular puncture

The right side of the neck is cleansed with antiseptic and draped in sterile fashion. Local anaesthetic is infiltrated into the soft tissues at the proposed site of the venous puncture.

1a, b The right internal jugular vein provides a direct route to the superior vena cava, right atrium and inferior vena cava and is the most suitable point of entry for TIPSS. Lying within the carotid sheath, lateral to the common carotid artery and below the angle of the mandible, the internal jugular vein comes to lie more anteriorly to the artery as it passes under the medial end of the clavicle to join the subclavian vein. To avoid puncturing the lung apex it is safest to site the point of entry just below the angle of the mandible, 1 cm lateral to the carotid pulse at an angle of 30° to the skin and directed towards the right nipple.

The Seldinger technique is used to catheterize the internal jugular vein, i.e. a needle is introduced into the vein and, when blood is aspirated, a guidewire is inserted and the needle is then withdrawn. The puncture site is progressively dilated to allow introduction of a 10-Fr 41-cm long sheath (included in the 'Rosch–Uchida Transjugular Liver Access Set'). This is advanced over the guidewire through the superior vena cava and right atrium to the inferior vena cava. A pressure measurement is then obtained. Occasionally the right internal jugular vein is small or absent. In this situation the left internal jugular vein can be successfully used for TIPSS.

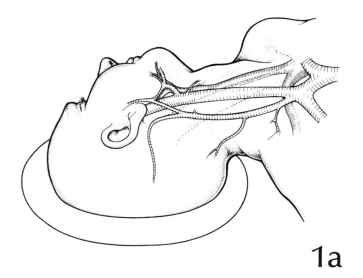

1a

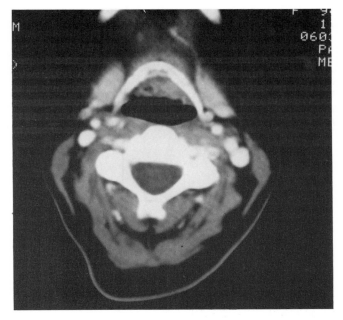

1b

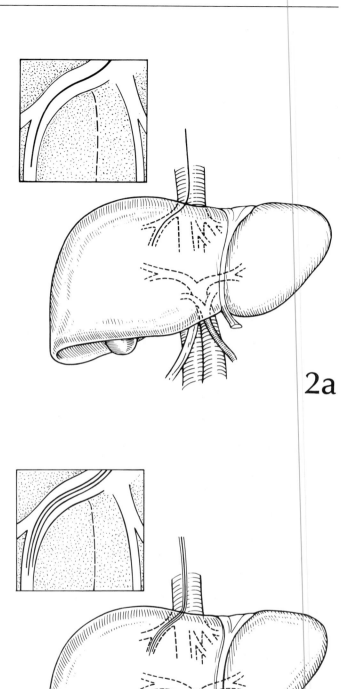

Placement of sheath in the hepatic vein

$2a, b$ The pattern of hepatic veins is variable but, in general, there are three veins: right, middle and left. The right vein is the largest, measuring 8–12 mm in diameter, and is therefore the one most frequently chosen for TIPSS. Under fluoroscopic guidance, using a preshaped catheter and guidewire introduced into the sheath, the right hepatic vein is selected. This allows passage of the sheath into the vein. The guidewire and catheter are then removed. The sheath is a vital component in all subsequent manipulations, providing access to the operation site and ensuring the safe and smooth introduction and retrieval of the instruments used.

2a

2b

Portal vein puncture

3 A curved or 'directional' needle is then introduced into the sheath and used to guide the puncture of one of the main branches of the portal vein using a fine stylet. The portal vein has right and left branches which subsequently divide to supply each segment. The right branch of the portal vein generally lies anteromedially and inferiorly in relation to the right hepatic vein. If the middle or left hepatic vein is used, the left branch of the portal vein generally lies posteromedially and inferiorly. Varying degrees of atrophy and hypertrophy may be present in cirrhosis and the normal orientation of the vascular structures may be disturbed, making the portal vein puncture more difficult. The directional needle is rotated appropriately and the sharp stylet is advanced in the direction of the portal branch. A puncture made through the capsule or into the extrahepatic portal vein may lead to intraperitoneal haemorrhage and care should be taken that the stylet does not extend outside the liver. Several punctures at different angles may be required to attain a safe and satisfactory entry into the portal system.

A metal marker may be applied to the skin surface at the level of the portal bifurcation using ultrasound guidance in order to aid the portal puncture. Alternatively, the venous phase of a splenic or superior mesenteric angiogram may be used to select the optimal direction for puncture. Many experienced interventional radiologists now omit preliminary imaging, favouring a technique similar to that used for transhepatic cholangiography.

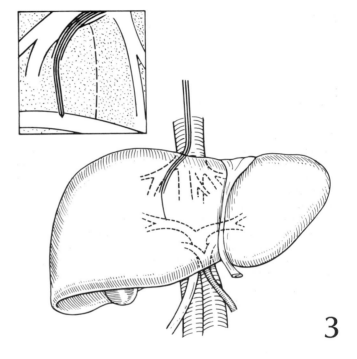

3

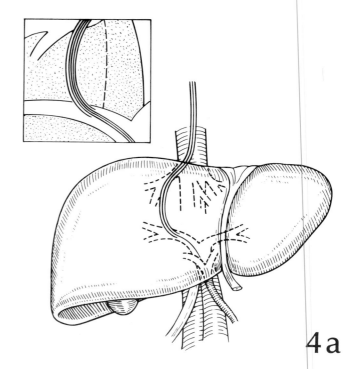

4a

4a, b The fine stylet used for the portal puncture has its own 5-Fr catheter. Once a puncture has been made, the stylet is withdrawn leaving the 5-Fr catheter at the site of puncture. This is slowly withdrawn, aspirating continuously. If blood is obtained, contrast medium is injected to outline the vessel which has been entered. If this vessel is a branch of the portal vein, a guidewire is advanced through the catheter into the portal system. This then supports the passage of catheter, directional needle and sheath into the portal vein. At this stage a pressure measurement is taken and a portogram performed. The portogram in *Illustration 4b* shows large varices filling from the left gastric vein. An inadvertent puncture of the biliary system provides a coincidental cholangiogram in the case illustrated.

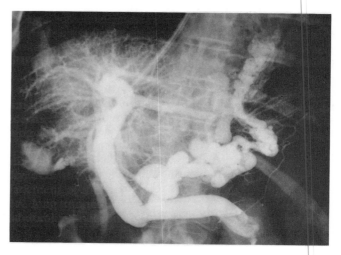

4b

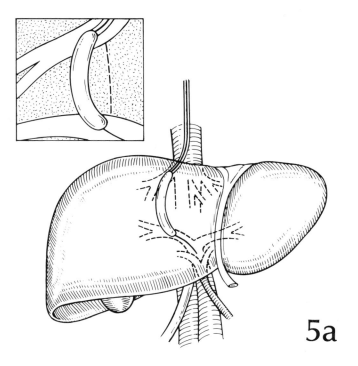

5a

Balloon dilation of shunt tract

5a, b Leaving the guidewire and sheath in the portal vein, an angioplasty balloon catheter is introduced through the sheath. The sheath is pulled back to the right atrium and the tract through the liver is dilated. During inflation of the balloon, a characteristic narrowing or 'waist' is observed at the entry point into the portal vein. This is due to the presence of dense periportal fibrous tissue. Dilatation of this area induces severe pain and analgesia should be administered in anticipation. A similar but less marked 'waist' is seen at the exit point from the hepatic vein. The diameter of the balloon catheter used depends on the diameter of stent chosen. In general a 10-mm or 12-mm diameter balloon with a 4-cm length is used. Pressure is maintained for a few minutes until the tract is fully dilated. The balloon is deflated and withdrawn through the sheath. The sheath is again advanced into the portal system.

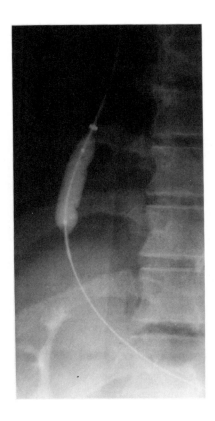

5b

Stent placement

6a, b A variety of stents can be used for TIPSS. The Palmaz stent was the first type to be used and is still favoured by some, but the Wallstent is now the most popular model[5]. The mode of stent deployment varies according to the design chosen. The Palmaz stent measures 3–4 cm in length. It is mounted on a balloon catheter and passed down the sheath to the distal end of the tract. The sheath is withdrawn and the balloon inflated to deploy the stent. Several overlapping stents may be required if the tract is long. The Wallstent is up to 9 cm in length, is self-expanding and covered with a 'rolling membrane'. Once in position the stent is released by simple withdrawal of the membrane.

Early shunt failure can occur if the tract is inadequately stented. It is important to ensure that the whole tract is lined. Hepatic vein stenosis can occur if the proximal stent does not extend up the hepatic vein to the inferior vena cava. It is preferable to have the stent lying in the long axes of the portal and hepatic veins. Stent positioning is critical in patients being considered for liver transplantation in that extension of the upper end of the stent into the inferior vena cava can interfere with the caval anastomosis. Similarly, placing the distal end of the stent too far down the portal vein may interfere with the portal vein anastomosis. Particular attention must be given to avoiding 'overstenting' in these patients.

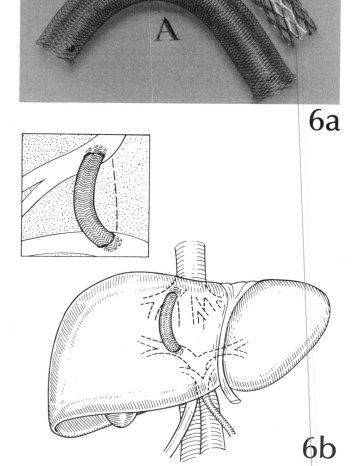

6a

6b

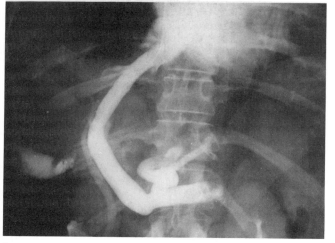

7

7 Following stent placement, a catheter is passed through the shunt to obtain a further portogram in which there should be reduced flow in the varices. The portal pressure measurement is repeated and the inferior vena cava pressure is also recorded (this tends to rise following TIPSS). The procedure is considered complete when there is good flow through the shunt and when there has been a satisfactory reduction in the portal pressure gradient. A final reading of 15 mmHg or less is desirable as variceal bleeding is unlikely to occur at this level.

Postoperative care

Pulse and blood pressure should be monitored to detect bleeding and the neck puncture site is checked regularly to detect haematoma formation. The temperature is monitored 4-hourly to detect infection. Hourly urine output is measured as a diuresis usually follows successful TIPSS insertion.

Complications

The procedural mortality reported with TIPSS is in the region of 1–2% and is mainly related to intraperitoneal haemorrhage from breach of the liver capsule or extrahepatic puncture of the portal vein.

Haemodynamic changes occur following TIPSS. Right atrial and wedged pulmonary artery pressures rise and cardiac output is increased. Pulmonary oedema and cardiac failure have also been reported.

Liver function tests show a deterioration following the procedure in about one-third of patients and in those with severe liver dysfunction the procedure may precipitate acute liver failure. Severe liver dysfunction is therefore regarded as a relative contraindication to TIPSS. However, in this group of patients it may be used as a bridge to transplantation.

Thrombosis within the portal system may be present from the outset or may develop during the procedure, particularly if it is prolonged. Thrombolytic agents may be used to good effect. Pulmonary embolus has also been reported in association with TIPSS. If shunt thrombosis occurs within a few days of the procedure, the most likely explanation is incomplete stenting of the tract. Portography will identify the site of the problem, and the shunt should be extended.

The two most serious complications of TIPSS are hepatic encephalopathy and shunt dysfunction. Encephalopathy develops for the first time in approximately 15% of patients. Most patients respond to medical treatment but in a small percentage a more radical remedy is required, namely reduction of the shunt diameter by placing a smaller calibre stent inside the original stent.

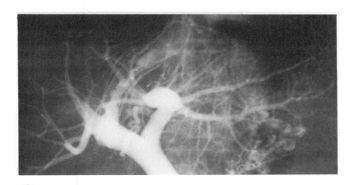

8

8 Intimal hyperplasia develops within the shunt in 20–30% patients within the first few months of TIPSS and may be responsible for recurrence of bleeding or ascites. Antiplatelet and anticoagulation therapy usually fail to prevent this hyperplasia but balloon angioplasty can be used to redilate the tract. This may be a recurring problem in a few patients. If regular surveillance is not carried out, the shunt may occlude completely. In this situation it may be necessary to create a second shunt in parallel. However, it makes more sense to provide regular surveillance (see below) and to make minor adjustments as required to maintain primary patency of the shunt, rather than to delay follow-up until radical rescue is required. It is hoped that the introduction of 'covered' stents will obviate the problem of intimal hyperplasia.

Stenosis can occur at the venous ends of the shunt and particularly affects the hepatic venous outflow. Extending the stent up the hepatic vein to the inferior vena cava prevents this complication. Problems relating to shunt dysfunction tend to occur within the first 6 months of the procedure. It is the author's policy to perform direct transjugular portography at 1 month and 6-monthly thereafter. If the clinical picture suggests shunt dysfunction, an earlier portogram should be performed. TIPSS is a technically demanding procedure and there is a distinct learning curve. In experienced hands, however, procedural complications are uncommon and, with regular follow-up, problems of shunt dysfunction can be detected and addressed early.

Outcome

The increasing experience and availability of TIPSS, together with the unequivocal reports of the success of the technique in comparative trials, have prompted a review of the management of patients with portal hypertension. There is a high technical success rate with this procedure, around 90%, and a low procedural complication rate[6]. It avoids major abdominal surgery and general anaesthesia. In many instances it is performed in patients who are otherwise unfit for surgery.

TIPSS not only controls bleeding but prevents rebleeding. It has been shown to be more effective than endoscopic sclerotherapy and banding, and is simpler, safer and less expensive than surgical alternatives. Surgical shunting does prevent rebleeding but the mortality of surgical shunting in patients with Child's grade C cirrhosis can reach 50% and there is a significant morbidity in terms of postoperative encephalopathy, which affects 10–45% of patients depending on the type of shunt performed. Liver transplantation also carries a high mortality if performed during an acute bleeding episode. Where there is severe liver dysfunction and the patient is considered for transplantation, TIPSS may be used to control bleeding and to allow the general clinical status to improve while a suitable donor organ is sought. In this way it acts as a bridge to transplantation. Drug therapies have had some success in the control of acute bleeding and prevention of rebleeding. However, there is no ideal drug available and long-term compliance may be a problem in this group of patients.

The majority of patients in all published series have alcoholic cirrhosis. However, as confidence in the technique grows, there are increasing reports of its use in less common conditions, e.g. in patients with the Budd–Chiari syndrome.

Since its inception in 1989, TIPSS has emerged as an essential component of the interventional repertoire in units which have a major interest in hepatobiliary disease and liver transplantation.

References

1. Rosch J, Hanafee WN, Snow H. Transjugular portal venography and radiologic portacaval shunt: experimental study. *Radiology* 1969; 92: 1112–4.

2. Colapinto RF, Stronell RD, Birch SJ *et al.* Creation of an intrahepatic portosystemic shunt with a Gruntzig balloon catheter. *Can Med Assoc J* 1982; 126: 267–8.

3. Richter GM, Noeldge G, Palmaz JC, Roessle M. The transjugular intrahepatic portosystemic shunt (TIPSS): results of a pilot study. *Cardiovasc Intervent Radiol* 1990; 13: 200–7.

4. Conn HO. Transjugular intrahepatic portal-systemic shunts: the state of the art. *Hepatology* 1993; 17: 148–58.

5. La Berge JM, Ring EJ, Gordon RL *et al.* Creation of transjugular intrahepatic portosystemic shunts with the Wallstent endoprosthesis: results in 100 patients. *Radiology* 1993; 187: 413–20.

6. Jalan R, Redhead DN, Simpson KJ, Elton RA, Hayes PC. Transjugular intrahepatic portosystemic stent-shunt (TIPSS): long-term follow-up. *Q J Med* 1994; 87: 565–73.

Ascites: peritoneovenous shunt

O. James Garden BSc, MD, FRCS(Ed), FRCS(Glas)
Senior Lecturer and Honorary Consultant Hepatobiliary Surgeon, University Department of Surgery and
Scottish Liver Transplantation Unit, Royal Infirmary, Edinburgh, UK

History

Although peritoneovenous shunting by means of an implanted device was first described in 1962[1], the technique did not achieve widespread popularity until LeVeen et al. developed an ingenious valve specifically for the drainage of ascites[2-5]. In recent years the role of peritoneovenous shunting has declined due to the more aggressive medical management of ascites, the selective use of surgical and transjugular portosystemic shunts, and the more widespread use of liver transplantation in patients with chronic liver disease and intractable ascites.

Principles and justification

1 Peritoneovenous shunts allow drainage of ascitic fluid from the peritoneal cavity into the intrathoracic central venous system. The shunts comprise (1) a fenestrated proximal catheter which is placed into the peritoneal cavity; (2) a unidirectional low pressure valve system; and (3) a distal venous catheter, the tip of which is placed into the superior vena cava or right atrium.

The pressure gradient and, as a result, the flow can be increased by using abdominal binders or deep breathing exercises. The author's preference is to use a Denver peritoneovenous shunt (illustrated) which, unlike the LeVeen shunt, has its valve mechanism housed in a flexible pump chamber of soft silicone rubber. The system can be flushed by compressing the chamber, thereby minimizing the risk of occlusion by debris. Flow through the shunt can be increased by pumping whenever spontaneous flow is insufficient to control ascites. Standard double-valve shunts are effective in most cases because of the lower risk of venous reflux, and the routine use of heparinized venous catheters minimizes the risk of thrombosis at the silicone rubber surface.

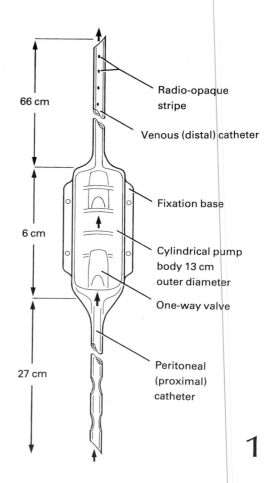

1

Indications

Peritoneovenous shunts are indicated in (1) intractable ascites in the cirrhotic patient which is refractory to medical treatment consisting of salt restriction, bed rest, diuretics and repeated paracentesis with replacement of protein as salt-poor albumin; (2) chylous ascites; and (3) malignant ascites. Although there is a potential risk of disseminating malignant cells in the ascitic fluid, this appears to be of little clinical relevance and good palliation is achieved in some patients.

Contraindications

Contraindications for the use of peritoneovenous shunts include (1) peritoneal sepsis; (2) severe hepatic insufficiency; (3) previous variceal bleeding not yet controlled by medical or surgical therapy; (4) acute tubular necrosis, although patients with hepatorenal failure may respond favourably to insertion of a shunt; and (5) patients being considered for liver transplantation.

Preoperative

Routine preoperative preparation should include measurement of body weight, full blood count and coagulation screen, measurement of serum urea, electrolytes, creatinine, albumin, protein and liver function. A sample of ascitic fluid should be submitted for bacteriological culture and cytological examination. Antibiotics are normally administered before surgery and are continued for 24 h after the operation to cover infections with Gram positive organisms, including staphylococci. The author's preference is for a combination of flucloxacillin and cefotaxime.

Anaesthesia

General anaesthesia with endotracheal intubation is preferred by the author. However, the procedure can be carried out under local anaesthesia with preoperative sedation and analgesia.

Operation

Position of patient

2 The patient is placed supine on the operating table with a rolled sheet or small pillow placed under the shoulder on the side in which the shunt is to be inserted. The head is turned away slightly from that side, although flexing of the head onto the opposite shoulder should be avoided since this may direct the venous catheter into the subclavian vein rather than into the superior vena cava.

Before insertion of the shunt it may be advisable to drain a proportion of ascitic fluid by paracentesis to reduce the risk of fluid overload and disseminated intravascular coagulation in the postoperative period.

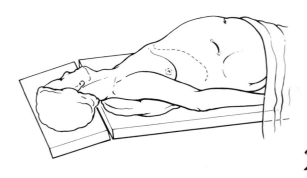

Incisions

The shunt may be inserted on the right or left side, but if the patient has had a prior shunt procedure which has failed because of thrombosis, use of the opposite internal jugular vein is contraindicated because of the risk of blindness, tongue oedema and facial oedema. In such patients the saphenous route of insertion is recommended. Previous abdominal operation scars should be avoided.

Supraclavicular incision

3 Although the cephalic or external jugular veins can be used, it is our preference to employ a direct approach to the internal jugular vein. A 5-cm incision is made 2–3 cm above the clavicle, extending laterally from the clavicular attachment of the sternomastoid muscle.

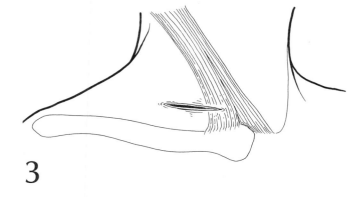

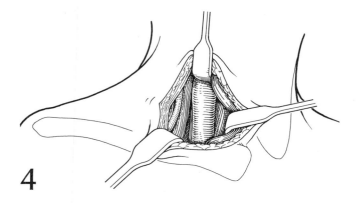

4 The internal jugular vein is exposed for a distance of 3 cm to facilitate insertion of the shunt and enable proximal and distal ligation with loop ties of 2/0 silk which are placed proximally and distally around the vein. The wound is loosely packed with a saline soaked swab and the abdominal part of the operation is commenced.

Abdominal incision

5 A 5-cm subcostal incision is made 5–7 cm below the costal margin in the right upper quadrant of the abdomen. The dissection is normally carried down lateral to the rectus sheath as a grid iron incision. The external and internal oblique fascia are split along their fibres, but the transversalis fascia should not be stripped from the peritoneum since the peritoneum would then be too thin to support purse-string sutures.

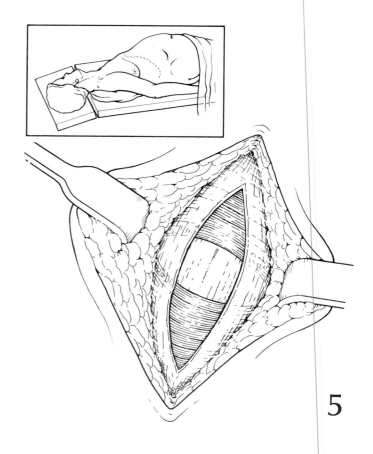

5

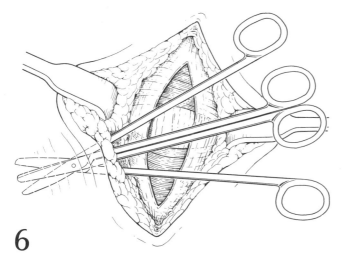

6

Tunnelling procedure and placement of shunt body

6 It is useful to tunnel the distal venous end of the shunt and to place the pump chamber in its final position before inserting the shunt into the peritoneal cavity.

Using the index finger a small tunnel is made superiorly and laterally over the costal margin of the chest wall to allow placement of the pump chamber in an intercostal space. A long tunnelling instrument is then passed from the abdominal incision to the cervical incision.

The venous end of the catheter can now be attached to a tunnelling instrument and pulled through. Alternatively, a heavy suture can be passed through and tied to the end of the shunt, which can then be pulled through with gentle traction on the suture. The pump chamber is secured in its final position with two non-absorbable sutures to fix it to the periosteum of the underlying ribs. The proximal end of the shunt is delivered through the layers of the abdominal wall at some distance from the abdominal incision. This manoeuvre minimizes postoperative leakage through the incision.

Establishing the shunt

7 Two purse-string sutures of 3/0 polypropylene (Prolene) are placed in the transversalis fascia and peritoneum. The transversalis fascia and peritoneum are incised in the centre of the sutures with a number 15 blade and the peritoneal catheter is inserted and directed into the right paracolic gutter. Once the purse-string sutures are tied and a water-tight closure obtained, ascitic fluid will pour from the distal venous end of the catheter. The valve chamber is pumped a few times to ensure that the shunt is cleared of all air bubbles and the peritoneal end of the catheter may be clamped to prevent leakage of fluid before the distal end is inserted into the vein.

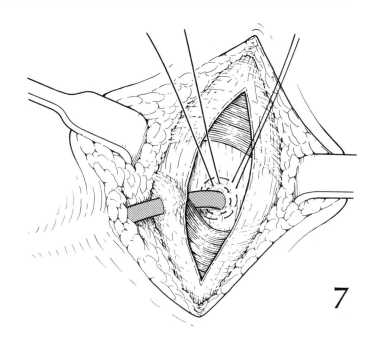

7

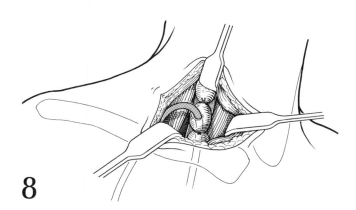

8

8 The upper venous ligature is tied to occlude the internal jugular vein and a longitudinal venotomy is then made between the two ligatures after placing the patient in a 15–20° head-down tilt. The venous catheter of the shunt is measured so that the tip can lie in the superior vena cava just above the level of the right atrium; this is usually 7 cm below the upper border of the sternum. The venous catheter is cut obliquely to facilitate insertion into the vein. The proximal ligature is tied, avoiding constriction of the shunt. The clamp on the peritoneal catheter is removed as the venous catheter is guided into the venotomy.

9 A chest radiograph is obtained on the operating table to confirm proper positioning of the venous catheter in the superior vena cava. The incisions are closed using non-absorbable sutures for the muscle and fascial layers, polyglycolic acid for the subcutaneous layer, and intracutaneous polypropylene to close the skin.

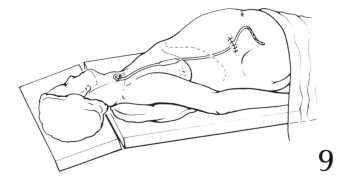

9

Postoperative care

In the recovery room the patient should be nursed with the head of the bed elevated to a 45° angle to minimize fluid overload. It may not be necessary to administer a diuretic routinely if paracentesis has been undertaken preoperatively, but if there is clinical evidence of fluid overload, or if urine output drops below 40 ml/h for two consecutive hours, it is the author's policy to administer frusemide 40–80 mg intravenously. A full blood count and a coagulation screen are undertaken in the immediate postoperative period. The pump chamber should be compressed once a day to check its patency and, after a week, regular pumping can be commenced. Incentive breathing exercises should be omitted in the immediate postoperative period since these may contribute to fluid overload, and it is advisable to discard any abdominal binder for the same reasons.

The patient is instructed in how to operate the shunt. The chamber should be compressed at a rate of approximately 10/min for maximal effect and two pumping sessions of 10–15 min/day are usually adequate.

Complications

The technical complications of malpositioning and obstruction of the venous catheter are usually avoided by careful insertion technique. Increasing abdominal girth and weight suggest shunt failure. Resistance to compression of the pump chamber indicates loss of patency in the venous catheter. Shunt occlusion can be assessed by injecting 5–10 ml of radio-opaque contrast medium with a 25 gauge needle into the pump chamber. Shunt failure due to clot formation has been treated successfully by infusion of streptokinase through the pump chamber, but re-exploration and partial or complete replacement of the shunt is usually required.

Wound infection and septicaemia unresponsive to aggressive antibiotic therapy may require removal of the shunt. Disseminated intravascular coagulation may occur due to the presence of procoagulants in the ascitic fluid. This complication is best avoided by the measures previously described, since treatment of established disseminated intravascular coagulation may be resistant to fresh frozen plasma and/or heparin. Massive tumour embolization has been described but is uncommon.

References

1. Smith AN. Peritoneocaval shunt with a Holter valve in the treatment of ascites. *Lancet* 1962; i: 671–2.

2. Lund RH, Newkirk JB. Peritoneo-venous shunting system for surgical management of ascites. *Contemp Surg* 1979; 14: 31–45.

3. Oosterlee, J. Peritoneovenous shunting for ascites in cancer patients. *Br J Surg* 1980; 67: 663–6.

4. LeVeen HH, Christoudias G, Ip M, Luft R, Falk G, Grosberg S. Peritoneovenous shunting for ascites. *Ann Surg* 1974; 180: 580–91.

5. LeVeen HH, Ip M, Ahmed N, Hutto RB, LeVeen EG. Coagulopathy post-peritoneovenous shunt. *Ann Surg* 1987; 205: 305–11.

Splenectomy, partial splenectomy and laparoscopic splenectomy

Miles Irving MD, ChM, FRCS
Professor of Surgery, University Department of Surgery, Hope Hospital, Salford, UK

Stephen Attwood MCh, FRCS, FRCS(I)
Consultant Surgeon, Department of Surgery, Hope Hospital, Salford, UK

David Gough FRCS, FRCS(Ed), FRACS, DCH
Consultant Paediatric Surgeon, Department of Surgery, Royal Manchester Children's Hospital, Salford, UK

Principles and justification

The principal indications for splenectomy are trauma, hereditary spherocytosis, immune thrombocytopenia (idiopathic thrombocytopenic purpura), cysts and tumours, and as part of radical upper abdominal surgery such as total gastrectomy. The operation is also selectively used in the management of patients with chronic lymphocytic leukaemia, chronic granulocytic (myeloid) leukaemia, the lymphomas and hypersplenism due to a variety of causes.

In parallel with the recognition of the benefits of splenectomy has come an awareness of the danger from serious infection (particularly pneumococcal) that may follow, even years later, in children and adults[1,2]. As a consequence, in those cases where splenectomy is not essential every effort should be made to conserve part or all the spleen. Whether this advice is always sensible in adults is a matter of judgement in the individual case. It may well be decided that the potential benefit of preventing death from overwhelming septicaemia is outweighed by the postoperative mortality and morbidity of attempts at splenic preservation. If total removal is unavoidable, prophylactic antibiotic treatment and vaccination are advisable (*see* below).

Indications

Trauma

Where the spleen is avulsed or fragmented, splenectomy is the only feasible treatment. However, where it is lacerated or only a segment is avulsed, conservative treatment or partial splenectomy should be attempted, even if splenectomy has to be resorted to in the end. Unrecognized traumatic splenic injury of mild degree has probably gone untreated for years without harm. Recent diagnostic methods have established that a planned non-operative approach for selected cases of traumatic splenic rupture is both safe and effective[3].

1 The relatively non-invasive investigations of ultrasonography and computed tomographic (CT) scanning have a high degree of sensitivity in revealing the presence of splenic injury and the associated haemoperitoneum. This allows a positive decision to be made to manage specific splenic injuries conservatively, such as that shown in the illustration of a patient who had major upper abdominal trauma with liver and splenic injury. The CT scan in *Illustration 1* shows a large fluid density collection in the left lobe of the liver consistent with a haematoma in the spleen which is displacing the stomach, filled with contrast medium to the left. A small amount of fluid is also seen lateral to the liver consistent with blood in the peritoneal cavity. The spleen is enlarged and is very heterogenous, particularly on its lateral aspect, consistent with splenic haematoma.

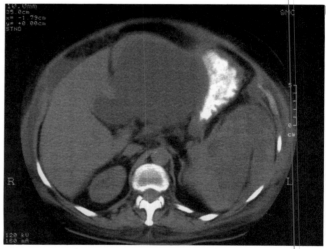

1

Because delayed splenic rupture is almost unknown in children, and in this age group the spleen is often the only organ injured, a policy of conservative management has always had considerable support among paediatric surgeons. With better imaging now available, increasing numbers of surgeons are adopting this policy in adults.

Autotransplantation of splenic fragments as free grafts can occur naturally after injury but is of no proven benefit as a planned surgical procedure.

Hypersplenism

In this state the spleen, which usually is enlarged, is destroying one or more components of the blood (e.g. erythrocytes, leucocytes and platelets) at a rate which exceeds the ability of the marrow to produce them. This may be the result of abnormalities of the cells which make them more easily destroyed than normally, or of enlargement of the spleen resulting in stagnation of blood cells and their premature destruction. Hereditary spherocytosis, sickle cell anaemia, immune thrombocytopenia, splenic anaemia due to portal hypertension and lymphomatous infiltration of the spleen can be classified as forms of hypersplenism.

A form of immune thrombocytopenia occurs in 5–10% of patients with the acquired immune deficiency syndrome (AIDS). With its rising prevalence, AIDS has become a more frequent indication for splenectomy.

Leukaemias

Haematologists now consider that certain cases of chronic lymphocytic leukaemia, chronic granulocytic leukaemia and variants such as hairy cell leukaemia can be treated more effectively if the spleen is removed. The operation has to be performed when the patient is in good condition and free from infection. It is contraindicated in acute leukaemias, blast crises, and when the patient is deteriorating and/or infected.

Upper abdominal surgery

Splenectomy is often necessary during major upper abdominal operations such as total gastrectomy or pancreatectomy, although when it is not essential for technical reasons the spleen should be left *in situ*.

Malignancy

While the nodes in the splenic hilum lie in the lymphatic drainage pathway from tumours of the lower oesophagus, stomach and pancreas, the benefits of splenectomy as part of a radical resection for these tumours has not been proven. The role of the spleen in immunity to malignancy is not known while, conversely, if lymph nodes in the splenic hilum are involved, the disease is at an advanced stage and carries a poor prognosis. It is therefore advisable to preserve the spleen in these operations as long as conservation does not compromise the clearance of overt malignant disease.

Giant splenomegaly

In some diseases such as myelofibrosis the spleen grows so large that its weight becomes unbearable and it becomes prone to repeated painful infarction. In these circumstances splenectomy is worthwhile.

Cysts, tumours, abscess, torsion, splenic artery aneurysm

In these rare conditions, splenectomy is necessary to establish the diagnosis as well as to treat the disease.

Staging laparotomy

Improvements in imaging and more effective treatment regimens mean that staging laparotomy, once an integral part of the effective treatment of Hodgkin's disease, is now redundant in most centres.

Preoperative

Close consultation with the haematologist and medical oncologist is essential in patients undergoing splenectomy for lymphoma or a haematological disorder. The surgeon should ensure that the haemoglobin, white cell and platelet counts have been measured recently and that the bone marrow has been assessed. Anaemia, leucopenia and thrombocytopenia are not in themselves contraindications to operation as long as the bone marrow shows evidence of its ability to produce these cells. There is rarely any benefit to be obtained from splenectomy for hypersplenism if the marrow is aplastic or totally replaced by tumour. If there is doubt about the role of the spleen in red cell or platelet destruction, survival studies with ^{51}Cr-labelled cells can be informative. In cases of haemolytic anaemia the gallbladder should be scanned with ultrasonography and, if gallstones are present, cholecystectomy is advisable at the time of splenectomy.

The surgeon should encourage colleagues to refer patients for splenectomy before the underlying disease and the associated cytopenias have progressed to the point where the patient is subject to serious infections. Splenectomy in infected hypersplenic patients almost never succeeds in improving their condition.

Before operation for uncomplicated splenectomy, two units of blood should be cross-matched. For large spleens, where there is a possibility of multiple vascular adhesions, up to six units of blood should be available. Platelet infusions should be ordered for severely thrombocytopenic patients but should not be given until the splenic artery has been tied. In cases of traumatic rupture of the spleen, preoperative colloid and blood transfusion is mandatory to resuscitate the patient.

The patient should be shaved from nipples to mid thigh and a nasogastric tube passed.

Anaesthesia

An endotracheal tube and muscle relaxation are essential. The anaesthetist should be warned that it may be necessary to divide the left costal margin and to open the thorax in difficult cases. Prophylaxis against venous thrombosis should be commenced before operation by prescribing subcutaneous heparin and is supplemented during operation by intermittent calf compression with pneumatic leg cuffs.

Operations

ELECTIVE SPLENECTOMY FOR NORMAL-SIZED OR SLIGHTLY ENLARGED SPLEEN

Incision

2 The patient is positioned supine on the operating table with a sandbag under the left lower ribs. A long midline or left subcostal muscle cutting incision is used.

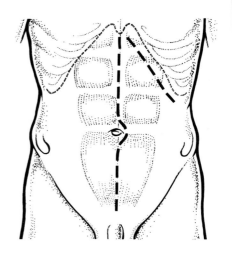

2

Exploration

General exploration commences with examination of the spleen, taking care not to tear any adhesions. The splenic hilum is palpated for lymph node enlargement and the liver examined for the presence of cirrhosis and tumour infiltration. The gallbladder is palpated and removed if it contains stones, a common finding in haemolytic anaemia.

The presence of accessory spleens is excluded by careful examination, paying particular attention to the gastrosplenic ligament, mesocolon and upper border of the pancreas.

Splenectomy

The operator's right hand is slid gently over the convex diaphragmatic surface of the spleen. In most cases it will slide without obstruction down to the lienorenal ligament. If adhesions are encountered they should not be broken down but dealt with in the manner described later.

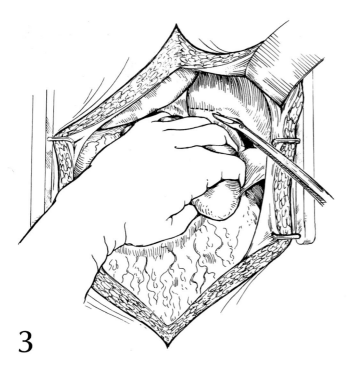

Mobilization of the spleen

3 The operator now substitutes his left hand for his right and gently pulls the spleen up towards the abdominal incision so that the taut posterior leaf of the lienorenal ligament is clearly demonstrated. This ligament is then incised with scissors along its full length allowing the posterior surface of the spleen and the contents of the hilum to be drawn up into the wound.

3

Division of vessels

4 At this stage a band of short gastric vessels passing to the upper pole of the spleen in the upper part of the gastrosplenic ligament may limit mobilization. These vessels are divided between artery forceps and ligated with 0 polyglactin (Vicryl) absorbable ligatures. Care must be taken not to include any of the stomach wall in the ligatures as this can lead to a gastric fistula. If difficulty is encountered because of the shortness of the ligament, it is often better to transfix and ligate the vessels on the gastric wall than to risk inclusion of gastric wall in the ligature.

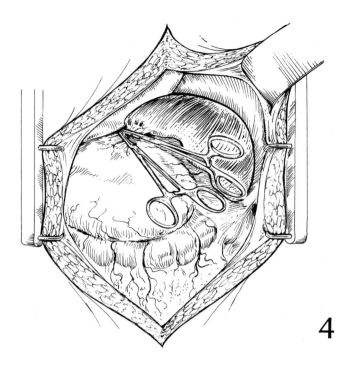

4

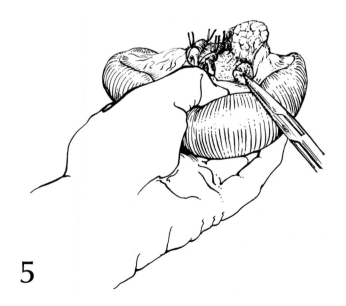

5

5 Attention is then turned to the posterior aspect of the splenic hilum. The tail of the pancreas is identified and carefully dissected from the hilum using scissors and gauze pledgets. Bleeding from small vessels can be arrested by diathermy coagulation or ligaclips. The splenic artery and vein become visible and can be dissected out and ligated in continuity with strong absorbable ligatures. The artery should be ligated before the vein. The vessels are then divided between the ligatures. In thrombocytopenic patients, platelet infusions should be given at this stage.

Division of the gastrosplenic ligament

6 The spleen is then turned over to demonstrate the gastrosplenic ligament and the attachments of the lower pole of the spleen to the splenic flexure of the colon, which are divided piecemeal between ligatures. This exposes the thin anterior leaf of the lienorenal ligament which, apart from a few small vessels, should be avascular. It is divided by dissection with the scissors, continued care being taken not to damage the pancreas. The spleen can now be removed. Haemostasis is secured by diathermy or suture ligation of any bleeding vessels in the splenic pedicle. If there has been extensive dissection in the left hypochondrium a low pressure suction drain should be placed in the subdiaphragmatic space.

The abdominal wall is then closed in layers.

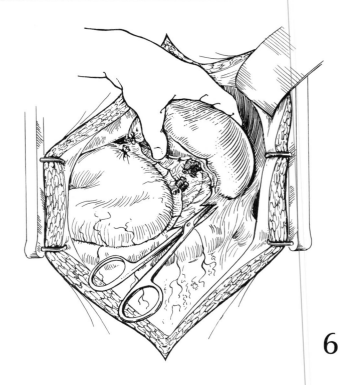

6

LAPAROSCOPIC SPLENECTOMY

Laparoscopic splenectomy is indicated for conditions such as immune thrombocytopenia or hereditary spherocytosis in which the spleen is usually of normal size or only slightly enlarged and where perisplenic adhesions are not a problem.

7 The patient is positioned head-up (anti-Trendelenburg) on the operating table in a partly chaired position and rotated 25–30° to the right. This allows gravity to assist with the retraction of the omentum and colon from the spleen. The patient's legs may be positioned in Lloyd-Davis supports. Some surgeons prefer to stand between the patient's legs while others prefer to stand on the patient's right side.

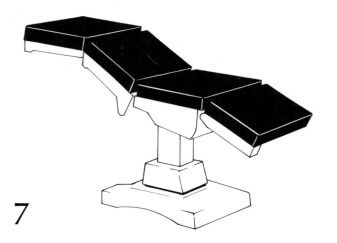

7

8 Port placements vary with the size of the spleen, the size of the patient and the view obtained at laparoscopy. A 10-mm port is first inserted above the umbilicus using a blunt entry technique to avoid damaging a large spleen. The peritoneum and spleen are assessed following insertion of the laparoscope and the degree of adhesion formation is evaluated. Two 12-mm ports are then inserted in the left side of the abdomen in the anterior axillary line below the costal margin, the other in the mid clavicular line at or above the level of the umbilicus. Two 10-mm ports are then inserted in the epigastrium and right upper quadrant.

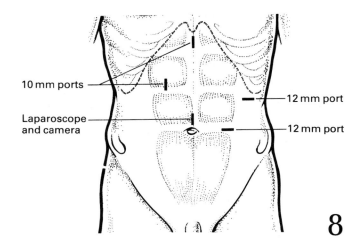

9 The anatomy of the upper abdomen is fully assessed using soft grasping instruments (Babcock forceps) to retract the stomach and lift the greater omentum. The splenic flexure of the colon and the spleen itself are assessed for adhesions posteriorly and accessibility to the splenic hilum is determined.

The operation commences with division of the attachments of the spleen to the splenic flexure of the colon, following which the spleen is retracted medially and the lienorenal ligament is divided. The use of clips is avoided if possible as these may interfere with subsequent application of the stapler. With very large spleens it may be difficult to see the upper half of the lienorenal ligament and a 30° telescope may help. The ligament is divided only as far as it can be clearly seen, leaving the rest until after division of the vessels in the splenic hilum.

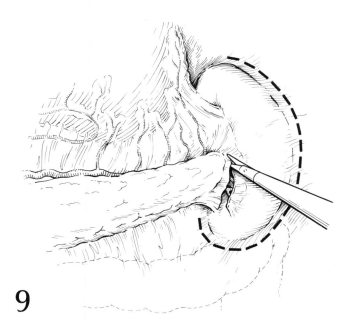

10 A 12-mm blunt probe such as the Endogauge is used to lift the splenic hilum forwards. A pair of dissecting forceps is used to clear any adhesions posteriorly and so create a space for a laparoscopic stapling device to be placed across the hilum.

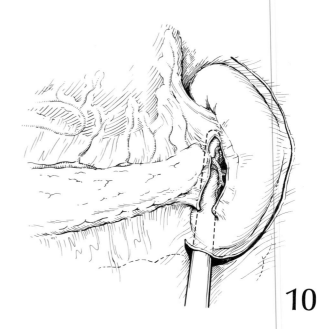

10

11 Vascular staples must be used and the stapler is fired two or three times until the hilum is fully divided.

11

12 Adhesions at the apex of the spleen and the upper remnants of the gastrosplenic and lieno-renal ligaments are then divided between clips or ties and the spleen is finally freed from all attachments.

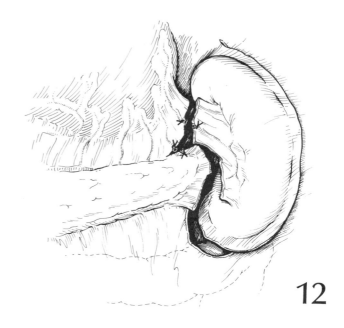

12

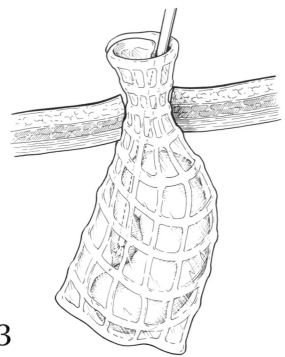

13

13 A sterile bag (Endobag) large enough to accommodate the whole spleen is introduced, the spleen is placed within it, and then macerated and aspirated. Maceration may be achieved with a liquidizing instrument, or by inserting the surgeon's finger into the bag, methodically fragmenting the spleen, and aspirating it with a large suction tube.

Haemostasis is checked, the presence of splenunculi is excluded, and the ports are removed.

MODIFICATION OF THE STANDARD OPEN TECHNIQUE FOR RUPTURED SPLEEN

The principles of the operation are the same as for elective splenectomy, with the additional problems of the initial control of haemorrhage, the detection of associated injuries, and the desirability of conserving the spleen where possible.

Incision

This should always be a long midline incision which allows free and rapid access to other viscera that may be damaged.

Control of bleeding

14 It is first necessary to remove blood and clot from the left hypochondrium by scooping, mopping and suction. The left costal margin is lifted with a retractor by the assistant and the surgeon's right hand is thrust down to the splenic hilum where, in cases of continuing vigorous bleeding, the vessels are grasped between finger and thumb.

If at this stage the patient is grossly shocked, compression should be maintained until the anaesthetist has corrected the hypovolaemia. Where prolonged compression is necessary it may be achieved by occluding all of the hilar structures with a non-crushing intestinal clamp.

Once the situation has stabilized and it is ascertained that the spleen is so badly damaged that no form of conservation or repair is possible, splenectomy is carried out in a manner as near as possible to that described for elective splenectomy. The surgeon should avoid the temptation to apply forceps in a blind fashion and to mass-ligature structures in the splenic hilum, as this may damage the gastric wall and pancreatic tail. However, in certain cases it can be very difficult to isolate and ligate the major vessels and in such cases the clamped tissues can be transfixed and ligated with strong sutures.

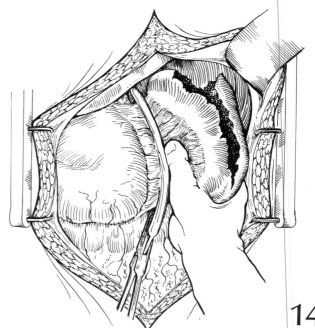

14

CONSERVATION, REPAIR AND PARTIAL SPLENECTOMY FOR RUPTURED SPLEEN

Conservative treatment

Although non-operative treatment of patients with splenic injury is well established, and it is now evident that, with careful observation and transfusion support, certain ruptured spleens can be left *in situ* to heal, it remains a difficult policy to adopt in patients with abdominal trauma. The hazards are obvious in that other injuries can be missed, bleeding can recur, and delayed rupture may occur. Splenic conservation does not simplify the treatment of injured patients but makes it more complex, and the policy must be abandoned where continuous bleeding is evident and other injuries are suspected.

15a, b The decision to leave the spleen to heal spontaneously can also be taken at operation. Where a minor splenic injury is seen and bleeding has ceased, the area can be inspected carefully by retraction and without dividing the lienorenal ligament. The lesser sac is entered to allow examination of the splenic hilum, pancreas and retroperitoneal tissues. If these areas are free from damage and haematoma, the spleen can be left *in situ* and the abdomen closed with low pressure suction drainage to the area. In some cases, persistent oozing of blood from the torn splenic substance may be controlled by the local application of dry microfibrillar collagen (Avitene) or calcium alginate (Kaltostat).

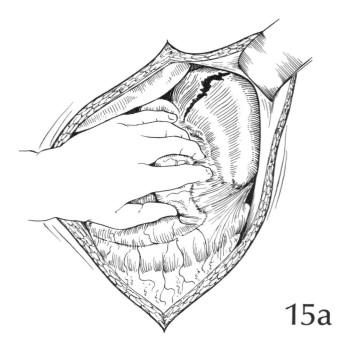

15a

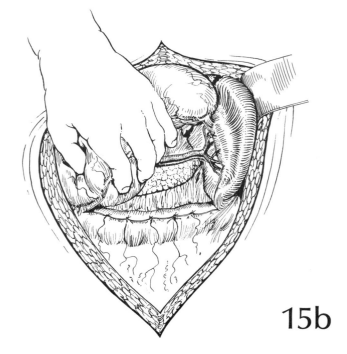

15b

Splenorrhaphy

16 Suture of splenic lacerations is advocated by some authorities, but where haemorrhage has ceased it is probably unnecessary and may even provoke rebleeding. However, bleeding from an easily accessible laceration in the lower pole of the spleen may be controlled by insertion of 0 polyglycolic acid sutures combined with ligation in continuity of the relevant polar artery. If active bleeding persists it is advisable to discontinue suturing and to perform total or partial splenectomy.

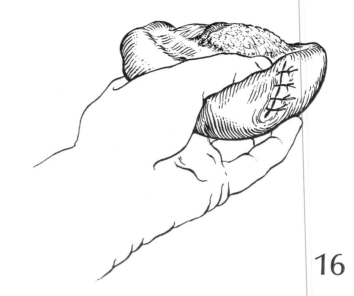

16

Partial splenectomy

If a fragment of spleen is completely or partially avulsed, usually at the upper or lower pole, then a different policy can be adopted. The main splenic artery usually divides before entering the splenic substance and the fact that these branches are end arteries allows partial splenic resection to be undertaken safely[4].

17 The spleen is fully mobilized as previously described by dividing the lienorenal and gastrosplenic attachments. The splenic pedicle is grasped by the assistant and compressed while the tail of the pancreas is dissected bluntly from the hilum and the vessels are exposed. Dissection close to the capsule exposes the relevant polar artery which is encircled and doubly ligated with a strong absorbable suture or occluded with metal clips.

17

18 Wedge resection is accomplished using cutting diathermy. Mattress sutures of an absorbable material such as 0 polyglactin are used to control oozing from the open edge. If the tissues are very friable the sutures can be inserted through collagen buttresses. After satisfactory haemostasis is obtained the abdomen is closed with suction drainage to the splenic area.

This procedure is probably only of value if more than half of the spleen is preserved.

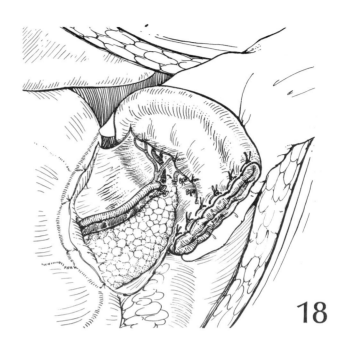

Splenic wrapping procedures

19 Major decapsulating injuries of the spleen are typically encountered in patients who present with delayed bleeding. In such individuals there is frequently a large subcapsular haematoma which, when evacuated, leaves an extensive area of denuded splenic pulp. Woven polyglycolic acid mesh is particularly helpful in achieving secure haemostasis in these cases. Topical haemostatic agents are applied to the bleeding areas and the entire spleen is encased in the mesh. The spleen is completely mobilized, attached only by its hilar vessels.

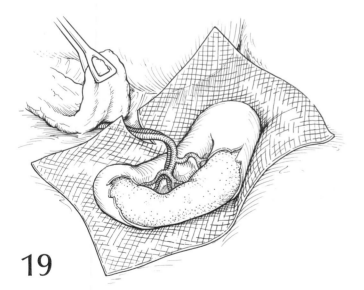

20 A window is fashioned in the mesh to accommodate the splenic artery and vein, and the spleen is enveloped by approximating the free edges of the mesh with polyglycolic acid sutures.

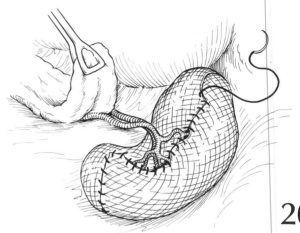

20

MODIFICATION OF OPEN TECHNIQUE FOR GIANT SPLEEN AND THE MANAGEMENT OF SPLENIC ADHESIONS

Providing they are mobile, huge spleens such as are found in myelofibrosis, chronic granulocytic leukaemia and the tropical splenomegalies are often easier to remove than small ones.

Incision

21 An oblique incision is made in the line of the ninth rib from the costal margin to the right iliac fossa. The incision may have to be very long to permit mobilization and delivery of the spleen.

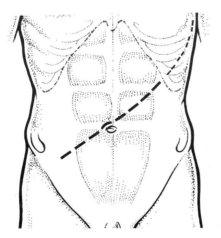

21

Mobilization

22 The abdominal section of the incision is opened and the surface of the spleen exposed. If the spleen is mobile and there are no adhesions the organ can usually be easily delivered from the abdomen because all the ligaments have been stretched. The technique of removal is then essentially the same as that already described for elective removal of a normal sized spleen.

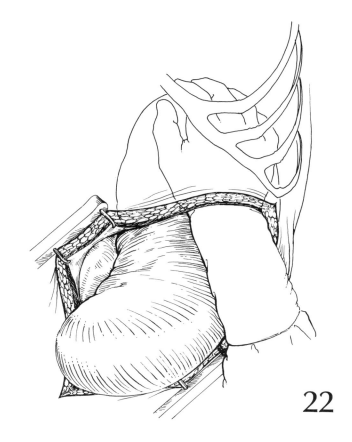

22

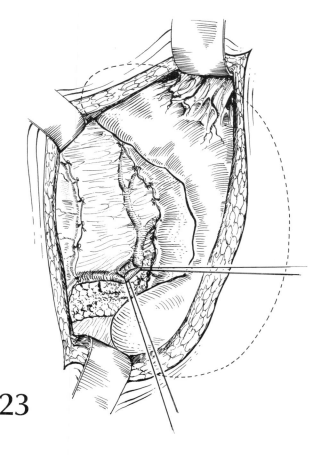

23

Management of splenic adhesions

Problems arise when the spleen is covered with vascular adhesions connecting it to the diaphragm and parietal peritoneum. In such circumstances the surgeon should not try to deliver the organ from the abdomen nor to break down the adhesions by blunt dissection.

23 The first step is to divide the gastrosplenic ligament, enter the lesser sac and expose the splenic artery at the upper border of the pancreas. The artery should be tied in continuity at the apex of one of its convolutions with strong linen thread ligatures (2 gauge) passed round it on an aneurysm needle.

24 The adhesions are then carefully assessed. If they are few and can be divided easily by electrocoagulation, laser, or between clamps under direct vision and without opening the chest, it is permissible to proceed.

If, however, there are many adhesions and they are thick and vascular, the incision should be extended, the costal margin divided, and the thorax opened through the bed of the ninth rib. The diaphragm is divided as far as is necessary to allow good access to the adhesions. The adhesions are divided and ligated individually until the lienorenal ligament is reached. Thereafter the operation proceeds as described above for elective splenectomy.

If such thick vascular adhesions are found at laparoscopic surgery they may be divided with diathermy scissors under vision. If this is difficult or the operative view poor, conversion to open surgery is indicated.

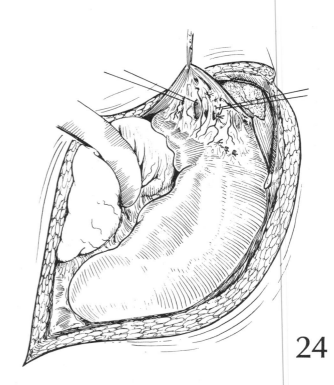

24

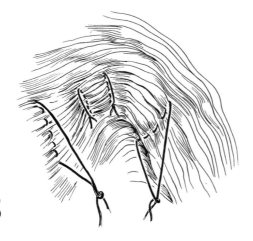

25

25 When a giant spleen with multiple adhesions is removed the surgeon may occasionally be left with a huge bed consisting of a large floppy diaphragm covered with raw oozing areas. This situation can be difficult to deal with and is virtually never completely controllable by diathermy coagulation, suction drains or haemostatic gauze. The most effective technique to control oozing is plication of the diaphragm with a series of firmly tied parallel 0 polyglactin sutures inserted at 5-cm intervals until bleeding is controlled.

Postoperative care

Most patients have an uncomplicated postoperative course following splenectomy or partial splenectomy. Suction drainage from the splenic bed usually diminishes to the point where the drains can be removed on the second postoperative day. A nasogastric tube is passed if the rare complication of acute dilatation occurs.

Intravenous infusion of crystalloids to maintain hydration is usually necessary for about 48 h and nasogastric suction can be discontinued after 24 h unless aspirates remain high. Skin sutures can be removed on the seventh day. Thrombocytopenic patients may develop considerable bruising of the skin around the wound, but this is usually of little consequence and resolves spontaneously. The thrombocytosis that follows splenectomy is no cause for alarm although, if the count goes above 1 million, it is reasonable to give aspirin by mouth until the count falls. Many patients develop some effusion and collapse of the left lower lobe of the lung which usually responds to physiotherapy.

It is now recognized that, even in adults, there is an increased risk of late systemic infection following splenectomy. Prophylaxis consists of vaccination against *Streptococcus pneumoniae* (and probably against *Haemophilus influenzae* type b and meningococcal strains A and C) as soon as is practicable after operation. Amoxycillin (250 mg daily) or phenoxymethyl penicillin (250 mg twice daily) is advisable although opinions are divided as to whether this should be prescribed for life or for periods of up to 5 years. Post-splenectomy patients are advised to seek medical advice promptly whenever infection is contracted or seems likely, and should avoid areas where malaria is endemic. The risks of overwhelming post-splenectomy infection are particularly high in children and young adults.

References

1. Singer DB. Post splenectomy sepsis. In: Rosenberg HS, Bolande RP, eds. *Perspectives in Pediatric Pathology*. Vol. 1. Chicago: Year Book Medical Publishers, 1973: 285–311.

2. Robinette CD, Fraumeni JF. Splenectomy and subsequent mortality in veterans of the 1939–45 war. *Lancet* 1977; 2: 127–9.

3. Shandling B. Splenectomy for trauma, a second look. *Arch Surg* 1976; 3: 1325–6.

4. Redmond HP, Redmond JM, Rooney BP, Duignan JP, Bouchier-Hayes DJ. Surgical anatomy of the human spleen. *Br J Surg* 1989; 76: 198–201.

Anatomy of the biliary tract

Sarah Cheslyn-Curtis MS, FRCS, FRCS(Gen)
Consultant Surgeon, Luton and Dunstable Hospital, Luton, UK

To operate safely on the biliary tree, the surgeon must have a thorough knowledge of biliary anatomy and its variations. Many intraoperative and postoperative complications occur as a result of inadequate exposure and misinterpretation of the anatomy, or because of lack of awareness of the anatomical variations that might be encountered.

The incidence of bile duct and vascular injuries during laparoscopic cholecystectomy has been higher than following open cholecystectomy. The increased frequency of these serious complications, which often have long-term morbidity and occasional mortality, may be due to inadequate training and limited experience with the laparoscopic technique. Alternatively, laparoscopic procedures may require a greater understanding of the anatomy than open operation. Laparoscopy provides a magnified image of the biliary region, but the image is two-dimensional, the field of view reduced and the surgeon is unable to palpate structures with his hands. It is particularly important for the laparoscopic surgeon to have a thorough knowledge of biliary anatomy and sufficient training to be able to appreciate the anatomy as viewed through a laparoscope.

Biliary tree

Intrahepatic biliary anatomy

1 The liver is divided into two major portions (right and left livers) and a dorsal lobe (caudate lobe or segment I). The main scissura dividing the right and left livers passes from the gallbladder fossa posteriorly to the inferior vena cava (*see* chapter on pp. 1–4). The intrahepatic ducts run throughout the liver as part of the portal triads with a tributary of the portal vein and a branch of the hepatic artery[1].

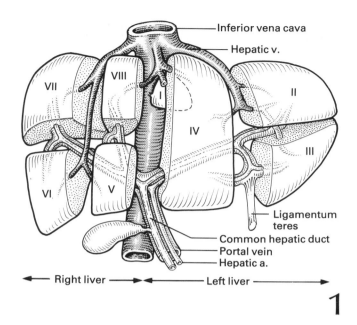

1

Hepatic ducts

The right hepatic duct drains the right liver. This duct is short and is formed by the union of the anterior and posterior sectoral ducts. The anterior sectoral duct drains segments V and VIII and has a vertical course, whereas the posterior sectoral duct drains segments VI and VII and has a more horizontal course. Surgical access to the right hepatic duct away from the hilus is difficult, but it can be approached through the gallbladder fossa.

2 The left hepatic duct drains the left liver which includes the lateral segment (segments II and III) and the quadrate lobe (segment IV). Unlike the right hepatic duct, the left hepatic duct is long and largely extrahepatic. It traverses superficially beneath the left liver at the base of the quadrate lobe in a groove between the quadrate and caudate lobes. The importance of this anatomical position is that the left duct can be exposed relatively easily along it course. The caudate lobe (segment I) usually drains by 2–3 ducts into both the right and left hepatic ducts.

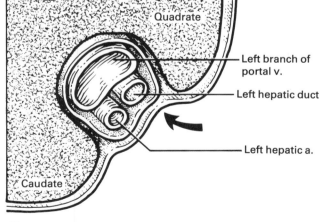

2

Confluence

3a,b The confluence of the right and left hepatic ducts overlies the right branch of the portal vein and is separated from the posterior aspect of the quadrate lobe of the liver (segment IV) by the hilar plate. The plate system is an important fascial layer formed by the fusion of connective tissue around the hepatic ducts and vessels within Glisson's capsule. The quadrate lobe may be extensively mobilized to reveal the confluence and left hepatic duct by incising the hilar plate and extending the incision into the umbilical fissure and gallbladder fossa. The technique of lowering the hilar plate is used to display dilated bile ducts above a bile duct stricture or hilar cholangiocarcinoma so that hepatojejunostomy can be performed.

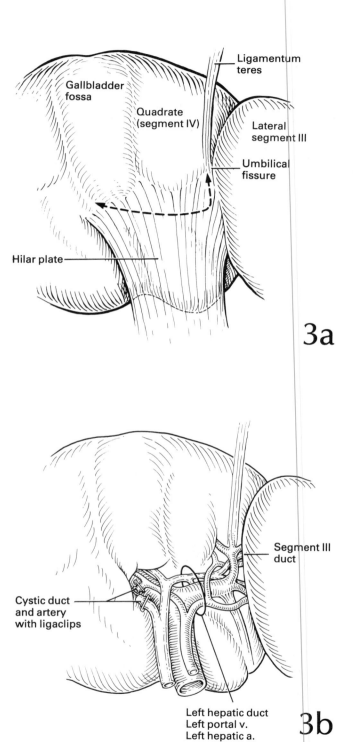

4 If access to the confluence is not possible because of tumour, a segment III intrahepatic bypass can be performed using a Roux loop of jejunum. The segment III duct is approached by tracing the ligamentum teres (obliterated umbilical vein) to its base where it connects to the portal vein. The segment III duct is exposed by a limited hepatotomy to the left of the base of the ligamentum teres and lies superficial to the left branch of the portal vein.

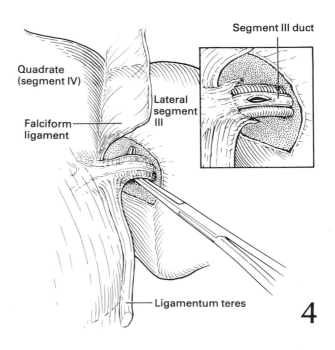

4

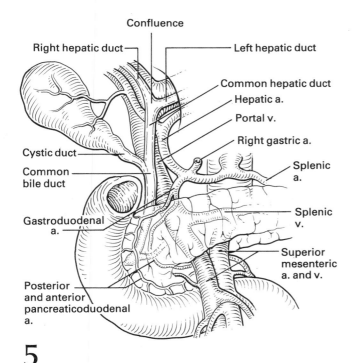

5

Extrahepatic biliary anatomy

5 The bile duct is divided in two by the cystic duct. The common hepatic duct is formed by the union of the right and left hepatic ducts at the confluence and is joined by the cystic duct to form the common bile duct. The common bile duct has supraduodenal and retropancreatic portions. The common hepatic duct and supraduodenal portion of the common bile duct run in the free edge of the lesser omentum lying anterior to the portal vein with the hepatic artery on the left. The retropancreatic duct passes through a groove or tunnel in the pancreas and runs parallel to the pancreatic duct for about 2 cm before reaching the second part of the duodenum. In 70–85% of patients these ducts have a common opening into the duodenum.

Gallbladder and cystic duct

The gallbladder acts as a reservoir and lies on the undersurface of the right lobe of the liver within the cystic fossa. It is sometimes deeply embedded in the liver (intrahepatic) and, occasionally, is suspended on a mesentery which predisposes to torsion. The gallbladder varies in size and has a neck, body and fundus. A stone impacted in the neck of the gallbladder creates a Hartmann's pouch which may obscure and become adherent to the bile duct making dissection hazardous during cholecystectomy. The fundus usually reaches the free edge of the liver.

6a–c

The cystic duct (1–3 mm in diameter) arises from the neck of the gallbladder and is of variable length. It joins the common hepatic duct supraduodenally in 75–80% of cases. In some patients the cystic duct has a low insertion into the common hepatic duct and these ducts may be bound together by connective tissue and pass retroduodenally or retropancreatic for a variable length before they unite. In a small number of subjects the cystic duct may spiral around the bile duct to enter it on the left side.

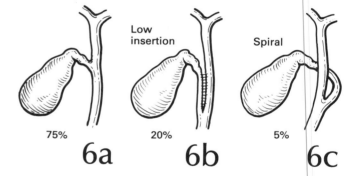

Low insertion   Spiral

75%   20%   5%

6a   6b   6c

Blood, lymphatic and nerve supply

Arterial

7 The blood supply of the bile duct can be divided into three segments:

(1) The hilar region has a rich supply from the right and left hepatic arteries.

(2) The main blood supply (60%) to the supraduodenal duct comes from below from various arteries, some 38% comes from above via the hepatic and cystic artery and only 2% comes from the hepatic artery lying to the left of the bile duct[2]. The supraduodenal portion is mostly supplied by axial arteries which run along the bile duct from above and below. On average there are eight small axial arteries which, if damaged (as when dissecting too close to the bile duct or as a result of flush ligation of the cystic duct with the bile duct), may result in ischaemia and subsequent stricture formation.

(3) The retropancreatic portion is surrounded by a rich network derived from the posterior pancreaticoduodenal artery.

The cystic artery arises from the right hepatic artery to the right of the hepatic duct within Calot's triangle and usually divides into anterior and posterior branches before reaching the gallbladder wall. The right hepatic artery is vulnerable during cholecystectomy.

Venous

The cystic vein, when present, runs parallel to the cystic artery and enters the right branch of the portal vein. Small veins from the bed of the gallbladder pass directly into the liver parenchyma. A venous plexus surrounds the hepatic and common bile ducts and drains into the liver, portal vein and posterior superior pancreaticoduodenal vein.

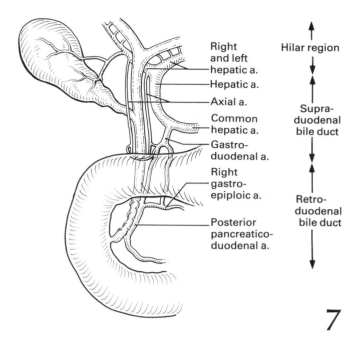

Right and left hepatic a.
Hepatic a.
Axial a.
Common hepatic a.
Gastro-duodenal a.
Right gastro-epiploic a.
Posterior pancreatico-duodenal a.

Hilar region
Supra-duodenal bile duct
Retro-duodenal bile duct

7

Lymphatics

8 Lymph drains from the liver, bile ducts and gallbladder to three chains of lymph nodes in the hepatoduodenal ligament (lesser omentum) as follows:

(1) Along the hepatic arteries which drain to the coeliac lymph nodes.

(2) Along the common bile duct which drains to the suprapyloric and subpyloric and the pancreatic or pancreaticoduodenal nodes which, in turn, drain to the coeliac nodes.

(3) To the gastric lymph nodes along the lesser curvature of the stomach and on to the coeliac nodes.

Lymph from the lower end of the common bile duct and papilla drains via the nodes in the pancreatic head to the mesenteric nodes. The cystic lymph node lies in Calot's triangle closely applied to the gallbladder neck or cystic duct and artery.

Nerves

The gallbladder and bile ducts have a rich nerve supply. The parasympathetic supply is from the vagus; the anterior vagus supplies the liver, gallbladder and bile ducts while the posterior vagus supplies the terminal segment of the bile duct. The sympathetic nerve fibres arise mainly from the coeliac plexus around the coeliac axis and accompany the hepatic and gastroduodenal arteries. Motility of the gallbladder and sphincter muscle tone is effected partly by the autonomic nervous system and partly by hormonal agents such as cholecystokinin. Sympathetic stimulation produces relaxation and parasympathetic stimulation causes contraction of the gallbladder. The cystic and common bile ducts do not undergo peristalsis, having no appreciable muscle coat. Pain is felt in response to traction or dilatation of the gallbladder and bile ducts via the autonomic nerves and phrenic nerve.

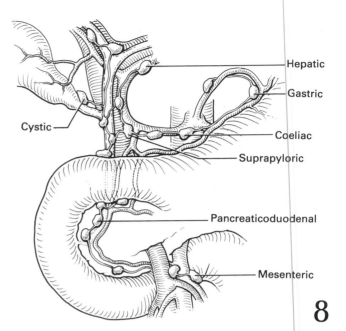

8

Anomalous anatomy of the biliary tract

There are wide anatomical variations in the extrahepatic biliary tree and adjacent hepatic artery and portal venous structures.

Ductal anomalies

9 The important ductal anaomalies are nearly all related to the manner of confluence of the right and left hepatic ducts and of the cystic duct with the common hepatic duct. The confluence is 'typical' in 57% of cases in that the right posterior and right anterior sectoral ducts join to form the short right hepatic duct which joins the left hepatic duct to become the common hepatic duct. A triple confluence may exist or the confluence may be absent. Other variations include the insertion of the right anterior or posterior sectoral duct separately into the common hepatic duct or left hepatic duct. If the right hepatic duct is absent the right posterior sectoral duct may drain into the cystic duct. These variants in right ductal anatomy have obvious implications for cholecystectomy.

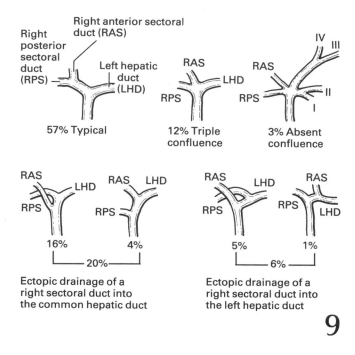

Ectopic drainage of a right sectoral duct into the common hepatic duct

Ectopic drainage of a right sectoral duct into the left hepatic duct

9

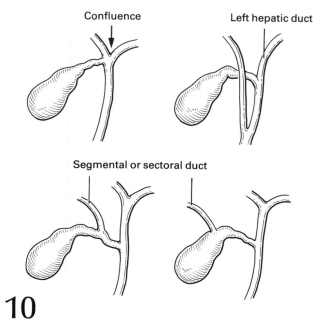

10 Several anomalies of drainage of the intrahepatic ducts and the cystic duct or gallbladder also exist. The cystic duct may drain into the confluence or left hepatic duct (absent confluence). A duct from the right liver (posterior sectoral or segmental duct) may drain anomalously into the cystic duct, the neck or body of the gallbladder. Cystohepatic ducts are ducts of the right liver which drain into the gallbladder or cystic duct. They may drain a subsegment, segment, sector or, rarely, the whole of the right liver. These ducts are particularly vulnerable during cholecystectomy and the seriousness of the injury depends on the extent of the liver that the damaged duct drains.

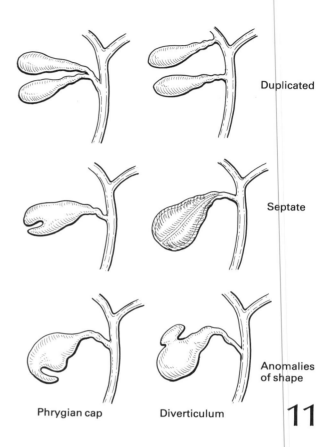

Duplicated

Septate

Anomalies
of shape

Phrygian cap   Diverticulum   11

Gallbladder anomalies

11 Anomalies of the gallbladder are interesting but rare. The gallbladder may be absent, bilobed with a single cystic duct and two fundi, duplicated with two cystic ducts and two fundi, septate, or have a congenital diverticulum. The cystic duct can be double.

Vascular anomalies

The important variations in vascular anatomy are the relationship of the hepatic arteries to the bile duct and portal vein, the variable origin of the hepatic arteries and the multiple cystic artery variations.

12 The most common configuration is for the right hepatic artery to pass posterior to the bile duct, but in 24% of patients it passes anteriorly. In at least 10–12% of patients the right hepatic artery (and occasionally the common hepatic artery) arises from the superior mesenteric artery and runs posterolateral to the bile duct in the free edge of the lesser omentum or in the groove between the bile duct and portal vein.

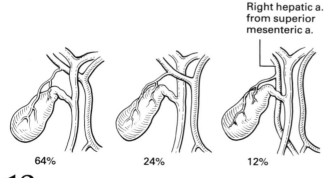

Right hepatic a.
from superior
mesenteric a.

64%   24%   12%

12

13 The right hepatic artery runs anterior to the portal vein in 91% of patients and posterior to the portal vein in 9%.

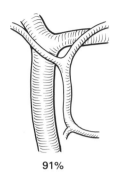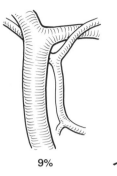

91%   9%   **13**

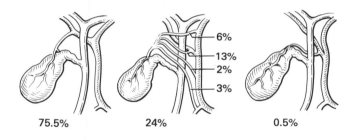

75.5%   24%   0.5%

14

14 The cystic artery typically arises from the right hepatic artery to the right of the bile duct in Calot's triangle. When the cystic artery arises to the left of the bile duct it almost always passes anterior, and only rarely passes posterior, to the bile duct. The cystic artery is occasionally double.

References

1. Couinaud C. *Le Foie. Etudes Anatomiques and Chirurgicales*. Paris: Masson, 1957.

2. Northover JMA, Terblanche J. A new look at the arterial supply of the bile duct in man and its surgical implications. *Br J Surg* 1979; 66: 379–84.

Preoperative assessment and preparation for biliary tract surgery

Attila Nakeeb MD
Surgical Resident, Department of Surgery, The Johns Hopkins Medical Institutions, Baltimore, Maryland, USA

Henry A Pitt MD
Professor and Vice Chairman, Department of Surgery, The Johns Hopkins Medical Institutions, Baltimore, Maryland, USA

Historically, the surgical treatment of biliary tract diseases has been associated with significant morbidity and mortality. This increased risk is often related to biliary tract obstruction, and a direct correlation between operative mortality and the degree of jaundice has been documented (*Table 1*). In recent years a better understanding of the pathophysiology of obstructive jaundice has led to advances in preoperative management that have resulted in improved operative survival[1]. This chapter will briefly review the pathophysiology of obstructive jaundice, the preoperative assessment of these patients, and the important factors in the preparation for surgery on the biliary tract.

Table 1 Correlation of serum bilirubin levels with postoperative mortality

Bilirubin (mg/dl)	Patients (no.)	Mortality (%)
< 1.5	61	3.3
1.5–5	40	2.5
5–10	23	8.7
10–20	22	18.2*
> 20	9	33.3*

Modified from Pitt et al. Am J Surg 1981; 141: 66.
*$p < 0.01$ vs patients with bilirubin < 5 mg/dl ≡ 85.5 µmol/l.

Pathophysiology of jaundice

Biliary obstruction produces local effects on the bile duct that lead to derangement of hepatic function and, ultimately, to widespread systemic effects. Patients who are jaundiced are at increased risk for developing hepatic dysfunction, renal failure, cardiovascular impairment, bleeding problems, infections, wound complications and nutritional deficits. Each of these abnormalities will be discussed in more detail.

Hepatobiliary dysfunction

The biliary system normally has a low pressure. In patients with complete or partial biliary obstruction the biliary pressure rises and the secretory, metabolic and synthetic functions of hepatocytes are altered. Raised biliary pressure results in diminished bile secretion. Similarly, jaundiced patients have a decreased capacity to excrete drugs, such as antibiotics, that are normally secreted into bile. The increased concentration of bile acids associated with obstructive jaundice results in inhibition of the hepatic cytochrome P450 enzymes and, therefore, in a decrease in the rate of oxidative metabolism in the liver. The synthetic function of the hepatocyte is also decreased with obstructive jaundice, as evidenced by decreased plasma levels of albumin, clotting factors and secretory immunoglobulins.

Renal failure

The association between jaundice and postoperative renal failure has been known for many years[1,2]. The incidence of postoperative acute renal failure in jaundiced patients is approximately 10%. Moreover, the mortality rate in jaundiced patients developing renal failure has been reported to be as high as 75%. Endotoxins probably play a significant role in the renal failure associated with jaundice. They are present in the peripheral blood of approximately 50% of patients with obstructive jaundice, probably because of a lack of bile salts in the gut lumen that normally prevent absorption of endotoxins and inhibit anaerobic bacterial growth. Endotoxin causes renal vasoconstriction, redistribution of renal blood flow away from the cortex, and activation of complement, macrophages, leukocytes and platelets. As a result, glomerular and peritubular fibrin is deposited. This factor, in combination with reduced renal cortical blood flow, results in the tubular and cortical necrosis observed in jaundiced patients with renal failure.

Cardiovascular impairment

In addition to the hepatic dysfunction and increased propensity to develop renal failure, obstructive jaundice is known to cause severe haemodynamic disturbances including (1) decreased cardiac contractility, (2) reduced left ventricular pressures, and (3) impaired response to β agonist drugs such as isoprenaline (isoproteranol) and noradrenaline[1,2]. The effect of obstructive jaundice on the peripheral vasculature is to cause a decrease in total peripheral resistance. In addition to the direct effects on the heart and peripheral vasculature, jaundice results in hypovolaemia. The increased serum levels of bile acids associated with obstructive jaundice have both a diuretic and natriuretic effect on the kidney. The combination of hyovolaemia, depressed cardiac function, and decreased total peripheral resistance probably accounts for the susceptibility of jaundiced patients to develop shock in the perioperative period.

Coagulation

Disturbances of blood coagulation are also commonly present in jaundiced patients[1]. The most frequently observed clotting defect in patients with biliary obstruction is prolongation of the prothrombin time. This defect results from impaired vitamin K absorption from the gut, secondary to a lack of intestinal bile. This coagulopathy is usually reversible by parenteral administration of vitamin K. Moreover, endotoxin release in jaundiced patients results in a low-grade disseminated intravascular coagulation with increased fibrin degradation products. Jaundiced patients with circulating endotoxin or increased levels of fibrin degradation product before surgery are at increased risk of developing haemorrhagic complications. In addition to problems with endotoxaemia, cirrhotic patients may have even more complicated clotting abnormalities such as problems with thrombocytopenia from hypersplenism and fibrinolysis.

Immune system

Surgery in the jaundiced patient is associated with a significant rate of septic complications[1]. Jaundiced patients have a number of defects in cellular immunity that make them more prone to infection. Several authors have demonstrated impaired T cell proliferation, decreased neutrophil chemotaxis, defective bacterial phagocytosis and altered delayed hypersensitivity in these patients. The ability of hepatic Kupffer cells to clear bacteria and endotoxin from the circulation is also reduced in obstructive jaundice. In addition, the absence of bile from the intestinal tract plays a role in the infectious complications seen in patients with obstructive jaundice. Bacterial translocation from the gut has been shown to be increased in the setting of bile duct obstruction. Obstruction causes a disruption of the enterohepatic circulation and results in the loss of the emulsifying anti-endotoxin effect of bile acids. A larger pool of endotoxin is therefore available within the intestine for absorption into the portal circulation. The combination of a lack of bile in the intestine and the impairment of cellular immunity and reticuloendothelial cell function is probably responsible for the observed increase in septic and infectious complications in jaundiced patients.

Wound healing

Delayed wound healing and a high incidence of wound dehiscence and incisional hernias have been observed in patients undergoing surgery for the relief of obstructive jaundice[1]. Patients with bile duct obstruction have decreased activity of the enzyme propylhydroxylase in their skin. Propylhydroxylase is necessary for the incorporation of proline amino acid residues into collagen. Thus, the rate of collagen formation is decreased and wound strength is diminished. An increased incidence of wound infection also contributes to the frequent wound problems observed in these patients.

Nutrition

Other problems that face jaundiced patients are anorexia, weight loss and resultant malnutrition[1]. Appetite is adversely influenced by the lack of bile salts in the intestinal tract. In addition, patients with pancreatic or periampullary malignant lesions may have partial duodenal obstruction or abnormal gastric emptying, perhaps secondary to tumour infiltration of the coeliac nerve plexus. Patients with pancreatic or periampullary tumours may also have pancreatic endocrine and exocrine insufficiency. This latter problem may further compound other nutritional defects that, in turn, may multiply the immune deficits of the jaundiced patient.

Preoperative assessment

When a patient presents with jaundice, the objective is to identify any potentially treatable causes. The most important distinction is whether the jaundice is caused by intrahepatic cholestasis or extraheaptic obstruction. Fortunately, the differentiation between 'medical' and 'surgical' jaundice can be made relatively easily with a careful history, physical examination, review of serum biochemistry and radiological evaluation[1]. An algorithm for the evaluation of the jaundiced patient is shown in *Figure 1*. The following discussion will present an approach to the jaundiced patient that will allow an accurate diagnosis to be made without subjecting the patient to needless risk, discomfort or expense.

Clinical

The first and most important step in the preparation of the patient who is to undergo biliary tract surgery is to obtain a careful history. Important historical points to consider include occupational exposure, travel history or contact with anyone who has had hepatitis or jaundice. Similarly, any exposure to transfusions, blood, tattoos or body fluids should be noted. The patient also needs to be questioned about drug ingestion, with special attention to alcohol and other hepatotoxins. A family history with respect to haemolytic anaemias or congenital hyperbilirubinaemias may also be helpful. Previous surgery, especially biliary, raises the suspicion of a benign biliary stricture or retained common duct stones. Hepatitis following transfusion or drug toxicity may also appear after a surgical procedure.

In the jaundiced patient the time of onset and progression should be determined and can often give a clue to the diagnosis. Viral hepatitis might be suspected if the jaundice presented with a rapid onset and was associated with nausea and anorexia. A history of biliary colic, on the other hand, suggests choledocholithiasis. Pancreatic cancer is more likely to present with progressive, painless jaundice and weight loss. A history of fever, chills and upper abdominal pain in addition to jaundice (Charcot's triad) is suggestive of cholangitis, which occurs more often in patients with choledocholithiasis than in those with malignant obstruction. Sepsis in patients with perihilar cholangiocarcinoma, underlying cirrhosis, liver abscesses and, especially, renal failure is associated with a very high perioperative mortality[3].

The colour of the patient's urine and stool should also be carefully noted. Total obstruction of the biliary tract results in acholic pale stools, increased amounts of

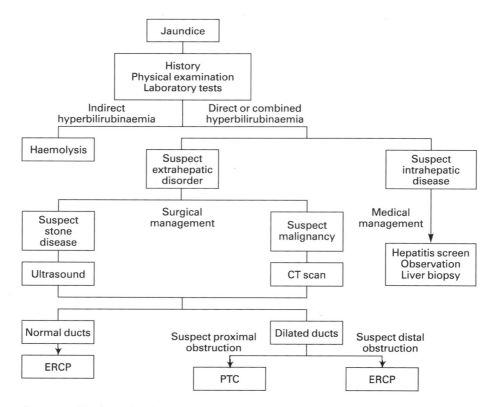

Figure 1   Algorithm for the management of the jaundiced patient. Reprinted with permission from Nakeeb and Pitt[1].

bilirubin in the urine, and absence of urine urobilinogen. If the urine is positive for bilirubin, then serum levels of conjugated bilirubin are usually raised. Stools that are black or silver suggest the presence of blood, which may indicate a periampullary lesion that is both bleeding and obstructing the distal bile duct.

On physical examination the abdomen should be carefully inspected, auscultated, percussed and palpated. A small liver may be discovered in patients with severe cirrhosis or hepatitis, a tender liver edge may be observed in those with hepatitis, congestive heart failure or alcoholic hepatitis, while a palpable, nontender gallbladder may be seen in patients with pancreatic or periampullary carcinoma (Courvoisier's sign). A tender gallbladder, on the other hand, may be palpated in cases of choledocholithiasis with associated cholecystitis (Murphy's sign). The stigmata of cirrhosis, such as ascites, spider naevi or periumbilical venous enlargement, should also be noted.

Biochemical assessment

In addition to the history and physical examination, biochemical evaluation is an integral part of the initial examination of the patient with biliary tract disease. The level of bilirubin can indicate the severity of the disease process, and bilirubin levels can be used to follow disease progression. The routine laboratory tests that should be performed on all jaundiced patients include direct (conjugated) and indirect (unconjugated) bilirubin, alkaline phosphatase, serum transaminases, albumin and amylase determinations. The urine also should be tested for bilirubin and urobilinogen, and coagulation studies should be performed.

Patients with haemolysis have an increase in the indirect (unconjugated) fraction of bilirubin, whereas the direct (conjugated) bilirubin level is normal (*Table 2*). The total bilirubin concentration in haemolysis rarely exceeds 4–5 mg/dl (68–85 µmol/l). Since unconjugated bilirubin is not excreted by the kidney, bilirubin is absent in the urine of patients with haemolysis.. If haemolysis is suspected, further laboratory tests should include a complete blood count, a blood smear, reticulocyte count, erythrocyte fragility test and a

Coombs test. The amino acid transaminases aspartate aminotransferase (AST) and alanine aminotransferase (ALT) are serum markers for hepatocyte damage. AST is found in liver, heart, kidney, skeletal muscle and brain tissue while ALT is found predominantly within hepatocytes, making it more specific for identifying liver injury.

Broad derangements of liver function tests are seen in patients with hepatic parenchymal disease (*Table 2*). The concentrations of both conjugated and unconjugated fractions of bilirubin are increased. With the increased level of conjugated bilirubin in the serum, bilirubinuria develops. In patients with acute hepatitis, serum levels of ALT and AST are markedly increased while alkaline phosphatase and bilirubin levels may be only slightly raised, and the serum amylase level is usually normal. The serum transaminases are also raised in alcoholic liver disease, with serum AST levels usually being more than twice the serum ALT levels. In the cirrhotic patient, serum bilirubin levels increase in proportion to the degree of parenchymal damage. Albumin and the coagulation factors V, VII, IX, X, prothrombin, and fibrinogen are all synthesized in the liver. The measurement of serum albumin levels and prothrombin time may therefore be helpful in assessing the degree of parenchymal liver injury.

In extrahepatic obstruction the fraction of direct bilirubin is significantly raised and the indirect bilirubin concentration is also moderately increased (*Table 2*). The highest elevations of bilirubin levels are usually found in patients with malignant extrahepatic obstruction where bilirubin levels may exceed 20 mg/dl (342 µmol/l). With malignant obstruction the alkaline phosphatase level is also increased to the same degree. Other liver function tests are usually normal or only slightly raised, and the amylase concentration is usually normal. Stones in the common bile duct, on the other hand, rarely cause an increase in the bilirubin level of more than 10–12 mg/dl (171–205 µmol/l). With choledocholithiasis, alkaline phosphatase levels are also usually increased to a moderate degree. As a gallstone passes through and momentarily obstructs the ampulla of Vater, serum transaminase levels may rise transiently. In this setting, hyperamylasaemia may also develop. If longstanding partial extrahepatic obstruction is present,

Table 2 Laboratory tests in the diagnosis of hepatobiliary disease

| Cause of jaundice | Serum bilirubin | | Serum alkaline phosphatase | Serum transaminases | Urine | |
	Conjugated	Unconjugated			Bilirubin	Urobilinogen
Haemolysis	↔	↑↑↑	↔	↔	0	↑↑
Hepatocellular dysfunction	↑↑	↑↑	↑	↑↑↑	↑↑	↑
Intrahepatic cholestasis	↑↑↑	↑↑	↑↑	↑↑	↑↑↑	0 or ↓
Extrahepatic obstruction	↑↑↑	↑↑	↑↑↑	↑	↑↑↑	0 or ↓

0, none; ↓, decreased; ↔, no change; ↑, mild elevation; ↑↑, moderate elevation; ↑↑↑, marked elevation.

liver damage and fibrosis can occur, resulting in a combined intrahepatic and extrahepatic biochemical profile.

Serum alkaline phosphatase is often a more sensitive indicator of obstruction, and levels may be increased when the bilirubin level is normal. This circumstance occurs most commonly with incomplete or partial obstruction. However, increased levels of alkaline phosphatase activity may also result from bone disease. If this possibility is suspected, serum 5'-nucleotidase or serum γ-glutamyl transpeptidase levels should be measured, since they both parallel changes in alkaline phosphatase from a hepatobiliary source and are not found in bone.

Radiological evaluation

The goals of the radiological evaluation of the jaundiced patient include (1) the confirmation of clinically suspected biliary obstruction by the demonstration of a dilated biliary tree, (2) the identification of the level and cause of extrahepatic biliary obstruction, (3) the selection of patients in whom surgical or interventional radiological or endoscopic treatment is indicated, and (4) the use of tests in a cost effective manner.

Abdominal plain radiographs

The likelihood of a plain abdominal radiograph providing diagnostic information in the patient with biliary obstruction is low. Abdominal radiography may reveal gallstones, a calcified gallbladder wall, or the outline of a distended gallbladder. Approximately 15–20% of gallstones are radio-opaque and can be visualized by radiography. However, cholangiography will still be necessary to determine whether common duct stones are present and to rule out other causes of jaundice such as hepatic parenchymal disease or an obstructing tumour. Plain radiographs may also be diagnostic of a spontaneous biliary fistula when air is present in the biliary tree or of emphysematous cholecystitis when air is noted in the gallbladder lumen or wall.

Ultrasonography

Ultrasonography (US) is commonly performed as the initial screening procedure in patients with biliary tract disease. It is non-invasive, inexpensive and widely available. Dilated intrahepatic bile ducts are a reliable sign of biliary obstruction, and most series report that ultrasonography can detect dilatation of the intrahepatic or proximal extrahepatic bile ducts with at least an 80% accuracy rate[1]. The normal extrahepatic bile duct diameter is less than 10 mm and normal intrahepatic ducts are less than 4 mm in diameter. Dilated ducts are easily detectable by ultrasonography and can often be identified before the onset of clinical jaundice.

Failure of ultrasonography to detect dilated ducts usually indicates a hepatic parenchymal source of jaundice. In this setting continued observation, screening tests for hepatitis, or liver biopsy may be indicated. However, the absence of ductal dilatation does not entirely rule out extrahepatic obstruction. In intermittent or partial obstruction the biliary tree may not be dilated. Likewise, in longstanding obstruction, especially if secondary biliary fibrosis or cirrhosis is present, dilated ducts may not be observed. In cases where extrahepatic obstruction is suspected despite negative ultrasonography findings, direct cholangiography, usually by the endoscopic route, may be indicated.

Ultrasonography can differentiate between extrahepatic obstruction and hepatocellular causes of jaundice in almost all cases[1], but it is limited in its ability to identify the cause and exact location of an obstructing lesion because it cannot visualize the entire common bile duct, especially the distal third, and it is unable to detect consistently stones in the common bile duct. Although ultrasonography is a valuable initial step in the evaluation of the jaundiced patient, further diagnostic studies such as computed tomographic scanning or direct cholangiography are therefore frequently necessary to identify the cause and exact location of the obstruction.

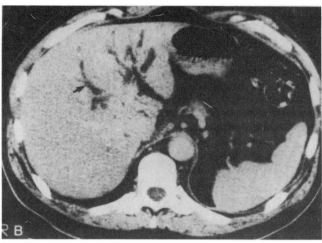

Figure 1(a)   CT scan in a patient with a perihilar cholangiocarci-noma demonstrating dilated intrahepatic ducts. The tumour cannot be differentiated from the liver parenchyma or portal vein in this scan with intravenous contrast medium.

Computed tomography

1a,b Computed tomographic (CT) scanning can also be used to differentiate between intrahepatic disease and non-dilated ducts from extra-hepatic obstruction[1], and it is more than 90% accurate in detecting the presence of ductal dilatation (*Illustration 1a*). The slightly higher success rate than with ultrasonography is because CT scanning provides better definition of anatomical structures and contrast media can be used to enhance delineations (*Illustration 1b*). CT portography or angiography and newer spiral or helical techniques have further improved the accuracy of this investigation in establishing the site and cause of biliary obstruction. In addition, CT scanning, especially with newer spiral techniques, can also provide highly accurate information regarding retroperitoneal extension, vascular invasion and spread to the liver in malignant causes of biliary obstruction.

CT scanning and ultrasonography therefore have similar utility in the diagnosis of biliary ductal dilatation. CT scanning may be the preferred initial screening procedure in obese patients, and most authorities agree that it is slightly more accurate in detecting the nature and anatomical level of obstruction. CT also has the advantage of being able to visualize the pancreas routinely and is therefore probably the screening procedure of choice if a pancreatic or periampullary malignancy is suspected. On the other hand, ultrasonography is less expensive, more widely available, and does not expose the patient to radiation; therefore, it should be performed initially if the clinical history suggests stone disease.

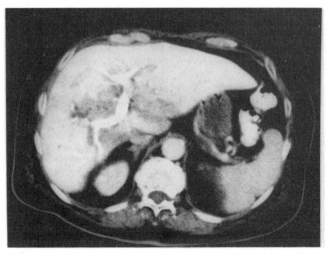

Figure 1(b)   CT angiogram in another patient with a perihilar cholangiocarcinoma. The tumour is clearly demarcated (dark) and the portal venous system is clearly visualized (white).

Magnetic resonance imaging

2a,b The use of magnetic resonance imaging (MRI) in the evaluation of the patient with biliary tract disease is relatively recent and the technique is still undergoing evaluation[1]. MRI is capable of detecting intrahepatic and extrahepatic biliary dilatation, but its sensitivity has not yet been compared with ultrasonography or CT scanning to determine its clinical usefulness. T2-weighted images in the coronal and sagittal planes may also be used to obtain a magnetic resonance cholangiogram. Initial studies suggest that MRI will identify a dilated biliary tree in approximately 85% of patients with obstructive jaundice, with the cause of obstruction being determined in approximately 60% of these patients. A more prominent role for MRI may be in its ability to define venous anatomy and identify the parenchymal extent of perihilar cholangiocarcinomas.

Biliary scintigraphy

Technetium-99[m] labelled iminodiacetic acid derivatives (HIDA, DISIDA, PIPIDA) are injected intravenously, rapidly extracted from the blood and excreted into the bile. These radionuclide scans provide functional information about the patient's ability to excrete radiolabelled substances from the liver into a non-obstructed biliary tree. Biliary scintigraphy is useful in the management of neonatal jaundice, the detection of bile leaks, and the diagnosis of acute cholecystitis. Cholescintigraphy also provides a non-invasive method with which to evaluate the patency and function of biliary-enteric anastomoses and to study the kinetics of bile flow when disordered biliary motility is suspected.

In comparison with ultrasonography, CT scanning and MRI, biliary scintigraphy plays only a limited role in the evaluation of a patient with jaundice[1]. The technique has been used to diagnose common bile duct obstruction. In this setting any appearance of the nucleotide in the gastrointestinal tract indicates patency of bile flow into the duodenum. However, other available non-invasive tests such as ultrasonography or CT scanning have generally been shown to be more accurate and are therefore preferred.

Percutaneous transhepatic cholangiography

Direct cholangiography is indicated if dilated bile ducts are visualized by ultrasonography or CT scanning, or if the clinical suspicion of biliary obstruction remains high despite a negative ultrasonographic or CT scan. Cholangiography may be performed percutaneously or endoscopically. With percutaneous transhepatic cholangiography (PTC) the intrahepatic bile ducts are cannulated with a thin, flexible Chiba needle under radiographic control, and contrast material is injected to

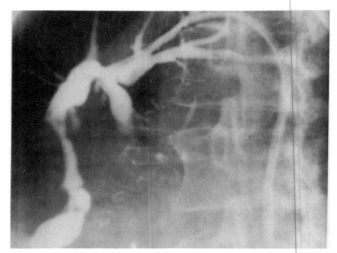

Figure 2(a) Cholangiogram demonstrating a perihilar cholangiocarcinoma.

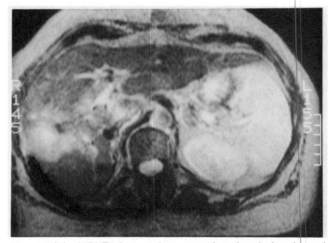

Figure 2(b) MRI T2 image demonstrating the cholangiocarcinoma (white) in an atrophied right lobe in the same patient.

outline the bile ducts. PTC is successful in differentiating intrahepatic from extrahepatic obstruction in up to 96% of cases[1].

Percutaneous cholangiography can define the site of an obstructing lesion in approximately 95% of patients and the cause of the obstruction in nearly 90% of cases (*Table 3*). Diagnostic cholangiography can also be combined with a series of therapeutic manoeuvres such as the insertion of biliary stents or endoprostheses, percutaneous stone extraction, biliary dilatation and cholangioscopy. In addition, cholangiography provides an anatomical road map of the biliary tree that is useful during surgical procedures. Thus, in the management of the jaundiced patient the advantages of PTC are the ability to (1) establish a diagnosis, (2) determine the site and cause of obstruction, and (3) provide specific anatomical detail.

Endoscopic retrograde cholangiography

Endoscopic retrograde cholangiography (ERC) is another option for direct visualization of the biliary system. The technique requires a skilled endoscopist who is capable of cannulating the sphincter of Oddi with a side viewing duodenoscope. The success rate is approximately 85–90% and improves with the experience of the endoscopist. ERC is able to define the site and cause of extrahepatic obstructive jaundice in 75–90% of patients[1]. As with PTC, the complication and mortality rates of ERC are acceptably low. The major complications of the procedure are sepsis, acute pancreatitis and duodenal perforation. Prophylactic antibiotics should be administered before either PTC or ERC if biliary obstruction is suspected.

In the patient with jaundice who has dilated ducts on ultrasonography or CT scanning, direct cholangiography by either PTC or ERC is the next procedure to be used. PTC is less expensive, more widely available, requires less expertise than ERC, and has a higher success rate if dilated ducts are present (*Table 3*). In patients with complete biliary obstruction, PTC provides the surgeon with information about the proximal biliary tree, whereas ERC frequently can only delineate the anatomy of the distal bile duct. PTC is the preferred

Table 3   Comparison of percutaneous transhepatic and Endoscopic cholangiography

Criterion	Transhepatic cholangiography	Endoscopic cholangiography
Success rate	>90% with dilated ducts, 70% with non-dilated ducts	80–90% with both dilated and non-dilated ducts
Identification of cause	90–100%	75–90%
Complications	5% (range 3–10%)	5% (range 2–7%)
Mortality	0.2–0.9%	0.1–0.2%
Expense	Less	More
Skill required	Less	More
Patient selection	Proximal lesions, altered gastroduodenal anatomy, failed endoscopic cholangiography	Distal lesions, pancreatic pathology, coagulopathy, ascites, failed transhepatic cholangiography

procedure for perihilar lesions if therapeutic manipulations such as biliary drainage, balloon dilatation or endoprosthesis placement are necessary. However, percutaneous cholangiography is contraindicated in patients with an incorrectable coagulopathy or with significant ascites.

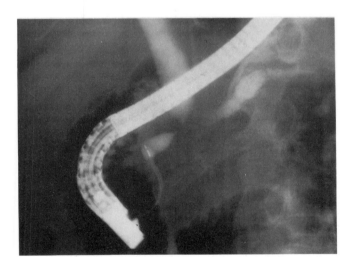

Figure 3   ERCP demonstrating obstruction of the bile duct and the pancreatic duct, 'double duct sign', in a patient with pancreatic cancer.

3 On the other hand, ERC is preferable to PTC in several instances. ERC allows endoscopic visualization of the upper gastrointestinal tract and ampullary region. Lesions can be biopsied and varices can be identified. Moreover, cannulation and injection of the pancreatic duct with contrast medium is often helpful in patients suspected of having pancreatic disease.

In patients with postcholecystectomy symptoms or sphincter of Oddi dyskinesia, ERC enables visualization and cannulation of the ampulla and manometric pressure recordings. As with PTC, therapeutic manipulations such as endoscopic sphincterotomy and stenting may be carried out in conjunction with ERC. However, ERC may be difficult or impossible to perform in patients with ampullary stenosis or in those who have altered gastrointestinal anatomy secondary to previous surgery.

The method of direct cholangiography should therefore be individualized in each case. In certain situations such as totally obstructing proximal lesions, PTC may be the procedure of choice. On the other hand, when non-invasive studies suggest periampullary or pancreatic pathology, ERC provides additional useful information. However, the final choice between these two procedures may ultimately be decided by the expertise of the radiologists and endoscopists at an individual institution.

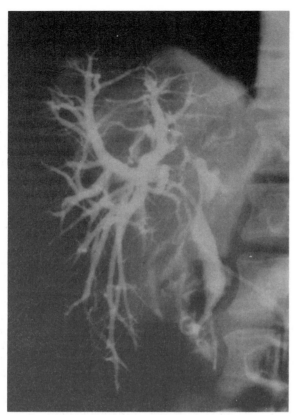

Figure 4(a)   Cholangiogram demonstrating a perihilar cholangiocarcinoma with extensive involvement of the right intrahepatic ducts and the common hepatic duct.

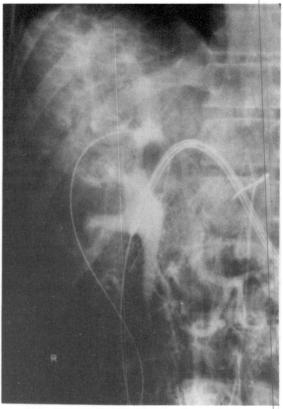

Figure 4(b)   Mesenteric angiogram demonstrating a patent main and left, but occluded right, portal vein branch in the same patient.

Angiography

4a,b Coeliac and superior mesenteric angiography is not a routine investigative procedure in the patient with biliary tract disease. Angiography is performed in cirrhotic patients with bleeding oesophageal varices prior to portosystemic or transhepatic shunts or for therapeutic infusion of intra-arterial vasopressin. In jaundiced patients with active gastrointestinal bleeding, haemobilia can be diagnosed and treated with selective embolization by skilled invasive radiologists. Angiography may also be of benefit in predicting resectability in patients with periampullary or perihilar neoplasms.

With a pancreatic or periampullary neoplasm a normal angiogram indicates that the tumour will be resectable in approximately 75% of patients[1]. If the angiogram suggests vascular encasement, approximately one-third of the tumours will still be resectable. However, if the mesenteric veins are occluded by the tumour, resection is usually not possible. Thus, major vessel occlusion rules out resection, and major vessel encasement makes resection less likely. However, angiography increases hospital cost and exposes the jaundiced patient, who is already at an increased risk of renal failure, to an additional contrast dye load. Angiography should therefore be used selectively.

Endoscopic ultrasonography

Endoscopic ultrasonography (EUS) is a relatively new investigation that may be of some benefit in the evaluation of the patient with biliary tract disease. A potential use is in the assessment of patients with malignant jaundice. Some reports suggest that endoscopic ultrasonography is able to predict resectability accurately in 85–90% of patients with pancreatic cancer[1]. A potential limitation of this technique, however, is that it may not be able to differentiate tumour infiltration of a vessel from simple compression. The addition of a pulsed Doppler may aid in this differentiation.

Advocates of endoscopic ultrasonography also claim that it can differentiate normal lymph nodes from those containing metastatic tumour. Normal lymph nodes are hyperechoic with indistinct margins, whereas lymph nodes containing cancer are hypoechoic with well defined margins. Preliminary studies suggest that endoscopic ultrasonography is 70–75% accurate in diagnosing lymph node metastasis[1]. Advocates further claim that, in patients with pancreatic cancer, it is superior to conventional ultrasonography, CT scanning and angiography in predicting resectability. Although promising, the ultimate role of endoscopic ultrasonography in the evaluation of patients with biliary tract disease must await further analysis.

Laparoscopy

Laparoscopy has recently been proposed as a useful technique for the staging of patients with suspected hepatobiliary and pancreatic tumours. Small liver and peritoneal metastases not detected by CT scanning or ultrasonography can be identified by direct examination. The addition of laparoscopic ultrasonography adds to the ability to assess mesenteric or portal vessel involvement as well as deeper liver lesions. Laparoscopy has been shown to be 65% accurate in predicting resectability (sensitivity 100%, specificity 50%) in patients with a pancreatic or periampullary malignancy without distant metastases. The addition of laparoscopic ultrasonography increased the accuracy of predicting resectability to almost 90%[1]. Thus, the combination of laparoscopy and laparoscopic ultrasonography is a valuable technique in staging patients with suspected pancreatic and periampullary malignancies. Whether it is as effective as the combination of CT scanning and angiography or spiral CT scanning in successfully predicting resectability has yet to be determined. Moreover, concerns about tumour implantation in port sites remains.

Liver biopsy

The application of ultrasonography and CT scanning has made percutaneous liver biopsy unnecessary in most cases of jaundice caused by extrahepatic obstruction. However, numerous indications for liver biopsy remain. If clinical and laboratory data indicate intrahepatic cholestasis and if dilated bile ducts are not present on ultrasonographic or CT scans, a liver biopsy is usually indicated. Liver biopsy may be useful if diagnostic studies are negative or equivocal or if parenchymal disease is suspected with extrahepatic obstruction.

Liver biopsy is relatively safe and reviews of very large series have reported mortality rates of 0.01–0.02% and a serious complication rate of 0.2–0.4%[1]. The most frequent complications of liver biopsy are haemorrhage and bacteraemia. This latter problem occurs most frequently in patients with chronic bile duct infections. Percutaneous liver biopsy is contraindicated if the patient is uncooperative or has an uncorrectable coagulation defect. If the patient has a prolonged prothrombin time or partial thromboplastin time or a diminished platelet count, attempts should be made to correct these abnormalities with vitamin K, fresh frozen plasma or specific component therapy. If the coagulopathy persists and liver biopsy is essential, laparoscopic or open liver biopsy may be indicated.

Assessment of risk

The morbidity associated with surgery in patients with biliary tract obstruction ranges from 30% to 60%, and the operative mortality varies between 2% and 15%[1]. Infectious complications including cholangitis, wound infections and intra-abdominal abscesses are the most common problems. Renal failure is a constant threat in the jaundiced patient. However, circulating endotoxin may also affect cardiac, pulmonary and hepatic function. As a result, multiple organ system failure is the most common cause of death in these patients.

A number of investigators have attempted to identify risk factors that may be associated with a poor prognosis. In various studies the risk factors that have been associated with increased mortality include: age greater than 60 years, malignant biliary obstruction, fever, haematocrit less than 30%, increased white blood cell count, hypoalbuminaemia, and elevations of serum bilirubin, alkaline phosphatase, blood urea nitrogen and creatinine levels. In multivariate analyses the assessment of nutritional status, renal function and underlying sepsis have been shown to be the most important factors in predicting which patients have a high operative risk[1]. Little[4] has devised a 'mortality index' which employs these factors to predict operative mortality in jaundiced patients (*Table 4*).

Table 4   Little's mortality index

Mortality index =

$$0.0016 \times \text{serum creatinine (}\mu\text{mol/l)}$$
$$- 0.0227 \times \text{albumin (g/l)}$$
$$+ 0.0641 \times \text{cholangitis score}$$
$$+ 0.6935$$

Cholangitis score:

0	if afebrile
1	if temperature < 37.5°C
2	if > 37.5°C without rigors
3	if > 37.5°C with rigors, right upper quadrant pain
4	if fever with shock and/or mental changes

An index of 0.4 or greater is associated with a high risk of death.

Preoperative preparation

Patients with obstructive jaundice and those with hepatocellular disease severe enough to cause jaundice are prone to develop many secondary problems. Jaundiced patients are at increased risk for the development of renal failure, gastrointestinal bleeding, infections and wound complications. Cardiac, pulmonary and renal function must be considered in every patient undergoing major abdominal surgery. In addition, special attention must be focused on the nutritional status, coagulability, immune function and presence or absence of biliary sepsis in the jaundiced patient. Patients with chronic liver disease and cirrhosis may also develop ascites and encephalopathy which may require specific treatment.

Cardiopulmonary

In assessing cardiopulmonary status, the patient's age, history of recent myocardial infarction, presence of congestive heart failure, significant valvular aortic stenosis, or a disturbance of normal cardiac rhythm have all been correlated with increased operative risk[1]. Patients with significant cardiac disease should have a complete evaluation before surgery. The examination may include an electrocardiogram, echocardiography, and/or stress testing. Efforts should be made to maximize cardiac function before surgery by treating heart failure and arrhythmias and optimizing fluid status. In addition, patients with severe pulmonary disease may not be candidates for extensive abdominal surgery. Pulmonary function tests which reveal values of forced vital capacity or forced expiratory volume in one second which are less than 50% of predicted indicate significant lung disease, and these patients are at high risk for developing complications. Preoperative pulmonary preparation should include cessation of smoking, instruction in deep breathing and incentive spirometry, and the administration of bronchodilators if indicated. If bronchitis is a problem, oral antibiotics may also be indicated.

Renal

Jaundiced patients, especially those with cirrhosis and cholangitis, are at increased risk of developing renal insufficiency[1,2]. The maintenance of adequate blood volume is extremely important if renal complications are to be avoided. However, fluid management can be quite complex in jaundiced patients. These patients often benefit from invasive haemodynamic monitoring with central venous catheters and, in some cases, pulmonary artery catheters to assist in assessing intravascular volume. Several trials with a small number of patients suggest that the preoperative administration of oral bile salts may be efficacious in preventing the development of postoperative renal dysfunction[1,2]. The perioperative use of mannitol, which results in an osmotic diuresis, and intravenous fluid have also been successful in protecting the kidneys in cases of obstructive jaundice.

Nutrition

Perioperative hyperalimentation has been shown to be of benefit in reducing morbidity and mortality rates associated with surgery in patients with severe malnutrition[1]. Characteristics of patients at risk include (1) serum albumin less than 30 g/l, (2) weight loss of 10–20% over several months, (3) serum transferrin levels of less than 200 mg/dl, (4) anergy to injected skin antigens, and (5) a history of functional impairment. Patients with these characteristics may benefit from nutritional repletion through either parenteral or enteral nutrition prior to surgery. Although most patients with benign biliary problems are adequately nourished, various degrees of malnutrition are frequently present in patients with malignant obstruction. Patients with malignant obstructive jaundice should therefore be evaluated for evidence of malnutrition, and nutritional support should be instituted if necessary.

Coagulation

Patients with obstructive jaundice, cholangitis, or cirrhosis are all prone to excessive intraoperative bleeding. The most common clotting defect in patients with obstructive jaundice is prolongation of the prothrombin time (PT), which is usually reversible by parenteral vitamin K.. Patients with severe jaundice and/or cholangitis may also develop disseminated intravascular coagulation (DIC) which may require infusion of platelets and fresh frozen plasma. Reversal of DIC also requires control of the underlying sepsis, which usually is due to cholangitis and requires biliary drainage and systemic antibiotics. In cirrhotic patients clotting abnormalities may be more complicated and include (1) thrombocytopenia secondary to hypersplenism, (2) prolongation of PT and partial thromboplastin time (PTT), and (3) fibrinolysis. Vitamin K should be administered if the PT is prolonged. If no effect is seen and/or the PTT is also prolonged, fresh frozen plasma should be given. Thrombocytopenia can usually be managed by intraoperative platelet infusions. If the patient has a shortened clot lysis time and hyofibrinogenaemia, ε-aminocaproic acid may be indicated.

Cholangitis

Biliary sepsis has also been identified as a major risk factor in the jaundiced patient[1,3]. Cholangitis may occur with either partial or complete obstruction of the bile duct, resulting in increased intraluminal pressure and infected bile behind the obstruction. Patients with uncomplicated cholangitis can usually be treated conservatively with appropriate antibiotics and fluid resuscitation. A subset of patients, however, will develop 'toxic' cholangitis (cholangitis plus hypotension and mental status changes). Patients with 'toxic' cholangitis have significant mortality when treated with antibiotic therapy alone and therefore require urgent biliary decompression.

Urgent surgical treatment is associated with significant morbidity and mortality. Both percutaneous and endoscopic biliary drainage have been proposed as effective treatment for the 5–10% of patients with 'toxic' cholangitis who are unresponsive to conservative treatment[1]. In patients with 'toxic' cholangitis and perihilar obstruction, percutaneous drainage by a skilled interventional radiologist is the procedure of choice, while in those with 'toxic' cholangitis due to distal obstruction by common duct stones, endoscopic sphincterotomy is the procedure of choice if an expert endoscopist is available.

Antibiotic coverage

Because of the depressed immune system that accompanies jaundice, adequate antibiotic coverage needs to be provided before any manipulation of the biliary tree as well as for the treatment of cholangitis. Under normal conditions, bile, the biliary tree and the liver are sterile. However, biliary stasis, obstruction, biliary-enteric anastomoses and foreign bodies predispose the biliary system to infection. The organisms most commonly isolated from the biliary tree include *Escherichia coli*, *Klebsiella pneumoniae*, enterococcus and, with increasing frequency, the anaerobe *Bacteroides fragilis*. Approximately two-thirds of patients with bactibilia will have Gram-negative aerobes, and 25–30% will have enterococci in their bile. Anaerobes are found in the bile of older patients, those with cholangitis and those with complex biliary problems and indwelling tubes[1].

Four factors must be considered when choosing antibiotics for the jaundiced patient: (1) the antibacterial spectrum of the antibiotic, (2) serum and liver concentrations, (3) biliary excretion and (4) toxicity. For many years the combination of a penicillin and an aminoglycoside has been recommended to cover the Gram-negative aerobes and enterococcus. However, concern about the nephrotoxicity of the aminoglycosides, especially in jaundiced patients, has led to a search for less toxic agents. Options include ureidopenicillins, third-generation cephalosporins and monobactams. The ureidopenicillins, such as piperacillin, have been shown to be effective in patients with cholangitis[1,5]. In a prospective, randomized study of 96 patients piperacillin was found to be as effective as the combination of tobramycin and ampicillin[5].

In patients with biliary obstruction and cholangitis serum levels of antibiotics are more important than biliary excretion. The biliary excretion of antibiotics is significantly reduced in biliary obstruction, making it difficult to achieve high bile levels of antibiotics in the situations where they are most needed. Antibacterial specificity and toxicity are therefore the most important factors to consider in the selection of antibiotic therapy.

Prophylactic antibiotics should be administered in all patients undergoing operative or non-operative manipulations of the biliary tree including cholangiography and sphincterotomy. In uncomplicated cases a broad-spectrum first-generation cephalosporin such as cefazolin usually provides adequate coverage. If bile culture data are available, antibiotics that are specific for the organisms present in the bile should be chosen. In more complicated cases where multiple organisms are likely to be present but have not been identified, broader antibiotic coverage may be indicated. In this setting the ureidopenicillins, which cover the Gram-negative aerobes, enterococci and, to some degree, the anaerobes, may be a good choice in the non-allergenic patient.

Preoperative biliary drainage

During the 1970s the surgical relief of biliary obstruction in severely jaundiced patients was associated with postoperative morbidity in 40–60% and mortality in 15–20% of patients[1,6]. During this same period, numerous authors reported that percutaneous transhepatic drainage could be performed with little morbidity[6]. For this reason, preoperative percutaneous transhepatic drainage was recommended and supported by retrospective and non-randomized studies. However, prospective randomized studies failed to demonstrate any advantage of preoperative biliary drainage by either the percutaneous or endoscopic technique (*Table 5*). Moreover, preoperative biliary tract drainage has been shown significantly to lengthen the hospital stay for

Table 5   Results of randomized trials comparing preoperative biliary drainage

Authors	No. of patients	Type of drainage	Postoperative mortality (%)	
			No drainage	Preoperative drainage
Hatfield et al. (*Lancet* 1982; 2: 896–9)	55	Transhepatic	15	14
McPherson *et al.* (*Br J Surg* 1984; 71: 371–5)	65	Transhepatic	19	32
Pitt *et al.* (*Ann Surg* 1985; 201: 545–53)	75	Transhepatic	5	8
Lai *et al.* (*Br J Surg* 1994; 81: 1195–8)	85	Endoscopic	14	15

these patients. Thus, although retrospective analyses suggested that preoperative drainage might be beneficial, prospective randomized studies have not supported this finding.

Although these data suggest that preoperative biliary drainage may not be of any benefit in the routine patient, this manoeuvre may have some value in selected patients. The combination of preoperative percutaneous biliary drainage and hyperalimentation in patients with advanced malnutrition has been shown to reduce the morbidity and mortality associated with surgery in the jaundiced patient. Patients with 'toxic' cholangitis should also undergo endoscopic or percutaneous decompression of the biliary tree prior to surgery. Preoperatively placed catheters are also of value in the operating theatre during difficult hilar dissections as well as in aiding in the placement of long-term transhepatic stents.

Summary

Biliary surgery, especially in the jaundiced patient, has been and continues to be associated with high postoperative morbidity and mortality. This phenomenon is due to a multitude of metabolic abnormalities that occur when the bile duct becomes obstructed. As a result, these patients are prone to sepsis with associated hepatic, renal, cardiac and pulmonary organ failure. In addition, their immune system is depressed, they are frequently malnourished, they often have coagulopathies, and their wounds do not heal normally. Preoperative assessment includes a careful history and physical examination, a complete biochemical evaluation, and a number or radiological studies. Laparoscopy and liver biopsy may also be indicated in selected cases.

Preoperative preparation must include treatment of underlying cardiac or pulmonary disease, maintenance of adequate blood volume, correction of coagulopathies and treatment of biliary sepsis. Antibiotic regimens that are not nephrotoxic are preferred, and non-operative biliary drainage may be required in patients with 'toxic' cholangitis. Selected patients with underlying renal disease and/or malnutrition may also benefit from a period of preoperative biliary drainage and hyperalimentation, preferably by an enteral route. Percutaneous transhepatic biliary drainage may be indicated before surgery in selected patients with perihilar obstruction in whom large-bore Silastic stents are to be placed intraoperatively.

References

1. Nakeeb A, Pitt HA. Jaundice. In: Polk HC, Gardner B, Stone HH, eds. *Basic Surgery.* 5th edn. St. Louis: Quality Medical Publishing, 1995: 558–78.

2. Green J, Better OS. Circulatory disturbance and renal dysfunction in liver disease and in obstructive jaundice. *Isr J Med Sci* 1994; 30: 48–65.

3. Gigot JF, Leese T, Dereme T, Coutinho J, Castaing D, Bismuth H. Acute cholangitis: Multivariate analysis of risk factors *Ann Surg* 1989; 209: 435–8.

4. Little JM. A prospective evaluation of computerized estimates of risk in the management of obstructive jaundice. *Surgery* 1987; 102: 473–6.

5. Thompson JE, Pitt HA, Doty JE, Coleman J, Irving C, Manchester B. Broad spectrum penicillin as an adequate therapy for acute cholangitis. *Surg Gynecol Obstet* 1990; 171: 275–82.

6. Nakeeb A, Pitt HA. The role of preoperative biliary decompression in obstructive jaundice. *Hepatogastroenterology* 1995; 42: 332–7.

Non-surgical management of gallstone disease: oral bile acids

Alberto Lanzini MD, PhD
Senior Registrar, Internal Medicine I, University of Brescia, Spedali Civili, Brescia, Italy

Timothy C. Northfield MA, MD, FRCP
Professor of Gastroenterology, St George's Hospital Medical School, London, and Consultant Gastroenterologist, St George's Hospital, London, UK

History

For more than 20 years, dissolution therapy with bile acids has provided an alternative to surgery for treating gallstones in selected patients. In the era of laparoscopic cholecystectomy[1], treatment of gallstones with bile acids is still indicated for a selected minority of symptomatic patients not fit for or afraid of surgery.

Principles and justification

Gallstones are very common in the general population and pose an important public health problem. The estimated overall prevalence in western countries is about 10%, and the incidence is about 3% per annum according to epidemiological studies using ultrasonography[2].

Patient selection criteria are based on information about the natural history of the disease. Morbidity is low in asymptomatic patients, with an estimated incidence of biliary pain of 2–5% during the first 5 years after diagnosis, and an annual complication rate of less than 1%. The consensus is that only symptomatic gallstones should be treated medically or surgically. The only symptom specific for cholelithiasis is biliary pain, i.e. a steady pain in the epigastrium and/or right hypochondrium lasting more than 2 h and unrelated to bowel movements. When applying this definition, only one-third of patients with gallstones identified in epidemiological studies are symptomatic. This observation implies that the majority of patients with gallstones do not need treatment.

The personal preference of patients with symptomatic gallstones is important in deciding which form of treatment they should receive. Laparoscopic cholecystectomy is now available in most clinical settings and has gained the favour of most patients. However, 5–20% of laparoscopic procedures require conversion to open surgery. This implies that patients not fit for open surgery, and some with previous upper abdominal surgery, are not suitable for laparoscopic cholecystectomy. These patients are among the selected minority suitable for medical treatment of gallstones and include the very elderly, those with concomitant diseases and those afraid of any form of surgery.

Potential candidates for bile acid therapy must satisfy two other absolute prerequisites. First, the gallbladder must opacify on oral cholecystography. This criterion is a proof of cystic duct patency and of the ability of the bile, modified by treatment, to enter the gallbladder and thus interact with the gallstones. Second, the gallstones must be composed of cholesterol monohydrate crystals to be dissolvable with bile acids. Of radiolucent stones seen on plane abdominal radiography, 85% are cholesterol-rich and thus potentially dissolvable, the remaining 15% being insoluble pigment stones. Computed tomographic (CT) scanning is more sensitive than conventional radiology for assessment of stone composition. Hyperdense stones and those with calcified rims are unlikely to dissolve completely with oral bile acid therapy. Frequent biliary pain and/or complications of cholelithiasis are also contraindications to treatment with bile acids.

Bile acid therapy

Available drugs

Chenodeoxycholic acid (CDCA) and ursodeoxycholic acid (UDCA) are two bile acids currently available for medical treatment of gallstones[3, 4]. Oral administration of these bile acids is accompanied by enrichment of the bile acid pool with the administered bile acid, and by decreased biliary cholesterol secretion relative to bile acid and phospholipid secretion. These effects result in reduced cholesterol saturation of gallbladder bile, a phenomenon associated with gallstone dissolution.

Response to treatment

Initial gallstone size is the main factor that affects the rate of gallstone dissolution during treatment with CDCA and UDCA. Stones with a pretreatment diameter of less than 6 mm reduce their volume by more than 50% after 6 months of therapy. By contrast, gallstones with a pretreatment diameter of more than 15 mm dissolve verly slowly and are not suitable for bile acid therapy. This effect of gallstone size on dissolution rate is attributed to the greater surface:volume ratio of small stones than larger ones.

The degree of bile desaturation is the second major factor that affects the dissolution rate. The degree of bile desaturation depends upon bile acid dose and is enhanced by bedtime administration and by the combined administration of CDCA and UDCA.

Consistent gallstone dissolution is associated with a reduction of the cholesterol saturation index to 0.80, a value achieved with 15 mg/kg/day CDCA and 8–10 mg/kg/day UDCA. Doses higher than these minimum effective doses are not recommended because they may cause diarrhoea and/or hypertransaminasaemia during CDCA therapy, or a rise in the cholesterol saturation index for UDCA at doses of more than 12 mg/kg/day. The combination of CDCA and UDCA (5–7 mg/kg/day each) is more effective than either CDCA or UDCA alone (10–15 mg/kg/day each) in reducing the cholesterol saturation index of gallbladder bile. This effect is attributed to the synergistic activity of bile acids with different mechanisms of action, since UDCA causes liquid crystal formation as well as micellar solubilization. Bedtime administration of CDCA and UDCA is more effective than mealtime administration in reducing the cholesterol saturation index of gallbladder bile.

This is attributed to the prevention of secretion of supersaturated bile that occurs at night when the bile acid secretion rate is low. Combination therapy is less expensive than UDCA monotherapy and has fewer side effects.

Clinical efficacy

Complete gallstone dissolution is dose-dependent for both CDCA and UDCA. At the optimum dose of 15 mg/kg/day CDCA, complete gallstone dissolution is achieved in about 40% of patients. This proportion can be raised to about 75% per annum by giving CDCA (15 mg/kg/day) at bedtime plus a low cholesterol diet (300 mg/day), and by selecting patients with small stones (< 15 mm diameter). Although the proportion of patients who achieve complete dissolution may be greater for UDCA than for CDCA during the first 6 months of treatment, equimolar doses of the two bile acids have broadly the same effect over a 1-year treatment period. In practice, combination therapy is now preferred.

In addition to the bile acid regimen chosen, the efficacy of treatment is largely dependent on patient selection. The efficacy is only about 40% in patients with radiolucent stones of any size in a functioning gallbladder treated with CDCA or UDCA. Efficacy rises to 70–80% for both CDCA and UDCA by selecting patients with small stones (< 15 mm diameter), by ensuring a high rate of compliance with long-term treatment, and by achieving unsaturated bile during treatment.

Side effects

CDCA may cause diarrhoea, a dose-related side effect which affects 30–60% of patients treated with the conventional dose of 15 mg/kg/day. This side effect requires treatment withdrawal in only about 5% of patients and usually settles spontaneously. Diarrhoea is infrequent during UDCA administration because this bile acid induces less inhibition of colonic absorption of sodium and water. CDCA may also cause mild hypertransaminasaemia in about 30% of treated patients. By contrast, UDCA can reduce hypertransaminasaemia, an effect attributed to the low detergency power of the bile acid pool enriched with UDCA. Acquired gallstone calcification occurs in about 10% of patients treated with UDCA and results in treatment failure, an effect that is rare during treatment with CDCA.

Recurrence following bile acid treatment

After dissolution of gallstones has been confirmed by ultrasonography, recurrence of the gallstones occurs in about 50% of patients within 10 years of stopping treatment[5]. The recurrence rate rises during the first 5–6 years after withdrawal of treatment and then reaches a plateau. The main risk factor for gallstone recurrence is the number of stones before treatment. Multiple stones are at greater risk of recurrence than solitary stones, probably because the former grow in bile containing a potent factor favouring cholesterol crystal nucleation.

Prevention or retreatment are the two strategies theoretically available for management of gallstone recurrence. Methods to prevent recurrence based on dietary manipulation (high fibre, low refined carbohydrates) or chronic administration of a small dose of CDCA or UDCA do not reliably prevent recurrence. Limited success may be obtained with UDCA (300 mg/day), but only in patients younger than 50 years. Patients taking non-steroidal anti-inflammatory drugs for arthritis may have lower recurrence rates, but the ability of these agents to prevent recurrence needs prospective evaluation.

Failing prevention, early retreatment of recurrent gallstones with bile acids provides a realistic alternative. It is theoretically predicted that, in a cohort of gallstone-free patients undergoing intermittent bile acid therapy (during gallstone recurrence), a steady state will develop with most of the patients being free from gallstones in the long term. This approach has been tested in a cohort of 150 patients with gallstone dissolution who were followed prospectively for 5 years with regular ultrasonography (every 6 months) and retreated with UDCA on recurrence. After 3 years a steady state was reached, and 80% of the population have remained gallstone-free during the subsequent 3 years of follow-up[6].

Overall strategy

The algorithm shown in *Figure 1* summarizes the authors' overall strategy in the treatment of gallstones. Asymptomatic patients should be followed with

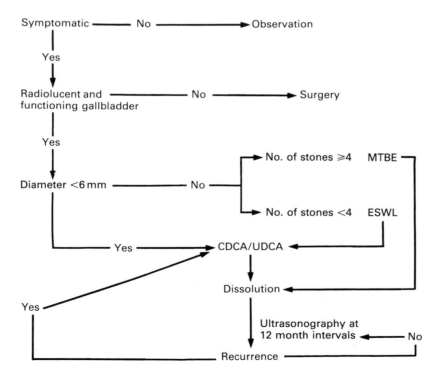

Figure 1   *Management of gallstones: alogorithm for overall strategy. ESWL, extracorporeal shock wave lithotripsy; MTBE, methyl-tertbutyl ether; CDCA, chenodeoxycholic acid; UDCA, ursodeoxycholic acid.*

observation alone. Laparoscopic cholecystectomy is the standard treatment for symptomatic patients. Medical treatment can be considered for a few symptomatic patients with radiolucent gallstones and radiologically functioning gallbladders who are unfit for or afraid of surgery. The choice of medical treatment depends mainly on gallstone size and number, and local expertise with each form of treatment. Small gallstones (<6 mm diameter) are ideal for bile acid therapy using a bedtime combination of CDCA and UDCA. Single stones up to 30 mm diameter or 2–3 stones with a cumulative volume of 15 ml are ideal for extracorporeal shock wave lithotripsy followed by bile acid therapy. Large single stones or multiple stones occupying more than 50% of the gallbladder volume are best treated by contact dissolution using methyl-tertbutyl ether. After gallstone dissolution has been confirmed, annual ultrasonography will allow early detection of recurrence and, thus, retreatment of small recurrent gallstones by bile acids.

References

1. Johnston DE, Kaplan MM. Pathogenesis and treatment of gallstones. *N Engl J Med* 1993; 328: 412–21.

2. Festi D, Barbara L, Frabboni R *et al.* Prevalence and incidence of gallstone disease: the Sirmione study. In: Capocaccia L, Ricci G, Angelico F, Angelico M, Attili AF, Lalloni L, eds. *Recent Advances in the Epidemiology and Prevention of Gallstone Disease.* Dordrecht: Kluwer Academic Publishers, 1991: 7–11.

3. Northfield TC. Review in depth: management of gallstones. *Eur J Gastroenterol Hepatol* 1994; 6: 849–84.

4. Lanzini A, Northfield TC. Pharmacological treatment of gallstones. Practical guidelines. *Drugs* 1994; 47: 458–70.

5. Lanzini A, Northfield TC. Management of recurrent gallstones. *Bailliere's Clinical Gastroenterology* 1992; 6: 767–83.

6. Petroni ML for the British Italian Gallstone (BIG) Study Group. Intermittent bile acid therapy for cholesterol gallstones: a 5-year prospective multicenter trial. *J Hepatol* 1995 (in press).

Illustrations by Peter Cox

Non-surgical management of gallstone disease: extracorporeal shock wave lithotripsy

F. B. V. Keane MD, FRCS, FRCSI
Associate Professor of Surgery, Dublin University, Meath and Adelaide Hospitals, Dublin, Ireland

Gallbladder stones

History

Extracorporeal shock wave lithotripsy (ESWL) was introduced as a possible alternative treatment to open cholecystectomy for symptomatic stones, given the morbidity, mortality and patient disability associated with surgical removal of the gallbladder. Dissolution therapy for gallstones had previously been disappointing when used alone, but the addition of ESWL offered the possibility of fragmenting stones and thus allowing the more rapid dissolution or passage of stone fragments out of the biliary system. Since 1980, ESWL has been used to treat kidney stones successfully, and the first large series reporting its use for gallstones was published in 1988[1]. However, ESWL has been found to have a limited role in the treatment of gallstones because only a minority of patients (10–20%) fulfil the required criteria of suitability. Complete clearance generally requires adjuvant bile salt dissolution therapy and may take up to 2 years. Even after successful clearance, the possibility of stone recurrence remains. Laparoscopic cholecystectomy has further limited the application of ESWL for gallbladder stones, and shock wave lithotripsy is not cost effective, except perhaps in elderly patients with a small stone load.

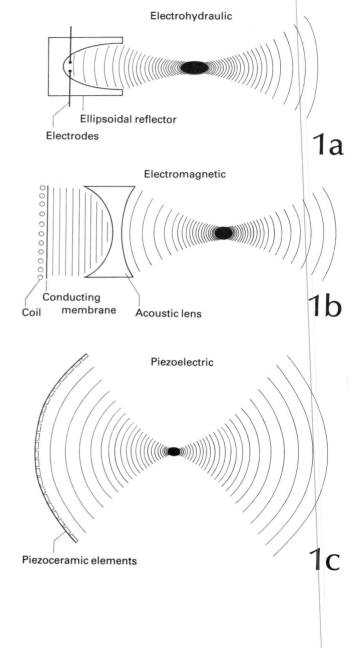

Electrohydraulic

Ellipsoidal reflector

Electrodes

1a

Electromagnetic

Coil   Conducting membrane   Acoustic lens

1b

Piezoelectric

Piezoceramic elements

1c

Principles

1a–c The fundamentals of shock wave production in lithotripsy are explained elsewhere in this series[2]. Shock waves can be generated by electrohydraulic spark-gap discharge, electromagnetic generation or piezoelectric generation. Commercial companies have produced a number of devices which use one of these three methods. The systems have not been compared directly; electromagnetic and piezoelectric systems give less discomfort and fewer complications but require more retreatments.

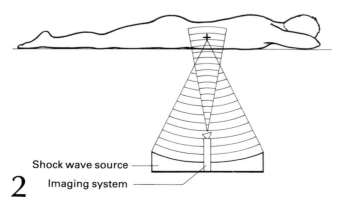

Shock wave source

Imaging system

2

2 Integral imaging systems for targeting the stones and assessing fragmentation are most commonly ultrasonographic, and the success of this therapy depends not only on appropriate patient selection and treatment schemes but also on the skill of the operator.

Patient selection and treatment

Patients with a 1–2-cm solitary radiolucent stone in a functional gallbladder benefit most from ESWL. While it remains possible to treat patients with multiple or calcified stones, the results become progressively poorer with increasing stone load and calcification[3]. Because alternative remedies are generally preferred, ESWL treatment is indicated only for patients at high surgical risk or for those who refuse operation.

Patients generally require 1–3 sessions of lithotripsy with the intention of reducing fragments to < 5 mm. Lithotripsy is generally performed as an outpatient procedure either with no sedation or mild sedation and analgesia. Concurrent bile acid therapy with cheno-deoxycholic acid or ursodeoxycholic acid (7–10 mg/kg/day), either alone or in combination, is usually continued from the outset of treatment until 3 months after complete gallbladder clearance of stone fragments has been confirmed.

Outcome and complications

Stone clearance rates at 1 year vary from 30% to 78% depending on the criteria used for patient selection. However, ESWL has also been shown to give good palliation by reducing episodes of biliary pain independent of complete stone clearance.

Complications during treatment are few and include episodes of biliary colic (20%), acute cholecystitis (4%), biliary obstruction or acute pancreatitis (3%). Side effects of bile acid therapy may also occur, but mortality as a consequence of ESWL is virtually unknown. A major drawback remains the risk of stone recurrence after treatment of approximately 20% at 4 years[4].

Common bile duct stones

Surgery or endoscopy are the preferred options in the management of most patients with common bile duct stones. However, in about 10% of cases endoscopic stone removal may not be possible because the stone may be too large, a duodenal diverticulum may increase the risk of sphincterotomy or altered anatomy following surgery prevents access to the common bile duct. ESWL may be useful in these circumstances, particularly for patients with a high operative risk and, perhaps, also for those with intrahepatic stones. Lithotripsy can be carried out under ultrasonographic guidance[5], but most consider that access to the common bile duct either endoscopically or percutaneously is a prerequisite in order to introduce contrast medium for fluoroscopic guidance, assess clearance and assist in the extraction of fragments[6]. Stone clearance rates of up to 88% have been reported with a low mortality rate of 0.5%. Complications include minor disturbances such as haematuria or haemobilia, or the more serious problem of cholangitis due to an exacerbation of pre-existing sepsis which may occur in up to 6% of cases.

References

1. Sackmann M, Delius M, Sauerbruch T *et al.* Shockwave lithotripsy of gallbladder stones. The first 175 patients. *N Engl J Med* 1988; 318: 393–7.

2. Coleman AJ. Fundamentals of shock wave production in lithotripsy. In: Whitfield HN, ed. *Rob & Smith's Operative Surgery: Genito-urinary Surgery*, 5th ed, 1992: 32–4.

3. Darzi A, El-Sayed E, O'Morain C, Tanner WA, Keane FB. Piezoelectric lithotripsy for gallstones: analysis of results in patients with extended selection. *Br J Surg* 1991; 78: 163–6.

4. Sackmann M, Niller H, Ippisch E *et al.* Gallstone recurrence after lithotripsy. *Gastroenterology* 1992; 102: A332.

5. Ponchon T, Martin X, Barkun A, Mestas JL, Chavaillon A, Boustiere C. Extracorporeal lithotripsy of bile duct stones using ultrasonography for stone localization. *Gastroenterology* 1990; 98: 726–32.

6. Sauerbruch T, Holl J, Sackmann M, Paumgartner G. Fragmentation of bile duct stones by extracorporeal shock-wave lithotripsy: a five year experience. *Hepatology* 1992; 15: 208–14.

Illustrations by Angela Christie

Non-surgical management of gallstone disease: endoscopic retrograde cholangiopancreatography and sphincterotomy

Kelvin R. Palmer MD, FRCP(Ed)
Consultant Physician, Western General Hospital, Edinburgh, UK

Principles and justification

Endoscopic retrograde cholangiopancreatography (ERCP) should only be undertaken if the equipment and expertise are available for therapeutic procedures such as sphincterotomy or stent insertion. It is the investigation of choice when choledocholithiasis is suspected, being more sensitive in this context than both transcutaneous ultrasound scanning and intravenous cholangiography. In practice, ultrasonography will usually have been performed before ERCP is undertaken. ERCP is also indicated in patients being considered for laparoscopic cholecystectomy who have presented with biliary pain, abnormal liver function or acute pancreatitis, and is a valuable method of evaluating post-cholecystectomy syndromes. It is performed urgently in patients who present with fulminant cholangitis or severe gallstone pancreatitis, once again providing that facilities for biliary sphincterotomy are available.

ERCP and drainage (following sphincterotomy or stenting) is used extensively to investigate and treat patients with jaundice due to malignant extrahepatic biliary obstruction. Percutaneous cholangiography and drainage are normally reserved for endoscopic failures.

Diagnostic ERCP can be complicated by acute pancreatitis and by cholangitis. Pancreatitis may follow repeated intubation of the pancreas and overfilling of the gland with contrast material. Cholangitis only occurs in the presence of choledocholithiasis or a stricture and should be treated by a drainage procedure such as endoscopic sphincterotomy or stenting.[1]

Preoperative

ERCP is usually performed on an outpatient basis although facilities for admission to hospital must be available in case a therapeutic procedure is performed or a complication occurs. If biliary sphincterotomy is likely to be needed, the prothrombin time and platelet count are checked and corrected if abnormal. The procedure is performed under sedation using a combination of pethidine and midazolam with an injection of hyosine or glucagon to paralyse the duodenum. Prophylactic antibiotics are given to jaundiced patients.

Operation

1a–c A side-viewing duodenoscope is passed under direct control into the second part of the duodenum with the patient lying in a supine position. The gastric loop is removed by withdrawing the instrument until the ampulla of Vater appears. A Teflon catheter, filled with contrast material, is passed through the biopsy channel of the endoscope and passed directly into the ampulla. An 'en-face' approach is used to cannulate the pancreas, while the cannula is directed towards an 11 o'clock position when attempting to intubate the biliary tree. Contrast material is then injected during fluoroscopy and radiographs are taken.

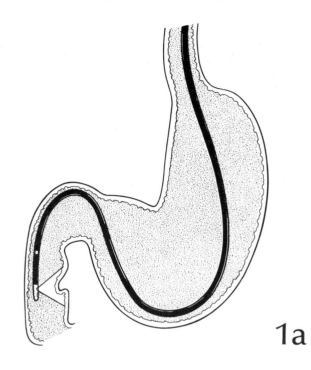

1a

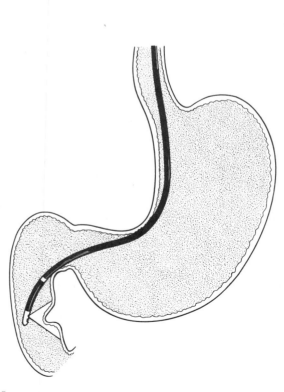

1b

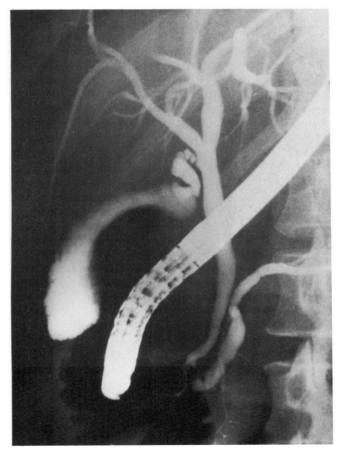

1c

Biliary sphincterotomy for choledocholithiasis

2a–c Diagnostic ERCP is first performed in the usual manner. A sphincterotome is then inserted into the biliary tree. The diagnostic catheter is usually removed before inserting the sphincterotome although it is possible to pass a guidewire into the biliary tree before removing a modified diagnostic cannula.

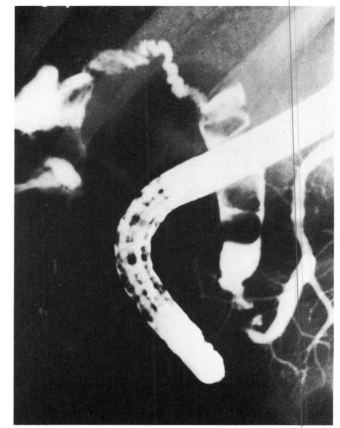

2a

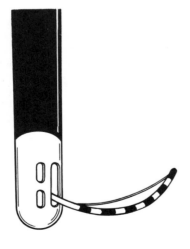

2b

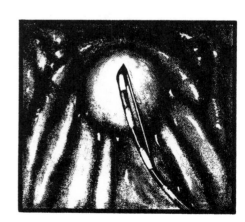

2c

3 After confirming radiographically that the sphincterotome is indeed within the biliary tree rather than the pancreas, the wire is positioned against the roof of the papilla. At the start of the procedure most of the wire should lie outside the ampulla; only the tip should lie within it at this stage.

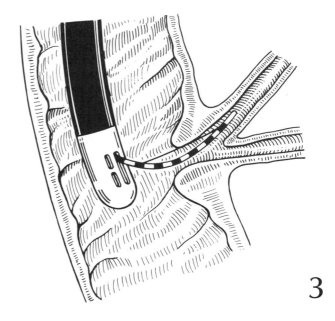

3

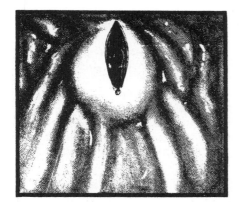

4

4 Diathermy blended current is applied to produce a cut approximately 15–20 mm in length. A spurt of bile indicates adequate division of the sphincter, and the cut should extend to the horizontal fold which passes above the papilla in the duodenal lumen.

5 When it proves impossible to cannulate the biliary tree using a standard sphincterotome, entry can be achieved using a 'needle knife'. This manoeuvre is used like a scalpel to cut in the line of the bile duct until bile appears. The sphincterotomy is then completed using a standard sphincterotome.

The risk of causing perforation and pancreatitis is increased by this technique, so needle knife sphincterotomy should only be undertaken by experienced endoscopists.

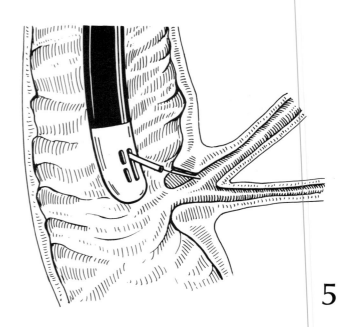

5

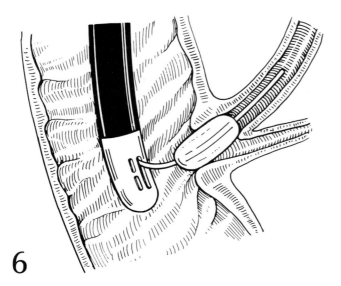

6

Balloon dilatation of the sphincter

6 This technique facilitates stone extraction without the potential hazard of bleeding induced by sphincterotomy. A low profile Gruntzig balloon is passed over a guidewire into the biliary tree. Balloons with inflation diameters of up to 20 mm are available and enable moderate-sized stones to be extracted. Larger calculi can be removed by this technique following fragmentation using mechanical lithotriptors.

Stone extraction after endoscopic sphincterotomy

7 Stones are removed after sphincterotomy or sphincter dilatation using balloon catheters or a Dormia basket.

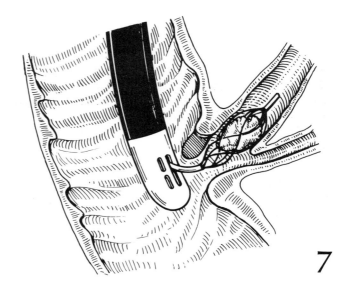

8 Large calculi can be fragmented using mechanical lithotriptors. The stone is caught within a strong metal basket and is crushed by forcing the basket into a metal overtube.

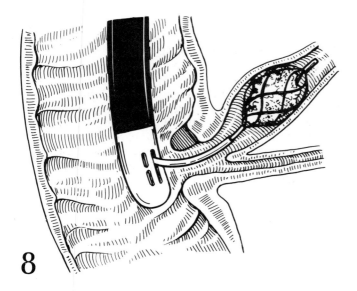

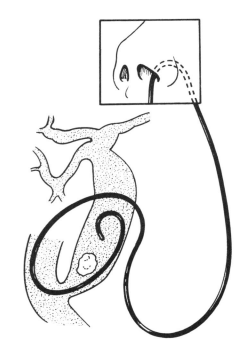

9a

9a, b If gallstone extraction is unsuccessful, a nasobiliary catheter is passed into the bile duct so that its tip lies above the stone. This catheter prevents cholangitis, enables cholangiography to be performed, facilitates dissolution therapy with solvents, and allows focusing for extracorporeal shock wave lithotripsy.

ERCP following gastric surgery

ERCP is much more difficult following Bilroth II gastrectomy, principally because the afferent loop is difficult to intubate.

When the papilla is found, endoscopic manoeuvres are reversed because the papilla is being approached in a retrograde direction. Biliary sphincterotomy is particularly awkward and is possible only using specially adapted sphincterotomes or a 'needle knife'.

Endoscopic stent insertion

Stents are usually employed to relieve malignant extrahepatic biliary obstruction but are sometimes used in patients with benign disease[2]. For example, strictures due to sclerosing cholangitis can be dealt with on a temporary basis by stenting. Biliary leaks complicating laparoscopic cholecystectomy will often close if pressure within the biliary system is lowered by stenting, and stenting can also be used as the definitive treatment for biliary obstruction caused by large common bile duct calculi which have not responded to other approaches in elderly, unfit patients.

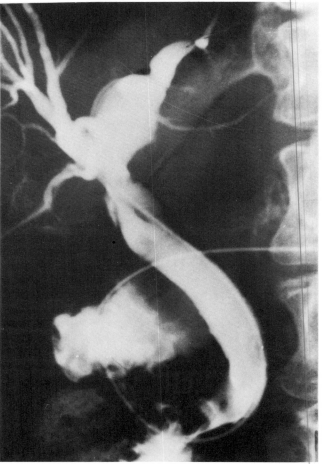

9b

Outcome

The success rate of endoscopic stone removal should exceed 90%. Failure is due to difficulty of access (e.g. duodenal diverticula or previous gastrectomy) or because stones are too large to pass and lithotripsy fails. Complications occur in approximately 10% of patients and there is an overall mortality rate of 1%[3]. The main complications are haemorrhage, acute pancreatitis, cholangitis, retroperitoneal perforation and stone impaction within a Dormia basket. Haemorrhage due to division of a major artery does not usually respond to conservative therapy (including endoscopic injection) and often requires a surgical operation to underrun the bleeding vessel. Cholangitis is treated by biliary drainage using stents or a nasobiliary tube. Pancreatitis and retroperitoneal perforation usually resolve with conservative therapy, and the demonstration of retro-duodenal air on a plain radiograph is not in itself an indication for surgery.

References

1. Cotton PB. Endoscopic management of bile duct stones. *Gut* 1984; 25: 587–97.

2. Dalton HR, Chapman RWG. Role of biliary stenting in the management of bile duct stones in the elderly. *Gut* 1995; 36: 485–7.

3. Neoptolemos JP, Davison BR, Shaw DE *et al.* Study of common bile duct exploration and endoscopic sphincterotomy in a consecutive series of 438 patients. *Br J Surg* 1987; 74: 916–21.

Minimally invasive surgery for gallstone disease: percutaneous techniques

R. C. G. Russell MS, FRCS
Consultant Surgeon, The Middlesex Hospital, London, UK

Principles and justification

The field of gallbladder surgery has been dominated by laparoscopic and mini-cholecystectomy, yet the percutaneous techniques developed during the 1980s continue to have a role in the management of certain patients who are unsuitable for general anaesthesia, or whose other medical problems preclude surgical intervention. For example, in patients who develop acute cholecystitis in conjunction with another illness, percutaneous techniques will, with time and therapy, enable them to be made fit for cholecystectomy. Such patients are ideally managed by a percutaneously placed drain using ultrasonographic control and local anaesthesia. A 9-Fr Cope catheter can satisfactorily drain an empyema and transform the condition of the patient. Similarly, a patient with severe coexistent disease in association with biliary colic can be cured using percutaneous cholecystolithotomy.

Percutaneous extraction of gallstones was first described in 1985 for the treatment of high-risk patients with acute cholecystitis and was performed in up to five stages using a percutaneous transhepatic tract[1]. In 1988 Kellett et al. adapted the technique of percutaneous nephrolithotomy for the extraction of gallstones[2]. This technique is indicated in ill patients with severe symptoms and young patients with functioning gallbladders who do not wish to lose their gallbladder.

Preoperative

Anaesthesia

The procedure can be performed under local or general anaesthesia. General anaesthesia is preferable as it allows the procedure to be done in one stage with minimum discomfort. If local anaesthesia is used, a staged procedure is necessary with puncture of the gallbladder, dilatation of the track and then stone extraction. The disadvantage of local anaesthesia is that some patients develop a profound vagal reaction with severe hypotension and bradycardia during the puncture.

Operation

Approach

The approach may be either transhepatic or transperitoneal. For simple puncture and drainage, the transhepatic approach is best; if dilatation is required, the transperitoneal approach is safer as the liver will tear if dilated beyond 12–15 Fr. Thus, if stone removal is required, the transperitoneal route is preferable, with a fundal puncture providing direct access to the whole of the gallbladder. The disadvantage of this approach is that a tube drain has to be left in the gallbladder for 10–14 days to enable the puncture track to heal without leakage.

Transperitoneal approach

1a, b Under ultrasonographic control the gallbladder is punctured with a Kellett needle (152 mm Longdwell sheathed needle). Contrast medium is injected into the gallbladder so that subsequent imaging is both by fluoroscopy and ultrasonography. If the initial puncture is not ideal, a second puncture is made in the fundus. A 0.89-mm wire with a floppy tip (Lunderquist) is introduced into the gallbladder and the needle is removed.

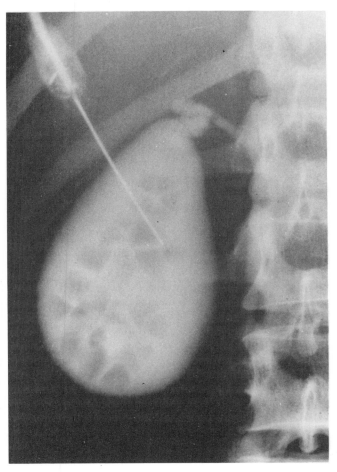

1a

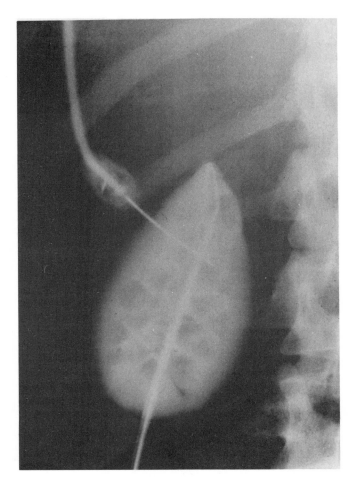

1b

Dilatation of the track

2   The track is dilated with Teflon dilators and rigid telescopic metal dilators (Olympus) are introduced in coaxial fashion. The tract is dilated to 30 Fr and a Teflon sheath of the same dimension is introduced coaxially. The metal dilators are removed.

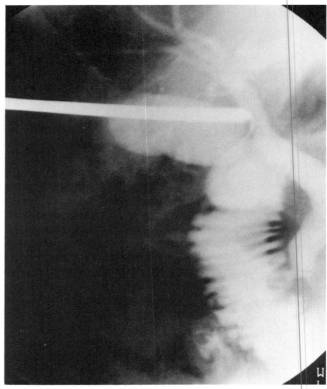

2

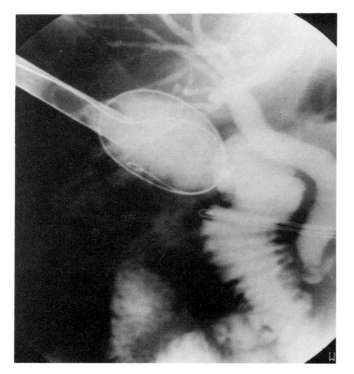

3

Preparation for endoscopy

3   In order to maintain a track in case the Teflon sheath becomes displaced during manipulation, a 0.89-mm wire with a J formation (3 mm in diameter) (Wilson Cook) is introduced so that its distal 5–10 cm is curled up within the gallbladder and the Lunderquist wire is removed. The J wire is left in place and held in position by an assistant to prevent displacement during stone extraction. With practice this wire can be used for hooking stones into a more convenient position for retrieval.

Endoscopy

4 The standard rigid straight viewing 26-Fr nephroscope with an 8-Fr working channel (Keymed) enables the interior of the gallbladder to be seen clearly and the stones retrieved. This procedure is aided by the use of a video camera with monitor allowing easier instrument manipulation. Continuous saline irrigation via the nephroscope is necessary to maintain a clear field of view.

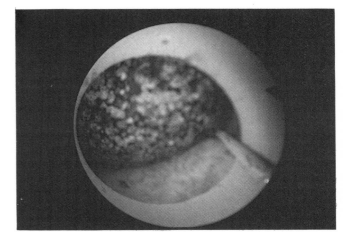

4

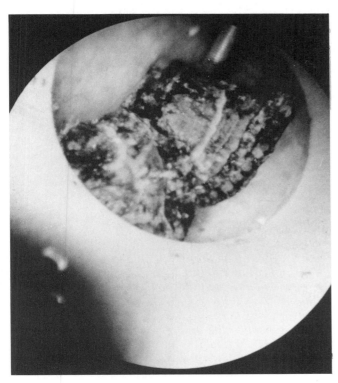

5

Removal of stones

5 Stones larger than 1 cm have to be broken before removal either by means of direct contact lithotripsy or using crushing baskets or forceps. Lithotripsy is performed under direct vision using either electrohydraulic, ultrasound or laser medium to shatter the stone. Ideally, the stone is broken up into larger fragments which can be picked out by triradiate forceps.

Clearance of the gallbladder

6a, b Once all the fragments have been removed, clearance is assessed radiologically (*Illustration 6a*). If the gallbladder is confirmed to be clear of stones, a 14-Fr or 16-Fr Foley catheter is introduced through the Amplatz sheath, the J wire is removed, and the balloon of the Foley catheter inflated. Gentle traction is applied to the catheter as the Teflon sheath is removed to minimize bile leakage. Contrast medium is again injected to ascertain clearance of all the stones (*Illustration 6b*).

Postoperative care

The Foley catheter is attached to a drainage bag and the patient returned to the ward. The patient is discharged on the second day and returns on the 14th day as an outpatient to have a contrast examination of the biliary tree. If no stones are seen, the Foley catheter is removed, but if stones are present, a guidewire is passed down the Foley catheter (the tip is always removed at the time of insertion) and an endoscopic removal of the residual stone is performed using the flexible choledochoscope.

Outcome

Patients rarely have symptoms following this procedure, and even non-functioning gallbladders return to function. Of 100 patients carefully followed for a mean of 24 months, 69 are stone-free and 31 have a recurrence of their stones[3,4]. Of those with stones, only 12 were symptomatic and required surgery, most of whom had their gallbladder removed laparoscopically. The incidence of recurrent stone formation is reduced with the use of bile acid therapy such as chenodeoxycholic acid.

References

1. Boland GW, Lee MJ, Leung J, Mueller PR. Percutaneous cholecystolithotomy in critically ill patients: early response and final outcome in 82 patients. *AJR* 1994; 163: 339–42.

2. Kellett MJ, Russell RCG, Wickham JEA. Percutaneous cholecystolithotomy. *BMJ* 1988; 296: 453–5.

3. Chiverton SG, Inglis JA, Hudd C, Kellett MJ, Russell RCG, Wickham JEA. Percutaneous cholecystolithotomy: the first 60 patients. *BMJ* 1990; 300: 1310–12.

4. Cheslyn-Curtis S, Gillams A, Russell RCG, *et al.* Selection, management and early outcome of 113 patients with symptomatic gallstones treated by percutaneous cholecystolithotomy. *Gut* 1992; 33: 1253–9.

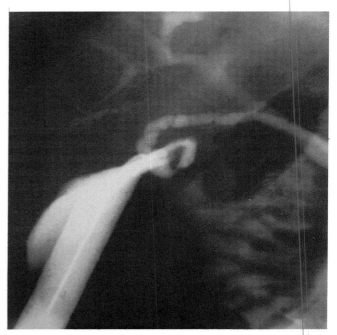

6a

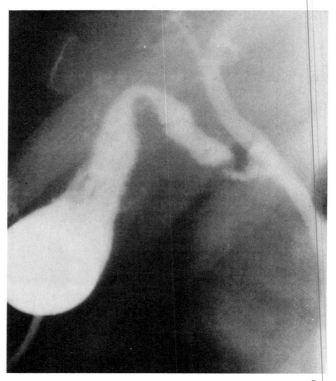

6b

Illustrations by Gillian Oliver and Gillian Lee

Minimally invasive surgery for gallstone disease: mini-cholecystectomy

R. C. G. Russell MS, FRCS
Consultant Surgeon, The Middlesex Hospital, London, UK

Principles and justification

Traditional cholecystectomy involved a large incision and a major laparotomy with consequent prolonged recovery. Before the era of laparoscopic cholecystectomy it was apparent that this approach was unnecessary, and a more limited procedure was adequate. Dubois *et al*. described a mini-cholecystectomy in 1981, and perfected this technique during the 1980s before developing the laparoscopic approach[1]. Despite the advances of laparoscopy, it is difficult to show that there are significant disadvantages for the mini-cholecystectomy approach in terms of ease of operation, length of hospital stay, recovery and return to work[2].

The indication for the procedure is the same as for any gallbladder operation, namely symptomatic gall-stones. It is not indicated for the removal of asymptomatic gallstones. It is essential to confirm the diagnosis by ultrasonography, to determine the thickness of the gallbladder wall, the presence of an empyema, the size of the duct and whether or not stones are present in the duct. Patients with stones in the duct, large ducts, an appropriate history for a duct stone and/or a history of previous obstructive jaundice are preferably managed with a preoperative endoscopic retrograde cholangiogram, and sphincterotomy if stones are found. The mini-cholecystectomy approach can be used for exploration of the duct, but preoperative clearance of the duct is advantageous. Provided the patient is well, admission on the day of operation is suitable.

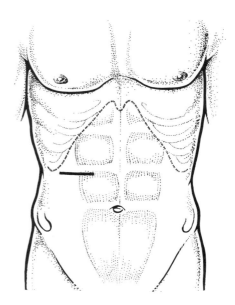

1a

Operation

Incision

1a, b A transverse incision about 6 cm in length is made, two-thirds of which is lateral to the lateral border of the rectus sheath. The oblique muscles and the anterior rectus sheath are divided. The rectus muscle is mobilized medially and not divided, so exposing the posterior rectus sheath and the peritoneum which is incised.

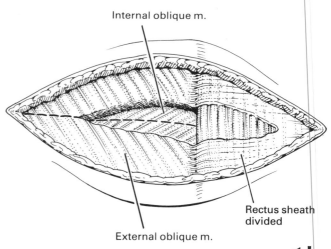

Internal oblique m.

Rectus sheath divided

External oblique m.

1b

Exposure of the gallbladder

2a, b   Once the peritoneal cavity is opened, it is important to locate the gallbladder and to assess the extent of the disease. It is not possible to perform a full laparotomy as the incision is too small to allow all but the smallest hand to enter the abdomen. Once the position of the gallbladder is defined, exposure by retraction is possible. Small standard retractors can be used, but the author's preference is for a stabilized ring retractor such as the Buchwalter retractor which enables retraction to be steady without relying on the foibles of an assistant[3]. A 4-cm blade is used to retract the liver upwards while a malleable 4-cm blade over a swab displaces the colon and omentum inferiorly, and a 2-cm malleable blade over a swab exposes the bile duct and porta hepatis. Exposure is further improved by a head-up position on the table with rotation of the patient away from the operator.

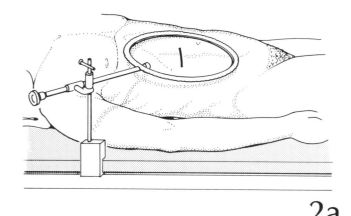

2a

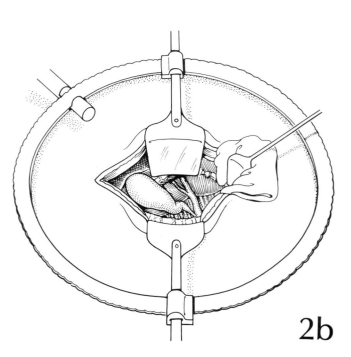

2b

Approach to the gallbladder

3 All adhesions on the inferior surface of the gallbladder are dissected away and, in particular, duodenal adhesions are separated with care so that the lower malleable retractor can be well positioned down in the hepatorenal pouch. If the gallbladder is distended, it is helpful to empty it completely by aspiration to prevent leakage during dissection. A fundus first approach is adopted taking the gallbladder away from the gallbladder bed. This must be carried out in as dry a field as possible to ensure that vision is not impeded. The laparoscopic diathermy hook is an ideal instrument for this procedure. As the gallbladder is dissected away from the liver, the position of the upper retractor is shifted to lie in the gallbladder bed.

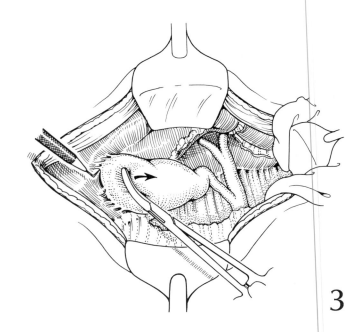

3

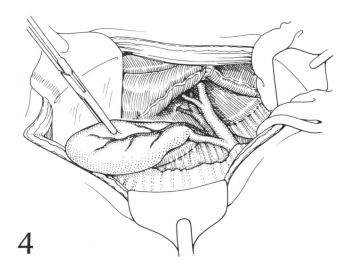

4

Dissection of the triangle of Calot

4 As the gallbladder is dissected away from the liver bed, the triangle of Calot is entered. To gain access and improve vision, the gallbladder is dislocated laterally, and the important structures of the porta hepatis are seen more clearly. The peritoneum covering the triangle of Calot is gently dissected with a hook away from the gallbladder to expose the cystic artery on the gallbladder. The artery is cauterized and divided. Often there is a posterior branch which is managed likewise. As the peritoneum is dissected away from Hartmann's pouch, the cystic duct is encountered.

Dissection of the cystic duct

5 The gallbladder is now separated from surrounding structures apart from the cystic duct; the cystic duct is often tortuous, may be dilated and may contain a stone. To prevent further problems, it is important to dissect the cystic duct until it is no more than 2 mm in diameter and will easily take a clip, preferably an absorbable one. A cholangiogram can be performed at this stage if desired. Once the duct has been clipped it is divided and the gallbladder removed. There is no indication for drainage provided haemostasis is precise.

Closure

Interrupted sutures of 1/0 polydioxanone (PDS) are used for mass closure. The fat is closed with a 3/0 polyglactin (Vicryl) suture and the skin with a subcuticular suture of 3/0 or 5/0 polydioxanone. A small dressing is applied.

Before closure of the skin, 30 ml of 0.5% bupivacaine with adrenaline is injected into the muscle above the wound to block the intercostal nerves. After closure is complete, a 100 mg diclofenac suppository is given.

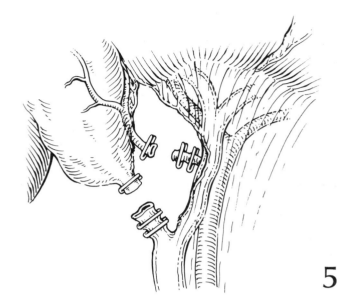

5

Postoperative care

It is important to emphasize early mobility and to get the patient out of bed the same day. Oral fluids may be given within 4 h and intravenous fluids discontinued within 12–24 h. A light diet is commenced on the first postoperative day and continued mobilization emphasized. The patient usually leaves hospital on the second postoperative day and returns to work within 2 weeks.

References

1. Dubois F, Icard P, Berthelot G, Levard H. Coelioscopic cholecystectomy: preliminary report of 36 cases. *Ann Surg* 1990; 211: 60–2.

2. McMahon AJ, Russell IT, Baxter JN *et al*. Laparascopic versus minilaparotomy cholecystectomy: a randomised trial. *Lancet* 1994; 343: 135–8.

3. Russell RCG, Shankar S. The stabilized ring retractor: a technique for cholecystectomy. *Br J Surg* 1987; 74: 826.

Minimally invasive surgery for gallstone disease: laparoscopic cholecystectomy

A. Cuschieri MD, ChM, FRCS, FRCS(Ed)
Professor and Head of Department, Department of Surgery, University of Dundee, Ninewells Hospital and Medical School, Dundee, UK

History

Some debate exists as to who performed the first laparoscopic cholecystectomy. Muehe was the first to describe the use of an operating proctoscope and carbon dioxide insufflation. The first series using dedicated laparoscopic instrumentation and ancillary equipment including a videocamera attached to the laparoscope was reported by Dubois *et al.* in 1989[1], while the first large retrospective series from a number of European centres was reported by Cuschieri *et al.* in 1991[2]. This report was soon followed by the prospective series reported by the Southern Surgeons Club[3]. Since then, laparoscopic cholecystectomy has become the standard surgical treatment for patients with symptomatic gallstone disease and can be used in over 95% of such patients.

Preoperative

Anaesthesia

Laparoscopic cholecystectomy is carried out under general anaesthesia. The patients are most commonly premedicated with benzodiazepines and some anaesthetists also give a long-acting 5-HT$_3$ antagonist to reduce the incidence of postoperative vomiting. Induction is carried out with thiopentone, and neuromuscular blockade is established using alcuronium or vercuronium in patients with hypertension. All patients are intubated with a cuffed endotracheal tube and ventilated mechanically. Nitrous oxide (66%), oxygen and enflurane are used to maintain anaesthesia with increments of alcuronium and fentanyl as required.

Monitoring during anaesthesia includes electrocardiography and measurement of blood pressure, oxygen saturation and end-tidal carbon dioxide (which is maintained at 30 mmHg). Fluid losses are replaced using Hartmann's solution. An intravenous injection of a cephalosporin (e.g. cephuroxime) is given at the start of the operation.

At the end of the procedure, neuromuscular blockade is reversed with neostigmine and atropine. Oxygen is administered for the first 3 h. Although potent opioid analgesics such as fentanyl are still used extensively to treat postoperative pain in the recovery room, increasingly many anaesthetists favour non-steroidal anti-inflammatory drugs, such as intravenous ketorolac, to minimize respiratory depression, nausea and sedation.

Operation

Laparoscopic cholecystectomy can be performed with the patient lying supine in either the classical or leg abduction position.

Leg abduction position

1 This position is favoured by many European surgeons. The patient is positioned supine on the operating table and the legs are abducted, preferably in the limb extension position and without the use of Lloyd-Davies stirrups. This position allows the surgeon to operate facing the patient's abdomen. The table is tilted 30° head up (reverse Trendelenburg position). The neutral electrosurgical pad is placed underneath the buttocks and connected to the electrosurgical generator. The assistant stands on the patient's right and the scrub nurse on the same side. The insufflator, suction/irrigation system, telescope heater, electrocautery unit and xenon light source are positioned on the right of the surgeon. The instrument trolley is placed on the left of the surgeon between him and the scrub nurse. The television monitor is placed on the right side of the patient such that the assistant and scrub nurse can clearly see the progress of the operation. Dual monitors are an advantage.

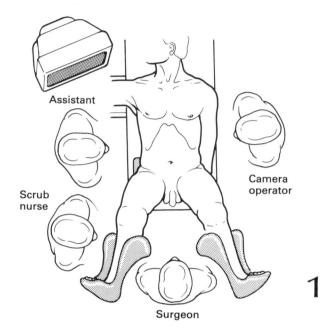

1

Classical supine position

2 This position is popular in North America and the United Kingdom. The patient is placed in the ordinary supine position with the table given a 30° reverse Trendelenburg tilt with the surgeon on the left and the assistant on the right of the patient. The classical supine position is less likely to cause compression trauma to the calf veins but two television monitors are required, one facing the surgeon and the other facing his assistant.

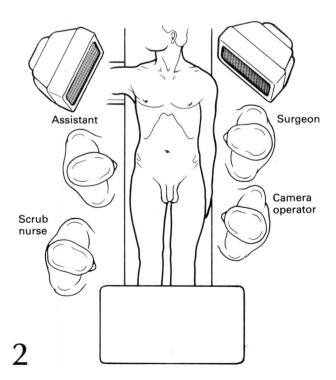

2

Nasogastric intubation and emptying of the bladder

A nasogastric tube is used to ensure complete gastric deflation during the procedure since a distended stomach and duodenal cap can obscure the operative field. The urinary bladder is emptied by a catheter (which is then removed) prior to the insertion of a Veress needle and creating a pneumoperitoneum. If catheterization is not practised routinely, it is important to percuss the suprapubic region to exclude a distended urinary bladder before inserting the Veress needle. The nasogastric tube is removed at the end of the operation.

Skin preparation and draping

The skin of the abdomen from the level of the nipple line to the pubic region is prepared with chlorhexidine soap followed by chlorhexidine-alcohol antiseptic solution (or suitable alternative). Standard drapes are used as for open cholecystectomy and some surgeons prefer to use disposable drapes. The edges of the drapes are sutured temporarily to the skin and skin clips should be avoided because of the anticipated need for intraoperative cholangiography.

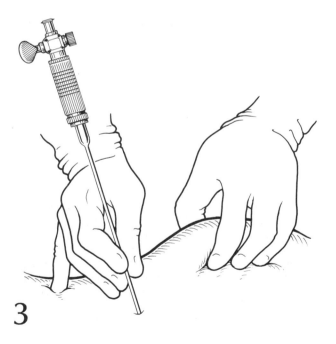

3

Access to the peritoneal cavity

Two techniques are available: (1) closed peritoneal insufflation followed by the insertion of the optical port (blind or visually guided); and (2) open laparoscopy using the modified Hasson's cannula.

Closed pneumoperitoneum followed by insertion of optical port

This technique entails the initial creation of a carbon dioxide pneumoperitoneum using a Veress needle and electronic insufflator. The function of the spring loaded snap mechanism of the Veress needle should be confirmed before initial insertion, as should its patency by checking gas flow through it. The Veress needle is most often inserted at the subumbilical site where the optical port will be introduced. A different site is chosen if subumbilical adhesions are suspected.

After the checks on the Veress needle, the palpation test is performed. This test provides the surgeon with a clear mental idea of the depth required for insertion of the needle tip and is achieved by finger pressure depression of the abdominal wall down to the aorta. This distance can be alarmingly short in thin individuals.

3   A small skin stab wound is made with a pointed scalpel and the Veress needle is inserted. The safest technique involves holding the Veress needle along its shaft at a distance from its tip which is roughly equal to the estimated abdominal wall thickness in the individual patient. Held in this manner, the needle is 'threaded through' the parietes as the abdominal wall is lifted up by hand. A definite click is felt as the anterior rectus sheath is penetrated. With care, a second click should be felt by the surgeon when the posterior sheath and peritoneum are breached.

At this point clues to safe and free penetration of the peritoneal cavity may be obtained as follows:
(i) *Syringe aspiration test*: isotonic saline (5 ml) is instilled into the peritoneal cavity via the Veress needle. If the needle tip lies freely, it should not be possible to aspirate the injected fluid; if the fluid can be aspirated, incorrect needle tip placement is likely. Aspiration of yellowish fluid (signifying contamination with bowel contents) or bloodstained fluid indicates needle misplacement.
(ii) *Drop test*: The tap on the Veress needle is closed, and its terminal hub is filled with saline which forms a convex droplet due to its surface tension. This drop disappears down the shaft as soon as the tap is opened if the needle tip is unobstructed.

(iii) *Negative pressure test*: the tubing leading from the insufflator is next connected to the Veress needle in order to measure peritoneal pressure prior to insufflation. This manoeuvre should reveal a slight negative pressure which is accentuated by elevation of the abdominal wall.

(iv) *Early insufflation pressures*: the next clue to correct positioning is the insufflation pressure (which should not exceed 8 mmHg at 1 l/min gas insufflation). The more recent electronic insufflators incorporate an automatic sensor system which gives an alarm when the tip of the needle is obstructed during insufflation.

Insufflation of the peritoneal cavity is then continued at an initial inflow rate of about 1 l/min. If this process proceeds smoothly without significant cardiovascular changes, the insufflator can be switched to high flow to allow complete filling of the peritoneal cavity to a pressure of approximately 10–15 mmHg. At this point the Veress needle is withdrawn. During the insufflation process, all quadrants of the abdomen are percussed to confirm uniform as distinct from localized distension.

If, during induction of the initial pneumoperitoneum, the needle tip is thought to be incorrectly positioned, the needle is simply withdrawn and reinserted. The number of passes required should be recorded in the operation note. If blood is aspirated, simple withdrawal of the needle and reinsertion is reasonable. However, if blood fountains back up the Veress needle, major vessel injury is likely, and laparotomy should be performed with the Veress needle *in situ*. If bowel content is aspirated, the needle is withdrawn and reinserted in another site. In this event, it is important to inspect the area of bowel injury when the laparoscope is first introduced. If the hole in the bowel consists of a simple puncture, the administration of antibiotics and local lavage/suction followed by careful postoperative observation may be all that is required. More extensive injuries, e.g. when bowel has been lacerated, require immediate suture repair (laparoscopically or at open operation).

Blind insertion of optical port

The cannula used for insertion of the videolaparoscope should have an external diameter of 11 mm (in preference to 10 mm) and can be reusable or disposable. The larger port, when used with a 10.5 mm reducer, results in a bigger space between the telescope and the inner surface of the cannula and so ensures larger gas flows and maintenance of the pneumoperitoneum during the operation. Although many types of disposable ports have outer protective shields to minimize the risk of visceral injury by the trocar during insertion, this risk is not abolished, especially if the technique of insertion is faulty. If a non-disposable cannula is used, the flap valve (trap door) variety rather than the trumpet valve variety should be used as the latter restricts movement of the telescope. The non-disposable metal trocars are hollow and have a hole near the pointed tip. This design provides an important safety feature during insertion.

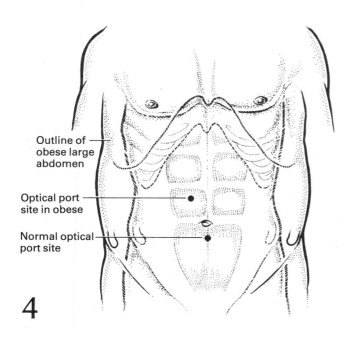

Outline of obese large abdomen

Optical port site in obese

Normal optical port site

4

4 The optimal site for insertion is the immediate subumbilical region. However, in large or obese individuals with a long distance between the umbilicus and the xiphoid process, the optical port should be sited at a higher level on either side of the umbilicus. If the subumbilical site is chosen, the skin incision used for insertion of the Veress needle is extended vertically or transversely to 1.5 cm and deepened to include the aponeurotic layer until the hiss of escaping gas is heard.

5 The trocar/cannula is held in the right hand with the butt firmly pressed against the palm and the index finger alongside the long axis of the shaft some 2.5 cm away from the tip. The periumbilical region is pulled firmly up by the left hand so that the abdominal wall is tented upwards, and the trocar/cannula is introduced through the subumbilical incision parallel to the axis of the aorta and pointing to the centre of the pelvis. Alternatively, two Littlewood's forceps are applied to the edges of the skin wound, and the abdominal wall is pulled upwards. Pressure from the wrist accompanied by to-and-fro rotational movement is used to 'ream' the trocar/cannula through the parietes. Pressure against the palm of the hand prevents the trocar from riding inside the cannula as it encounters the resistance provided by the abdominal wall. The tip of the index finger against the long shaft of the assembly acts as a safety stop in case of sudden give. With the disposable sheathed cannulae, a click is heard due to snapping of the sheath over the trocar point as soon as the peritoneal lining is breached. By contrast, with the non-disposable type, the perforation near the tip of the trocar leads to a sudden escape of gas with a resultant audible hiss as soon as complete penetration of the abdominal wall is achieved. The trocar is withdrawn before the cannula is advanced further. The gas line is then connected to the side port of the cannula, and the tap is opened to maintain insufflation of the peritoneal cavity.

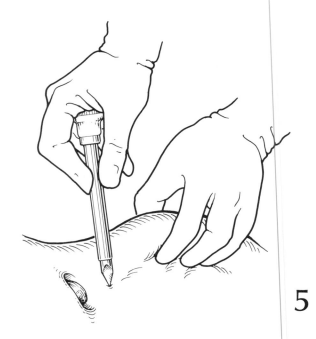

5

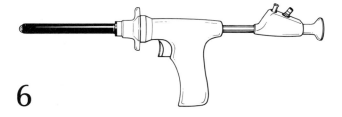

6

Visually guided insertion of the optical port

6 In this method the optical cannula is inserted under vision once the pneumoperitoneum has been created. This technique is possible using reusable or disposable equipment. The reusable device is known as the optical scalpel and is manufactured by Olympus (Japan). The disposable equipment is manufactured by United States Surgical Corporation (Norwalk, Connecticut, USA) or Ethicon (Cincinnati, USA).

All of the systems work on the same principle — an integral blade can be deployed to cut the abdominal layers under visual control until a safe window of parietal peritoneum (transparent as opposed to opaque) is created. These visual systems are undoubtedly safer and are recommended in difficult cases (obese patients and those with scars from previous surgery).

Open laparoscopy

Open laparoscopy dispenses with prior insufflation of the peritoneal cavity. The cannula is introduced through a small wound into the peritoneal cavity. After the cannula is fixed to the parietes with sutures to ensure an air tight seal, insufflation of the peritoneal cavity is commenced through the gas inlet of the cannula. Although open laparoscopy can be performed using an ordinary reusable or disposable port, the Hasson's cannula designed specifically for this purpose (initially for gynaecological laparoscopy) is better.

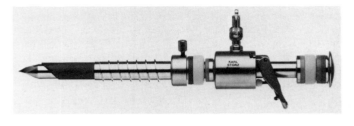

7   The modern versions of this device have three components: (1) a sliding olive which allows for variation in the length of the cannula inside the peritoneal cavity; (2) fixation suture wings attached to the olive; and (3) a blunt obturator.

Open laparoscopy virtually abolishes the risk of major vascular injury although injuries to the bowel may still occur.

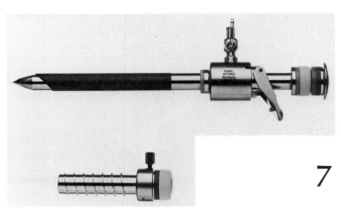

7

Insertion of the telescope

The previously heated 10 mm laparoscope (0° or 30°) is attached to the endocamera (sterile or inside transparent sterile plastic sleeve), the light cable is attached to the telescope, and the system is 'white balanced'. The telescope is then inserted down the optic port.

Insertion of operating and assisting ports

These ports are all placed under vision. If reusable cannulae are used, they should be equipped with flap valves in preference to trumpet valves as the latter require depression before instruments can be moved inside the cannula. Jamming of instruments inside the port not only slows down the procedure but carries the risk of stab injuries as increased force is needed to advance the instrument. Cannulae with trumpet valves damage the insulation of instruments used for electrosurgery and, for this reason, should not be used with these instruments. Another occurrence which is encountered frequently with both disposable and reusable cannulae is dislocation of the access port during

instrument manipulation due either to valve sticking or the presence of congealed blood between the instrument and the cannula. With reusable cannulae, an external spiral screw relief can minimize this problem. Plastic cannulae fixation outer screws must not be used if the port consists of electroconductive material, since this results in electric isolation of the port from the abdominal parietes. In this situation, capacitance current from the electrode (each time this is activated) accumulates in the cannula as it cannot discharge to the abdominal wall. The cannula effectively becomes a charged electric capacitor and, if its tip then touches any tissue inside the abdomen, a high density current is discharged at the point of contact causing a burn.

In the majority of patients undergoing laparoscopic cholecystectomy, three accessory cannulae are needed. The location of these ports depends on the technique used to expose the triangle of Calot; North American or French. The North American exposure is easier provided the right lobe of the liver is not rigid and the quadrate lobe is not hypertrophied. Otherwise, the French exposure provides more adequate access.

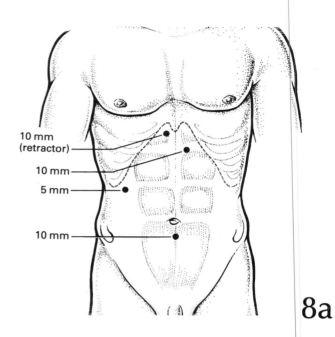

8a

French approach

8a,b The liver is retracted upwards by a medially placed retractor. The port sites for this technique are 10 mm upper left paramedian (for electrosurgical hook knife, scissors, etc.), 10 mm upper medial subcostal (for retraction, suction/irrigation) and 5 mm lower right hypochondrial just lateral to linea semilunaris (for grasping forceps).

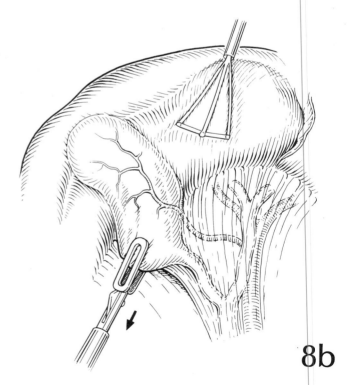

8b

North American approach

9a,b The cystic pedicle is exposed by grasping the gallbladder fundus which is then lifted together with the right lobe and rotated backwards. The following placements are used with this technique: 10 mm left upper paramedian (or just to the right of the midline avoiding the falciform ligament), 5 mm right upper midclavicular and 5 mm right lower axillary. The left upper paramedian cannula is placed about 1 cm lateral to the linea alba and 3 cm below the left costal margin. Some prefer to insert this cannula just to the right of the falciform ligament to obviate any entanglement in this structure. However, this position may result in crowding of instruments in the subhepatic pouch. The right upper cannula is best sited by reference to the gallbladder fundus using the finger depression technique for precise localization. This port must enter the parietes just below the liver edge. The right lower cannula is more laterally situated along the anterior axillary line some 4 cm below the costal margin. This cannula just skims the hepatic flexure and must be introduced with great care to avoid colonic injury.

With either the French or American approach the prescribed positions need to be adjusted in accordance with the build of the patient and, in particular, with the anatomy of the liver. An important consideration is the avoidance of placement of the ports above the inferior margin of the liver.

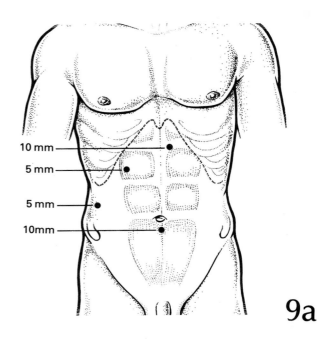

9a

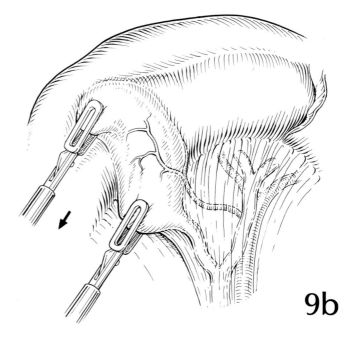

9b

Laparoscopic inspection

The initial laparoscopic inspection has three objectives: (1) detection of inadvertent injuries caused during insufflation and insertion of the main trocar/cannula; (2) exclusion of additional unsuspected intra-abdominal pathology; and (3) assessment of the feasibility of laparoscopic cholecystectomy.

A systematic inspection of the contents of the four quadrants and pelvis is undertaken. This step is equivalent to exploratory laparotomy during open cholecystectomy. Apart from excluding unsuspected disease, this inspection should rule out any significant trauma perpetrated during creation of the pneumoperitoneum or insertion of the first cannula.

To a large extent, the decision on the technical feasibility of the procedure is influenced by the experience of the surgeon in laparoscopic surgery. The situations which may be encountered are 'easy' cases, 'more difficult' cases, cases of 'uncertain feasibility' and unsuitable cases

'Easy' cases

10 There is minimal intraperitoneal fat and the gallbladder is floppy and non-adherent. When the gallbladder is lifted and retracted upwards by a pair of grasping forceps, the cystic pedicle (fold of peritoneum covering the cystic artery, duct and lymph node) is readily identified as a smooth triangular fold between Hartmann's pouch and the common bile duct.

'More difficult' cases

These include obese patients in whom the cystic pedicle is fat-laden. A gallbladder containing a large stone load may be difficult to grasp and this causes problems with retraction and exposure. The gallbladder may be distended due to cholecystitis or because of a stone impacted in the neck or Hartmann's pouch. Difficulties may also be encountered due to adhesions from previous surgery or abnormal anatomy of the hepatic arteries or extrahepatic biliary system. Provided the surgeon is experienced and is prepared to proceed slowly, these patients can undergo laparoscopic cholecystectomy with safety and a good outcome.

Cases of 'uncertain feasibility'

Trial dissection is indicated in such cases. This group includes patients with dense adhesions, those in whom the cystic pedicle cannot be visualized and patients with contracted fibrotic organs where the neck or Hartmann's pouch appears to be adherent to the common bile duct. In all these situations, the feasibility of the procedure becomes apparent as a careful trial dissection

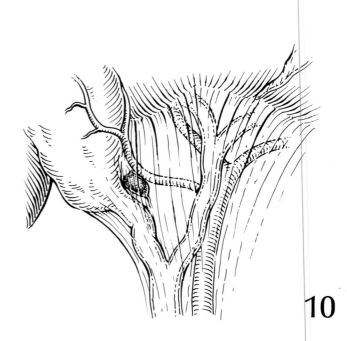

10

proceeds. In adopting this approach, common sense must prevail, and trial dissection should not be equated with a long hazardous procedure. If the surgeon cannot for any reason clearly identify and expose the structures of the cystic pedicle in the triangle of Calot in reasonable time, the case is converted to open surgery. Elective conversion must not be equated with surgical failure, and results in a much better clinical outcome than persistence with the laparoscopic approach in the presence of technical difficulties, which often result in iatrogenic injury and enforced conversion with enhanced morbidity.

Unsuitable cases

These include patients with severe acute cholecystitis with gangrenous patches or gross inflammatory phlegmon obscuring the structures of the porta hepatis, a chronically inflamed gallbladder with its neck adherent to the common bile duct (indicative of Mirizzi syndrome), and patients with advanced cirrhosis and established portal hypertension who have large high pressure varices surrounding the gallbladder and cystic pedicle.

In patients with severe acute cholecystitis which precludes safe dissection, a laparoscopic cholecystostomy may be performed with interval cholecystectomy at a later date.

Exposure of the subhepatic region and cystic pedicle

In the French technique a retractor is inserted through the upper medial right subcostal cannula and used to elevate the quadrate lobe. With an atraumatic grasper, introduced through the lower right port, the neck of the gallbladder is grasped and pulled anteriorly and downwards to display the cystic pedicle and the contents of the triangle of Calot (*see Illustration 8b*).

In the North American technique a gallbladder holding forceps is introduced through the right lower assisting port and is used to grasp the gallbladder fundus which is lifted in a lateral direction and rolled backwards to expose the subhepatic pouch. A second atraumatic grasper, inserted through the right upper cannula, is applied to the neck which is lifted upwards and anteriorly (*see Illustration 9b*). Although capture and retraction of the floppy non-inflamed gallbladder presents no problems, this step may be difficult in patients with a contracted fibrotic organ or if the gallbladder is distended or tightly packed with stones. Aspiration of the gallbladder by reducing the distension will permit a better grasp. A stone impacted in Hartmann's pouch may render capture of the neck of the organ very difficult. Attempts to dislodge the stone into the body of the organ, if successful, will greatly facilitate the dissection.

Dissection of the cystic pedicle

With both techniques, the cystic pedicle is inspected by advancing the telescope to obtain a closer view. In thin patients, this pedicle appears as a triangular fold between the neck of the gallbladder and the common bile duct which is often readily identified, especially if a forward oblique (30°) viewing telescope is used. The cystic pedicle outlines the margins of the triangle of Calot and contains between its superior and inferior leaves the cystic duct (usually anteriorly), the cystic artery (above and behind the duct) and the cystic lymph node which is closely applied to the neck of the gallbladder between the duct and the artery. The prominent anterior free edge of the cystic pedicle is formed as the peritoneum folds over the cystic duct. Dissection will prove difficult if the cystic pedicle is foreshortened or fat-laden.

The dissection of the cystic pedicle can be performed with scissors, electrosurgical hook knife or by teasing with fine pointed atraumatic graspers. In practice a combination of these techniques is often employed. Irrespective of the technique used, the first step consists of division of the superior leaf of the cystic pedicle.

The blunt teasing technique consists of stripping the peritoneum covering the cystic duct and artery in a medial direction towards the common duct against countertraction provided by a grasping forceps on the neck of the gallbladder. Oozing is controlled by soft coagulation, and the area is irrigated to maintain a clear view of the anatomy.

11a,b With the scissors technique, favoured by the author, the gallbladder is held retracted by an atraumatic grasper applied to its neck. The superior leaf of the cystic pedicle is divided from its free edge along the base of the triangle of Calot, keeping close to the medial aspect of the gallbladder as far as the liver. The dissection is kept superficial, dividing only the peritoneal covering and teasing it from the underlying structures. When the dissection has been completed, the cystic duct and artery become obvious, and dissection is then continued close to the cystic duct, mobilizing its posterior aspect with division of the inferior leaf of the cystic pedicle. The curved dissecting grasper is then employed to open the window between the cystic duct and the cystic artery. The tip of the instrument is placed in the cleft, and its jaws are opened gently and parallel to the two structures to commence the separation. This procedure has to be repeated several times until sufficient posterior mobilization has been achieved and a clear window is obtained. A fairly constant branch of the cystic artery traverses this window to supply the gallbladder neck. If identified, this branch is coagulated before division by the scissors. If oozing is sufficient to obscure the view at this stage, the area is irrigated, and minor bleeders are coagulated. When this has been completed, a gap becomes visible between the cystic duct in front and the artery behind. This gap is opened further by grasping and lifting the cystic duct anteriorly. A few fibrous attachments on either side of the gap are divided. Finally, the cystic duct is cleared of any residual extraneous tissues. In most patients, it is possible to isolate a 1.5–2-cm segment of the cystic duct. It is much safer to gain length by extending the dissection towards the gallbladder neck than extending medially.

The electrosurgical hook dissection is favoured by many surgeons. The instrument consists of a hollow insulated probe with a hook (J- or L-shaped) at the functional end. The other end is connected to the diathermy leads and also incorporates a suction/irrigation port which is controlled by a trumpet valve at the external end to release smoke and permit irrigation.

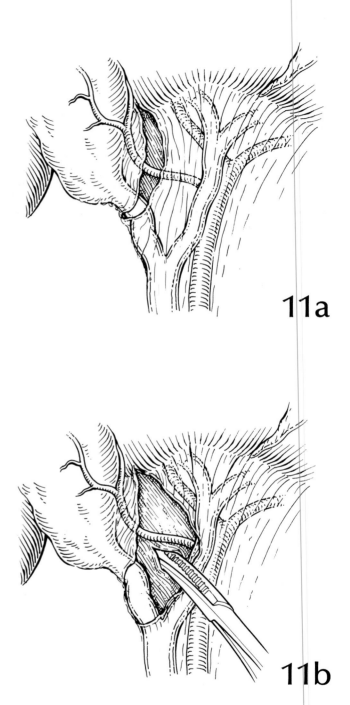

11a

11b

12 The technique entails lifting the peritoneum of the cystic pedicle from the underlying structures with the hook and then applying blended current to cut the lifted peritoneal covering. Tenting of the tissue is essential before activating the current for three reasons: (1) it limits the electrosurgical burn to the tissue constricted by the hook; (2) the cut is facilitated by the tension on the tissue; and (3) the gap between the tissue and the underlying structures increases the safety margin against collateral thermal injury.

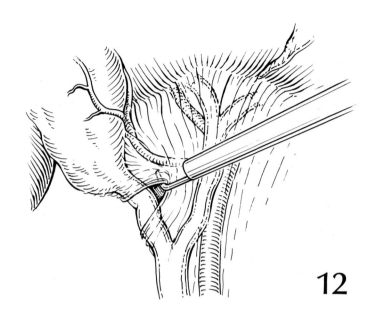

12

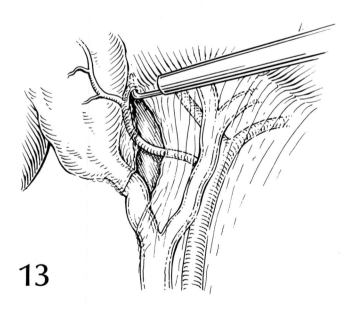

13

13 The dissection starts on the superior leaf of the cystic pedicle, proceeds laterally towards the neck of the gallbladder, and then curves upwards to the liver. The gap between the cystic duct and artery is identified.

14 Thereafter, the heel of the hook is inserted into this space and pushed backwards and medially before it is elevated in a forward direction to pick up the intervening tissue which is then cut by blender current. The inferior peritoneum of the cystic pedicle is divided using the same technique, keeping close to the neck of the gallbladder.

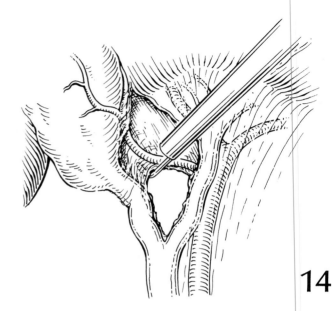

14

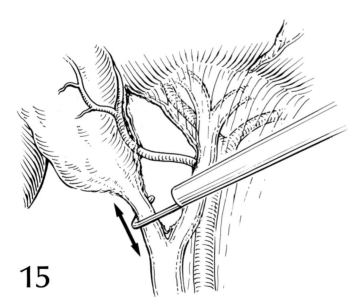

15

15 Eventually, it should be possible to place the hook around the mobilized cystic duct and to slide it up and down to separate any residual loose fibrous attachments.

The main disadvantage of electrosurgical dissection is the excess smoke generation. In addition, this technique causes considerable charring and some contraction of tissue planes.

The mobilized cystic duct must be clearly shown to be continuous with the neck of the gallbladder. Sometimes, an anomalous anterior cystic artery may be mistaken for the cystic duct and, as the cystic pedicle is under tension as a result of retraction of the gallbladder, pulsation may not be detected. Whenever this suspicion is raised, the telescope is advanced closer to the structure, and the retraction on the gallbladder is relaxed. This simple manoeuvre may restore obvious pulsations and help to resolve the problem.

Ligature/clipping and division of the cystic artery

16 The dissected cystic artery should be well displayed and shown to be terminating in the gallbladder. Anomalies of the cystic artery are common and have to be identified or excluded in every case. The most common anatomical arrangement is for the cystic artery to originate from the right hepatic artery as a single branch.

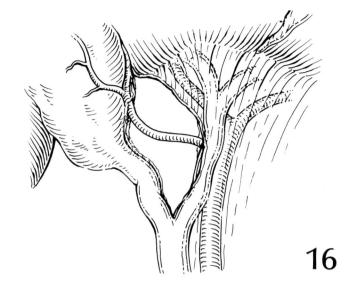

16

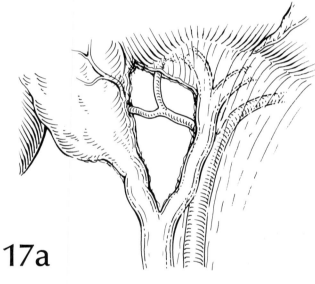

17a

17a,b The most dangerous variant is a looped right hepatic artery which can easily be mistaken for the cystic artery. Other important anomalies include early division of the cystic artery and aberrant origin of the right hepatic artery from the superior mesenteric artery.

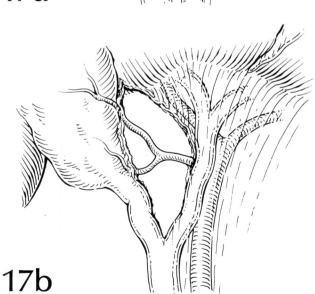

17b

18 A good length of cystic artery, at least 1 cm, should be mobilized if possible. Again, it is safer to gain the desired length by extending the dissection laterally towards the gallbladder neck. Most commonly, the fully mobilized artery is doubly clipped proximally. Although it is an end artery, its distal end should also be clipped before division by hook scissors at a safe distance from the proximal double clipped end.

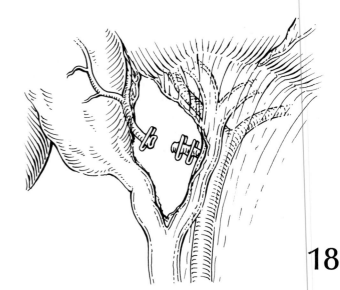

18

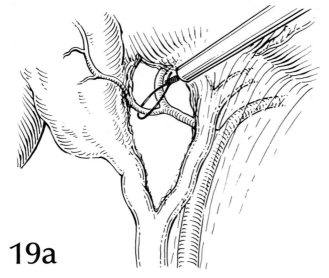

19a

19a,b Sufficient length of cystic artery for secure clipping may not be obtained when the artery divides early into anterior and posterior branches or when a short cystic artery arises from a looped right hepatic artery. In these situations, the safest technique is proximal ligature in continuity using 2/0 chromic catgut and a Roeder slip knot[4]. The distal end(s) may be secured by clipping.

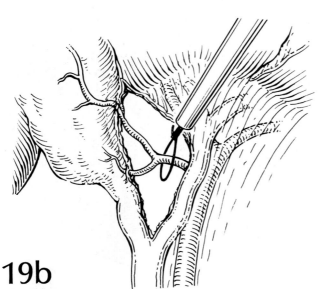

19b

Cholangiography

The need for operative cholangiography during laparoscopic cholecystectomy remains controversial. Some dispense with it altogether and others advocate a selective policy. The consensus view has changed in recent years in favour of routine intraoperative cholangiography for the following reasons:

1. Cholangiography provides a road map that identifies anomalies of the biliary tract which are especially relevant to safe ligature/clipping and division of the cystic duct.
2. Regular usage results in proficiency of cannulation of the cystic duct and in optimal interpretation of cholangiographic appearances. In this respect, the selective policy is counterproductive because the surgeon has difficulty in executing the procedure when he needs it most.
3. Cholangiography detects associated pathology including unsuspected stones.
4. Experience with and proficient use of intraoperative cholangiography is essential if a surgeon intends to progress to laparoscopic treatment of ductal calculi.

20a,b Laparoscopic cholangiography can be performed either by injecting contrast medium into the gallbladder (cholecystocholangiogram) or into the cystic duct using a modern C-arm image intensifier to allow detailed fluoroscopy. This technique is far preferable to the use of portable X-ray machines with blind exposure of three films after successive injections of contrast medium[5]. Unless the cystic duct anatomy is grossly disturbed (e.g. suspicion of a Mirizzi syndrome), a cystic duct cholangiogram is usually preferred.

The gallbladder end of the cystic duct is clipped but not the medial end. A cut is made on the anterior wall of the cystic duct by fine pointed curved microscissors and deepened until the lumen is entered.

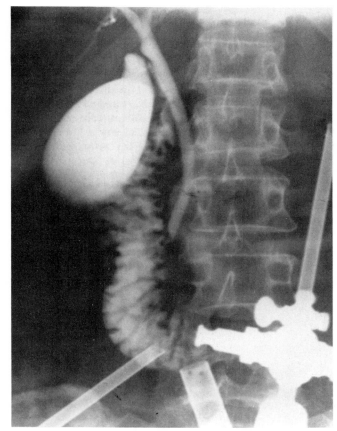

20a

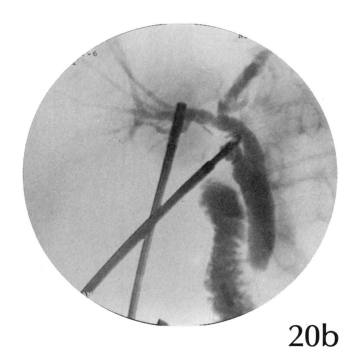

20b

21 Cannulation of the cystic duct (most commonly with a Cook ureteric catheter, 4–5 Fr) is considerably simplified by the use of a carrier device such as the cholangiograsper. The catheter is connected via a three-way tap to saline- and contrast-filled syringes (20 ml), and is inserted inside the cholangiograsper. The cholangiograsper loaded with the ureteric catheter is then introduced into the peritoneal cavity through the right upper port. With the jaws of the instrument open, the catheter is threaded inside the cystic duct. This step is greatly facilitated by steady injection of saline through the catheter to lift up the mucosal folds of the cystic duct.

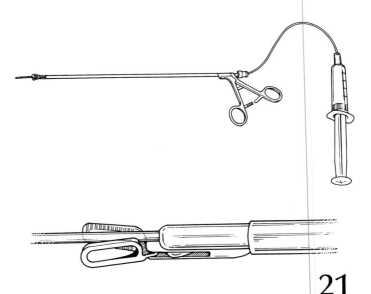

21

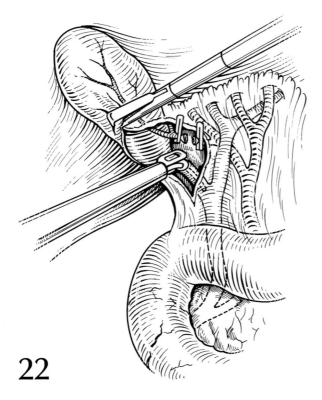

22

22 Once an adequate length is in place, the cholangiograsper is tilted medially and its jaws closed over the cystic duct and catheter. Contrast is injected slowly during image intensification to record the early phases of the duct filling.

On completion of the cholangiogram, the jaws are released, and the cholangiograsper and catheter are withdrawn. Fluorocholangiography performed in this manner should be completed within 10 minutes.

Closure and division of the cystic duct

Four techniques are available for securing the medial end of the cystic duct: (1) it can be clipped (metal or polydioxanone), (2) ligated in continuity, (3) secured by a preformed endoloop, or (4) closed by suture.

Medial clipping of the cystic duct

23   Most commonly, metal clips (titanium), usually double, are used although absorbable polydioxanone (Absolok, Ethicon) are preferred by some and do not carry the risk of stone formation. Both types of clip require specific applicators. It is important to apply the clips at right angles to the long axis of the duct and to ensure that the lateral wall of the common bile duct is not included in the clip. This problem may easily arise as upward and lateral displacement of the gallbladder often leads to tenting of the junction of the cystic and common bile duct. Although clipping of the cystic duct is the most popular method, this technique has certain disadvantages. In the first instance, clipping requires more duct length than ligature in continuity. Unless clips are applied at right angles to the axis of the duct, they are prone to slip and bile leakage postoperatively has a median reported incidence of 3%. Metal clips also may become internalized in the bile duct and form calculi.

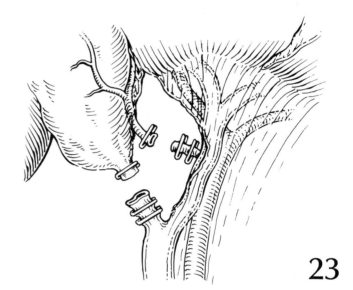

23

Medial ligature in continuity

24a–d This method involves ligature with an external Roeder slip knot after passing a 2/0 catgut around the cystic duct. The knot is fashioned externally and then slipped down and locked on the cystic duct close to the common bile duct. Dry chromic catgut (1.5 m in length) is best and is available commercially already mounted in a push rod. Alternatively, alcohol-packed material of suitable length is wiped clear of alcohol and left exposed on the sterile trolley to dry for at least 10 min. Ideally, this should be done by the scrub nurse at the start of the procedure.

The end of the catgut projecting beyond the bevelled tip of the push rod is grasped in a 3 mm needle holder and inserted inside a suture applicator passed through the left upper paramedian cannula. The end of the ligature is passed around the back of the cystic duct from above (*Illustration 24a*). The ligature is then grasped by the 5 mm needle holder (inserted through the right upper port) below the duct and transferred back to the 3 mm needle which is used to externalize the ligature (*Illustration 24b*). In order to prevent the ligature serrating the duct, closed forceps are inserted inside the loop to take up the tension (*Illustration 24c*). The Roeder knot is fashioned once the end of the ligature is exteriorized, and the knot is then slipped inside the abdomen by the push rod.

The resulting 'noose' is placed by the push rod a few millimetres medial to the opening of the cystic duct before it is locked tightly in place (*Illustration 24d*). The push rod is then withdrawn a few centimetres and the knot and its position on the duct are inspected.

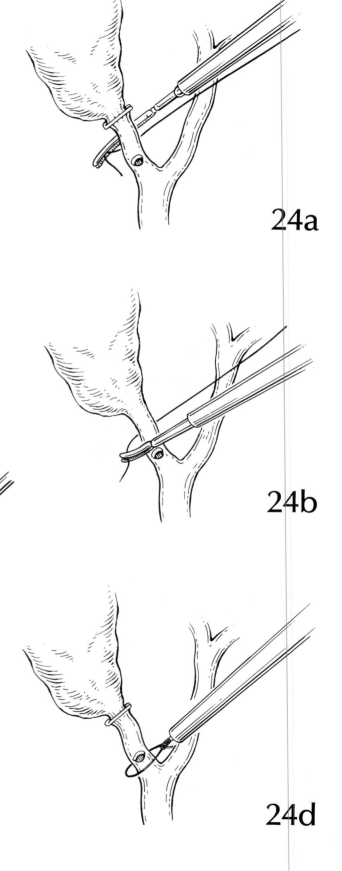

24a

24b

24c

24d

25 If considered satisfactory, the duct is then cut by claw scissors, and the excess suture, push rod and suture applicator are removed.

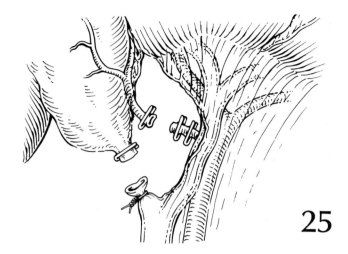

25

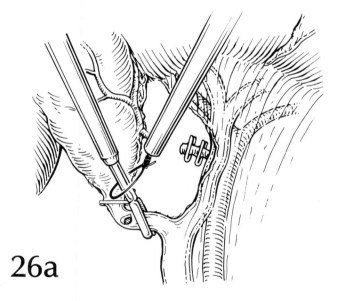

26a

Ligature by endoloop

26a,b An atraumatic grasper is passed through a preformed endoloop and used to grasp the cystic duct. The cystic duct is then divided just lateral to where it is grasped. The loop is threaded beyond the grasper, and the knot is tightened medial to the instrument before this is released.

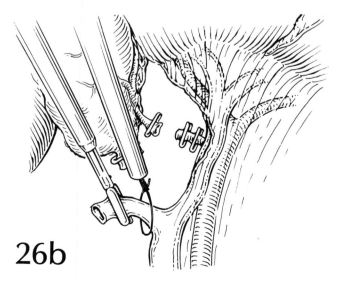

26b

27 After clipping and dividing the cystic duct, some surgeons apply an endoloop just medial to the proximal clip.

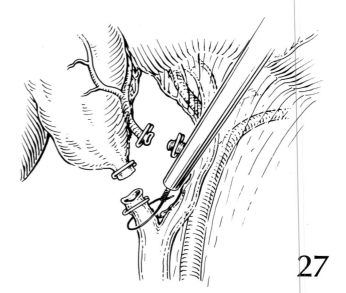

27

Suture closure of the cystic duct

28 This technique is necessary when the cystic duct is very short, and the opening is close to the common bile duct. A 3/0 catgut or synthetic absorbable atraumatic suture (Polysorb or coated Vicryl) is used to close the duct by a Z suture with intracorporeal knotting using a surgeon's knot. Closure and cutting of the cystic duct completes the detachment of the gallbladder from the structures of the porta hepatis.

28

Separation of the gallbladder from the liver bed

The plane of dissection is in the loose fibrous layer which separates the gallbladder from the subjacent fascia covering the liver bed. This plane is easy to find and follow in non-inflamed gallbladders, but can be difficult in cases with fibrous contracture. In any event, the dissection must not be carried through the superficial layers of the hepatic parenchyma as this causes excessive bleeding and may damage superficial bile ductules (including the ducts of Luschka) with the likelihood of postoperative bile leakage[6].

In non-fibrotic cases separation of the gallbladder from the liver can be carried out with electrosurgical, scissor or laser dissection.

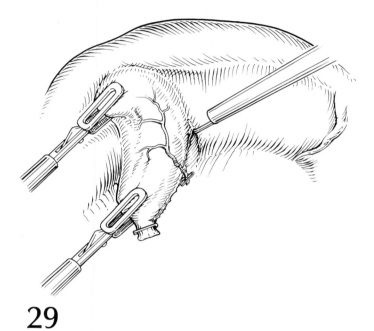

29 The detachment starts by separation of the gallbladder neck and infundibulum as the organ is held by an atraumatic grasper by the cut cystic duct. In non-adherent cases, this step should open up the loose areolar tissue plane between the gallbladder and the subjacent hepatic fascia. The gallbladder is held on the stretch by two grasping forceps, one on the fundus (assistant) and the other on the detached neck (surgeon's left hand). A pledget swab mounted on the appropriate laparoscopic holder is then used to separate, by blunt dissection, the undersurface of the gallbladder from the liver. This very efficient procedure mobilizes about 70% of the gallbladder in suitable cases and leaves only the lateral margins and the fundus still attached by their peritoneal reflections. These are then best divided by the electrosurgical hook.

29

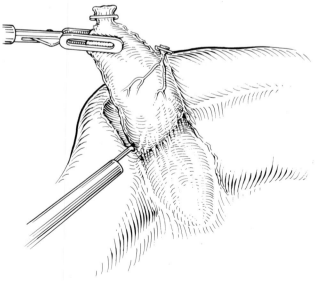

30 Following mobilization of the neck of the organ, the serosal lining on either side is divided with the electrosurgical hook-knife a few millimetres from the liver margin until the fundus is reached. Thereafter, with the gallbladder lifted upwards and held on the stretch in this position, the central dense fibrovascular attachments between the inferior surface of the gallbladder and the liver are divided with coagulation of any bleeding points. In these cases, particular attention is needed to ensure that the line of separation is not carried too deeply into the hepatic parenchyma. This problem should be suspected if excessive bleeding is encountered. Once separation of the gallbladder is complete, the fundus is grasped by the assistant until the organ is extracted.

30

31 When the fundal attachments are reached, reversal of the hold on the gallbladder facilitates the final separation. A grasper is placed on the fibrous tissue layer on the edge of the right lobe, just above the fundus, and used to elevate the liver as the gallbladder is allowed to hang down. It is steadied in this position by the other grasper held by the surgeon. The residual fundal attachments are then divided.

This technique is unsuitable for adherent contracted gallbladders or those which are deeply embedded in the liver substance.

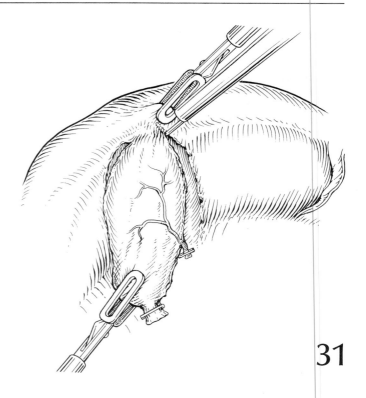

31

Extraction of the gallbladder

The gallbladder may be extracted through the left upper paramedian or umbilical incision. If the latter site is chosen, the telescope is removed from the umbilical port and reinserted through the left upper paramedian port.

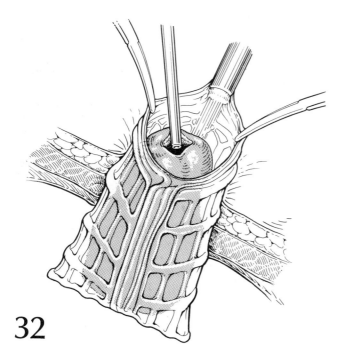

32

32 Several instances of tumour implantation have now been reported in the exit wound in patients with unsuspected gallbladder cancer undergoing laparoscopic cholecystectomy for symptomatic gallstones[7]. For this reason, unprotected extraction is ill advised, and every gallbladder should be extracted inside a rip proof bag. Several types of bag are available, but the easiest to deploy is that marketed by Advanced Surgical which opens up following insufflation of its two constituent layers and, moreover, closes completely by means of a drawstring once the gallbladder is placed inside it.

A rip proof bag also solves the problem of extraction in the presence of a large stone load. When the neck is exteriorized, the bag is opened, and the edges are held up above the wound. The fluid contents of the gallbladder are aspirated through a small opening which is enlarged to crush and remove the stones by means of a Desjardin forceps. This technique has replaced all others, including ultrasonic or electromechanical rotary lithotripsy.

Inspection, suction/irrigation and haemostasis

Any clots are evacuated. The subhepatic region and the gallbladder bed are irrigated and sucked dry. Any bleeding points in the gallbladder fossa are electrocoagulated to ensure a dry operative field. The liver surface is closely inspected for any accidental stab wounds or minor lacerations. The suphrenic space and the right paracolic gutter are next irrigated and aspirated until the fluid is clear and any debris and clots have been evacuated. Finally, the rest of the peritoneal cavity including the pelvis is inspected. A subhepatic drain is not needed after routine laparoscopic cholecystectomy unless the dissection has proved difficult with oozing and some bile leakage, in which case a silicon subhepatic drain attached to a closed suction system is inserted.

Desufflation and removal of ports

It is important that the access cannulae are removed under vision to ensure that there is no abdominal wall bleeding from any of the wounds. Unless recognized and dealt with, this problem may result in significant postoperative morbidity. The desufflation of the pneumoperitoneum must be as complete as possible to reduce the amount of postoperative shoulder pain.

Suture of the stab wounds

The wounds are infiltrated with long acting local anaesthetic (bupivacaine) before closure. All 10 mm (or larger) wounds require closure of the aponeurotic layers because of the risk of hernia formation. Smaller wounds require superficial approximation only (subcuticular absorbable sutures or skin tapes).

Postoperative care

Following reversal of neuromuscular blackade and extubation, an oropharyngeal airway is inserted, and oxygen is administered by mask for the first 3 h. The patient is nursed on the side. Analgesia is administered as required. The majority of patients are ready for discharge the next day. Although day-case laparoscopic cholecystectomy is practised in some centres, this practice must be backed up with effective nursing care.

Acknowledgement

Illustrations 3 and *5* have been reproduced with permission from Cuschieri *et al* (ed.) *Laparoscopic Biliary Surgery*, 2nd edn, published by Blackwell Science Ltd, Oxford.

References

1. Dubois, F, Berthelot G, Levard H. Cholecystectomy by coelioscopy. *Presse Med* 1989; 18: 980–2.

2. Cuschieri A, Dubois F, Mouiel J *et al*. The European experience with laparoscopic cholecystectomy. *Am J Surg* 1991; 161: 385–7.

3. The Southern Surgeons Club. A prospective analysis of 1518 laparoscopic cholecystectomies. *N Engl J Med* 1991; 324: 1073–8.

4. Nathanson LK, Easter DW, Cuschieri A. Ligation of the structures of the cystic pedicle during laparoscopic cholecystectomy. *Am J Surg* 1991; 161: 350–4.

5. Cuschieri A, Shimi S, Banting S, Nathanson LK, Pietrabissa A. Intraoperative cholangiography during laparoscopic cholecystectomy. Routine versus selective policy. *Surg Endosc* 1994; 8: 302–5.

6. Deziel DJ, Millikan KW, Economou SG, Doolas A, Ko ST, Airan MC. Complications of laparoscopic cholecystectomy: a national survey of 4292 hospitals and an analysis of 77 604 cases. *Am J Surg* 1993; 165: 9–14.

7. Clair DG, Lautz DB, Brooks DC. Rapid development of umbilical metastases after laparoscopic cholecystectomy for unsuspected gallbladder carcinoma. *Surgery* 1993; 113: 355–8.

Illustrations by Patrick Elliott

Minimally invasive surgery for gallstone disease: choledocholithiasis

George A. Fielding FRACS, FRCS
Visiting Surgeon, Royal Brisbane Hospital, Wesley Medical Centre, Auchenflower, Queensland, Australia

Principles and justification

Since the development of laparoscopic cholecystectomy, there has been continuing controversy over the correct management of common bile duct stones[1]. After initial enthusiasm for preoperative endoscopic retrograde cholangiopancreatography (ERCP)[2] or intravenous cholangiography[3], studies showed only a modest rate of detection of stones based on preoperative indications of choledocholithiasis. Efforts were then turned to developing technology of common bile duct exploration at the time of laparoscopic surgery. This advance, it is hoped, will allow management of gallbladder and ductal stones in one procedure, thus saving the patient repeat admission to hospital and avoiding more than one procedure. These techniques depend on the ability to perform cholangiography. For the best results, fluoroscopy with an image intensifier is needed with the ability to store images.

Preoperative

Anaesthesia

A general anaesthetic is used. A nasogastric tube and urinary catheter are not necessary in most patients. All insufflation is created using an open Hasson technique at the umbilicus.

Equipment

The essential equipment for the operation includes a laparoscope (30° viewing angle preferable), camera equipment, fluoroscope, standard laparoscopic cholecystectomy equipment, an Olsen–Reddick cholangiography cannula, short-tipped No. 4 Dormia basket (four wires), No. 4 or 5 ureteric catheter (end hole only), flexible choledochoscope (optional) and second camera, video mixer (optional), needle holder, T tube and suction drain.

An experienced assistant and theatre staff dedicated to laparoscopic surgery make the procedure much easier.

Operation

Position of patient

The patient is placed in a slight reverse Trendelenburg position with the right side slightly forwards. This position throws the colon and duodenum off Calot's triangle, although occasionally an extra port is needed to retract a bulky omentum and transverse colon.

Laparoscopy

1a, b A 30° telescope provides a better view than a standard 0° telescope, particularly of the common hepatic duct and subhepatic anatomy. Four ports are used in most cases. The lateral placement of the Hartmann's pouch retractor port allows this port to be used for cholangiography, and facilitates exposure of Calot's triangle.

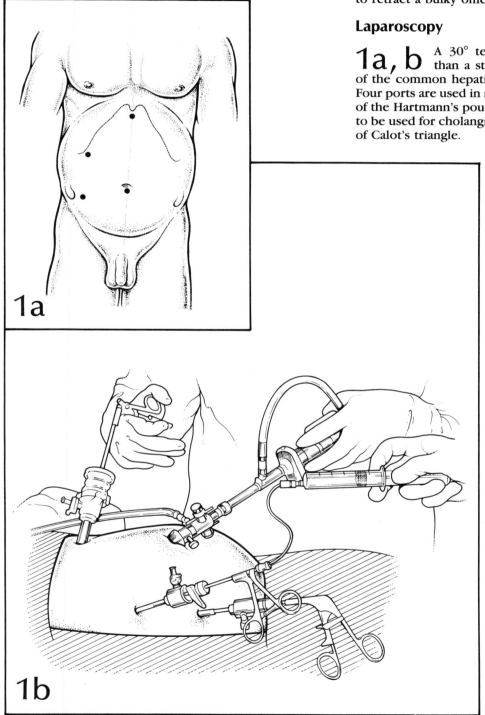

1a

1b

Dissection

2 Calot's triangle is dissected to expose two smaller spaces, between the cystic duct and cystic artery, and between the cystic artery and the liver. A second cystic artery may also be present. This mobilization is made easier by first dissecting the posterior peritoneal surface of the gallbladder, which frees up Hartmann's pouch and the cystic duct. No clips are placed until this dissection is complete. It is not necessary to dissect out the T junction of the cystic and hepatic ducts, and it is safest to stay close to the gallbladder at all times.

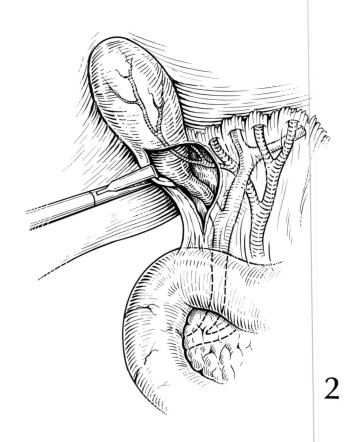

2

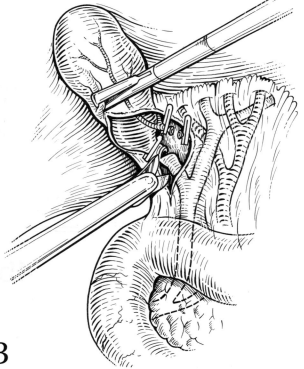

3

3 The cystic artery is clipped and divided, and a clip is placed just below Hartmann's pouch. The grasper is then removed from the right upper quadrant and inserted through the sub-xiphoid port to grasp Hartmann's pouch and retract laterally. The scissors are then inserted via the right upper quadrant port and used to divide the cystic artery and incise the cystic duct just below the clip.

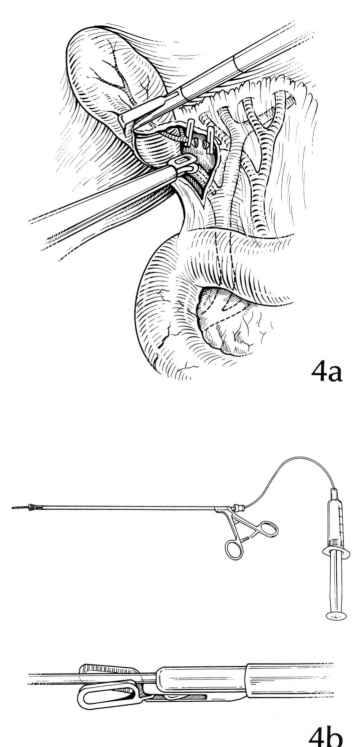

4a

4b

Cholangiography

4a, b The scissors are removed, and the Olsen–
Reddick cholangiography forceps are inserted through the right upper quadrant port. A No. 4 or 5 ureteric catheter, with an end hole only, is inserted into the cystic duct via the cholangiography forceps. The cholangiography forceps are then closed over the cystic duct, and cholangiography is performed.

A C-arm fluoroscopy unit with the ability to store images provides instant information concerning flow of contrast medium, distal biliary anatomy and the presence of stones in the common duct. It also allows monitoring of stone removal and easy clearance after cholangiography.

If stones are seen distal to the cystic duct and less than 1 cm in diameter, then basket extraction via the cystic duct is used under fluoroscopy or at choledochoscopy. Stones proximal to the cystic duct and more than 1 cm in diameter or multiple stones (> 10) are removed by choledochotomy.

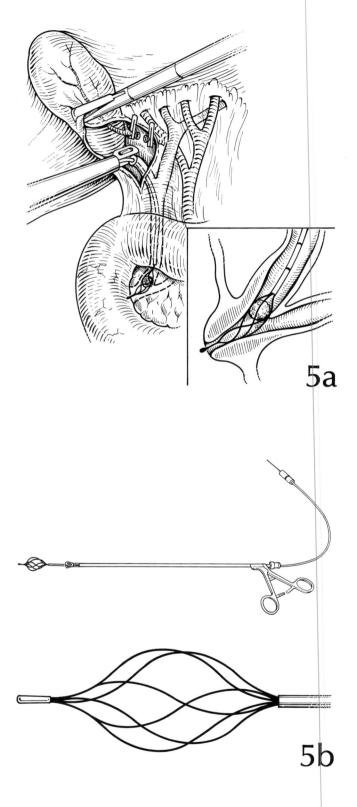

5a

5b

Dormia basket extraction

5a, b For basket extraction via the cystic duct, the cholangiography catheter is first removed leaving the forceps in place. A No. 4 Dormia basket (short tip, four-wire) is inserted into the cystic duct using cholangiography forceps and passed down the common bile duct to the ampulla. Fluoroscopy is used to check the position of the basket.

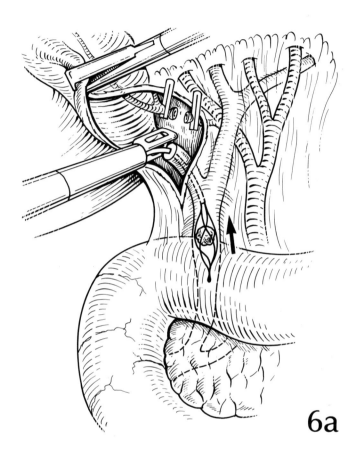

6a

6a, b Under fluoroscopy, the basket is opened and the stone or stones are snared. Without closing the basket, the wire is pulled back via the cystic duct, removing the stones. If small stones are lost from the basket it is repassed, the stones are snared and the basket is then closed. Leaving the basket open allows it to deform more readily as it passes into the cystic duct, reducing the chances of impaction at this junction.

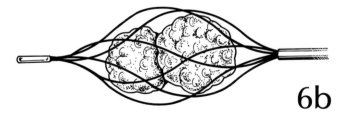

6b

7 Check cholangiography is then performed. The cystic duct is closed with clips or an endoloop if it is large. The gallbladder is then removed along with any stones that may be loose in the subhepatic space. Copious lavage is performed. A drain is not usually inserted.

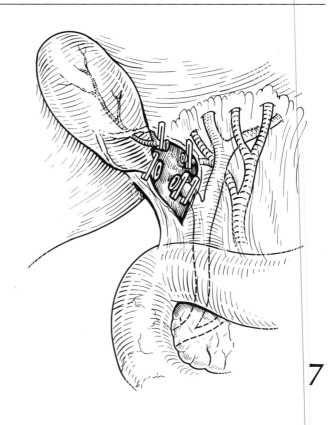

7

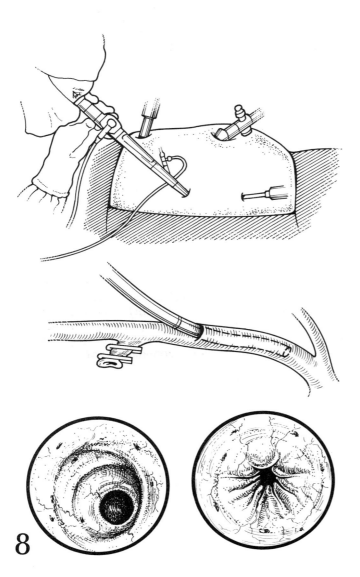

Choledochoscopy

8 A 3-mm choledochoscope can be passed via the right upper quadrant port or a 5-mm choledochoscope inserted through the subxiphoid port. The choledochoscope is inserted through the cystic duct, the stone is identified, and a basket is passed down the working channel. The stone is snared, and the choledochoscope, basket and stone are removed as one. The stones can be dropped into a bag or into the subhepatic space for later retrieval. The manoeuvre is repeated until all stones have been withdrawn. The stones and gallbladder are then removed from the abdomen. The choledochoscope can be connected to a second camera and then to a mixing device to allow simultaneous viewing of both laparoscopic and choledochoscope images. Alternatively, the image can be viewed directly through the choledochoscope without a camera.

8

Choledochotomy

9 If multiple, large or hepatic stones are present, the T junction of the cystic duct with the common duct is dissected. The cystic duct is divided, but the gallbladder is left *in situ* for retraction. The anterior surface of the common bile duct is dissected, and a 2-cm incision line is marked out with cutting diathermy, using low voltage. This method minimizes bleeding from surface veins on the common bile duct.

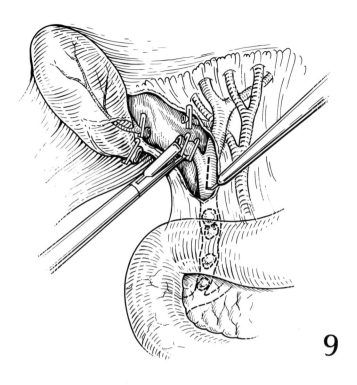

9

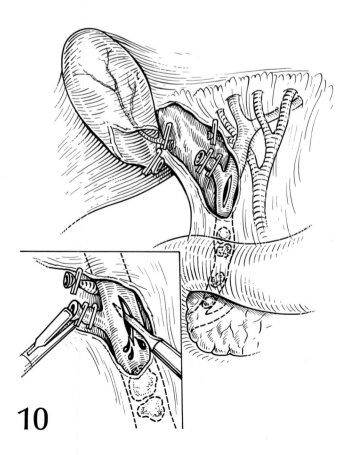

10

10 A fifth port (5 mm) is inserted in line with the umbilicus for retraction and suturing. The common bile duct is incised which may result in a sudden flow of bile and occasionally of stones. However, it is more common for stones not to appear, probably due to the increased intra-abdominal pressure.

11a, b Under fluoroscopic guidance, the Olsen–Reddick forceps are inserted via the subxiphoid port. A Fogarty balloon (long catheter, not the small biliary balloon) is inserted through the forceps into the common duct and passed beyond the stones. The balloon is inflated (usually with a 2-mm syringe) and withdrawn, bringing the stones with it.

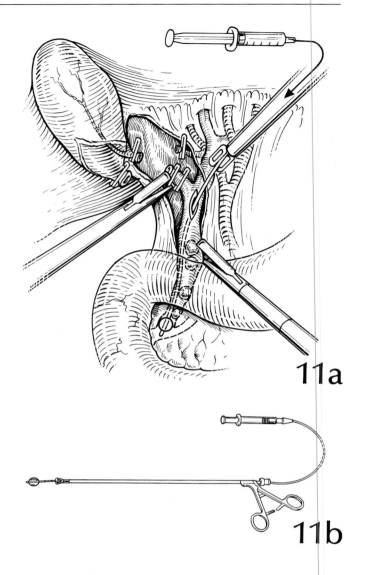

11a

11b

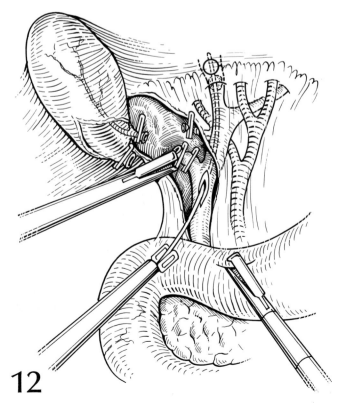

12

12 If hepatic stones are present, the balloon is passed into the hepatic ducts and the procedure is repeated. Lateral traction on the cystic duct and inferior retraction on the duodenum aid this procedure.

If stones are difficult to dislodge, a Dormia basket may be helpful. For stones impacted at the ampulla, a lithoclast lithotripter may help to shatter the stones to allow their removal with a basket. A contact laser may also be used in this setting. If a choledochoscope is available, these procedures may be performed under direct vision rather than under fluoroscopic control.

At completion, cholangiography of the upper and lower biliary tree is performed using the Olsen–Reddick forceps to occlude the choledochotomy around the cholangiography catheter. Cholangiography supplements choledochoscopy, especially in patients with multiple and intrahepatic stones.

Insertion of T tube

13a–d A No. 12 or 14 T tube is prepared, cut to the correct length and filleted. The T tube is then inserted through the subxiphoid port using an appendix introducer. The tips of the tube are delivered to the choledochotomy. Using graspers inserted in the right upper quadrant port, the tips are inserted into the common bile duct and then pushed up and down the duct. The introducer is removed, and the long end of the T tube is brought into the abdomen.

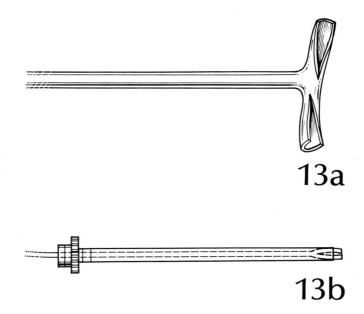

13a

13b

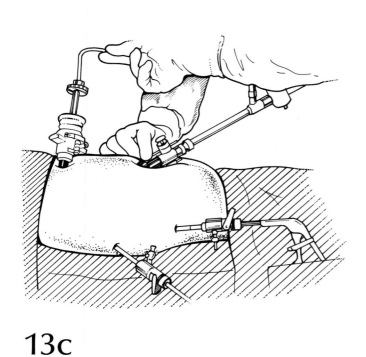

13c

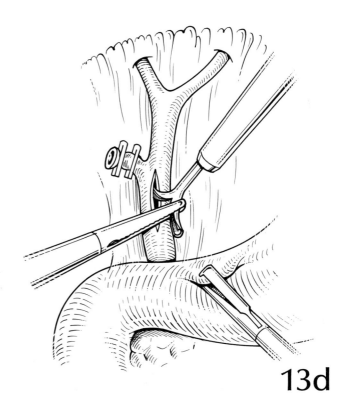

13d

14 The T tube is pushed to the top or bottom of the choledochotomy which is then sutured with a running 4/0 absorbable polydioxanone (PDS) suture. Cutting the suture length to 15 cm or less facilitates easy knot tying. This suture is then backloaded into an introducer and inserted completely into the abdomen.

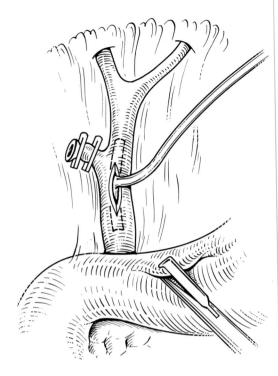

14

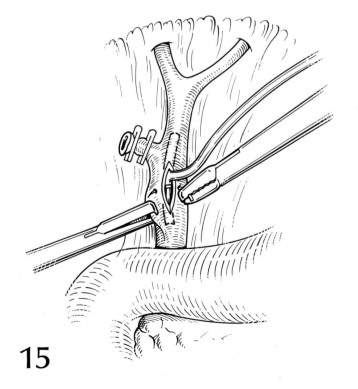

15

15 The choledochotomy is closed with a continuous suture starting adjacent to the tube. It is easier to come down the common bile duct from above and have the assistant follow the suture with a grasper inserted through the extra right upper quadrant port. Usually, 2–3 sutures are required, and the end is tied to itself. The needle holder is best inserted through the subxiphoid port, and the operator should have another grasper for retraction which is inserted through the right upper quadrant port. Two-handed operating is essential for suturing techniques.

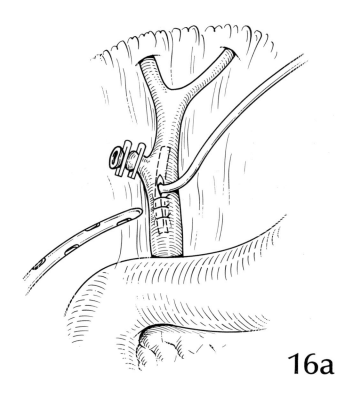

16a

16a, b
A suction drain is inserted through the right upper quadrant port, and the T tube is removed via the extra port in this quadrant.

The wounds are closed with subcuticular sutures and Steri-Strips and may be infiltrated with bupivacaine. An indomethacin suppository may also be given.

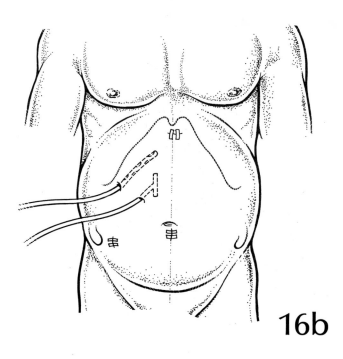

16b

Postoperative care

If the transcystic duct approach has been used, patients behave as if they have had a laparoscopic cholecystectomy in that most are able to go home the next day. If patients have had a choledochotomy, most are discharged between the second and fourth days. The suction drain is removed on the day after surgery. Patients are sent home with a T tube draining into the bile bag. They are seen 1 week after the operation and, if they are well, the tube is clamped. A T tube cholangiogram is performed after 3 weeks and, if it is clear, the T tube is removed and the patient discharged.

The most common complication is bile leakage around the choledochotomy (which usually persists for 2–3 days), and accidental removal of the T tube. These complications can also occur after open choledochotomy and are dealt with in the same way.

Outcome

This procedure allows management of cholelithiasis and choledocholithiasis in one sitting and minimizes the need for preoperative or postoperative ERCP. It can be done without extra equipment such as a choledochoscope and a second set of cameras, by using fluoroscopy to guide stone removal. However, choledochoscopy adds to the efficacy of the procedure.

A total of 129 such cases have been managed by the author[4]. Fifteen had saline flushing alone with a 73% success rate, but this technique is no longer used.

Dormia basket extraction was used in 79 cases with 96% success and with a median operating time (including cholecystectomy) of 55 min. A further 35 patients have had choledochotomy with a 91% success rate and a median operating time of 120 min. The median hospital stay was 2 days for Dormia basket extraction and 4 days for choledochotomy. Overall, 119 patients (92%) had successful stone removal, six had postoperative ERCP, two had open surgery after failed choledochotomy, and two had retained stones on T tube cholangiography. These results are in accord with those of other published series[5,6].

References

1. Perissat J, Huibregste K, Keane FB, Russell RCG, Neoptolomos JP. Management of bile duct stones in the era of laparoscopic cholecystectomy. *Br J Surg* 1994; 81: 799–810.

2. O'Rourke NA, Askew AR, Cowen AE, Roberts R, Fielding GA. The role of ERCP and sphincterotomy in the era of laparoscopic cholecystectomy. *Aust NZ J Surg* 1993; 63: 3–7.

3. Alinder G, Nilsson U, Lunderquist A, Herlin P, Holmin T. Pre-operative infusion cholangiography compared to routine operative cholangiography at elective cholecystectomy. *Br J Surg* 1986; 73: 383–7.

4. Rhodes M, Nathanson L, O'Rourke N, Fielding G. Laparoscopic common bile duct exploration – lessons learned from 129 consecutive cases. *Br J Surg* 1995; 82: 666–8.

5. Petelin JB. Laparoscopic approach to common duct pathology. *Am J Surg* 1993; 165: 487–91.

6. Stoker ME, Leveillee RJ, McCann JC, Maini BS. Laparoscopic common bile duct exploration. *J Laparoendosc Surg* 1991; 1: 287–93.

Illustrations by Gillian Lee

Cholecystectomy, cholecystostomy and exploration of the bile duct

David C. Carter MD, FRCS(Ed), FRCS(Glas), FRCS, FRSE
Regius Professor of Clinical Surgery, Royal Infirmary, Edinburgh, UK

S. Paterson-Brown MS, MPhil, FRCS(Ed), FRCS
Consultant Surgeon, University Department of Surgery, Royal Infirmary, Edinburgh, UK

Principles and justification

Open cholecystectomy was until recently the commonest major general surgical operation and approximately 500 000 operations were undertaken annually in the USA and some 40 000 in the UK. The reported incidence of common bile duct stones in these patients varied from 6% to 19% with a mean incidence of just over 10%[1]. Large series of patients undergoing open cholecystectomy without mortality have been reported[2], but it is well recognized that patients undergoing emergency surgery are at greater risk, as are those having concurrent exploration of the common bile duct. Experience in specialist centres may fail to reflect national or regional experience. In the decade up to 1989, the annual mortality rate for cholecystectomy alone in the Lothian region of Scotland fell consistently below 1%, averaging some 0.6%, while the mortality of cholecystectomy with bile duct exploration fell from around 3% to fluctuate around 1%. In some years, cholecystectomy with bile duct exploration incurred no mortality, and this undoubtedly reflected the increasing use of endoscopic papillotomy in high-risk patients with choledocholithiasis, jaundice and cholangitis.

Since the advent of laparoscopic cholecystectomy in 1987 the number of patients undergoing open cholecystectomy has fallen sharply. In one large study involving seven European centres, only 4% of patients scheduled for laparoscopic cholecystectomy required conversion to open operation[3]. However, it is clear that the ability to perform open cholecystectomy is still an essential part of the surgeon's armamentarium and, in many areas of the world, lack of resources means that this is still the standard method of removing the gallbladder.

Indications for cholecystectomy

The indications for cholecystectomy have not changed substantially with the advent of laparoscopic cholecystectomy.

Gallstone disease

Cholecystectomy is indicated in patients with biliary colic or acute cholecystitis and can be undertaken early in the acute admission or as an elective procedure in patients who have had previous attacks. While the basis of pain in biliary colic and acute cholecystitis is relatively easy to understand, there is less certainty about the association between flatulent dyspepsia and gallstones and whether this symptom complex is in itself a sufficient basis for cholecystectomy. In general, the prevalence of flatulent dyspeptic symptoms is similar when individuals with and without gallstones are compared[4]. Cholecystectomy does not always relieve symptoms, and about one-third of patients consult their general practitioner because of recurrent pain in the year following cholecystectomy. Asymptomatic gallstones are no longer regarded as an indication for cholecystectomy as they remain asymptomatic in the great majority of cases; exceptions may be made in the case of younger patients with multiple small stones (and a potential risk of gallstone pancreatitis), diabetics (who are more liable to life-threatening complications if cholecystitis develops), patients receiving immuno-suppression, and those receiving long-term parenteral nutrition.

Acute acalculous cholecystitis

This relatively rare condition accounts for up to 5% of all cases of acute cholecystitis; it is usually associated with critical and prolonged illness such as that seen with multiple trauma, major burns and sepsis, and may be commoner in patients having multiple transfusions and/or total parenteral nutrition. Emergency cholecys-tectomy is indicated as the condition frequently progresses to gangrenous cholecystitis.

Acalculous biliary pain

There is greater uncertainty about the role of cholecys-tectomy in patients thought to have acalculous biliary pain. The pain is similar to that found in symptomatic gallstone disease but occurs in the absence of gallstones or proven gallbladder disease. The patients are predomi-nantly young or middle-aged women. The decision to undertake cholecystectomy is a matter for clinical judgement in individual patients, although some con-sider that a positive response to a cholecystokinin provocation test may help to identify patients likely to benefit from cholecystectomy. Cholecystectomy fails to relieve symptoms in about 50% of patients, and not all accept that a functional disorder of the gallbladder is a satisfactory explanation for pain. It is conceivable that a functional disorder of the sphincter of Oddi causes pain in some patients and that cholecystectomy is in-appropriate if sphincter dysfunction is proven at manometry.

'Prophylactic' cholecystectomy

On rare occasions, cholecystectomy is undertaken 'prophylactically' in patients having a catheter inserted into the hepatic artery for hepatic perfusion chemo-therapy.

Gallbladder cancer

Cholecystectomy for gallbladder cancer is discussed in the chapter on pp. 407–416.

Preoperative

Many patients undergoing cholecystectomy are elderly and have intercurrent diseases that require full assess-ment and may benefit from preoperative management. Many are obese and weight reduction is advisable whenever possible to minimize the difficulty of surgery and risk of complications.

Postoperative wound infection is largely preventable by prescribing perioperative antibiotics such as tazobac-tam. Up to one-third of patients have infected bile, and the risk of infective complications in such individuals is increased. Risk factors include age over 50 years, history of jaundice, tender palpable gallbladder with fever or leucocytosis, a non-functioning gallbladder on cholecystography, abnormal liver function tests, and abnormalities of the common bile duct (notably ductal stones). When three or more of these factors are present or the patient has obvious infection, antibiotic therapy may be advisable for 5–7 days. The common infecting organisms are *Escherichia coli* and *Streptococcus faecalis* and appropriate antibiotics are tazobactam or cefotaxime and amoxycillin, the objective being to produce high blood and tissue levels rather than high levels in the bile.

The patient's blood should be grouped and a sample saved so that compatible blood can be released quickly if transfusion is necessary. An intravenous line is established before anaesthesia, and a catheter is advisable in jaundiced patients to monitor hourly urine output. A nasogastric tube is not inserted routinely.

Anaesthesia

General anaesthesia is employed, the objective being to render the patient unconscious and provide adequate analgesia and good muscle relaxation. If a nasogastric tube has been passed, its tip should be withdrawn well into the stomach so that it does not obscure the bile duct and affect the interpretation of operative cholangiograms.

Operations

CHOLECYSTECOMY

Position of patient

1 A C-arm to allow fluoroscopy is highly desirable. If fluoroscopy facilities are not available, the patient is placed supine on a cassette changer top so that the tip of the ninth costal cartilage is opposite the centre of the grid. Foam wedges or small bolsters are placed under the lower left rib cage and left buttock so that the common bile duct is not superimposed on the lumbar spine during cholangiography. The plane of the grid remains at right angles to the X-ray beam in order to give clear definition. A foam pillow or water-filled balloon (or gloves) is placed under the ankles to avoid calf compression during surgery. Subcutaneous heparin is used to reduce the risk of deep venous thrombosis.

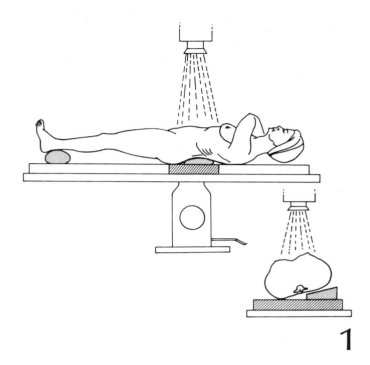

1

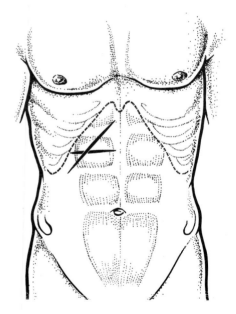

2

Incision

2 A Kocher's right subcostal or upper right transverse incision is used in preference to a vertical midline or right paramedian incision. Incision length is dictated by the patient's habitus and by the exposure needed once the peritoneal cavity has been entered and the findings assessed. Although incisions as small as 5 cm have been advocated for 'minicholecystectomy' and may provide adequate exposure in thin patients, failure to provide adequate access remains one of the major risk factors in cholecystectomy. The skin incision should be as long as is necessary for safe surgery. In the following description, a subcostal incision has been employed.

The surgeon normally stands on the patient's right with his assistant on the other side. The abdomen and lower chest is prepared and draped in the usual manner, but towel clips are avoided as they can obscure operative cholangiography. An adhesive skin drape is desirable to minimize wound infection. The subcostal incision is placed 4 cm below and parallel to the right costal margin and usually extends from close to the midline to the eighth or ninth costal cartilage.

3a–c Once the skin and subcutaneous tissue have been incised, the anterior rectus sheath is divided with a scalpel in the line of the skin incision. Diathermy is then used to cut through the rectus abdominis, coagulating or ligating any vessels. A Mayo or Roberts forceps can be passed behind the muscle so that it is placed on a slight stretch to facilitate the identification of vessels and their formal coagulation or ligation before they retract into the muscle. The peritoneum is next opened with a knife between forceps. The incision can then be lengthened with scissors or diathermy; if exposure is inadequate the muscle layers can be divided laterally with diathermy taking care to avoid damaging the ninth intercostal nerve.

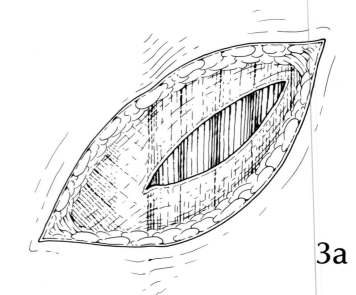

3a

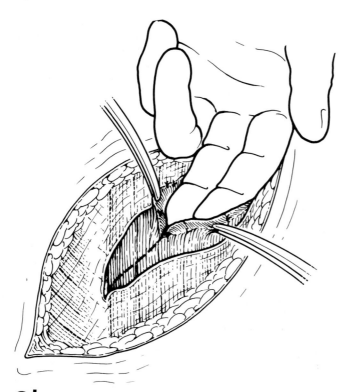

3b

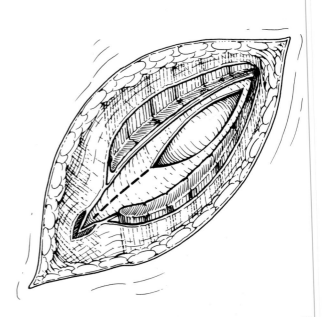

3c

Exploration

The peritoneal cavity is explored systematically paying particular attention to the oesophageal hiatus, stomach, duodenum, liver, gallbladder, small bowel and colon. The pancreas, spleen, kidneys, uterus and ovaries are not normally visualized but are palpated to detect any abnormality.

Exposure

The right hand is passed over the liver to introduce air so that the liver can descend into the wound. The gallbladder is grasped with two pairs of Mayo forceps or sponge-holding forceps, one pair being applied to the fundus and the other to Hartmann's pouch. This enables the gallbladder to be retracted downwards and laterally. Any adhesions are divided using dissecting scissors, taking care to avoid damage to the hepatic flexure of the colon or duodenum. Vascular adhesions involving the omentum may require ligature or diathermy.

4 Two moist packs are then inserted. The first packs the colon downwards and prevents bowel from entering the operative field. The second is placed so that the duodenum, stomach and free edge of the lesser omentum can be retracted to the left throughout the operation. These packs can be kept in place by Deever's retractors fixed to a retraction system such as an Omnitract or ring system, or held by assistants. In the past, a third assistant was often used to retract the costal margin upwards, but this can now be achieved by a short-bladed retractor fixed to a retractor system or taped under tension to a vertical pole attached to the table and hidden beneath the drapes. If only one assistant is available, his left hand may be used instead of a Deever retractor to retract the lesser omentum to the left.

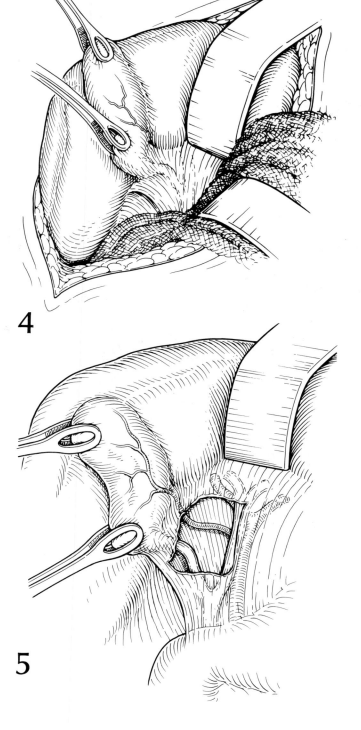

4

5 The peritoneum overlying the cystic duct is then incised using dissecting scissors, the incision being extended into the peritoneum overlying the common hepatic duct. The anatomy of the biliary tree is assessed carefully, noting the diameter of the cystic duct and common hepatic/common bile duct. A pledget held in a pair of Mayo or Robert's forceps is used to sweep adventitial tissues carefully away from the cystic duct and so display the triangle bounded by the cystic duct, common hepatic duct and inferior edge of the liver. This manoeuvre usually brings the cystic artery into view.

5

6 At every stage, one must remember that variations in the anatomy of the bile ducts and hepatic arteries are common. Common pitfalls are to mistake a small calibre common bile duct for the cystic duct (a potentially catastrophic cause of bile duct injury which is a particular problem in young slim women), failure to appreciate a low junction of the right and left hepatic ducts (the cystic duct in such cases may enter the right hepatic duct or one of its sectoral branches and the junction of right hepatic duct and left hepatic duct may be mistaken for the junction of the cystic duct and common hepatic duct), and failure to appreciate that the cystic duct is absent or very short. A common problem with arterial anatomy is posed by a right hepatic artery which swings far to the right before giving off a short cystic artery and multiple cystic arteries. The surgeon must have a clear picture of the anatomy before dividing any arterial or ductal structure; failure to appreciate the anatomy is the major cause of injury to the biliary tree or hepatic arterial supply.

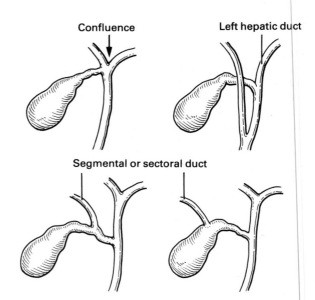

6

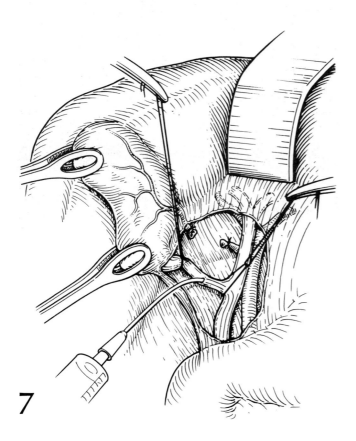

7

Operative cholangiography

There has always been (and probably always will be) controversy about the need for routine operative cholangiography. The authors undertake operative cholangiography routinely as a means of confirming ductal anatomy, avoiding ductal injury and detecting ductal stones.

Insertion of catheter

7 Many methods are available for operative cholangiography. The authors prefer to clear a length of cystic duct, tying a ligature around it just after it leaves the gallbladder and loosely encircling it with another ligature as it courses to join the common hepatic duct. A small scalpel (blade size No. 15) is used to incise, but not transect, the duct between these ligatures. A sample of bile is sent for bacteriological culture, and a fine cannula (e.g. Stoke or Trent cannula or ureteric catheter) is passed into the cystic duct and on into the common bile duct. Adhesions or mucosal valves which prevent ready passage can be broken down gently with a fine probe. It is important not to insert so much cannula that it passes into the duodenum and fails to provide a cholangiogram. A syringe of isotonic saline is used to flush all air from the cannula before its insertion to avoid air bubbles being mistaken for gallstones on the operative cholangiogram.

Once the cannula has been inserted and its patency confirmed by aspirating bile, the loose ligature around the cystic duct is tied to prevent leakage of contrast during cholangiography. Alternatively, metal clips (Ligaclips) can be used to occlude the cystic duct.

Exposure of films

All instruments and packs are removed from the abdomen and the wound is covered with a sterile towel. As indicated earlier, the patient lies on a cassette exchanger unless facilities for fluoroscopy and image intensification are available. If the patient has not been positioned with the left side raised by about 10–15°, the table can be tilted to make sure that the image of the bile duct is not obscured by being superimposed on the vertebral column. The saline-filled syringe is replaced by one containing 25% Hypaque or similar solution, again taking meticulous care to avoid introducing air bubbles during the exchange. Three films are then taken after introducing 2–3 ml, 4–6 ml and 7–10 ml of contrast medium respectively, the amount being influenced by the size of the duct system. The theatre is cleared momentarily of all personnel during exposure of the films, and the anaesthetist arrests ventilatory movement while the films are being exposed.

8 There are five criteria for a normal cholangiogram and these should be documented: (1) no filling defects in the biliary tree; (2) normal width of the common bile duct (opinions vary as to whether a diameter of up to 8 or 10 mm is normal at the level of insertion of the cystic duct); (3) gentle tapering of the common bile duct as it comes into proximity with the duodenum and enters its lumen; (4) free flow of contrast medium into the duodenum; and (5) normal filling of both the left and right hepatic ducts.

Once a cholangiogram has been obtained, the surgeon has three options: (1) to proceed with the operation if the cholangiogram is of acceptable quality and normal; (2) to proceed with duct exploration if a filling defect(s) is seen; and (3) to repeat the cholangiogram if the films are inadequate.

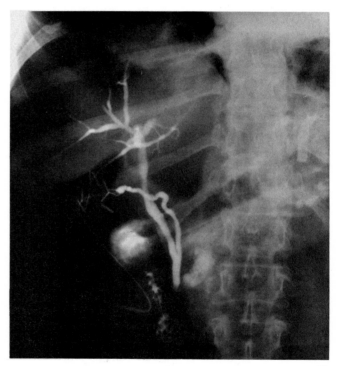

8

Removal of the gallbladder

9 Assuming that the cholangiogram is normal, the cannula is removed and the cystic duct is then securely tied with an absorbable ligature. The cystic artery is also doubly ligated and both structures are then divided.

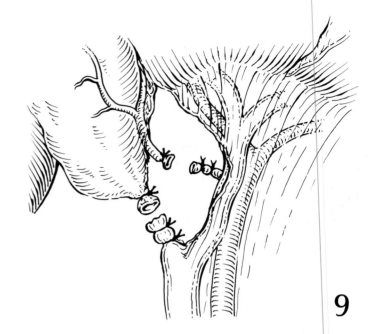

9

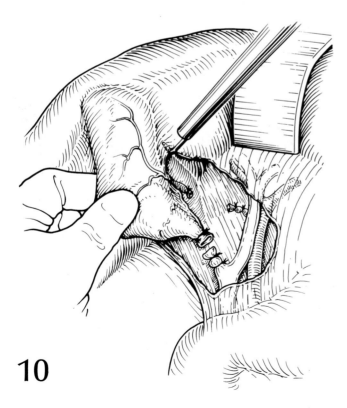

10

10 The gallbladder is kept under tension by gentle traction from the surgeon's left hand, and the fold of peritoneum attaching the gallbladder to the liver is divided using a combination of sharp dissection and electrocoagulation.

11a,b

On occasion, it may be safer to remove the gallbladder using a 'fundus first' approach, particularly when inflammation or adhesion formation makes it difficult to display the common bile duct, cystic duct and cystic artery. If the 'fundus first' approach is adopted it is important to establish the correct plane between the gallbladder and its bed; dissecting too deeply will enter the liver parenchyma, while dissecting too superficially risks entering the gallbladder lumen. Dissecting too close to the gallbladder is the lesser of the two evils. A combination of sharp dissection, diathermy dissection and blunt dissection with a pledget is often needed, and the suction apparatus is often a surprisingly useful tool for blunt dissection. Care must be taken as the dissection approaches the main biliary tree and when displaying the cystic duct and cystic artery. It may be safer to leave a small oversewn cuff of Hartmann's pouch rather than to attempt hazardous dissection to free an adherent gallbladder and cystic duct from the common hepatic duct.

Partial cholecystectomy is also a sensible option in patients with cirrhosis and/or portal hypertension.

Regardless of whether the gallbladder is removed fundus first or by the more conventional method, a small swab is placed in the gallbladder bed to control oozing. Any small bleeding vessels are coagulated, and if bleeding is troublesome and persists, a gauze swab or small pack is left in the gallbladder bed for 3–5 min. If this does not produce adequate haemostasis, underrunning of the bleeding points with a fine absorbable suture may be needed.

Once haemostasis is achieved, the right upper quadrant is lavaged with warm saline which is then removed. A drain is not inserted routinely, although many surgeons use a small suction drain (e.g. Redivac) if there are lingering anxieties about haemostasis. The incision is closed using a mass suture technique, and the skin edges are approximated with metal clips.

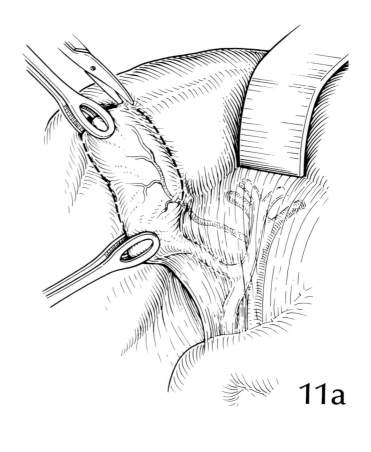

11a

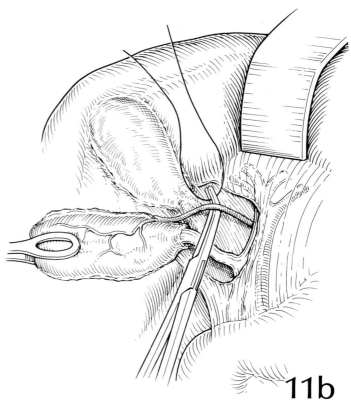

11b

CHOLECYSTOSTOMY

Drainage of the gallbladder is occasionally indicated when cholecystectomy proves unduly difficult and potentially hazardous, and may be undertaken by an open or percutaneous technique. Open cholecysto-stomy will be described here and percutaneous cholecystostomy is described on page 290.

12 If trial dissection indicates that cholecystectomy is impractical, the fundus of the gallbladder should be packed off from the surrounding tissues. The fundus is then incised between stay sutures or within a purse-string suture so that the lumen is entered and its contents evacuated. Alternatively, a trocar and cannula can be used with suction applied to the side arm of the cannula to empty the gallbladder of its contents. Large stones are sometimes difficult to extract, but every effort must be made to ensure that the gallbladder is emptied completely.

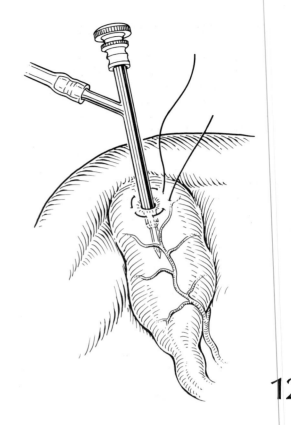

12

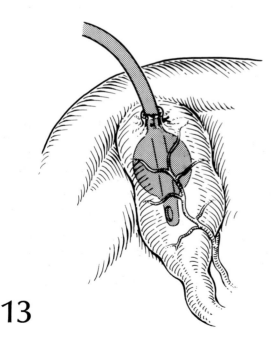

13

13 The cholecystotomy is next closed around a Foley catheter of appropriate size, after first passing the catheter through a small stab incision to one side of the main wound. The gallbladder wall is snugged around the emerging catheter using resorbable suture material, and most surgeons prefer to use a purse-string suture rather than interrupted sutures.

If possible, up to four interrupted sutures are then used to approximate the gallbladder wall to the peritoneum around the site of the stab incision. However, this may not be feasible if the gallbladder is not of sufficient size to lie comfortably against the peritoneum of the anterior abdominal wall.

EXPLORATION OF THE COMMON BILE DUCT

The decision to explore the common bile duct rests on the demonstration of stones on operative cholangiography or on palpation. Postoperative endoscopic retrieval of stones now offers an alternative approach which may be considered in a younger patient with a small calibre common bile duct and small stones. On the other hand, an elderly patient with large stones in a distended common bile duct is best served by operative exploration at the time of cholecystectomy. In general, a good reason is required not to proceed to explore the duct if stones have been demonstrated, and it should be borne in mind that endoscopic removal is not always successful and is not without risks.

14 Having removed the gallbladder and made the decision to explore the common bile duct, the second part of the duodenum is then mobilized by division of the lateral leaf of its peritoneal covering (Kocher manoeuvre). This allows the surgeon's hand to pass behind the duodenum and head of the pancreas to palpate the lower common bile duct. The anterior surface of the common duct is then cleared of its peritoneal covering and needled to obtain a specimen of bile for bacteriological examination.

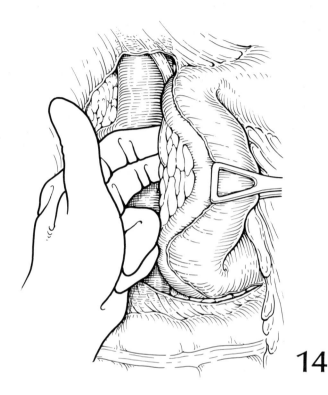

14

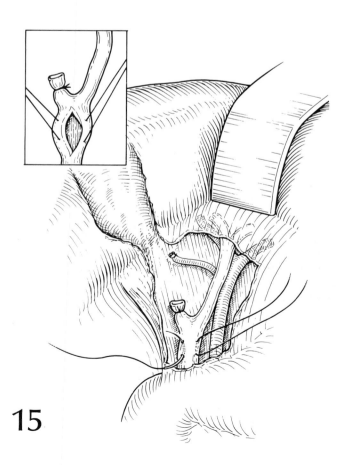

15

15 The duct is then incised between stay sutures using a size 15 blade and the longitudinal choledochotomy is enlarged using angled dissection scissors. The size of the opening is dictated by the size of the stones but it is usually about 15–20 mm long. Care must be taken when extending the incision upwards not to damage the hepatic arterial tree, and the right hepatic artery is often at particular risk as it loops in front of the bile duct. Similarly, care should be taken when extending the choledochotomy downwards not to damage the numerous small veins running on to the duodenum and so encounter troublesome bleeding.

16a–d

A fine catheter may be inserted into the bile duct at this stage and warm saline is used to try to flush out any small stones and debris. A flexible choledochoscope then offers the ideal method of inspecting the biliary tree from within and it should be passed down as far as the ampulla and upwards as far as the right and left hepatic ducts. Any residual stones are removed by further flushing with warm saline or by using a biliary Fogarty balloon catheter. The catheter is first passed into the duodenum and the balloon is carefully inflated. The catheter is then gently withdrawn allowing the balloon to deflate so that it passes through the papilla of Vater and sphincter of Oddi without undue force. Once above the sphincter region, the balloon is reinflated so that stones can be seen in the choledochotomy and withdrawn from the duct. A similar manoeuvre is used to extract any residual stones from the upper reaches of the biliary tree.

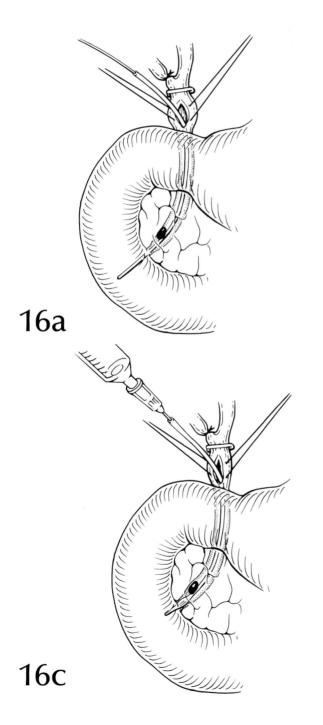

16a

16c

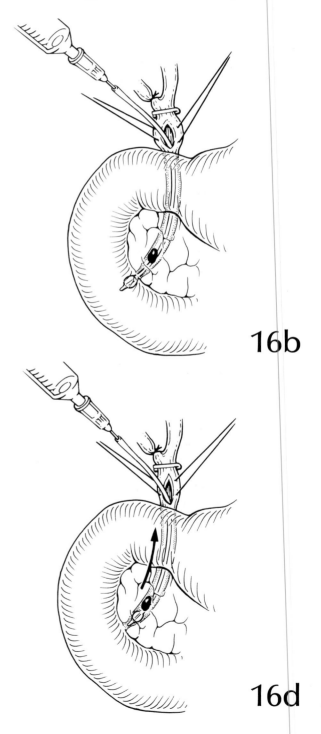

16b

16d

17 If these measures fail, Desjardin's forceps can be inserted into the duct system to grasp any stones that are visible. Repeated attempts to grasp stones 'blindly' with Desjardin's forceps can damage the duct and should be avoided.

Stones which have not been retrieved at this stage can sometimes be recovered under choledochoscopic guidance using a Dormia basket.

A stone which is trapped at the lower end of the bile duct and cannot be dislodged can pose particular difficulties. Large stones can sometimes be retrieved if the choledochotomy is extended a little more distally so that the stone comes into view. Failing this, the surgeon can elect to open the duodenum and remove the stone following sphincterotomy (*see* pp. 282–290), or to carry out a choledochoduodenostomy (*see* pp. 351–353) leaving the stone in place. Simply closing the duct and relying on postoperative endoscopic retrieval is not an option as the chances of successful endoscopic extraction are poor when the stone has been found to be impacted at open operation. Transduodenal extraction is the method of choice provided the surgeon is sufficiently experienced and the general condition of the patient permits, and a sphincteroplasty (*see* pp. 354–361) should be performed once the offending stone has been removed.

Confirmation that the bile ducts have been cleared is obtained by choledochoscopy. If a choledochoscope is not available, post-explorative cholangiography can be performed using a Fogarty catheter with its balloon inflated to prevent leakage of dye while films are taken first of the upper reaches of the bile duct and then of its lower portion.

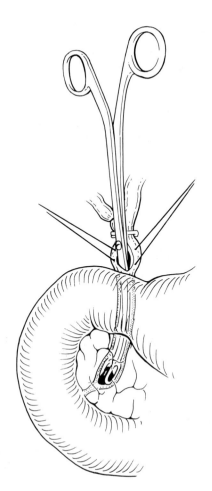

17

18 Once duct clearance has been confirmed, a rubber T tube (size 14−16 Fr depending on duct size) is inserted after trimming the ends of its short arm to an appropriate length and guttering this part of the tube. The choledochotomy is closed snugly around the T tube using interrupted 3/0 absorbable sutures such as polydioxanone (PDS). The T tube is brought out through the abdominal wall at a convenient point away from the main wound, taking care to ensure that it runs perpendicular to the axis of the bile duct. An anchoring suture to the skin is used to prevent the T tube from falling out prematurely.

Some surgeons do not insert a T tube after exploring the bile duct, but the authors insert one routinely and use it to obtain a check cholangiogram 5−7 days after the operation. Premature removal of the T tube may allow biliary leakage and biliary peritonitis and most surgeons do not remove the tube for at least 7−10 days.

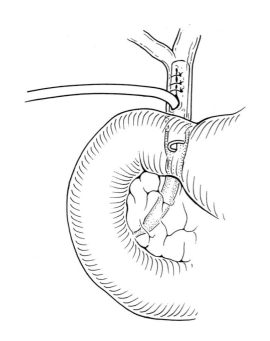

18

Postoperative care

Following cholecystectomy, patients are maintained on intravenous fluids for the first 12 h. Oral intake is resumed on the first postoperative day according to the clinical condition of the patient, and early mobilization is encouraged. After uneventful elective cholecystectomy, many patients are ready for discharge from hospital within a few days.

References

1. Menzies D, Motson RW. Choledocholithiasis − detection and open management. In: Paterson-Brown S, Garden OJ, eds. *Principles and Practice of Surgical Laparoscopy*. Philadelphia: WB Saunders, 1994: 81−104.

2. Clavien PA, Sanabria JR, Mentha G *et al*. Recent results of elective open cholecystectomy in a North American and a European center. Comparison of complications and risk factors. *Ann Surg* 1992; 216: 618−26.

3. Cuschieri A, Dubois F, Mouiel J *et al*. The European experience with laparoscopic cholecystectomy. *Am J Surg* 1991; 161: 385−7.

4. Banting S, Carter DC. Expectations of cholecystectomy. In: Paterson-Brown S, Garden OJ, eds. *Principles and Practice of Surgical Laparoscopy*. Philadelphia: WB Saunders, 1994: 53−66.

Choledochoduodenostomy

R. C. G. Russell MS, FRCS
Consultant Surgeon, The Middlesex Hospital, London, UK

History

This operation was introduced in 1892 by Riedel, and since then has waxed and waned in popularity as a result of its potential for stenosis with consequent infection within the pancreatic portion of the bile duct. Its significant advantage now is that it provides access to the biliary tree for the endoscopist.

Principles and justification

Choledochoduodenostomy is indicated in the management of both benign and malignant disease, but only if the common bile duct is dilated to 12 mm or more. This operation should never be performed if the duct is small. For benign disease, the indications are now rare as the majority of common bile ducts can be cleared endoscopically or by combination with an operation. The only indication for stone disease is in elderly patients who do not have endoscopic access to the biliary tree because of a previous partial gastrectomy or a diverticulum at the ampulla of Vater which may make sphincterotomy difficult or dangerous. In the presence of stone disease and poor drainage a choledochoduodenostomy is ideal in the older person, but in the younger patient an end-to-side choledochojejunostomy is preferable.

In patients with oriental cholangitis or multiple intrahepatic stones, a choledochoduodenostomy can provide good drainage and direct access to the biliary tree for the endoscopist. However, it is rarely required as the percutaneous approach to the intrahepatic ducts is easier and more successful for clearing stones from the biliary tree, especially with the development of improved choledochoscopes.

The commonest indication for choledochoduodenostomy is malignant obstruction by pancreatic tumours. Provided the anastomosis is performed in the mid bile duct, recurrence of jaundice is rare (less than 10% in a series reported by Smith et al.[1]).

Preoperative

These patients are usually ill, infected and jaundiced, so they require careful preoperative preparation. Coagulation must be checked and corrected and vitamin K should be given. An intravenous infusion should be commenced the previous evening to ensure adequate hydration and a good urine output. The bladder is catheterized preoperatively. If the patient has malignant disease, thrombolic prophylaxis with TED stockings and low-dose subcutaneous heparin should be instituted. Antibiotics are given as appropriate. It is presumed that endoscopy and, if malignancy is suspected, spiral computed tomographic scanning has defined the disease preoperatively and the operation plan is clear.

351

Operation

Incision

This is a minimally invasive procedure and, thus, the principles for such operations should be followed. A transverse 6-cm incision is adequate both to undertake a cholecystectomy and to perform the procedure, together with a gastrojejunostomy if required.

Exposure

The gallbladder is assessed as for a mini-cholecystectomy and removed both to increase exposure and prevent late sepsis subsequent to blockage of the cystic duct by tumour. The nature of the pathology is determined, and the preoperative findings are confirmed. To expose the bile duct and the duodenum, the fascia which binds the hepatic flexure to the duodenum is divided to enable adequate exposure of the subhepatic space, the bile duct and duodenum. Mobilization of the duodenum is unnecessary. A stabilized ring retractor is used to facilitate the exposure.

Dissection

1 The cystic duct stump is followed to the bile duct, and the peritoneum over the bile duct is dissected to explore the wall of the duct and ensure that there is no tumour involvement. The first part of the duodenum is mobilized by dividing the branches of the right gastric artery and the adjacent peritoneum. These vessels are usually small and can be cauterized safely. This manoeuvre enables the first part of the duodenum to be brought up to the mid position of the bile duct without tension.

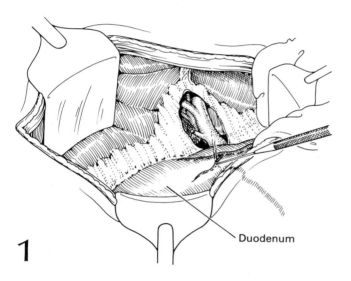

Duodenum

1

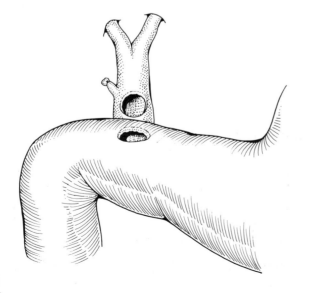

2

Formation of stoma

2 A disc of mid common bile duct, 1 cm in diameter, is removed from the anterior surface of the bile duct, and a similar disc, 1 cm in diameter, is removed from the superior surface of the duodenum.

Anastomosis

3a–c The two holes are approximated and sutured with interrupted 3/0 polyglactin (Vicryl) or 4/0 polydioxanone (PDS) sutures incorporating all layers. It is easiest to start laterally and then to place the posterior sutures. Sutures should be placed 3 mm apart and 3 mm deep to ensure an even closure. The sutures are tied after all the posterior layer has been completed. The anterior layer is then completed, and the sutures are tied at the end. An outer or covering layer is not necessary.

Closure

Meticulous haemostasis is ascertained, and the wound is closed without drainage as for a mini-cholecystectomy. Again, the muscle is infiltrated with 20–30 ml bupivicaine and adrenaline. The skin is closed with a subcuticular suture of 3/0 polydioxanone. A diclofenac suppository (100 mg) is given at the end of the procedure.

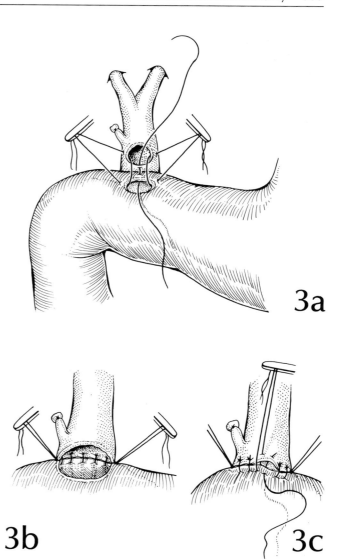

3a

3b

3c

Postoperative care

These patients are ill and often have extensive malignant disease. They are thus prone to complications. Renal failure must be avoided by measurement of urine putput on an hourly basis, and appropriate action should be taken if the output falls below 30 ml/h. If there was evidence of biliary infection, appropriate antibiotics should be administered while the results of bile culture are awaited.

Oral fluids may be commenced the following day, and the intravenous infusion can be discontinued as soon as there is an adequate oral intake. Mobilization should start immediately, and care must be taken to avoid chest infection.

Outcome

For benign disease, the morbidity should be less than 10% and the mortality below 1% but, for malignant disease, the outcome is less good with a 30-day mortality of 15% and a significant morbidity of 30%.[2] Unfortunately, these patients are often regarded as having a terminal malignancy and do not receive the care they require, with the result that the ideal results achieved by some are not attained by many.[3]

References

1. Smith AC, Dowsett JF, Russell RC, Hatfield AR, Cotton PB. Randomised trial of endoscopic stenting versus surgical bypass in malignant low bile duct obstruction. *Lancet* 1994; 344: 1655–60.

2. Bramhall SR, Allum WH, Jones AG, Allwood A, Cummins C, Neoptolemos JP. Treatment and survival in 13560 patients with pancreatic cancer, and incidence of the disease in the West Midlands: an epidemiological study. *Br J Surg* 1995; 82: 111–15.

3. Lillemoe KD, Sauter PK, Pitt HA, Yeo CJ, Cameron JL. Current status of surgical palliation of periampullary carcinoma. *Surg Gynecol Obstet* 1993; 176: 1–10.

Transduodenal sphincteroplasty and exploration of the common bile duct

Charles M. Ferguson MD
Assistant Professor of Surgery and Associate Visiting Surgeon, Massachusetts General Hospital, Harvard Medical School, Boston, Massachusetts, USA

Andrew L. Warshaw MD
Harold and Ellen Danser Professor of Surgery, Chief of General Surgery and Associate Chief of the Surgical Services, Massachusetts General Hospital, Harvard Medical School, Boston, Massachusetts, USA

Principles and justification

Transduodenal sphincteroplasty is, in essence, a side-to-side choledochoduodenostomy performed through the duodenal lumen. As such, this operation is useful in removal of an impacted common duct stone and in the treatment of stenosis of the papilla or muscular dysfunction of the sphincter of Oddi. While the majority of common duct stones can be easily removed through a choledochotomy at or just below the confluence of the cystic and common ducts, a stone in the ampulla can be particularly difficult to remove, despite the use of stone forceps, balloon catheters, or choledochoscopy. Transduodenal sphincteroplasty may find its greatest use in removal of these stones.

More controversial is the use of transduodenal sphincteroplasty for stenosing papillitis or dysfunction of the sphincter of Oddi. Patients with this disorder present with recurrent episodes of severe upper abdominal pain, occasionally with low grade fever and abdominal tenderness or acute pancreatitis with hyperamylasaemia. They rarely have jaundice or other abnormalities of liver function tests, and dilatation of the biliary or pancreatic ducts is infrequent. While some have suggested that delayed emptying of the common duct following cholangiography, reproduction of the pain on cannulation of the papilla, or raised serum levels of liver or pancreatic enzymes are diagnostic, most patients will not have these findings. Similarly, provocative testing with morphine-prostigmine or secretin has not become widely accepted because of difficulty with reproducibility. While transampullary manometry seems a logical method to diagnose ampullary stenosis, insufficient experience is available to accept these results as diagnostic or reproducible in practice. Thus, when dealing with ampullary stenosis or dysfunction, one is often left with unexplained episodic abdominal pain in a patient who has previously undergone cholecystectomy for similar symptoms, and without another explanation for the symptoms. Because of this lack of specificity in diagnosis, relief of pain is uncertain, and the decision to operate requires mature surgical judgement.

Preoperative

No special preoperative preparation is required. Patients with obstructive jaundice should have coagulation studies performed and any abnormalities corrected by the administration of vitamin K. Preoperative visualization of the common duct by endoscopic retrograde or transhepatic cholangiography may alert the surgeon when an impacted stone is present and may require sphincteroplasty. In practice, however, the information may not be available before the operation, and a judgement must be made at the time of surgery. Common duct stones, even those impacted in the ampulla, can frequently be released and extracted by endoscopic techniques. Nasobiliary catheters or endoprostheses can be inserted into the bile duct to effect preoperative biliary drainage when stones are too big or too impacted to remove by endoscopic techniques. This strategy may be particularly useful in patients with acute cholangitis in order to help control infection before surgical intervention.

Preoperative administration of antibiotics is absolutely indicated in patients with clinical infection. Because the biliary tree is more likely to be contaminated when stones or obstruction are present, prophylactic antibiotics are indicated in most patients. The authors' preference is to prescribe a single dose of antibiotic appropriate principally to Gram-negative enteric organisms, such as a cephalosporin or the combination of ampicillin and gentamicin. Before sphincteroplasty for ampullary stenosis, it is important to exclude other causes for the pain.

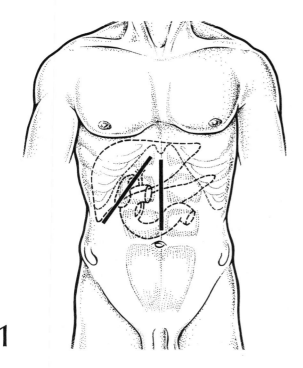

1

Operation

1   A right subcostal or midline incision may be used. Both provide excellent access to the biliary tree without limiting exposure in the way that a paramedian incision does. The abdominal cavity is explored to exclude other pathology.

2 The hepatic flexure of the colon is mobilized to expose the first, second and proximal third portion of the duodenum. The head of the pancreas is likewise exposed. If the gallbladder has not previously been removed, it should be removed at this point both to eliminate a source of stones and a potential future suspect if pain persists or recurs. Furthermore, the gallbladder will not fill following sphincteroplasty and, therefore, has no further function.

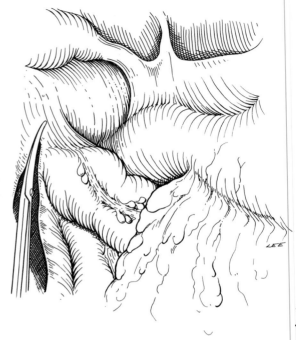

2

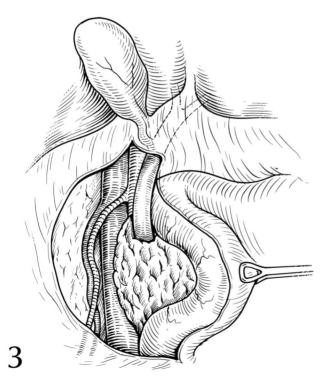

3

3 A wide Kocher manoeuvre is performed, freeing the duodenum and head of the pancreas from their retroperitoneal attachments. This manoeuvre should be carried medially to the aorta so that the entire pancreatic head is free and can be brought up into the wound.

4 The left hand is placed behind the head of the pancreas, and the papilla is identified by palpation of the medial wall of the duodenum. The papilla is particularly easy to identify in patients with an impacted stone, but may be more difficult to find in others. When the location of the major papilla is uncertain, a catheter (5-Fr Fogarty or paediatric feeding catheter) may be passed down the common duct (via the cystic duct or choledochostomy) to help find the choledochoduodenal junction. If the gallbladder is being removed, the cystic duct provides convenient access for the catheter.

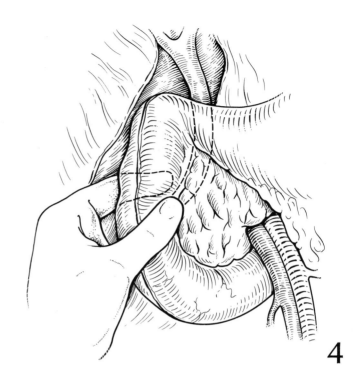

4

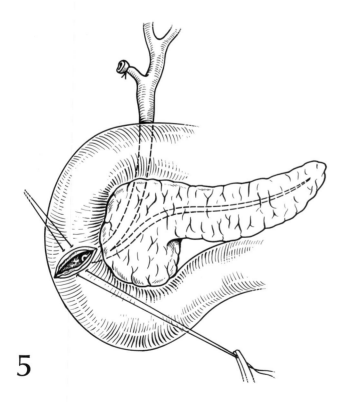

5

5 Once the papilla is identified, stay sutures are placed in the free wall of the duodenum directly opposite it. A tranverse or oblique incision is made opposite the papilla, centred on the papilla, and 2–4 cm in length. The transverse orientation is less likely to lead to duodenal stenosis than a longitudinal incision and provides equivalent exposure. The major papilla is located by inspection or by seeing the catheter exiting through it, by palpation, or by tracing the stream of bile coming from it.

6 A stitch or atraumatic clamp is placed below the papilla for traction, and the papilla is drawn out of the duodenum in the direction of the right iliac crest. Exposure is improved by placing a small retractor on the superior margin of the duodenostomy. A 5-Fr feeding tube is placed through the papilla. Free flow of bile confirms that it lies in the common duct. If clear fluid returns, the catheter lies in the pancreatic duct (as happens very frequently). Because the bile duct always lies superolateral to the pancreatic duct, the surgeon has the choice of replacing the catheter, directing a second catheter into the bile duct, or beginning a sphincterotomy to search for the bile duct lumen.

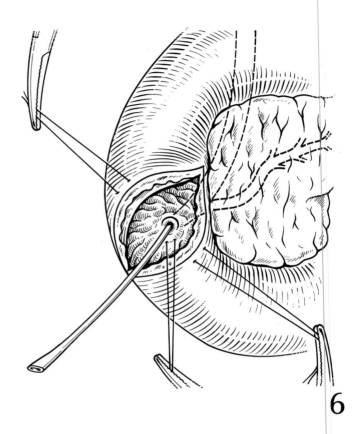

6

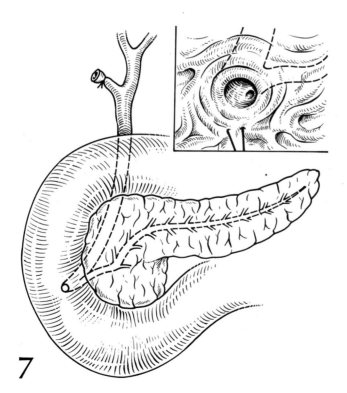

7

7 While the pancreatic duct and bile duct are together at the point of entry into the duodenum, they rapidly diverge when traced away from the duodenal lumen. The bile duct proceeds almost vertically, but the pancreatic duct soon takes a more medial course and then veers to the left. Magnification loupes (2.5 ×) may be helpful in identification of the duct and in the subsequent accurate placement of stitches.

8 When a stone is impacted in the ampulla, the sphincterotomy can be initiated by cutting down directly onto the stone and extracting it. Otherwise, it is desirable to have a guide within the lumen so that the incision is directed accurately. This guidance can be accomplished with a small catheter, fine haemostat or grooved director. If a catheter has been threaded down from above, it can be grasped with the haemostat and then pulled back so that the haemostat is guided into the lumen. Once the haemostat is within the papilla, its jaws are opened and the papilla is divided using a pair of Pott's scissors or knife. The initial incision in the papilla should be 2–3 mm in length and placed at 11 o'clock (anterior cephalad aspect of the papilla). Holding the Pott's scissors upside down often provides a better angle to insert them into the duct lumen.

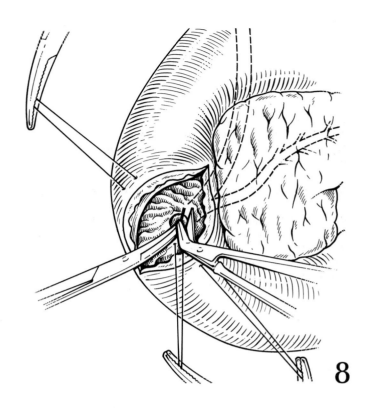

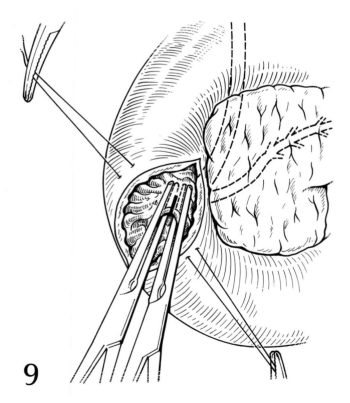

9 Small haemostats are applied with one blade in the bile duct lumen and one in the duodenum to grasp 3–5 mm of the full thickness of the papilla along the long axis of the common bile duct, and the intervening tissue is divided with a pair of Pott's scissors.

10 The mucosa of the common bile duct and duodenum are approximated with interrupted stitches using 4/0 synthetic absorbable material. This division is continued at least until the effective lumen of the choledochoduodenostomy is equivalent to the full diameter of the common bile duct. To ablate the sphincter mechanism entirely, it is necessary to divide 2–3 cm of the ampullary wall. In so doing, the anastomosis will extend through the wall of the duodenum, and one must take care to ensure careful approximation of the duodenum and common bile duct. The apex stitch must be placed with particular care to preserve the maximum size of the lumen. The lumen size should be calibrated with an instrument to ensure that no sutures have inadvertently compromised it.

The pancreatic duct is easily identified on the posterior aspect of the lower common bile duct at the 5 o'clock position, near the ampullary-duodenal junction. If there is any difficulty in identifying the pancreatic duct, intravenous secretin (1 unit/kg) will cause the prompt flow of pancreatic secretion and help to point out the orifice. Absence of flow should raise the suspicion of pancreas divisum with an absent duct of Wirsung.

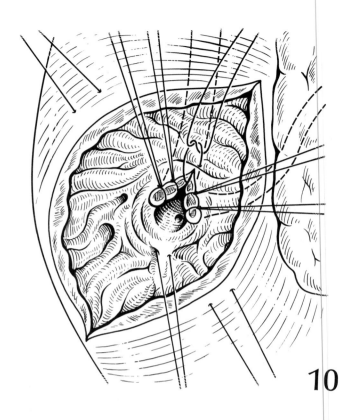

10

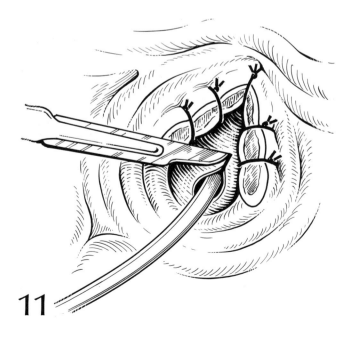

11

11 If septoplasty is to be performed, a small probe or feeding tube is placed in the lumen of the pancreatic duct and the septum is simply incised with a no. 15 knife for 1 cm. Personal preference may dictate that fine absorbable sutures are used to approximate the mucosa of the pancreatic duct to that of the bile duct (septoplasty).

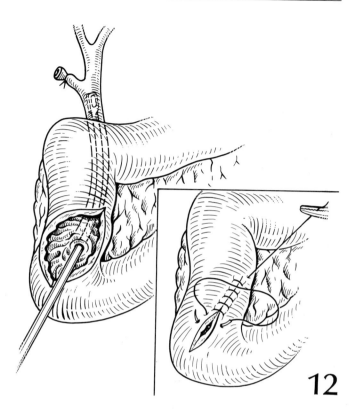

12 Once the sphincteroplasty is completed, wide access to the common duct is available for passage of stone forceps, Fogarty catheters and a choledochoscope. Most stones are easily removed.

After clearing the common duct of stones, the duodenotomy is closed in the same direction in which it was opened (transversely or obliquely) in order to avoid narrowing the duodenum. The authors prefer to use two layers of sutures, one of continuous absorbable material and one of interrupted silk. A complementary gastrostomy may be added to anticipate and treat delay in gastric emptying, a finding which is not uncommon following sphincteroplasty, perhaps because of mild pancreatitis or oedema. The T tube is not normally inserted unless a choledochotomy was performed. Drainage of the duodenal suture line or subhepatic space is not advised. The abdominal wall is closed according to the surgeon's preference.

Postoperative care

The patient is maintained on intravenous fluids and kept fasting until the return of peristalsis. The stomach is kept decompressed by the gastrostomy (if inserted) or by nasogastric suction. The antibiotics used for preoperative prophylaxis are continued for a single postoperative dose.

Complications

Postoperative complications of sphincteroplasty are quite uncommon, but those that do occur are generally a consequence of misadventure or technical deficiency. Suture line bleeding, either from the sphincteroplasty or duodenal closure, will usually subside but can require reoperation and suture-ligation. Leakage from the duodenotomy closure almost always requires re-exploration and thorough external drainage. The resulting fistula has a good chance of healing with gastric decompression and provision of intravenous nutrition. Pancreatitis may occur from injury to the pancreatic duct or partial occlusion of the duct by sphincteroplasty. Care must be taken to ensure that no sutures impinge on its opening.

Further reading

Jones SA. Sphincteroplasty (not sphincterotomy) in the prophylaxis and treatment of residual common duct stones. In: Maingot R, ed. *Abdominal Operations.* 6th edn. New York: Appleton-Century-Crofts, 1974: 1044–54.

Moody FG, Vecchio R, Calabuig R, Runkel N. Transduodenal sphincteroplasty with transampullary septectomy for stenosing papillitis. *Am J Surg* 1991; 161: 213–18.

Nussbaum MS, Warner BW, Sax HC, Fischer JE. Transduodenal sphincteroplasty and transampullary septotomy for primary sphincter of Oddi dysfunction. *Am J Surg* 1989; 157: 38–43.

Toouli J. Clinical relevance of sphincter of Oddi dysfunction. *Br J Surg* 1990; 77: 723–4.

Choledochal cyst

R. Peter Altman MD
Professor of Surgery and Pediatrics, Columbia University, College of Physicians and Surgeons, and Surgeon-in-Chief, Babies' Hospital, Columbia-Presbyterian Medical Center, New York, USA

Barry A. Hicks MD
Assistant Professor of Surgery, Division of Pediatric Surgery, The University of Texas Southwestern Medical Center, Dallas, Texas, USA

Principles and justification

Choledochal cyst was initially recognized by Douglas in 1852. In the clinical series reported over 100 years later, Alonso-Lej *et al.* described a classification system and suggested approaches to treatment[1].

1a–e
Descriptions based on the anatomy of the cyst and distribution within the hepatobiliary tree have since been offered. The type I choledochal cyst is the most common. It is solitary and characterized by fusiform dilation of the common bile duct. The gallbladder and cystic duct, almost invariably dilated, enter the cyst. Choledochal cyst is not an isolated defect restricted to the bile duct, but is more appropriately regarded as part of a constellation of pathological anomalies in the pancreaticobiliary system[2]. Types II (diverticulum of the common bile duct) and III (choledochocele) are less commonly encountered. In type IV, the second most common variant, both intrahepatic cysts and a choledochal cyst are present. Caroli's disease (type V) is characterized by intrahepatic biliary cystic disease with no choledochal cyst. The hepatic histology varies from normal in some patients to advanced fibrosis and cirrhosis in others.

Aetiology

The aetiology of choledochal cyst remains speculative. It has been proposed that the cause is distal narrowing of the bile duct originating *in utero*. A more commonly accepted explanation is that an abnormal junction of the bile duct with the pancreatic duct creates an anatomically common channel which allows reflux of pancreatic juice into the bile duct, thereby weakening its wall by enzymatic destruction resulting in inflammation,

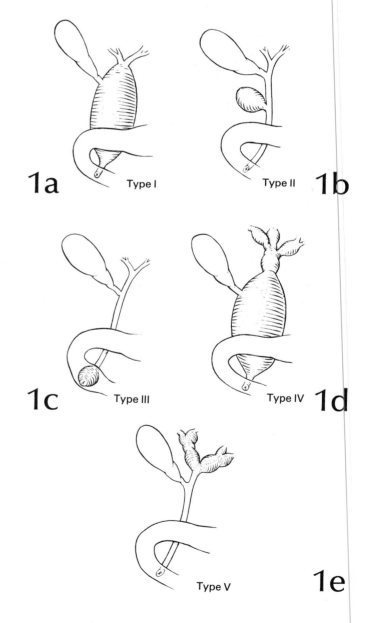

1a   Type I

1b   Type II

1c   Type III

1d   Type IV

1e   Type V

dilatation and cyst formation[3]. A 'common channel' is not found in all patients with choledochal cyst, however, and is found in some normal individuals. It is likely that multiple factors contribute to the formation of choledochal cysts and that the cysts are a component of the spectrum of anomalies within the pancreatico-biliary system. Regardless of the cause, the resulting dilatation and stasis leads to infection and hepatic cirrhosis unless remedied surgically.

Clinical features

Symptoms often present during the first decade of life. Girls are more often affected than boys (ratio 4:1). The classic symptom complex of pain, abdominal mass and jaundice is, in fact, uncommon. With the wide use of prenatal ultrasonography, choledochal cysts are diagnosed or suspected in the antenatal period. In older patients the usual presentation is recurrent abdominal pain, sometimes associated with minimal jaundice, which may not be readily apparent. Recurrent episodes of pancreatitis or presentation with acute cholecystitis is also frequent in adults[4]. In younger patients, and particularly in infants, the obstructive component predominates so that the common presentation is jaundice with an abdominal mass.

Diagnosis

2, 3   With contemporary imaging techniques confirmation of the diagnosis is now readily obtained. In previous years, an upper gastrointestinal contrast study demonstrating a mass effect and distortion of the duodenum was the standard test. This has been replaced by ultrasonography (*Illustration 2*) or computed tomography (*Illustration 3*). Both studies clearly define the dimensions of the cyst and the extent of intrahepatic ductal involvement.

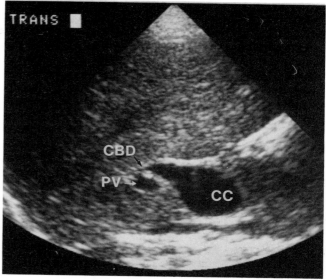

CBD = common bile duct; PV = portal vein; CC = choledochal cyst

2

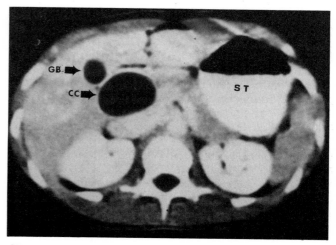

GB = gallbladder; CC = choledochal cyst; ST = stomach

3

4 Nuclear scanning with ^{99m}Tc-labelled IDA may demonstrate the extrahepatic biliary dilatation. In patients with high-grade distal ductal obstruction, no radionuclide is identified in the gastrointestinal tract.

If the regional anatomy remains obscure after these non-invasive studies, endoscopic retrograde cholangiopancreatography is a useful adjunctive procedure. In adults percutaneous transhepatic cholangiography may also be required to define the intrahepatic ductal anatomy. Because of the risk of precipitating cholangitis, antibiotic cover is recommended before cholangiography.

Treatment

Internal drainage of the cyst by cystenterostomy was the traditional surgical approach. Resectional procedures were regarded as having an unacceptably high mortality rate. The long-term morbidity from cystenterostomy, however, has proved to be excessive. The cyst wall is composed of thick fibrous tissue devoid of mucosal lining, and even after drainage the cyst persists as a receptacle for stagnant bile. Anastomotic stricture and bile stasis result in cholangitis, stone formation and biliary colic, so that many patients require subsequent surgery for management of these complications. Furthermore, it has been shown that cholangiocarcinoma may develop in the retained cyst wall[2, 5]. The incidence of neoplasm in the remaining abnormal duct is reported to be between 3% and 20%. Surgical resection of the choledochal cyst is the treatment of choice.

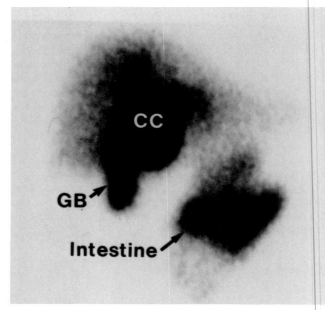

GB = gallbladder; CC = choledochal cyst

4

Operations

5 In children who have not had preoperative cholangiography, operative cholangiography is essential in planning the resection and reconstruction. After aspirating the gallbladder and cyst, contrast medium is instilled through a catheter placed in the gallbladder. The entire extrahepatic biliary ductal anatomy is thus visualized. It is important to identify the junction of the pancreatic and bile ducts in order to protect the pancreatic duct as the distal common bile duct is transected.

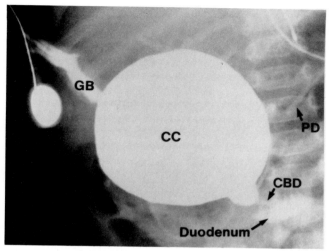

GB = gallbladder; CBD = common bile duct;
CC = choledochal cyst; PD = pancreatic duct

5

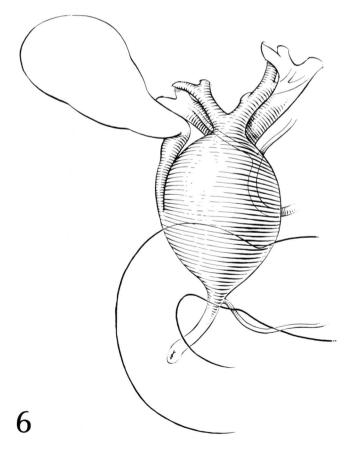

6

CIRCUMFERENTIAL DISSECTION

The choice of procedure depends on the degree of inflammatory reaction encountered at the porta hepatis. If the regional anatomy is readily defined, dissection of the gallbladder and choledochal cyst from the intimately associated vascular structures proceeds rather easily.

6 The cystic artery is divided and the gallbladder mobilized from its bed, leaving the cystic duct in continuity with the choledochal cyst from which it invariably arises.

As the dissection proceeds, the cyst is mobilized by separating the medial and posterior aspects from the portal vein. When scarring and inflammation render dissection behind the cyst hazardous, an alternative technique for resection is proposed (*see below*). Once the distal extent of the cyst has been mobilized, the common bile duct is transected and secured by suture. Care is taken to ensure that pancreatic duct drainage is unimpaired should this duct enter the common bile duct to form a common channel.

7 The transition from abnormal cyst to normal-calibre hepatic duct is then identified as the distal cyst is elevated and the remaining posterior dissection completed proximally.

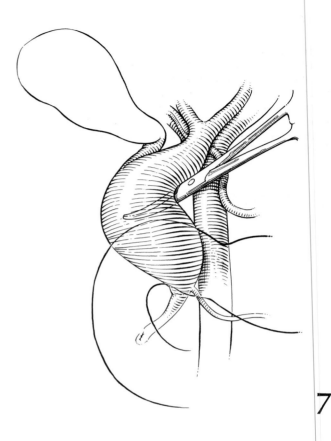

7

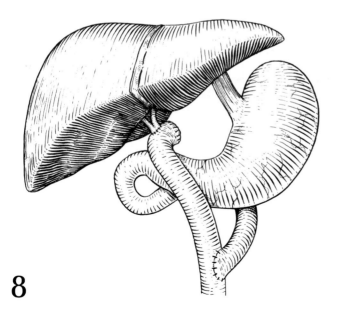

8

8 The hepatic duct is divided at this point, and biliary drainage is established with a retrocolic Roux-en-Y hepaticojejunostomy.

In children an alternative conduit may be created with a valved jejunal interposition hepaticoduodenostomy, on the presumption that this more closely approximates the normal gastrointestinal physiology[6].

ALTERNATIVE TECHNIQUES

If the pericystic inflammation obscures the anatomy, circumferential dissection of the cyst can be hazardous and may result in unacceptable blood loss, particularly if there is already established liver disease and portal hypertension. For such patients, a technique of resection may be used in which the plane between the posterior wall of the cyst and the underlying portal vein need not be disturbed.

9 The regional anatomy is defined by either pre-operative or operative cholangiography. The gall-bladder and cystic duct are then mobilized as described above. The anterior cyst wall is incised transversely and the cyst contents evacuated.

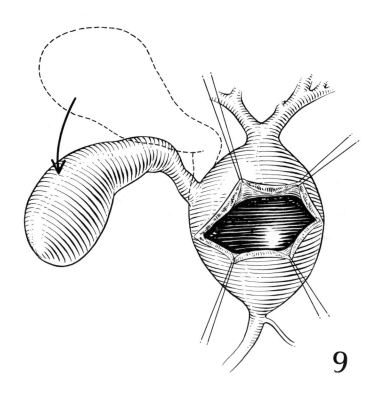

9

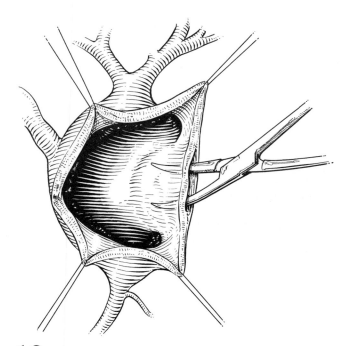

10

10 A plane is developed by dissection within the cyst wall in a posterior direction. This technique establishes an intramural separation of the thick inner cyst lining from the thinner exterior cyst wall, immediately under which lies the portal vein.

11 After developing the plane within the cyst posteriorly, the cyst lining is divided. Intramural dissection is continued cephalad and caudad as the remainder of the cyst is mobilized anterolaterally to the point at which the hepatic duct and common bile duct assume normal or near normal dimensions.

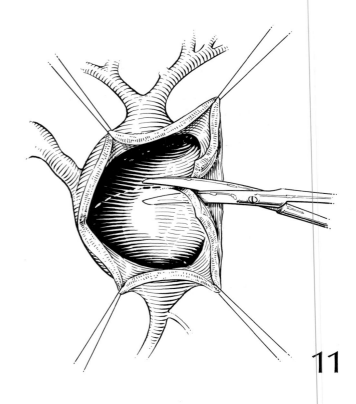

11

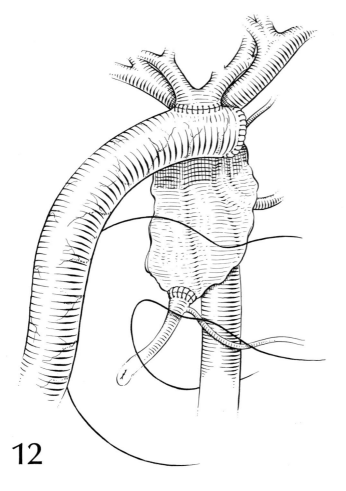

12

12 The cyst with attached gallbladder is resected and the distal common bile duct oversewn. By this technique, the cyst and its lining are removed, but a portion of the outer posterior wall remains. This avoids the hazardous dissection between the densely inflamed back wall of the cyst and the portal vein. Biliary drainage is re-established with a retrocolic Roux-en-Y hepatico-jejunostomy.

If dilation of the choledochal cyst extends distally into the duodenum, it may be necessary to divide the distal cyst leaving some residual expanded common duct (cyst) cephalad to the duodenum. The cyst lining is readily stripped and removed before the walls are approximated and secured. Care should be taken to avoid injury to the pancreatic duct. Dilation may also extend proximally along the common hepatic duct to involve one or both of the hepatic ducts within the liver. In such patients the resection is extended, removing as much of the involved ductal structure as possible.

Outcome

The prognosis after choledochal cyst resection varies considerably. For some children, particularly older children with established liver disease, the prognosis is guarded. In most adults without an associated malignancy the prognosis is good. However, cyst excision does not completely eliminate the risk of malignancy. None the less, the outcome is generally favourable.

Acknowledgement

Illustrations 6, 7 and *9–12* have been redrawn from originals by J. K. Karapelou.

References

1. Alonso-Lej F, Rever WB Jr, Pessagno DJ. Congenital choledochal cysts, with a report of two and an analysis of 94 cases. *Int Abstr Surg* 1959; 108: 1–30.

2. Iwai N, Yanagihara J, Tokiwa K, Shimotake T, Nakamura K. Congenital choledochal dilatation with emphasis on pathophysiology of the biliary tract. *Ann Surg* 1992; 215: 27–30.

3. Babbitt DP. Congenital choledochal cysts: new etiological concept based on anomalous relationships of the common bile duct and pancreatic bulb. *Ann Radiol* 1969; 12: 231–40.

4. Lipsett PA, Pitt HA, Colombani PM *et al.* Choledochal cyst disease: a changing pattern of presentation. *Ann Surg* 1994; 220: 644–52.

5. Ozmen V, Martin PC, Igci A *et al.* Adenocarcinoma of the gallbladder associated with congenital choledochal cyst and anomalous pancreaticobiliary ductal junction. Case report. *Eur J Surg* 1991; 157: 549–51.

6. Cosentino CM, Luck SR, Raffensperger JG, Reynolds M. Choledochal duct cyst: resection with physiologic reconstruction. *Surgery* 1992; 112: 740–8.

Benign biliary stricture

Henry A. Pitt MD
Professor and Vice Chairman, Department of Surgery, The Johns Hopkins Medical Institutions, Baltimore, Maryland, USA

History

Benign biliary strictures occur most commonly following operations on the gallbladder and bile ducts. Since the first cholecystectomy was performed more than a century ago, the challenge of reconstructing the injured biliary tree has also faced surgeons. By the 1980s, Roux-en-Y hepaticojejunostomy had become the surgical treatment of choice, and percutaneous and endoscopic management options had been developed[1,2]. In this era before laparoscopic cholecystectomy the incidence of biliary stricture after cholecystectomy was only one or two per 1000, and the most common presentation was jaundice and/or cholangitis, usually occurring weeks or months after surgery. However, with the introduction of laparoscopic cholecystectomy the incidence has increased to 3–5 per 1000, and these patients are now more likely to present with unusual pain in the early postoperative period due to a biloma or bile ascites[3]. Nevertheless, the principles of management have not changed significantly in the 1990s.

Principles and justification

Benign biliary strictures can result from a variety of clinical problems. In addition to those occurring after biliary surgery, injury to the bile ducts may also follow gastrectomy, pancreatic procedures, hepatic resection, portal decompressive procedures and hepatic transplantation. Strictures may also occur in a prior biliary-enteric anastomosis or following trauma. A number of inflammatory conditions may also lead to stricturing of the bile duct. A distal bile duct stricture secondary to chronic pancreatitis is the most common non-operative cause. Occasionally, a gallstone eroding into the common bile duct (the Mirizzi syndrome) or choledocholithiasis with recurrent cholangitis will lead to a bile duct stricture. Stenosis of the sphincter of Oddi may also cause a ductal stricture. In addition, duodenal pathology such as peptic ulcer disease or Crohn's disease may lead to narrowing of the distal bile duct. This discussion, however, will focus on strictures following cholecystectomy which usually involve the more proximal biliary tree.

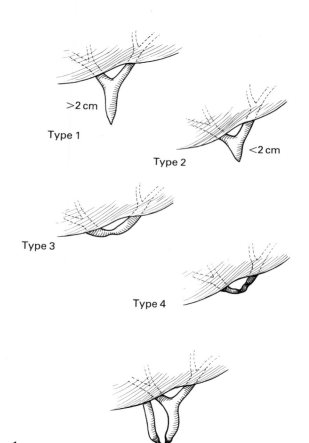

1

1 Postoperative strictures have been classified by Bismuth[4] into five types. Type 1 includes all strictures more than 2 cm below the hepatic duct bifurcation; type 2 includes strictures that are less than 2 cm below the hepatic duct bifurcation which, in most reports, is the most common type; type 3, which is a stricture at the hilum, is also common; type 4 strictures separate the right and left hepatic ducts and are more difficult to repair; and type 5 strictures involve a branch of the right hepatic duct while the common hepatic duct may or may not be involved

Occasionally a subsegmental duct, which is usually less than 2 mm in diameter, or a small duct entering directly into the gallbladder (duct of Lushka) may be injured. Treatment in these rare situations only requires simple ligation. However, treatment of most benign biliary strictures will be more involved and usually requires a team with expertise in endoscopy and interventional radiology as well as reconstructive surgery.

Interestingly, only a few of these problems are recognized by the operating surgeon[1–3]. When the injury is recognized during surgery, the temptation to attempt a complex repair is great. However, external drainage and referral to a team of experts may be in the patient's best interest. Repair of a partial injury over a T tube brought out of the bile duct through a separate choledochotomy will usually have a good result. However, primary end-to-end repair of a complete transection rarely leads to a good long-term outcome, especially if a segment of the bile duct is missing. Most patients with benign postoperative bile duct strictures present early after their initial operation, and over 80% develop symptoms within 1 year of surgery[1]. However, presentation may be delayed for many years. Thus, the preoperative assessment and preparation may vary somewhat depending on the type and timing of presentation.

Preoperative

When a patient presents early after laparoscopic cholecystectomy, many studies are available to confirm that a bile duct problem exists. Liver function tests should be performed, but major abnormalities may not be present if bile is leaking rather than obstructed. Similarly, with partial obstruction the only abnormality may be an elevated serum alkaline phosphatase level.

2   To determine whether a biloma, bile ascites or biliary obstruction is present, ultrasonography, computed tomographic (CT) scanning or cholescintigraphy may be performed. Each of these studies has advantages and disadvantages. Ultrasonography will detect a fluid collection and the presence of dilated bile ducts but usually does not give a complete anatomical picture of the problem. CT scanning (illustrated) provides the same information with a more complete and clear picture but does not give biliary anatomical or functional information. Cholescintigraphy will usually demonstrate a bile leak and determine whether bile is entering the duodenum, but anatomical detail of the bile ducts and any fluid collections is often lacking.

Cholangiography is usually required to determine the anatomy of the bile leak or stricture. Options include endoscopic retrograde cholangiopancreatography (ERCP) and percutaneous transhepatic cholangiography (PTC). Again, both options have advantages and disadvantages. ERCP may be most helpful if a cystic duct leak is suspected by the presence of a localized subhepatic bile collection. In this situation endoscopic sphincterotomy, usually with the addition of an endoscopic stent, will be sufficient to solve the problem. However, with most bile duct injuries, ERCP will only demonstrate a normal biliary tree below a surgical clip or a leaking common bile duct and will not provide a picture of the proximal biliary tree

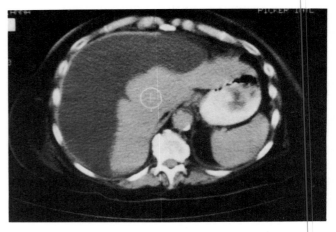

Computed tomographic scan of a patient with a large postoperative bile collection. Reprinted with permission of Lillemoe et al.[3].

2

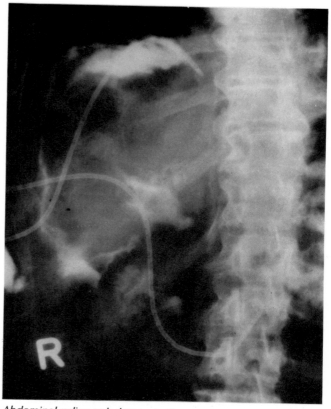

Abdominal radiograph demonstrating one percutaneous drainage catheter in the subphrenic space and a second through the liver and biliary system into the duodenum. Contrast is leaking from the injured bile duct into the subhepatic space. Reprinted with permission from Lillemoe et al.[3].

3 PTC has the advantage of providing a picture of the ducts above the problem but may be technically difficult in the presence of a biloma and the absence of dilated ducts. However, percutaneous drainage of both the bile collections and the biliary tree will usually avoid the need for emergency surgery. Moreover, the chance of being able to perform a definitive repair is increased if the surrounding area is not inflamed by a bile collection or an abscess. If biliary drainage can be achieved and sepsis controlled by percutaneous drainage, surgical reconstruction can be performed electively 6–8 weeks later when inflammation has subsided and the patient's overall health has improved.

In situations where the biliary tree or a prior anastomosis is strictured but not leaking, the initial placement of a percutaneous transhepatic drainage catheter may also be useful. If the stricture can be transversed, balloon dilatation becomes an option. Even if the catheter cannot be passed beyond the stricture, the catheter can be quite helpful intraoperatively for identifying the injured bile duct and in the placement of large Silastic transhepatic stents. The use of stents in these patients remains controversial, but many experts employ them with the most proximal, complex strictures. Further details of preoperative management regarding the treatment of cholangitis and the correction of the coagulopathy as well as fluid and electrolyte balance are discussed in the chapter on pp. 262–274.

Anaesthesia

Most endoscopic or percutaneous drainage procedures can be performed with a combination of intravenous sedatives and narcotics. Balloon dilatation, on the other hand, may be quite painful and sometimes requires a general anaesthetic. Definitive surgery must also be done under general endotracheal anaesthesia. If stenosis or stricture of the sphincter of Oddi is suspected, anaesthetic regimens that include a narcotic should be avoided because these agents will cause further obstruction of the sphincter. In addition, in patients with recent or ongoing biliary obstruction, drugs that can cause cholestasis or hepatotoxicity should be avoided.

3

Operation

Incision

4 Most patients who have undergone an open cholecystectomy have had a right subcostal incision. Re-entering this old incision has advantages in terms of cosmesis; however, lysis of adhesions may be more difficult and retrieval of adequate jejunum to create a Roux-en-Y limb may also be hampered by limited access from the right upper quadrant. The use of an old incision is less of an issue when the stricture follows laparoscopic cholecystectomy. An upper midline incision has versatility for exposure of the liver and the biliary strictures as well as the jejunum. Moreover, ideal placement of a large-bore Silastic transhepatic stent in the right upper abdomen is not restricted by a midline incision.

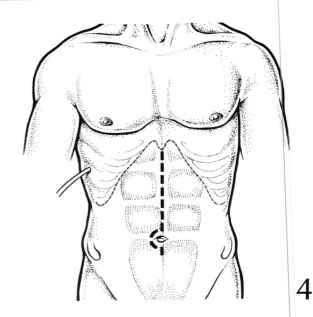

4

Removal of adhesions

5a,b Regardless of the incision used, the first step is to take down adhesions around the liver. Detachment of the falciform ligament from the anterior abdominal wall facilitates exposure of the liver. Lysis of successive layers of adhesions from left to right will eventually expose the hilar structures. Care must be taken in this process to avoid injury to the hepatic artery. Preoperative placement of a transhepatic (Ring) catheter will also aid in the identification of the strictured and scarred bile duct.

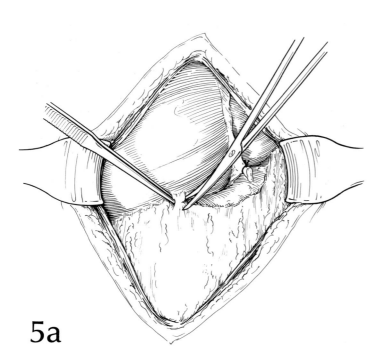

5a

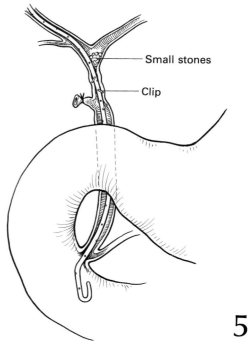

Small stones

Clip

5b

Exposure of proximal duct

6 Once the extrahepatic biliary tract has been identified, it is mobilized and encircled with a vessel loop. Care must be taken during this process to avoid injury to the hepatic artery and the portal vein. Dissection is then continued toward the hilum which is frequently surrounded by a dense inflammatory reaction. However, as the dissection continues proximally, an undisturbed plane is often encountered and this normal tissue is where the anastomosis should be performed. At this level, a transverse incision is made in the bile duct and the Ring catheter is retrieved. The case illustrated is a Bismuth type 2 stricture and the proximal extent is just below the hepatic duct bifurcation. If the stricture had been a Bismuth type 3 or 4 stricture, individual hepaticojejunostomies would have to be performed to the right and left hepatic ducts. In this situation, bilateral Ring catheters should be placed before surgery and each anastomosis stented with a separate Silastic stent.

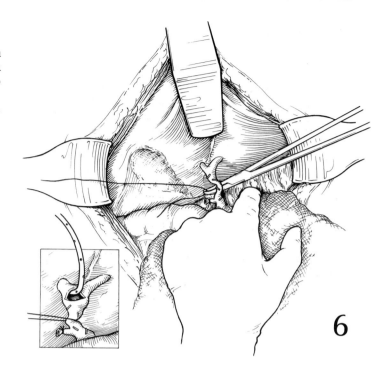

6

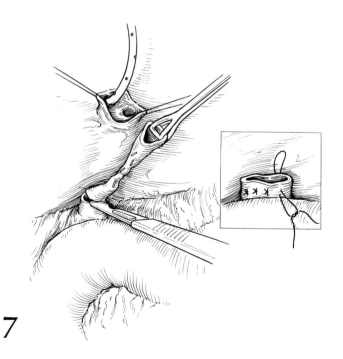

7

Resection of stricture

7 After placement of stay sutures in the proximal biliary segment, the back wall of the common hepatic duct is divided. The strictured segment is mobilized from the portal vein and right hepatic artery (behind) and from the left and common hepatic artery on the patient's left. Vascular anomalies and injuries must also be considered during this dissection. When the entire stricture has been dissected free, the duct is divided and the distal end is oversewn. The specimen should be submitted for pathological examination even though the likelihood of discovering a malignancy is extremely low. However, the presence of a neuroma in up to 15% of patients may provide insight into the pathogenesis of the problem[2].

Placement of the transhepatic stent

8a–d To facilitate placement of the large-bore Silastic transhepatic stent, the preoperatively placed 8.3-Fr Ring catheter is further retrieved into the abdomen and the curved end is cut off. A guidewire is placed through the residual Ring catheter to avoid losing the tract if a catheter should break during the exchange process. A 12-Fr Coudé catheter with the tip cut off is then sutured to the residual Ring catheter and passed through the biliary tree and liver parenchyma over the guidewire. Counterpressure with an empty sponge forceps will help prevent tears in the liver parenchyma during this catheter exchange process. A 14-Fr Coudé catheter is passed in a similar fashion before a 16-Fr Silastic catheter is sutured to the flanged end of the Coudé catheter. Once the Silastic catheter is in place, a heavy chromic mattress suture should be placed around the exit site of the catheter from the liver to prevent bile leakage.

If a Ring catheter has not been placed before the operation, a no.3 Bake's dilator may be passed out of a bile duct branch and through the liver parenchyma, and a no.2 suture is tied to the dilator. After pulling this suture through the tract, it is then sewn to an 8-Fr Coudé catheter which is pulled through the tract along with a guidewire. Once this tract has been established, progressively larger Coudé catheters are passed and a Silastic stent is placed. This process is identical to that described above when a Ring catheter has been placed before surgery. Having the Ring catheter in place usually minimizes operative trauma as long as the catheter enters a bile duct peripherally, away from the hilum. Regardless of how the Silastic stent is placed, it should be positioned so that the portion with the side holes lies in the bile duct and jejunum. The portion of the stent that exits the liver and traverses the peritoneum and abdominal wall should not have any side holes.

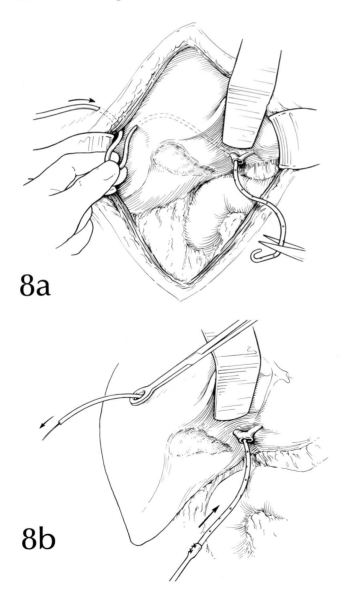

8a

8b

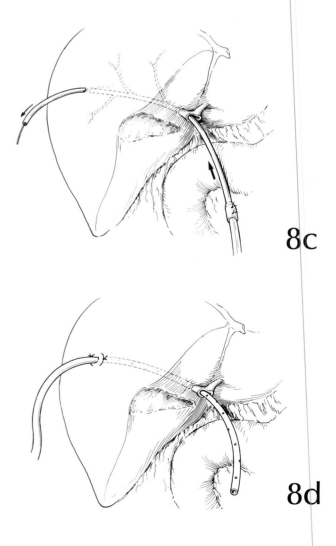

8c

8d

Division of jejunum

9a,b To create the Roux-en-Y limb, the jejunum is divided approximately 30 cm from the ligament of Treitz. Ideally, the site chosen for division will have a gap in the arcade of the mesenteric vessels so that sufficient collaterals exist and that the distal end can be easily mobilized to the hepatic hilum. The jejunum can be divided with either a gastrointestinal stapler or between occluding intestinal clamps, and the mesentery is also divided. The distal end of the jejunum is oversewn before it is brought through the mesocolon. To bring the distal end of the jejunum to the hepatic hilum in a dependent, retrocolic fashion, the right colon needs to be mobilized from the head of the pancreas and the duodenum. A defect is then made in the mesocolon to the right of the middle colic vessels, and the distal end of the jejunum is brought through this defect.

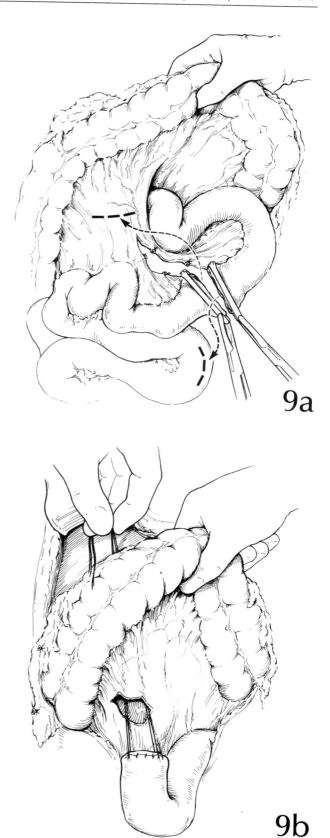

9a

9b

Hepaticojejunostomy

10a–f The Roux-en-Y loop should reach the hepatic hilum comfortably and without tension. The hepaticojejunostomy can be performed in one or two layers. In the example shown, a two-layer anastomosis is being performed. The outer layer of 4/0 non-absorbable sutures is inserted between the back wall of the bile duct and the jejunum. After making the enterotomy in the jejunum and excising a small ellipse of mucosa, an inner layer of 4/0 absorbable sutures approximates the bile duct and jejunal mucosa. The Silastic biliary stent is then passed through the anastomosis in the jejunum and the anterior inner row of 4/0 absorbable sutures is inserted. The anterior outer row of 4/0 non-absorbable sutures is then completed. Operative fluorocholangiography via the transhepatic stent is used to check its position within the biliary tree and to detect any leakage at the anastomosis.

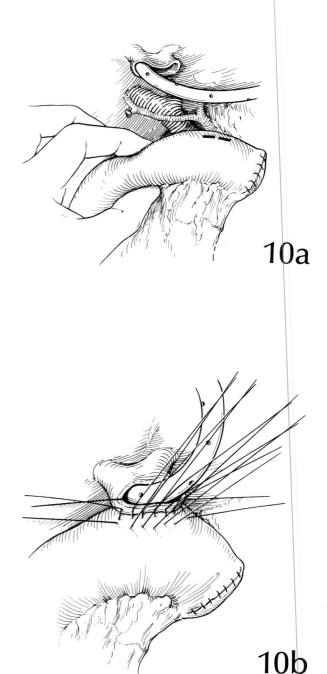

10a

10b

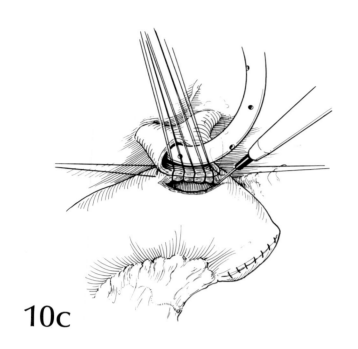

10c

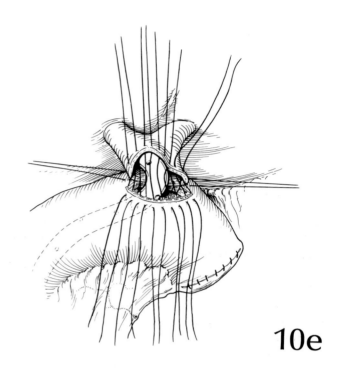

10e

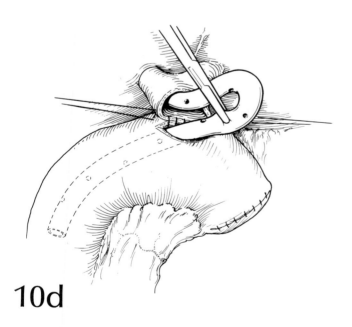

10d

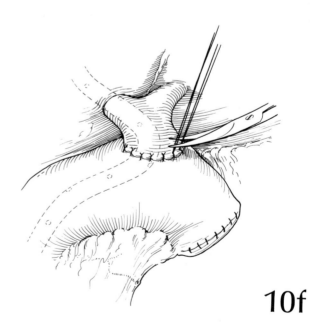

10f

Completion of Roux-en-Y

11 Enteric continuity is re-established by performing an end-to-side jejunostomy, approximately 50–60 cm distal to the hepaticojejunostomy. This standard intestinal anastomosis is performed in two layers. The inner continuous layer is performed with a 3/0 absorbable suture and the outer interrupted layer with 3/0 non-absorbable sutures. Mesenteric defects are closed with 3/0 non-absorbable sutures to prevent internal herniation. The Roux-en-Y limb may be tacked to periportal tissues to further ensure that there is no tension on the hepaticojejunostomy.

Closed suction drains are placed adjacent to the hepaticojejunostomy as well as at the exit site of the transhepatic Silastic stent from the liver. These drains and the Silastic stent are all brought through separate stab incisions in the abdominal wall. Care should be taken to assure that the path of the Silastic stent is straight to facilitate subsequent changes and that the stent is placed in a comfortable position for the patient. The drains and stent are sutured to the skin and the abdominal wall is closed in a standard fashion.

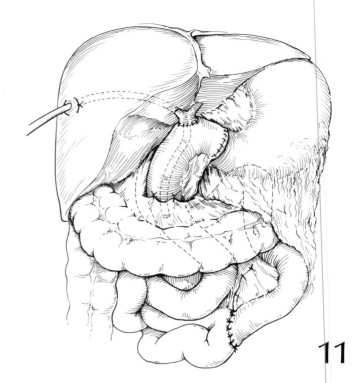

11

Postoperative care

The Silastic stent is attached to a bile bag and left on gravity drainage in the early postoperative period. Perioperative prophylactic antibiotics are continued for at least 48 h, which is longer than usual because cholangitis and bacteraemia are common after intraoperative placement of large-bore transhepatic stents. The nasogastric tube is removed and feeding is commenced when intestinal function returns. A tube cholangiogram is performed on the fifth or sixth postoperative day. Antibiotic prophylaxis directed at the organisms cultured from the patient's bile are given before and for 24 h after the cholangiogram to prevent cholangitis. If the cholangiogram demonstrates no leaks and good stent position, and if the patient has no cholangitis after the procedure, the bile bag is removed on the next day. If no bile is seen in the drains after the stent has been closed, the drains may be removed.

The stent is capped with a heparin lock. The patient is taught to flush the stent with 10 or 20 ml of saline twice a day to prevent the build-up of biliary 'sludge'. Even a 16-Fr Silastic stent which is flushed regularly will become occluded with 'sludge' in 4 months, so stents that are to be left in for more than 3 months are changed before the patient develops problems with obstructive jaundice or cholangitis. This procedure can be performed on an outpatient basis by an interventional radiologist. Simply, a guidewire is passed through the old stent which is then removed. A new stent is passed over the guidewire which, in turn, is removed when proper positioning has been checked with cholangiography. The new stent is resutured to the skin and the patient is observed for a few hours for signs of cholangitis prior to discharge.

Both the use of stents and the length of stenting remain controversial. Those who believe that long-term stenting is beneficial argue that scar formation is a 9–12 month process. One of the last phases of this process is scar contraction. Thus, to have a stent through the anastomosis during scar contraction may prevent restricturing and improve the long-term outcome. The decision to remove the stent is based on the patient's clinical course, liver function tests, cholangiography and the Whitaker test[5]. This test is performed by the interventional radiologist at the time of a stent change. First, careful cholangiography is performed with the stent pulled back to be sure that no stricture is present. In addition, saline is perfused across the anastomosis at increased rates while pressures are monitored. If pressures remain low and other parameters are satisfactory, the stent may be removed. A clinical trial with the stent positioned above the anastomosis before removal may also be employed.

Outcome

To determine the result of any treatment for a benign bile duct stricture, sufficient follow-up is necessary. Most authorities have stated that a minimum of 5 years of follow-up is required to assess accurately the long-term results. The technique of hepaticojejunostomy with long-term transhepatic stenting described here has been reported to provide a successful outcome in 85–90% of patients[2,3]. Similar results have been reported with the Hepp–Couinaud technique which involves a long unstented anastomosis to the left hepatic duct[6]. However, this technique is not applicable to the Bismuth types 4 and 5 strictures which often have the worst results. Moreover, to date, no randomized data exist comparing the methods described in this chapter with the Hepp–Couinaud technique in similar patients. Until prospective, randomized trials are performed, debate will persist regarding the use of stents and the optimal length of time for which stents should be employed.

In general, the results of balloon dilatation of proximal strictures have not been as good as those of surgery[2,3]. Balloon dilatation may be performed by either a percutaneous transhepatic or an endoscopic technique. However, only the percutaneous method is applicable if the patient has had a prior biliary-enteric anastomosis. On the other hand, the results of balloon dilatation have been best in patients who have not had a prior anastomosis and in those with distal strictures[3]. Another option is the use of indwelling, expanding metallic stents. However, this method cannot be recommended for patients with benign strictures because these stents eventually become occluded and complicate subsequent surgery. Nevertheless, balloon dilatation can be recommended for carefully selected patients and for those who are unwilling to undergo further surgery. However, the patient should understand that the long-term results of surgery are better than those of non-surgical treatment.

References

1. Pitt HA, Miyamoto T, Parapatis SK, Tompkins RK, Longmire WP. Factors influencing outcome with postoperative biliary strictures. *Am J Surg* 1982; 144: 14–21.

2. Pitt HA, Kaufman SL, Coleman J, White RI, Cameron JL. Benign postoperative biliary strictures: operate or dilate? *Ann Surg* 1989; 210: 417–27.

3. Lillemoe KD, Pitt HA, Cameron JL. Current management of benign bile duct strictures. *Adv Surg* 1992; 25: 119–74.

4. Bismuth H. Postoperative strictures of the bile duct. In: Blumgart LH, ed. *The Biliary Tract*. Edinburgh: Churchill Livingstone, 1982: 209–18.

5. Savader SJ, Cameron JL, Pitt HA *et al*. Biliary manometry versus clinical trial: value as predictors of success following treatment of biliary tract strictures. *J Vasc Intervent Radiol* 1994; 5: 757–63.

6. Hepp J, Couinaud C. L'abourd et l'utilisation du canal hépatique gauche dans les réparations de la voie biliare principale. *Presse Med* 1956; 64: 947–8.

Recurrent pyogenic cholangitis

S. T. Fan MS, FRCS(Glas), FACS
Professor, Department of Surgery, The University of Hong Kong, Hong Kong

John Wong PhD, FRACS, FRCS(Ed), FACS
Professor and Head, Department of Surgery, The University of Hong Kong, Hong Kong

History

In 1930 Digby[1] described eight cases of 'common duct stones of liver origin'. These cases presented with symptoms of recurrent biliary sepsis and, at operation, soft stones were found in the common bile duct which Digby concluded had formed in the liver. In 1954 Cook et al.[2] first used the name 'recurrent pyogenic cholangitis' to describe this peculiar pathological entity which is prevalent in south-east Asia. In 1962 Ong[3] decribed this condition in detail and laid the foundation for its surgical treatment.

Principles and justification

The primary pathological changes of recurrent pyogenic cholangitis are in the biliary tract, with secondary inflammatory changes in the liver. The common bile duct may be markedly dilated and filled with stones that are composed mainly of calcium bilirubinate, with varying amounts of cholesterol. The intrahepatic ducts are also thickened and dilated. There may be multiple stenosis, and stones may be found in the dilated portion of the duct system. In long-standing cases a segment or lobe of the liver may be completely destroyed, and in about 3% of cases cholangiocarcinoma may develop. The left lobe of the liver is usually more involved by the disease than the right. When the right lobe is involved, the posterior segment is commonly affected.

Recurrent pyogenic cholangitis is prevalent in south-east Asia, but whereas the disease accounted for 50% of all of the biliary stones in the 1950s and 1960s, it has accounted for only 10% of stones in Hong Kong in recent years[4]. Accompanying the reduction in incidence is a shift of peak age from the third to the seventh decade, and the complexity of the disease has increased in individual patients as a consequence of progression and the effects of previous operations. These changes may reflect the fact that an increasing proportion of patients survive surgery only to experience recurrence later in life. Fortunately, there has been significant progress in radiology, endoscopy, lithotripsy and general anaesthesia, and new surgical techniques are available to manage this difficult condition.

Approximately 60% of the patients present initially with acute cholangitis[4]. With conservative treatment about 70% of these patients recover, and elective operations can be undertaken when all the symptoms have subsided. In 30% of cases clinical deterioration is manifested by rising body temperature, tachycardia, shock and signs of spreading peritonitis, and emergency intervention becomes necessary.

Preoperative

Patients presenting with acute cholangitis should be given broad-spectrum antibiotics, e.g. a second or third generation cephalosporin or a broad-spectrum penicillin immediately after blood has been taken for culture. In the event that the patient has undergone a bilioenteric anastomosis, coverage for anaerobic bacteria is also needed. Adequate hydration and mannitol infusion is necessary when the patient is jaundiced. Vitamin K may be beneficial, but the availability of sufficient fresh frozen plasma, platelet concentrates and blood is more important if the patient has a coagulopathy. Correction of any electrolyte abnormality is mandatory. In shocked patients, inotropic support may be necessary in the perioperative period.

Ultrasonography, computed tomographic scanning, direct cholangiography (T tube cholangiography, transhepatic cholangiography or endoscopic retrograde cholangiopancreatography) are complementary in delineating the site of biliary strictures, in localizing stones, and in defining segmental liver atrophy in patients presenting in the quiescent phase. These findings are important in planning of surgical treatment. The preoperative preparation of the patient is similar to that for the acute situation.

Operation in the acute phase

Decompression of the biliary tract

The aim of emergency operation is to decompress the biliary tract. If the condition of the patient is not satisfactory, the operation time should be as short as possible. Complete removal of stones is not mandatory if adequate biliary drainage can be achieved by a T tube or transhepatic tube. Residual stones can be removed subsequently by choledochoscopy through the T tube tract or transhepatic tract.

Incision

1 A subcostal or a right paramedian incision is used.

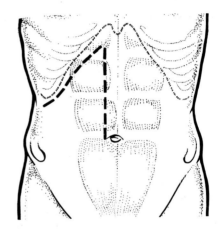

Exploration

2 The common bile duct will be found to be markedly dilated, and soft stones are palpable. In patients with long-standing disease or previous operations, exposure of the common bile duct may be difficult. In such cases, care must be taken to avoid damage to the hepatic artery, portal vein, duodenum and hepatic flexure of the colon. In patients with concomitant portal hypertension or portal vein thrombosis, dilated veins may be present around the bile ducts and are liable to damage and uncontrollable bleeding.

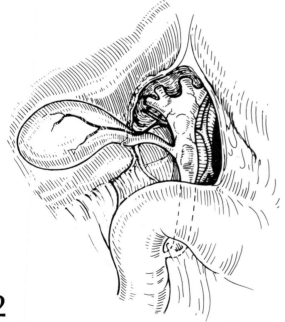

Exploration of common bile duct

3 A longitudinal choledochotomy is made. Purulent bile or pus will escape under tension. Stones that are easily removed are evacuated using stone forceps. The length of the choledochotomy should be generous to enable large stones to come out of the common bile duct easily. If the common bile duct is huge, exploration using a finger is useful to assess the right and left hepatic duct and distal common bile duct and to fragment or evacuate soft stones. Passage of a biliary sound up into the right and left hepatic ducts is a useful means of detecting stones and strictures and confirming patency, but forceful passage of a biliary sound through the ampulla of Vater is not encouraged. Forceful irrigation of the upper part of the biliary tract with normal saline is dangerous in that it may induce bacteraemia, but flushing of the lower end of the common bile duct is a safe and effective method of removing stones from this end of the common bile duct. Similarly, choledochoscopy should be confined to the lower end of the common bile duct, the instrument being inserted through a large choledochotomy and irrigation pressure being kept to a minimum. However, when the condition of the patient is poor, choledochoscopy should be avoided.

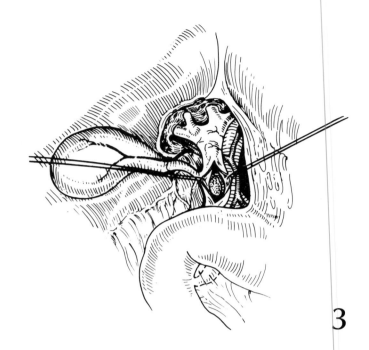

3

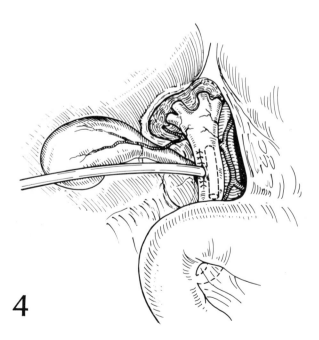

4

Insertion of T tube

4 A large-bore T tube is inserted and the choledochotomy is closed around it using absorbable sutures. A large-bore T tube will allow mud and thick bile to egress. Caution is necessary to avoid kinking of the T tube inside the peritoneal cavity or at the abdominal wall.

Transhepatic biliary drainage

When strictures are found in the right or left hepatic duct, a graduated sound can be passed to dilate the narrowed areas. To ensure adequate biliary drainage of the intrahepatic ducts proximal to the strictures, transhepatic biliary drainage can be performed.

5 The first step is to force a biliary sound through the intrahepatic bile duct, liver parenchyma and liver capsule.

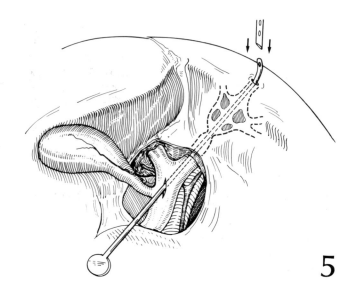

5

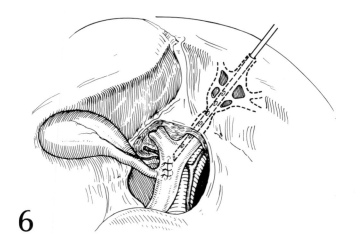

6

6 A latex tube with side holes is then tied to the biliary sound which is drawn back through the common bile duct to bring the transhepatic tube into the correct position. Kinking must be avoided when bringing the transhepatic tube through the abdominal wall.

Cholecystectomy

Cholecystectomy may prolong the operation in a critically ill patient and is not indicated during the acute attack unless the condition of the patient is satisfactory or when there is an empyema with perforation or gangrene.

Operations in the quiescent phase

Exploration and cholecystectomy

Adhesiolysis is sometimes necessary to allow thorough examination of the liver and bile duct and to determine the operative procedures. Intraoperative ultrasonography is helpful in the detection and localization of intrahepatic stones and abscesses. Intraoperative ultrasonography is best performed before exploration of the common bile duct because air in the biliary tract makes interpretation of the ultrasound image very difficult.

Cholecystectomy should be performed in the elective situation whether gallstones are present or not.

Exploration of common bile duct

The operative steps are as described in the acute situation except that choledochoscopy of the entire biliary tract is mandatory to confirm the presence of any abnormality seen on preoperative radiological studies. When impacted stones are found and cannot be removed by the usual methods, electrohydraulic lithotripsy can be employed. The tip of the electro-

hydraulic probe is passed through the working channel of the choledochoscope and brought into contact with the stone under direct vision. The power output of the electrohydraulic lithotripter is set to 100 volts. The tip of the probe should be at least 1 cm from the end of the choledochoscope before pressing the footswitch in order to prevent damage to the choledochoscope by the spark.

Internal biliary drainage

The rationale of internal biliary drainage in recurrent pyogenic cholangitis is to provide unimpeded passage of thick bile, mud and small stones into the bowel. Internal biliary drainage is indicated when recurrence is deemed likely. Sphincteroplasty, choledochojejunostomy or hepaticojejunostomy are commonly performed. The indications for sphincteroplasty include stenosis at the ampulla of Vater or impaction of a stone at the lower end of the common bile duct. Choledochojejunostomy or hepaticojejunostomy are indicated when the common bile duct is grossly dilated and thickened, or when a stricture is present in the common bile duct. These surgical techniques are described in the chapters on pages 594–609 and 370–381.

HEPATICOCUTANEOUS JEJUNOSTOMY

This operation is an extension of hepaticojejunostomy and is indicated when it is anticipated that many sessions of postoperative choledochoscopy will be needed to deal with intrahepatic stones and strictures and when recurrence of the disease is likely. In the presence of intrahepatic strictures, hepaticojejunostomy alone will not provide effective biliary drainage and prevent recurrence. Reoperation for recurrence of the disease can be difficult and hazardous, especially during an acute attack. Hepaticocutaneous jejunostomy can provide percutaneous access to the biliary tract if the need arises.

7 Two stay stitches are first placed over the supraduodenal portion of the common bile duct.

7

8 A transverse incision is then made in the common bile duct and bile is aspirated and all stones are removed. When all of the biliary mud has been washed away, the duct is transected.

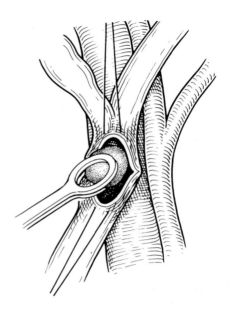

8

9 The duct wall is carefully separated from the portal vein which lies immediately posterior to it and is then transected by cutting around its whole circumference. This step is best performed with a pair of scissors. Arterial bleeding occurs at the 3 and 9 o'clock positions and haemostasis is achieved by fine sutures rather than by electrocautery.

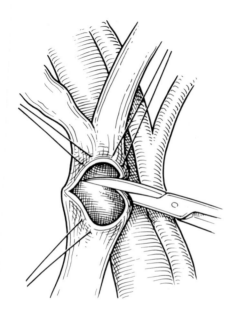

9

10 The lower end of the divided duct is closed with a single layer of interrupted sutures. The upper end is next dissected from its bed, taking care to avoid extensive dissection which could compromise the ductal blood supply.

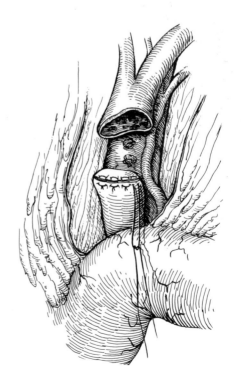

10

11 The arterial arcades of the jejunum are then studied, and the jejunum is divided at about 45 cm from the duodenojejunal junction, along with one or two feeding jejunal vessels. This loop will serve as a Roux loop and now derives its blood supply via the arterial arcades. In obese patients the arterial pattern is better seen following transillumination through the mesentery.

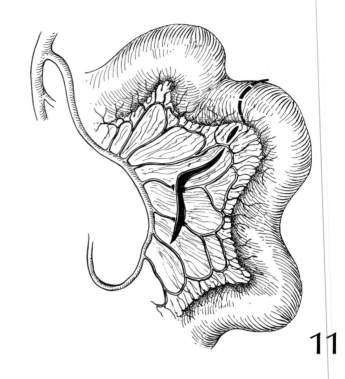

11

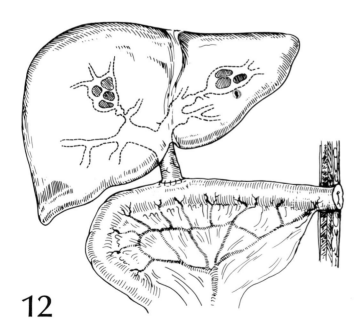

12

12 A bilioenteric anastomosis is then constructed using the common duct, confluence of right and left hepatic ducts, left hepatic duct or left lateral inferior duct, depending on the site of biliary stricture and the ease of exposure of the bile duct. The proximal end of the Roux loop is brought to skin level and opened as a cutaneous stoma. The location of the stoma is dictated by the need to avoid previous abdominal scars and the need to provide a straight route for postoperative choledochoscopy.

Choledochoscopy can be safely performed 2 weeks after operation if there is no evidence of anastomotic leakage. Compared with choledochoscopy via a T tube tract, choledochoscopy via a cutaneous stoma is much less painful and avoids the risk of disruption of the tract or loss of stones in the abdominal cavity. After satisfactory dilatation of strictures and complete eradication of stones, aided by electrohydraulic lithotripsy if necessary, the stoma can be closed and buried in the subcutaneous space. If the disease recurs the jejunal loop can be retrieved, and the stoma is reconstructed for choledochoscopy.

STRICTUROPLASTY

Strictures of the common bile duct or left hepatic duct are treated by choledochojejunostomy or hepatico-jejunostomy, the anastomoses being constructed proximal to the stricture. In the case of stricture of the right segmental duct orifice, stricturoplasty can be performed.

13 The anterior surface of the common hepatic and left hepatic ducts are dissected clear and the location of the hepaticodochotomy is planned.

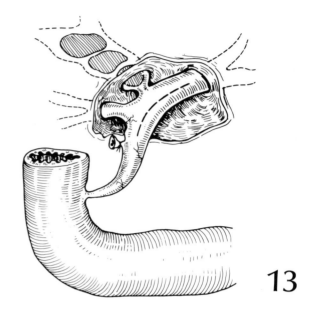

13

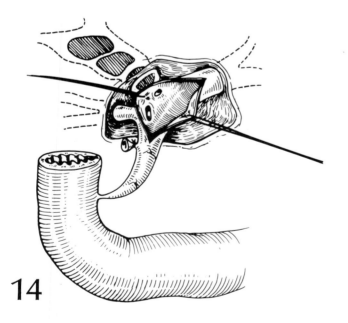

14

14 The orifice of the right segmental duct is exposed after extending the hepaticodochotomy up to the left duct. Any major branch of the hepatic artery crossing in front of the common hepatic or left hepatic duct should be protected.

15 The right segmental duct stricture is enlarged by excision of the septum and resuturing of the edges.

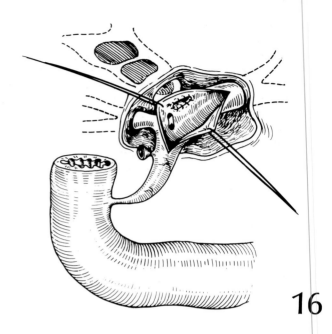

16

16 After complete eradication of stones inside the intrahepatic ducts, a hepaticojejunal anastomosis is made using the full length of the hepaticodochotomy and a hepaticocutaneous jejunostomy is fashioned.

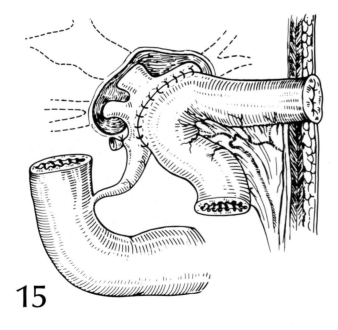

15

HEPATECTOMY

Hepatectomy is indicated when a liver segment or lobe is grossly atrophic secondary to repeated infection in the presence of strictures or impacted stones. It is also indicated when the affected liver segment is involved by multiple cholangitic liver abscesses even though the volume of the liver segment is not reduced, or when concomitant intrahepatic cholangiocarcinoma is diagnosed preoperatively. Left lateral segmentectomy is the commonest type of hepatic resection performed for recurrent pyogenic cholangitis followed by left hepatic lobectomy and, less commonly, by right hepatic lobectomy.

Left lateral segmentectomy

Incision

17 A vertical midline or bilateral subcostal incision is made.

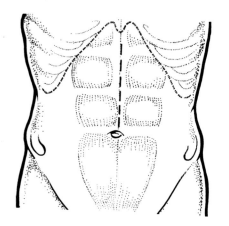

Mobilization of the left lateral segment

18 The left lateral segment is mobilized by division of the left triangular ligament. The left diaphragmatic vein may be adherent to the inflamed liver, and care must be taken to avoid damaging it, especially at its junction with the left hepatic vein. Further dissection is then carried out to separate the left lateral segment from the stomach and spleen. Dense adhesions may be present due to concealed abscesses around the left lateral segment. These abscesses are the result of rupture of cholangitic liver abscesses.

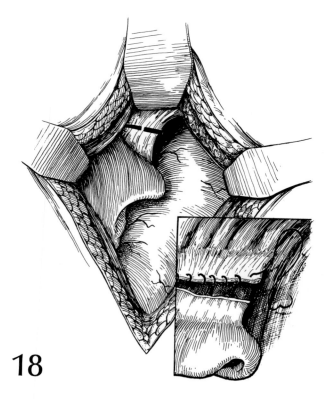

Dissection of the left hepatic vein

19 Completion of the mobilization of the left lateral segment will help in the identification and encircling of the left hepatic vein. Excessive efforts to encircle the left hepatic vein are not encouraged when inflammatory adhesions are dense and when the left hepatic vein has a short portion. In this situation, the left hepatic vein is better controlled inside the liver during the process of parenchymal transection. If the left hepatic vein is injured, the injury is usually in the form of a nick. If bleeding is difficult to control by suturing, the tips of a broad-blade vascular clamp are applied to the nick, and it is sutured after removing the left lateral segment.

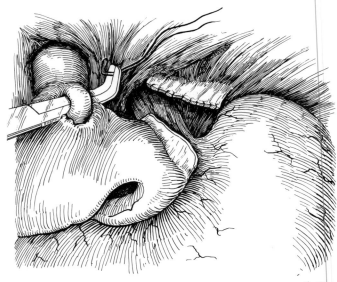

19

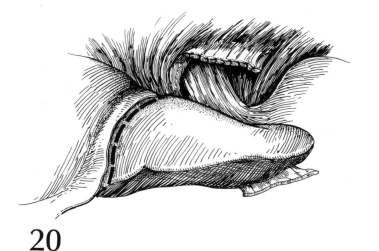

20

Transection of the liver

20 For left lateral segmentectomy, transection of the liver can follow dissection of the left hepatic vein without the need for hilar dissection. Dissection at the umbilical fissure may actually increase the chance of injury to the branches of the hepatic duct and vascular supply to the left medial segment. The transection line is marked on the surface of the left lateral segment about 0.5 cm to the left of the falciform ligament. Vascular inflow is then occluded using the Pringle manoeuvre, and outflow is occluded by applying a vascular clamp to the left hepatic vein if it has been encircled. The liver parenchyma is transected using a pair of crushing clamps or an ultrasonic dissector.

Identification of subsegmental vascular pedicles

21 The two subsegmental vascular pedicles are exposed near the umbilical fissure and are divided between clamps and transfixed. The Pringle manoeuvre must be released immediately after control of the two subsegmental pedicles has been achieved. When the left lateral segment is atrophic, bleeding from the transected surface is usually not severe, and the Pringle manoeuvre may not be necessary.

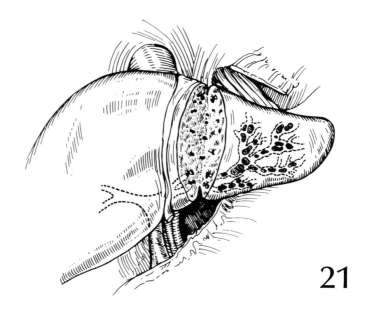

21

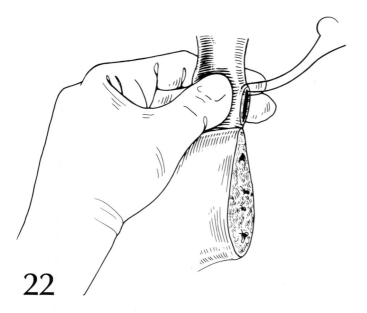

22

Control of the left hepatic vein

22 Life-threatening bleeding may occur if the left hepatic vein slips from the vascular clamp or ligature after division, and a defect appears in the left side of the inferior vena cava. In this situation, it may be impossible to apply a vascular clamp to the side wall of the cava due to limitation of space. Blind insertion of large bite stitches may lead to partial occlusion of the inferior vena cava. To achieve complete control it is necessary to clamp inflow vessels, the infrahepatic inferior vena cava and the suprahepatic vena cava (in the pericardial cavity). An alternative is to first encircle the suprahepatic portion of the inferior vena cava with the left index finger while the right index finger and thumb occlude the defect of the inferior vena cava. The defect is then controlled with the left thumb in front and the left index and middle fingers behind. Accepting that the control may be incomplete, running sutures can be inserted quickly to close the defect.

Control of bleeding and bile leakage from resected liver edge

Bleeding from the resected liver edge is easily controlled by individual suture. A high incidence of subphrenic abscess secondary to bile leakage has been observed. This complication is perhaps due to the fact that minute bile duct openings may remain open because of chronic inflammation of the ductal wall. To prevent bile leakage from such minute bile duct openings on the transected surface, fibrin glue can be sprayed on to the surface. A drain is left in the left subphrenic space, and the abdomen is closed.

Left hepatic lobectomy

Left hepatic lobectomy in recurrent pyogenic cholangitis is performed in the standard fashion.

Right hepatic lobectomy

Incision

23 A bilateral subcostal incision with an upward midline incision is used. If the right lobe is atrophic and the left lobe hypertrophic, the liver hilum may rotate towards the right subphrenic space. In this situation a thoracoabdominal incision may be a better choice.

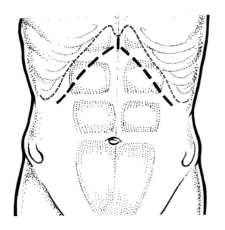

23

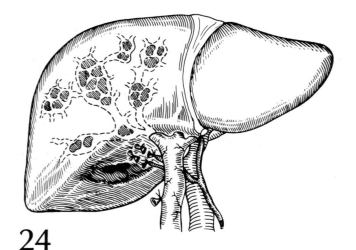

24

Dissection of the right hepatic artery and right portal vein

24 After cholecystectomy the tissue plane between the common hepatic duct and portal vein is opened. The right hepatic artery is dissected, encircled, ligated and divided at a point overlying the caudate process. Further separation of the plane between the common hepatic duct and the anterior surface of the portal vein exposes the junction of the right and left portal vein. The right portal vein is encircled at the level of the caudate process, taking care to avoid damage to branches of the caudate lobe. The vein is then ligated and divided. If the right portal vein is too short for safe division, a further length of vein can be obtained at the time of parenchymal transection, and the vein can be divided at that stage. The right hepatic duct can be dissected at this time, but complete encircling may be easier to accomplish using the ultrasonic dissector at the stage of parenchymal transection.

Mobilization of the right lobe

25 The right lobe of the liver is mobilized by division of the triangular ligament followed by ligation and division of the short venous branches that drain from the posterior surface of the liver into the inferior vena cava. The right hepatic vein is then controlled extrahepatically, divided between vascular clamps, and sutured. Dense inflammatory adhesions may limit mobilization of the right lobe of the liver, and the diaphragm may be injured and the right pleural cavity entered. Immediate suturing of the diaphragmatic defect is advisable to reduce bleeding into the right pleural cavity. If there is difficulty in encircling the right hepatic vein, the procedure should be abandoned as the right hepatic vein can be controlled at the time of parenchymal transection.

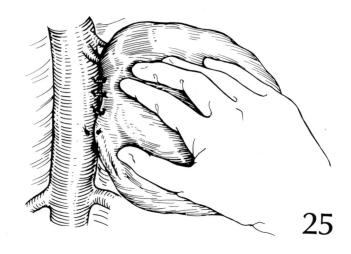

25

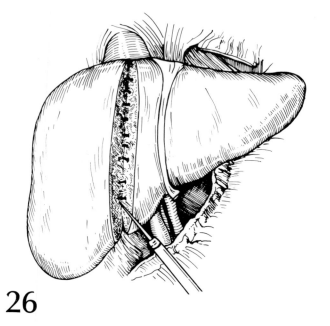

26

Transection of the liver

26 The line of transection is marked on the surface of the liver by diathermy after the middle hepatic vein is located by intraoperative ultrasonography. The parenchyma can be transected using a pair of crushing clamps, finger fracture or, preferably, in this situation with thick liver parenchyma, by the ultrasonic dissector. The power output of the ultrasonic dissector is set to about 40% of the maximum or higher depending on the texture of the liver. With the tip of the probe moving horizontally, ductal and vascular structures are exposed. If they measure 1 mm or less, they are dealt with by diathermy. If larger, they are clipped or ligated. The caudate process is then transected, and completion of the parenchymal transection and control of the right hepatic vein allows delivery of the specimen.

The transected hepatic duct is sutured with absorbable material. Fibrin glue is then sprayed on to the cut surface and hilum to conceal minute bile duct openings. Methylene blue can be injected into the common bile duct via a T tube to check for leakage from the hepatic duct or smaller duct openings on the transected surface of the liver. A drain is left in the right subphrenic space, and the abdomen is closed.

Postoperative care

Broad-spectrum antibiotics, such as a second or third generation cephalosporin or a broad-spectrum penicillin, are given for 1 week. In patients with previous bilioenteric anastomosis, anaerobic bacteria may be present in the bile and this necessitates anaerobic coverage. Intravenous fluid is given until oral intake is sufficient. The output from the T tube is monitored and replaced accordingly. When hepatectomy has been carried out, albumin infusion may be needed for 3–5 days.

Stomahesive is applied to the stoma so that the skin will not be excoriated by the bile.

Complications

T tube drainage

Absence of bile flow indicates that the T tube is kinked or dislodged from the common bile duct. Before a cholangiogram is performed, the T tube must be examined by taking away the dressing to be certain that the tube is not kinked at the skin exit site because of an anchoring stitch or folding in the dressing. Copious output from the T tube can be caused by obstruction of the lower end of the common bile duct or infestation by *Clonorchis sinensis*. In cases of impaction of a stone at the lower end of the common bile duct, consideration should be given for early endoscopic papillotomy and stone extraction to reduce morbidity secondary to loss of fluid and electrolytes. In *Clonorchis* infestation, praziquantel is prescribed. A T tube cholangiogram under antibiotic cover is performed about 2 weeks after the operation. If stones or strictures are found, choledochoscopy via the T tube tract is performed about 6 weeks after the operation.

Hepaticocutaneous jejunostomy

There are few complications peculiar to hepaticocutaneous jejunostomy. The jejunal loop is sometimes too redundant to allow passage of the choledochoscope and identification of the hepaticojejunal anastomosis. Even if the hepaticojejunal anastomosis is reached, not enough length of the choledochoscope may be left for passage into the intrahepatic duct. Careful planning of the length of the jejunal loop is therefore necessary.

Excoriation of the skin by bile may occur, particularly if there is irregularity of the skin due to a previous abdominal scar. The location of the stoma should be determined preoperatively to avoid such a problem, and the patient should understand the rationale of hepaticocutaneous jejunostomy. When closing the cutaneous stoma, inadequate mobilization of the jejunal loop from the abdominal wall may lead to failure and fistula formation.

Hepatectomy

Compared with hepatectomy for neoplasia, hepatectomy for recurrent pyogenic cholangitis carries a higher incidence of postoperative intra-abdominal sepsis[5]. This difference is related to the presence of infected bile and abscesses in this condition. Prevention of bile leakage and antibiotic cover are mandatory to reduce the incidence of sepsis.

Outcome

Although the operations are described separately in this chapter, many patients with complicated disease are treated by a combination of two or more methods in order to optimize the result. For intrahepatic disease, partial hepatectomy together with other procedures can achieve long-term symptomatic relief in 84% of patients. Better results are expected in patients with extrahepatic involvement only. Recurrence is likely in those with complicated intrahepatic disease. While it may not be possible to prevent recurrence, percutaneous access to the biliary tract by hepaticocutaneous jejunostomy substantially facilitates overall management and reduces the need for subsequent open operations.

References

1. Digby KH. Common-duct stones of liver origin. *Br J Surg* 1930; 17: 578–91.

2. Cook J, Hou PC, Ho HC, McFadzean AJS. Recurrent pyogenic cholangitis. *Br J Surg* 1954; 42: 188–203.

3. Ong GB. A study of recurrent pyogenic cholangitis. *Arch Surg* 1962; 84: 199–225.

4. Fan ST, Choi TK, Lo CM, Mok FP, Lai EC, Wong J. Treatment of hepatolithiasis: improvement of result by a systemic approach. *Surgery* 1991; 109: 474–80.

5. Fan ST, Lai EC, Wong J. Hepatic resection for hepatolithiasis. *Arch Surg* 1993; 128: 1070–4.

Endoscopic choledochoscopy and endoscopic intrahepatic stone treatment

A.R.W. Hatfield MD, FRCP
Consultant Gastroenterologist, The Middlesex Hospital, London, UK

Principles and justification

When therapeutic endoscopic retrograde cholangiopancreatography (ERCP) was first established a significant failure rate occurred when in dealing with large bile duct stones, very tight or multiple bile duct strictures, stones above strictures and, especially, intrahepatic stones above high bile duct strictures[1]. With improvements in both endoscopes and accessories, particularly the development of low-profile, high-pressure dilating balloons and mechanical lithotriptors, a much higher success rate with endoscopy has evolved when dealing with these difficult problems[2]. However, a small proportion of patients still remains in whom therapeutic ERCP fails, and open surgery would then be the only other option. As many of these patients have had previous and often difficult biliary surgery or are elderly and medically unfit, more sophisticated non-operative endoscopic techniques have been developed.

The development of small diameter, highly flexible and manoeuvrable endoscopes for percutaneous use stems from experience in the bronchial tree and renal tract. At a time when percutaneous cholecystolithotomy was in vogue and extensively performed, small percutaneous endoscopes for biliary use were developed, particularly for extracting stones jammed in Hartmann's pouch or the cystic duct. These endoscopes were developed with direct contact lithotripsy in mind, and accessories were fashioned for the removal of small stones and small fragments via the gallbladder and percutaneous tract. With the further development of laparoscopic cholecystectomy, percutaneous chole-cystolithotomy has, by and large, been abandoned but the prototype endoscopes developed have proved to be of enormous use for percutaneous choledochoscopy. Olympus Tokyo have developed a series of percutaneous choledochoscopes (XCHF), the latest being 60 cm long and 12 Fr in diameter. A side channel can be used for irrigation and instrumentation taking accessories up to 3 Fr.

Methods of access

In the immediate postoperative period, for patients in whom a T tube or other surgical drain of at least 12 Fr diameter has been inserted in the biliary tree, instrumentation with the choledochoscope can be safely performed after 10 days. In the majority of cases where the patient presents after the immediate postoperative period, a new access tract into the biliary tree has to be created. This tract is invariably via the percutaneous transhepatic route. After conventional transhepatic cholangiography, the intrahepatic duct system can be punctured, the tract dilated and a 12-Fr catheter left *in situ* for 10 days before choledochoscopy. If immediate biliary treatment is required, the choledochoscope can be inserted into the biliary tree transhepatically via a 'peel-away' sheath without waiting for the tract to become established.

In patients who have already undergone hepaticojejunostomy and in whom transhepatic access is contraindicated or impossible, direct radiological puncture of the jejunal loop and access to the anastomosis from below is possible and will be described later in this chapter.

Technique

The procedure is performed under sterile conditions with intravenous antibiotic cover and light intravenous sedation. The introduction of the endoscope down an established tract is usually not painful, but intravenous sedation may be necessary for manipulations such as balloon dilatation and direct contact lithotripsy of gallstones.

If the percutaneous tract has been established for some time, introduction of the endoscope is usually very straightforward. The endoscope can usually be inserted under direct vision into the liver or bile duct but, if the tract is difficult or tortuous, it may be wise to remove the biliary drain over a guidewire so that the endoscope can be inserted easily under radiological control over the same guidewire. This step reduces the risk of damaging the tract and causing leakage or rupture, risks which might be incurred if the tract was angulated or tortuous. Once in the biliary tree, a slow infusion of saline ensures a good view. Radiological contrast media can be injected down the channel of the instrument leading to very precise and often selective opacification of the entire biliary system. This combination of an endoscopic view and radiological screening gives a most accurate assessment of stones, strictures and possible tumours. Defects that radiologically are thought to be stones can be confirmed as air bubbles when seen endoscopically and any doubt is instantly resolved. Strictures can be viewed directly and suspicious lesions brushed and biopsied down the side channel.

Strictures that are too tight to allow the endoscope to pass or a gallstone to be retrieved can be dilated. It is a simple matter under endoscopic and/or radiological control to pass a guidewire through a stricture, remove the endoscope and then dilate the stricture with low-profile high-pressure balloons of differing diameters. The choledochoscope is then inserted back over the guidewire. This process of removing the endoscope, balloon dilatation and repositioning the endoscope over a guidewire is very rapid and multiple introductions of the endoscope can be made safely in a short period without any discomfort to the patient.

Therapeutic options

1a, b Small stones in the intrahepatic or extrahepatic ducts can be removed through the tract with a basket or balloon. In the majority of cases the size of the gallstone precludes this method of retrieval and, as most patients have already undergone unsuccessful ERCP, sphincterotomy and attempted gallstone removal, the presence of a patent sphincterotomy allows a larger stone to be shattered with lithotripsy so that fragments can be pushed or flushed into the duodenum from above.

If the gallstone lies above a bile duct stricture, the stricture is first dilated with a balloon, the stone is then either pushed through intact or shattered under direct vision, and the fragments are pushed through the stricture from above. In some cases the fragments may be extracted through the liver as well.

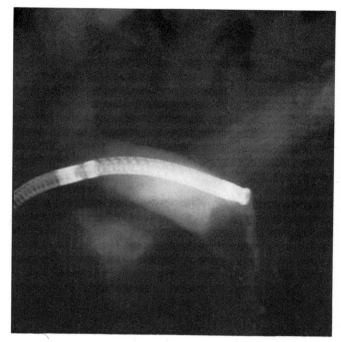

1a

Intraductal lithotripsy

Electrohydraulic lithotripsy or a YAG or pulsed dye laser can be used for direct contact lithotripsy[3]. The pulsed dye laser has the advantage of being completely safe in that its wavelength can be adjusted so that stones are fragmented without damaging the bile duct mucosa. Unfortunately, these lasers are extremely expensive, temperamental and difficult to maintain. Electrohydraulic lithotripsy is, however, much cheaper and very simple to use. A flexible probe can be placed directly on the stone, and an electrical impulse generates a powerful shockwave if the probe and gallstone are surrounded by fluid and not air. This results in successful fragmentation of the stone. Electrohydraulic lithotripsy can easily damage the bile duct wall, causing a small leak or perforation, if the probe slips off the stone and an impulse is triggered when the tip of the probe is on or adjacent to the bile duct wall. Because of the cost factor alone, most centres use electrohydraulic lithotripsy but with great caution.

Good irrigation is essential to clear the murky view which is invariable during fragmentation. These small endoscopes have the disadvantage of possessing only one port for intubation and irrigation, so that irrigation is necessarily reduced when the probe is in place during lithotripsy. As it is very simple and rapid to remove and reintroduce the endoscope, a good view is obtained once the probe has been removed, the murky bile aspirated and the bile duct irrigated afresh. Sludge and biliary debris can be flushed past the stone into the duodenum or allowed to drain outwards via the transhepatic tract if the endoscope is removed.

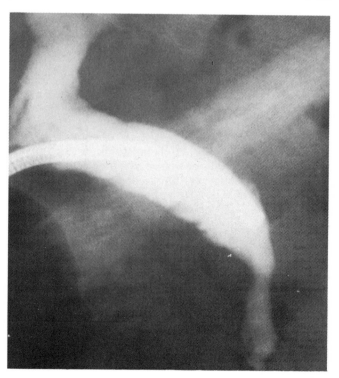

1b

Multiple gallstones

More complicated cases with multiple stones may need several sessions of lithotripsy and fragment or stone removal. If there are multiple stones above a stricture or above a sphincterotomy, clearly the uppermost stone is fragmented first and these fragments may temporarily impact in the bile duct, making it more difficult to approach more distally placed stones. In this situation, a drainage catheter is placed in the biliary tree over a guidewire once the endoscope has been withdrawn and a further procedure(s) are scheduled. Such reinterventions can be undertaken after 1–2 days and during the same admission or the patient can be readmitted a week later depending on the clinical situation. The procedure is very well tolerated and multiple short sessions to clear numbers of stones are much more acceptable than multiple, more lengthy and complex therapeutic ERCP sessions.

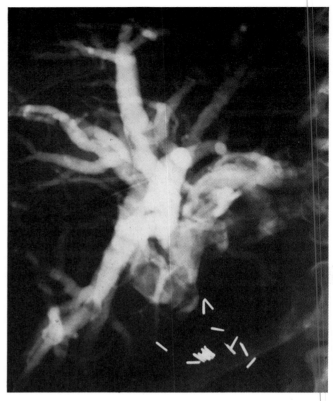

2a

2a–c A transhepatic cholangiogram in a patient who had had a bile duct repair to correct previous surgical transection is shown. An ERCP had demonstrated the complete block in the mid bile duct and, when seen from above, the intrahepatic ducts were full of stones above a very tight stricture. Following establishment of a transhepatic tract, choledochoscopy and lithotripsy had already cleared many of these stones. The biliary stricture was dilated (*Illustration 2b*) and only some stones still remain. After four sessions of choledochoscopy with lithotripsy and stricture dilatation, the biliary tree was clear of stones (*Illustration 2c*) and the transhepatic access tube was removed.

Once the bile duct has been completely cleared of stones, the transhepatic catheter can be removed following a final tube cholangiogram. If the biliary stricture has been dilated before gallstone removal and a follow-up is necessary, this check can always be achieved by ERCP at a later stage.

Multiple intrahepatic stones

When stones are present in both the left and right sides of the liver, a single transhepatic puncture into either side of the liver usually allows access to both sides, since the endoscope is so manoeuvrable that it can easily pass from right to left or vice versa. If multiple sessions are anticipated and a drainage catheter may have to be left in place between procedures for some time, a left lobe puncture is preferred as the patient is more comfortable when a catheter is left emerging from the abdominal wall than between the ribs (which would be the case following a right lobe puncture). Even if stones lie behind strictures in both lobes of the liver, a single puncture allows access to both sides when the endoscope is retroverted at the hilum, having dilated the stricture at the origin of the right and left ducts accordingly.

In some complex cases, multiple small stones fill the peripheral intrahepatic ducts and are impossible to clear initially or are not visible on cholangiography. In such patients treatment with oral ursodeoxycholic acid for a month before re-examination may allow further peripheral stone clearance. The transhepatic drainage catheter can also be used to irrigate the bile duct when small fragments remain, providing a patent sphincterotomy is present below.

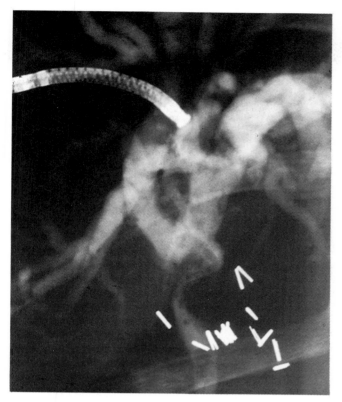

2b

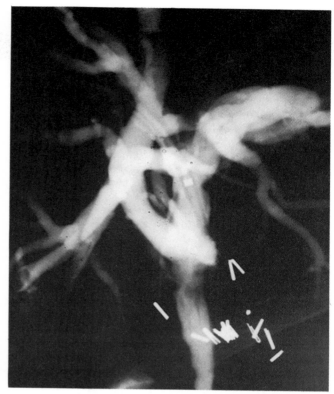

2c

Management after hepaticojejunostomy

Traditionally, jaundice and/or cholangitis secondary to stricturing of a hepaticojejunostomy has been managed by the radiologist with transhepatic puncture and balloon dilatation of the stricture. Such patients often progressively develop secondary biliary cirrhosis and abnormal clotting can create difficulties for further transhepatic manoeuvres, particularly if multiple procedures are required over a number of years. The intrahepatic ducts may also get progressively smaller and fail to dilate due to the cirrhosis, even in the presence of biliary obstruction. Additionally, stricturing of the origins of the right and left hepatic ducts at the anastomosis means that bilateral right and left punctures have to be performed to catheterize each side selectively. If multiple procedures are envisaged, transhepatic catheters have to be left *in situ* and clearly this has the disadvantage of discomfort and potential for sepsis. Furthermore, patients may find transhepatic catheters difficult to endure and cope with at home between admissions. Being of small calibre, they often block or slip out. Although anastomotic strictures can be dealt with in this way, the intrahepatic calculi, which

are so often present, can make radiological management alone difficult.

In patients with cirrhotic livers with small ducts, radiological methods to puncture the jejunal loop below the anastomosis have been developed and guidewires and balloons can then be passed through strictures from below under radiological control[4]. However, difficulties may be encountered when negotiating long jejunal loops and identifying and traversing very tight anastomotic strictures. This technique has now been further developed to allow puncturing of the jejunal loop, insertion of a catheter to create an access tract, and then instrumentation of the loop with a choledochoscope[4]. Some patients will have had a jejunal access loop with some sort of marking system attached to the undersurface of the abdominal wall at the time of hepaticojejunostomy. However, most patients will not have had this specific procedure. The jejunal loop has therefore to be identified by ultrasonography and, in some cases, transhepatic cholangiography.

3 Superficial loops are easier to puncture but jejunal loops which lie more deeply sometimes have to be distended with contrast medium or saline instilled at percutaneous transhepatic cholangiography or through a transabdominal needle. The loop can then be punctured more securely, often with the aid of percutaneously placed fixation devices which are sutured to the abdominal wall. The tract can then be dilated to take a 12- or 14-Fr self-retaining Cope catheter which is left in place for 14 days.

Again, if instant biliary instrumentation is required, access to the jejunal loop can be obtained immediately via a 'peel-away' sheath system.

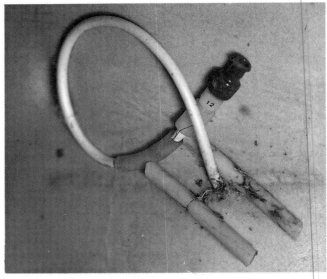

3

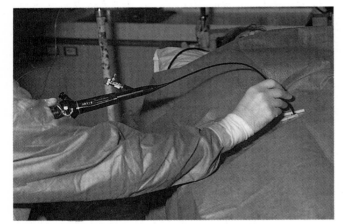

4

4 A combination of direct vision and radiological imaging can be used to advance the endoscope up the jejunal loop and identify the hepaticojejunostomy.

5a–d The strictured anastomosis can be cannulated from below, contrast medium injected and the intrahepatic duct system visualised. The strictured anastomosis is cannulated with a guidewire, the choledochoscope is removed, and a balloon catheter is positioned within the stricture. Once the anastomosis has been dilated, any stones lying above the anastomosis can be removed under endoscopic and/or radiological control with baskets or balloons.

With this type of problem repeat dilatations are likely to be necessary, and a catheter can be left in the jejunal loop to maintain access. A 'gastrostomy button' can also be used to help to maintain the access. This method is better tolerated by patients, obviates the need for dressings over a catheter site, and allows the patient to bath normally. Such devices can be left in place for months or years.

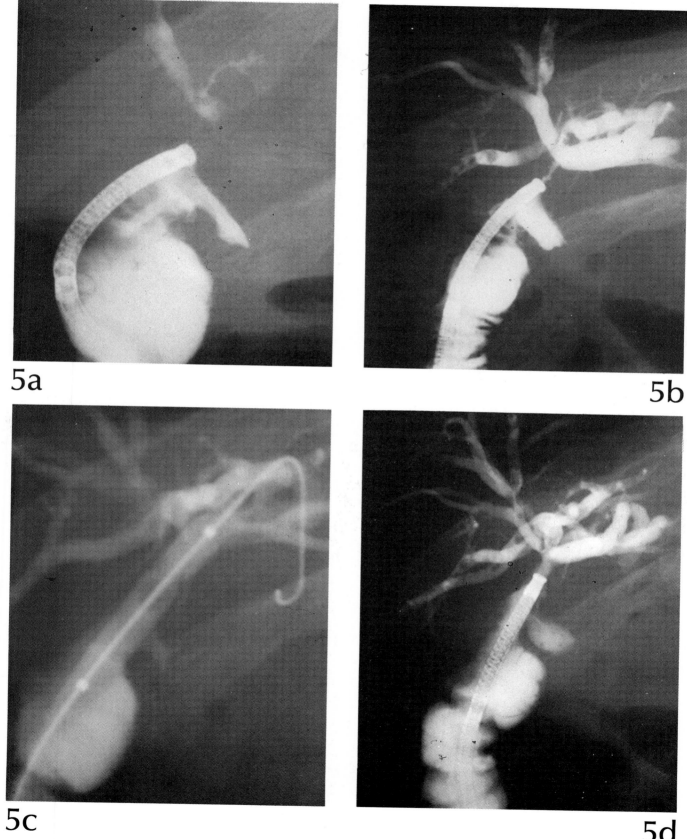

5a

5b

5c

5d

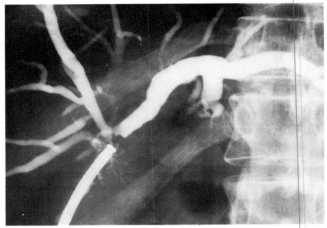

6a,b Separate strictures of both right and left intrahepatic ducts can easily be dilated individually by selective cannulation from below. In the case illustrated, guidewires have been passed selectively into the left and right intrahepatic duct systems and, once the choledochoscope is removed, both strictures can be separately dilated. At the bottom of the radiograph the site of jejunal loop puncture can be seen where there are two metal markers which represent the T piece of the anchor sutures.

6a

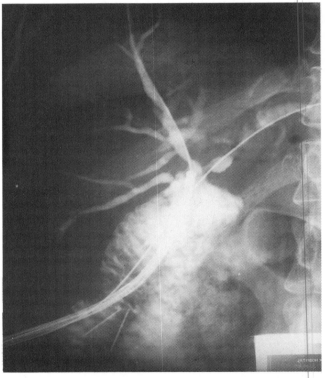

6b

Other conditions

The technique of percutaneous choledochoscopy can be very useful in the assessment and management of choledochal cysts, particularly when the cyst has been incompletely resected and/or drained at previous surgery. If choledochal cysts extend into the liver, high bile duct anastomoses can stricture and lead to stasis with stone formation within the cystic chambers in the liver as well as in the true intrahepatic ducts. Such patients can be very difficult to manage by further open surgery, and it is usually possible to clear all stones from the cyst(s) and duct system with a transhepatic and/or transjejunal approach. Filling defects within choledochal cysts, which often are due to debris or stones, can be mistaken for tumour radiologically. This distinction is very important as the risk of tumour development within a choledochal cyst increases with age, and direct inspection and biopsy via the choledochoscope will clarify the situation.

Smaller choledochoscopes can be passed along tortuous surgical drainage or fistula tracts when it is desirable to insert a percutaneous drain into an intra-abdominal viscus or abscess cavity. This approach has been particularly useful in patients with complete bile duct obstruction after cholecystectomy where the upper biliary tree has been opacified and intubated via a fistula tract, thus avoiding the need for transhepatic puncture and drainage before reconstructive surgery.

Comparison with other non-operative techniques

Percutaneous choledochoscopy often avoids the need for multiple and difficult transhepatic manoeuvres and, once a tract has been established, further interventions can be performed easily and safely. The alternative method of performing therapeutic endoscopy within the bile duct itself involves peroral choledochoscopy, the so-called 'mother and baby scope' technique[5].

7   A small 12-Fr endoscope can be passed down the side channel of a therapeutic duodenoscope at the time of ERCP and then passed through a small sphincterotomy into the bile duct from below. Once in the bile duct, stones can be identified and shattered with lithotripsy and strictures and suspicious areas can be identified and biopsied.

The 'mother and baby scope' technique is time consuming, extremely complex, and needs two expert endoscopists. The equipment is expensive, it is often difficult to introduce the endoscope into the bile duct. In addition, if multiple stones or fragments have to be dealt with after lithotripsy, it is very time consuming to keep passing the endoscope in and out of the biliary tree. Percutaneous choledochoscopy offers a greater degree of freedom of instrumentation and multiple stones can be more rapidly cleared from the biliary tree. Although the 'mother and baby scope' technique avoids the need for a transhepatic puncture, it is more suitable for patients with solitary stones.

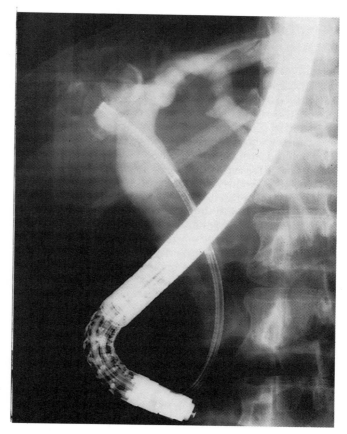

7

Results, complications and outcome

Percutaneous choledochoscopy is a new technique and has been used in very few centres[6]. At the Middlesex Hospital, 56 patients have been treated over the last 6 years. The majority have been patients with large gallstones located above strictures, and many have had intrahepatic stones which have not been dealt with successfully by therapeutic ERCP. In all patients large stones have been shattered and removed from the biliary tree after dilating the strictures. In some patients with very small intrahepatic stones, tiny stones have been left in the peripheral intrahepatic ducts and the patients have remained on bile acid therapy.

Complications have included minor discomfort during the initial transhepatic manoeuvres to establish the tract, and during choledochoscopy when strictures are dilated or intraduct lithotripsy is employed. More discomfort can be experienced after creation of a jejunal loop access, but this usually settles rapidly within 48 h. Post-procedure sepsis is remarkably uncommon as the patients are on antibiotics and are always left with an effective drainage tube following the procedure. In 40 of the 56 patients, direct contact electrohydraulic lithotripsy was used and bile duct perforation was observed in only one patient. This led to localized pain and peritonitis which settled with conservative management over 2–3 days. Many patients having repeat procedures at regular intervals to remove or flush out stones shattered at a prior procedure often need no sedation.

In many cases follow-up ERCP procedures have been performed in patients with biliary strictures and, in the majority, once all gallstones have been removed, strictures have resolved spontaneously. If necessary, further balloon dilatation of strictures can be performed at ERCP, reducing the likelihood of further stasis and gallstone formation.

The long-term outlook for patients with a strictured hepaticojejunostomy treated by repeated transjejunal endoscopic dilatation is still being assessed. Many of these patients have established secondary biliary cirrhosis at the time of presentation with jaundice or cholangitis. In such patients with cirrhosis and coagulation problems, the transjejunal approach is far safer than the transhepatic route and avoids the risk of bleeding and septicaemic episodes which may occur during transhepatic puncture. However, in patients who present relatively early after initial surgery and before cirrhosis is established, repeated dilatations at regular intervals may slow or avoid the progression towards biliary cirrhosis.

References

1. Persson B. Relation of size and number of common duct calculi to success of sphincterotomy and stone extraction. *Gastrointest Radiol* 1991; 16: 212–4.

2. Schneider MU, Matek W, Bauer R, Domschke W. Mechanical lithotripsy of bile duct stones in 209 patients: effect of technical advances. *Endoscopy* 1988; 20: 248–53.

3. Neuhaus H, Hoffmann W, Zillinger C, Classen M. Laser lithotripsy of difficult bile duct stones under direct visual control. *Gut* 1993; 34: 415–21.

4. Rottenberg GT, Hatfield ARW, Lees WR. Percutaneous jejunostomy formation for antegrade endoscopic access to the postoperative biliary tree. *J Intervent Radiol* 1994; 9: 143–6.

5. Leung JWC, Chung SSC. Electrohydraulic lithotripsy with peroral choledochoscopy. *BMJ* 1989; 299: 595–8.

6. Hatfield ARW, Craig P, Lanzon-Miller SL *et al*. Percutaneous choledochoscopy in the management of benign biliary disease. *Gut* 1992; 33(Suppl. 1): S34.

Gallbladder cancer

Henry A. Pitt MD

Professor and Vice Chairman, Department of Surgery, The Johns Hopkins Medical Institutions, Baltimore, Maryland, USA

History

Gallbladder cancer was first described by Maximillian de Stoll in 1777[1]. More than a century later, Keen was the first to perform a liver resection for gallbladder cancer in 1891[1]. The association between gallstones and gallbladder cancer was made by Mayo in 1903[1]. The high incidence of gallbladder cancer in rubber industry workers and in southwestern American Indians was first reported in the 1960s[1]. The realization that an anomalous pancreaticobiliary duct junction may play a role in the pathogenesis was appreciated in the 1980s[2]. An understanding of oncogene expression, tumour DNA content, and cellular antigen expression have all been described in the 1990s[1].

Principles and justification

More than 80% of gallbladder cancers are adenocarcinomas[1]. Gallbladder carcinomas may be of several histological types including papillary, nodular, tubular, poorly differentiated and combinations with varying degrees of invasion[1]. The histological grade has significant prognostic implications as does the presence or absence of adjacent metaplasia. Well differentiated tumours and those with adjacent metaplasia have a better prognosis[3]. The next most important pathological classification is the gross anatomical form which includes papillary, tubular and nodular. In general, papillary tumours have a better prognosis whereas nodular tumours are the most likely to involve the liver and have lymph node metastases.

The degree of invasion is an important factor in staging, in the success of an operative procedure and in predicting survival. T_1 tumours involve the mucosa or muscle layer, T_2 tumours extend into the perimuscular connective tissue, T_3 tumours perforate the serosa and/or directly invade one adjacent organ, and T_4 tumours extend more than 2 cm into two or more adjacent organs. As with other tumours, the presence of lymph node or distant metastases affects stage, resectability and prognosis. Cell turnover characteristics are another factor. The majority of gallbladder cancers are aneuploid, and these tumours tend to be poorly differentiated, to invade beyond the muscularis propria, and to have a poor prognosis.

The majority of patients with gallbladder cancer present with advanced disease. Common presenting symptoms include pain, weight loss and jaundice. In many of these patients the tumour extends beyond the gallbladder into the adjacent liver, extrahepatic bile ducts, regional lymph nodes or distant sites. If metastatic disease is documented, non-operative palliative measures are indicated. Many patients who present with extrahepatic bile duct obstruction also have encasement of the portal vein and/or hepatic artery which prevents resection. In these patients percutaneous or endoscopic placement of an endoprosthesis will palliate the jaundice. However, some patients also have duodenal obstruction which may require surgical palliation.

Between 10% and 20% of patients with gallbladder cancer present with biliary symptoms due to associated gallstones[1]. After undergoing elective cholecystectomy, pathological examination of the gallbladder reveals an adenocarcinoma. The management of these patients with 'incidental' gallbladder cancer depends upon the degree of invasion of the tumour. If carcinoma *in situ* or a tumour localized to the mucosa is identified, no further treatment may be necessary. In early stage tumours the position of the tumour within the gallbladder may be important. If the gallbladder cancer is superficial (T_1) and not adjacent to the liver, cholecystectomy may be an adequate operation. However, if the tumour is adjacent to the liver, the chance of local recurrence is increased, and an 'extended cholecystectomy', which includes resection of the gallbladder bed, may be indicated.

Hepatic resection and regional lymphadenectomy may also be appropriate for patients with more deeply invading (T_3 and T_4) but localized tumours[4]. Local invasion of the transverse colon may also warrant segmental colon resection. Tumours that invade both the liver and the duodenum or pancreas may require a combined liver resection and pancreaticoduodenectomy to achieve negative margins[5]. Most of these tumours also involve hilar vessels and are not therefore resectable. In addition, the mortality rate in patients who undergo hepatopancreatoduodenectomy is high, especially in those who are jaundiced and malnourished. Careful patient selection and preoperative preparation should therefore be undertaken if a radical operation is contemplated. Although a patient may be explored with an intent to resect, palliative procedures to relieve biliary obstruction and prevent duodenal obstruction and pain may be more appropriate.

Preoperative

Gallbladder cancers occur most commonly in elderly women with gallstones. Abdominal pain is the most common complaint, and biliary colic or acute cholecystitis are often part of the initial presentation. Almost half of the patients present with jaundice due to tumour invasion of the common hepatic duct. Most patients also have nausea, anorexia and weight loss. In patients who present with jaundice, a typical profile of significant elevation of bilirubin and alkaline phosphatase and a slight increase in transaminase levels is observed. Some patients have a modest increase in carcinoembryonic antigen (CEA) levels. However, the incidence of raised CEA levels is low and the specificity is poor. Thus, CEA and other tumour markers are not good screening tests for gallbladder cancer.

1a–d

Plain abdominal radiography, ultrasonography, computed tomography (CT), magnetic resonance imaging (MRI), cholangiography and angiography have all been employed to evaluate patients with gallbladder cancer. The presence of a 'porcelain' gallbladder on a plain abdominal radiograph should alert the clinician to the possibility of gallbladder cancer. Compared with the newer spiral CT and MRI techniques, ultrasonography is useful in documenting associated gallstones or gallbladder polyps but not in staging the disease. Spiral CT scanning will demonstrate the extent of the tumour, vascular encasement and liver metastases. If the patient presents with obstructive jaundice, cholangiography usually demonstrates a long stricture of the common hepatic duct which sometimes also involves the right and left hepatic ducts (*Illustration 1a*). The presence of a long common channel on endoscopic retrograde cholangiopancreatography also suggests that a gallbladder cancer may be present. Newer MRI techniques are able to provide a cholangiogram and are best at demonstrating the extent of the tumour including parenchymal and vascular invasion as well as liver metastases. The magnetic resonance scans in *Illustrations 1b–d* show gallbladder cancer adjacent to the right portal vein with invasion of the liver and portal structures.

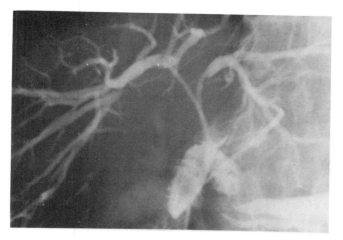

1a

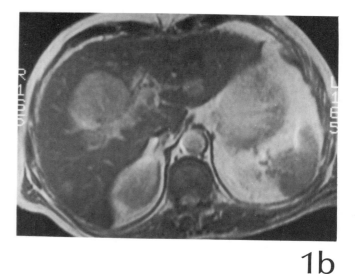

1b

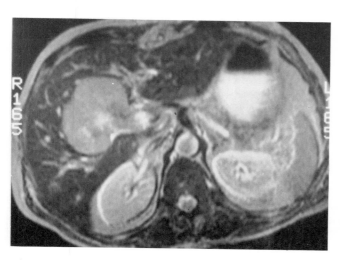

1c

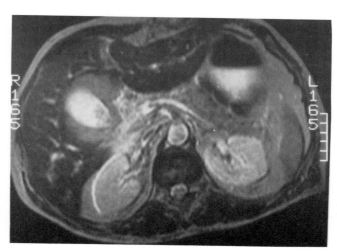

1d

Over the past decade, many groups have routinely employed angiography to stage these patients. However, spiral CT scanning and MRI are now providing as much or more information, and routine angiography may no longer be necessary. Endoscopic ultrasonography (EUS) has also been proposed to stage patients with biliary and pancreatic malignancies. However, whether EUS adds anything to a state-of-the-art CT or MRI scan has yet to be proven. Laparoscopy, on the other hand, will demonstrate liver and peritoneal metastases that are not detected by CT or MRI scanning. The addition of ultrasonography to laparoscopy significantly increases the accuracy of this procedure in staging. Metastatic or unresectable tumours may also be biopsied during laparoscopy. If non-invasive studies suggest unresectable disease, and if surgical palliation is not required, ultrasonographic or CT-guided needle biopsy may be appropriate to establish the diagnosis and avoid exploratory surgery.

Local invasion of the adjacent liver is a common finding that can sometimes be managed with wedge resection. More extensive involvement of the liver may require resection of segments IV, V and VI, the right lobe, or the right lobe and a portion of segment IV. If right lobectomy is required, encasement or occlusion of the main portal vein, the common hepatic artery or the left hepatic artery will preclude resection. On the other hand, encasement of the right portal vein or the right hepatic artery does not prevent resection if right hepatic lobectomy is contemplated. Moreover, a few metastatic nodules in the right lobe adjacent to the gallbladder may not preclude resection. However, multiple bilateral liver, peritoneal or distant metastases are contraindications to resection.

In addition to a full assessment of the extent of the tumour, a number of patient characteristics must also be considered in preparing these patients for surgery. Factors such as age, obesity, diabetes and hypertension should be considered but, by themselves, are rarely a contraindication to surgery. On the other hand, recent myocardial infarction, major valvular heart disease, congestive heart failure, severe pulmonary insufficiency, chronic renal failure and pre-existing cirrhosis, especially with associated portal hypertension, may dramatically increase the risk of surgery. Obstructive jaundice affects organ and immune function and should be relieved before surgery if liver resection is contemplated. Biliary sepsis, impaired renal function and poor nutritional status are also associated with a poor outcome after surgery (see chapter on pp. 262–274). In comparison, preoperative preparation is minimal for non-jaundiced, healthy patients found to have an 'incidental' gallbladder cancer. In this setting, the preoperative administration of a single dose of a first generation cephalosporin for wound infection prophylaxis may be all that is necessary.

Anaesthesia

Non-operative palliation of obstructive jaundice due to a gallbladder cancer may be achieved with either percutaneous transhepatic biliary drainage or an endoscopically placed endoprosthesis. Both procedures can usually be performed with intravenous sedation and narcotics. Similarly, staging these patients with angiography or endoscopic ultrasound can normally be done with sedation and minimal or no analgesia. On the other hand, laparoscopic staging usually requires a general anaesthetic. In addition, laparotomy performed for either resection or palliation is carried out under a general endotracheal anaesthetic. With all of these procedures, especially in jaundiced patients, drugs which may cause cholestasis, coagulopathy or renal insufficiency should be avoided.

Operation

Incision

2a,b The incision should be individualized according to the procedure that is most likely to be performed. If the patient has been diagnosed by prior laparoscopic removal of the gallbladder and 'extended cholecystectomy' is contemplated, a midline incision which includes excision of the laparoscopic ports should be performed. In this clinical situation, excision of the umbilicus may be indicated if the gallbladder had been removed through the umbilical port. This manoeuvre is precautionary because metastases have been reported at the port site[1]. On the other hand, if the diagnosis is suspected before surgery and resection of a portion or all of the right lobe of the liver is contemplated, an extended right subcostal incision will provide excellent exposure. This incision extends from the xiphoid in the midline, along the costal margin and around the lower border of the rib cage in the right flank.

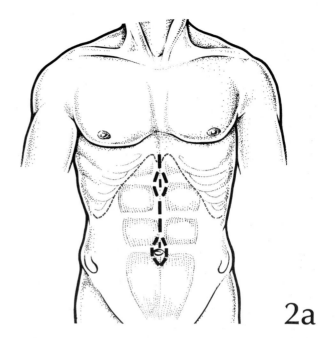

2a

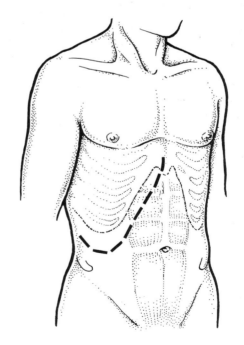

2b

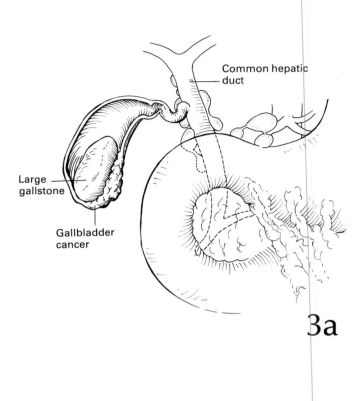

3a

Exploration and Kocher manoeuvre

3a,b A complete exploration of the abdomen should be undertaken whenever gallbladder cancer is suspected. Factors which raise the level of suspicion that a gallbladder cancer may be present, include a single large gallstone, a 'porcelain' gallbladder, gallbladder polyps and a long common channel between the bile and pancreatic ducts. Metastases may be found on the surface of the liver as well as on the peritoneum adjacent to the gallbladder and along the right paracolic gutter. Direct invasion of the right transverse colon, the duodenum or head of the pancreas should also be anticipated. If laparoscopic cholecystectomy has been performed, adhesions will have to be divided to make this determination. Performance of a Kocher manoeuvre including release of the duodenum, hepatic flexure and reopening of the foramen of Winslow, if occluded by adhesions, is the next step. This mobilization will help to determine whether the tumour has invaded the portal vein or head of the pancreas.

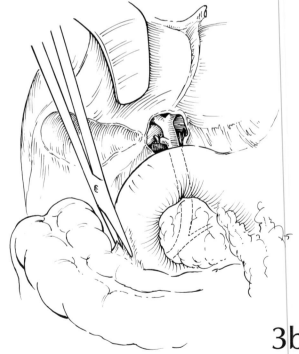

3b

Extended cholecystectomy

4a–c If there is no invasion of the extrahepatic bile ducts, hilar vessels, colon, duodenum or pancreas, and if distant metastases are not present, extended cholecystectomy may be indicated. The depth of invasion and position of the tumour in the gallbladder must also be considered. If the tumour has not invaded deeply into the gallbladder or was confined to its surface away from the liver, extended cholecystectomy should be performed. Intraoperative ultrasonography may be helpful in determining the depth of invasion into the liver and also in detecting small liver metastases. To perform an extended cholecystectomy, whether the gallbladder has previously been removed or is still *in situ*, the common hepatic duct is exposed, and the liver around the gallbladder bed is scored with electrocautery. A wedge resection of this triangular section of the liver may be performed with a Cavitron ultrasonic dissector or by placing large chromic overlapping 'liver' sutures. The resection is then completed with electrocautery. Haemostasis is achieved with electrocautery or sutures as necessary, or the argon beam, if available.

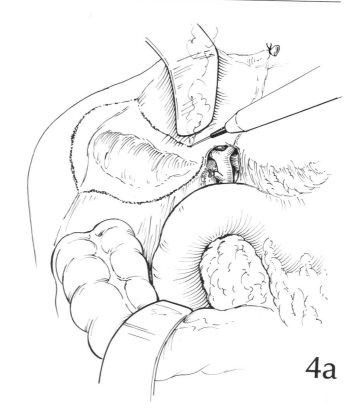

4a

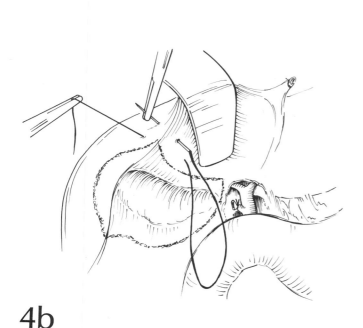

4b

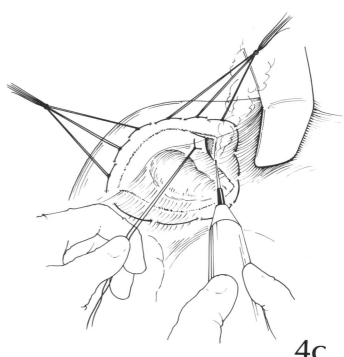

4c

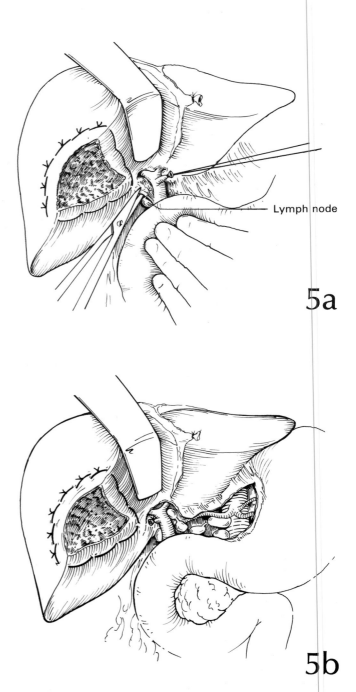

Lymph node

5a

5b

Regional lymphadenectomy

5a,b After completing the wedge resection of the liver, a regional lymph node dissection is performed. This dissection begins at the surface of the liver. All of the lymphatic tissue in the hepatoduodenal ligament is dissected free leaving only the bile duct, portal vein and hepatic artery. The dissection is continued into the retroperitoneum behind the head of the pancreas as well as along the hepatic artery and cephalad edge of the body of the pancreas to the coeliac axis. The lymph nodes around the origin of the left gastric and splenic arteries should also be excised.

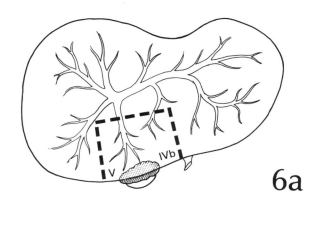

6a

Segmental liver resection

6a–c If the tumour extends more deeply into the liver, segmental resection of segments IVb and V, which surround the gallbladder, may be required to achieve an adequate margin (*Illustration 6a*). If the tumour extends even more deeply into the liver, preservation of the blood supply to segment VI may not be possible and resection of segments IVb, V and VI may therefore be necessary (*Illustration 6b*). Tumour involvement of the right portal vein or right hepatic artery may necessitate resection of segments IVb, V, VI, VII and VIII (*Illustration 6c*) (*see* chapters on pp. 30–45 and 46–55).

Occasionally, a wedge or segmental liver resection along with excision of the extrahepatic bile ducts may be indicated (*see* chapter on pp. 437–446). Rarely, a wedge or segmental liver resection in combination with pancreaticoduodenectomy may be the only way to achieve a negative margin (*see* chapter on pp. 528–543 and 610–623).

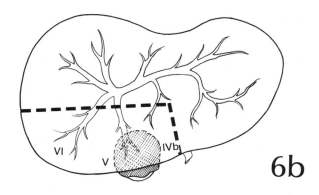

6b

Palliation

The majority of patients with gallbladder cancer will be undergoing palliative treatment. If preoperative assessment demonstrates unresectable disease and the only problem is jaundice, non-operative palliation with percutaneous or endoscopic stents will usually suffice (*see* chapter on pp. 417–419). If duodenal obstruction is also a problem or if exploration is required to determine resectability, surgery is indicated even though the likelihood that the tumour can be resected is low. In this setting, the gallbladder is usually removed to prevent acute cholecystitis, a biliary bypass procedure and a gastrojejunostomy are performed, and an alcohol splanchnicectomy may also be done to treat or prevent pain (*see* chapter on pp. 570–575). If widespread peritoneal metastases are present, a preoperatively placed biliary stent may be left in place, and the biliary bypass procedure is not undertaken because of the patient's short life expectancy. On the other hand, if the tumour is localized but unresectable, a Roux-en-Y choledochojejunostomy with large-bore Silastic stents may be performed caudal to the tumour. Alternatively, if the hilar area is completely involved by the tumour, a segment III bypass may be performed (*see* chapter on pp. 430–436).

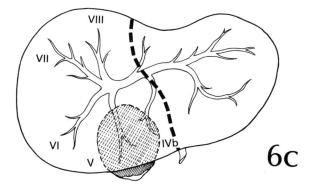

6c

Postoperative care

When an extended cholecystectomy with regional lymph node dissection is performed, gastric emptying may be delayed in the early postoperative period due to partial denervation of the gastric antrum. Thus, a nasogastric tube may be necessary until residual aspirates decrease in volume. The use of a prokinetic agent may also be helpful in the early postoperative period. The risk of liver failure will depend upon the degree of preoperative biliary obstruction, the amount of parenchyma resected and the degree of fibrosis in the residual liver. If a major resection has been performed in an obstructed or fibrotic liver, careful monitoring of the liver function is important. On the other hand, liver failure is hardly a consideration if only a wedge resection of the gallbladder bed is performed and blood flow to the remaining liver is not compromised.

The use of closed suction drains placed along the cut edge of the liver is controversial. Advocates claim that the morbidity of a bile leak is lessened if a drain is in place. If a drain has been placed, it should be left in until bile flow has been stimulated by food intake. The drain can usually be safely removed if no bile is observed after oral intake has been initiated. The management of large-bore Silastic transhepatic stents that may be used for palliation is discussed in detail elsewhere (*see* chapter on pp. 420–429). With an extended cholecystectomy or a more significant liver resection, prophylactic antibiotics are discontinued rapidly after the operation. However, if a jaundiced patient needs a transhepatic stent for palliation, antibiotic treatment may be required for 48 h or longer to treat cholangitis. In these patients antibiotics should also be given before and after tube cholangiography.

Outcome

The morbidity and mortality of extended cholecystectomy are quite acceptable[1,3]. However, the addition of a major liver resection dramatically increases 30-day mortality to as high as 15–18%[1,3]. The combination of liver and a pancreatic resection is also associated with high mortality[1,4,5]. In general, the survival rates of patients with gallbladder cancer have been poor, with the exception of those with stage I tumours discovered incidentally. Most patients have advanced disease at the time of presentation and, as a result, less than 5% of all patients with gallbladder cancer are alive after 5 years.

With this dismal outlook a variety of chemotherapeutic and radiation therapy protocols have been tried. In general, the response rates to chemotherapy have been low[1]. In addition, no randomized data have proven a survival advantage with external beam radiation alone. On the other hand, reports of small numbers of patients receiving intraoperative radiotherapy have been encouraging[1,6]. Nevertheless, the effect, if any, of combined radiation and chemotherapy needs to be tested in patients with malignancies of the biliary tree.

Survival depends on the stage of the tumour as well as the operation that is performed. Patients with stage I lesions who undergo a simple cholecystectomy should have a 5-year survival rate of more than 85%. In comparison, 5-year survival rates for patients with stage II, III and IV disease are approximately 25%, 10% and 2%, respectively. However, patients with stage II malignancies treated with an extended cholecystectomy may expect up to a 65% 5-year survival rate. In addition, patients with stage III and IV tumours treated by liver resection can be expected to have a survival rate of 15–25% at 5 years. The quality of survival of these patients must also be addressed. Factors to consider include pain, jaundice, pruritus, nausea and vomiting.

References

1. Pitt HA, Dooley WC, Yeo CJ, Cameron JL. Malignancies of the biliary tree. *Curr Probl Surg* 1995; 32: 1–90.

2. Tanaka K, Nishimura A, Yamada K, *et al*. Cancer of the gallbladder associated with anomalous junction of the pancreatobiliary duct system without bile duct dilatation *Br J Surg* 1993; 80: 622–4.

3. Sumiyoshi K, Nagai E, Chijiiwa K, *et al*. Pathology of carcinoma of the gallbladder. *World J Surg* 1991; 15: 315–21.

4. Ogura Y, Mizumoto R, Isaji S, *et al*. Radical operations for carcinoma of the gallbladder. *World J Surg* 1991; 15: 337–43.

5. Nimura Y, Hayakawa N, Kamiya J, *et al*. Hepatopancreato-duodenectomy for advanced carcinoma of the biliary tract. *Hepatogastroenterology* 1991; 38: 170–5.

6. Todaroki T, Iwasaki Y, Oril K, *et al*. Resection combined with intraoperative radiation therapy for stage IV gallbladder carcinoma. *World J Surg* 1991; 15: 357–66.

Non-surgical relief of malignant extrahepatic biliary obstruction

Kelvin R. Palmer MD, FRCP(Ed)
Consultant Physician, Western General Hospital, Edinburgh, UK

Stents are usually inserted to palliate malignant extra-hepatic biliary obstruction, but are sometimes used as a temporary measure to relieve jaundice before potentially curative radical surgery. Endoscopic insertion is preferred, but when this proves impossible for technical reasons, stents can be inserted by a percutaneous transhepatic approach. In general, obstructing lesions in the distal common bile duct can usually be stented endoscopically whereas lesions in the upper biliary tree are more likely to require a transhepatic approach. In some cases a 'rendevous' technique can be employed in which a guidewire is passed down the biliary tree from above so that the endoscopist can then pass a stent upwards from the duodenum so that it lies across the obstructing lesion.

Endoscopic insertion of stents

1   The patient is prepared for diagnostic endoscopic retrograde cholangiopancreatography (ERCP) and stenting as described on pp. 282–290. Diagnostic ERCP is first undertaken to define the nature, site and length of the stricture. A guidewire within a plastic sheath is then passed through the stricture. Prior sphincterotomy is unnecessary although a needle knife incision is needed occasionally to gain access to the biliary tree (*see* page 286).

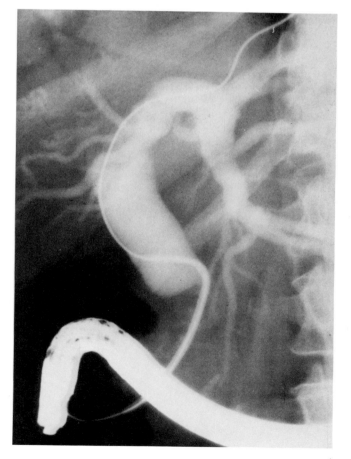

1

Choice of stents

A choice of plastic and metal stents is available. Plastic stents are usually 10–12 Fr in diameter, are straight with no side holes, and have proximal and distal flanges to prevent displacement. Double pigtail 7-Fr stents can be used but are normally only employed in the conservative treatment of choledocholithiasis. Plastic stents are cheap and can be removed. They are used when the prosthesis is only needed as a temporary measure or when palliating advanced malignant disease in patients with a short life expectancy. Plastic stents generally remain patent for 3–6 months before the return of obstructive jaundice and/or cholangitis signals the need for stent replacement.

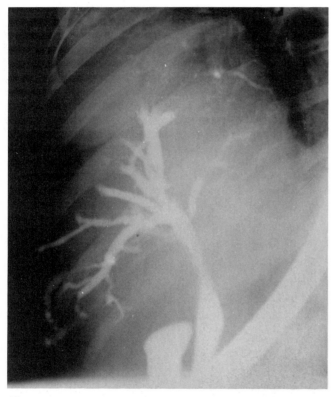

2

2   Metal stents expand to 2 cm in diameter and are deployed using specialized introducers. They are much less likely to occlude but are much more expensive than plastic stents, and are used for palliation in patients whose life expectancy is more than a few months. Tumour ingrowth through the interstices of the expanded stent can pose problems.

3a, b

The stent chosen is positioned across the stricture. With plastic stents, the shortest stent which adequately traverses the stricture is used, and the distal end of the stent is left within the duodenum. This facilitates removal if the stent blocks. Care should be used in positioning metal stents because these shorten after insertion and may then fail to maintain a patent channel through the obstructing lesion.

Results

Biliary stenting is successful in approximately 80% of cases. Failures are due principally to access difficulties posed by duodenal infiltration with tumour. Tight stenoses can be dilated and tortuous strictures intubated using floppy hydrophilic guidewires. Success rates are highest for common bile duct strictures, while tumours at the bifurcation of the biliary tree or within the liver are more difficult to stent and palliation is less effective.

Complications

The principal early complication of biliary stenting is cholangitis. This only occurs if the biliary tree is incompletely drained; prophylactic antibiotics are normally used to cover the procedure and reduce the risks of biliary sepsis.

The major late complication is stent occlusion leading to ascending cholangitis and recurrence of jaundice. Plastic stents become occluded by bacterial adherence to the stent lumen followed by deposition of bile salts and biliary debris. Long-term administration of antibiotics or choleretic agents does not prevent this complication. Metal stents occlude less frequently and recurrent jaundice is usually due to tumour ingrowth through the stent.

Management of blocked stents

Occluded plastic stents can be removed using a Dormia basket or specialized forceps. Restenting is then performed using the standard technique. Alternatively, the occluded stent can be removed over a guidewire to facilitate insertion of a new stent.

Tumour ingrowth through the interstices of a metal prosthesis is simply treated by passing a plastic or metal prosthesis through the blocked stent.

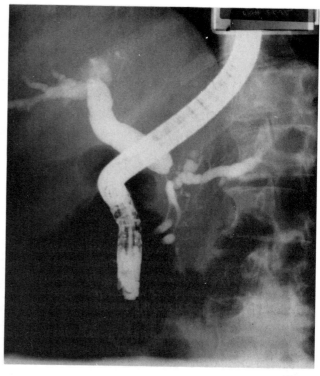

3a

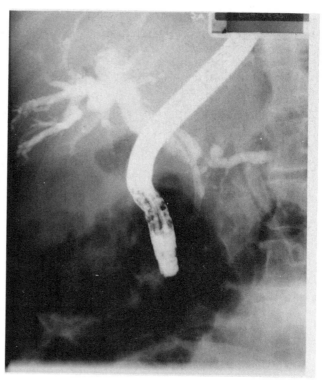

3b

Bile duct cancer: palliative management

Henry A. Pitt MD
Professor and Vice Chairman, Department of Surgery, The Johns Hopkins Medical Institutions, Baltimore, Maryland, USA

History

Cancer of the bile ducts was first described over a century ago. By 1960, more than 1000 cases of this rare malignancy had been reported[1]. However, the fact that the majority of these lesions occur in the perihilar region, as opposed to the intrahepatic or distal bile ducts, was not appreciated for many years. In 1965 Klatskin[2] reported 13 patients with cancers of the hepatic duct bifurcation. This report and the develop-ment of endoscopic and percutaneous cholangiography in the 1970s stimulated interest in this uncommon malignancy at the hepatic duct bifurcation which many now call 'Klatskin' tumours. Since approximately 70% of cholangiocarcinomas occur in the region of the hepatic duct bifurcation, this chapter will focus on palliation of these perihilar tumours.

Principles and justification

Improved diagnosis of perihilar cholangiocarcinomas and lower procedure-related mortality has led to increased enthusiasm for resecting these tumours. Resection remains the only treatment that offers the possibility, albeit low, for cure. However, in most series only a few patients with perihilar cholangiocarcinomas are able to have a potentially curative resection with all margins microscopically free of tumour, so in most patients the aim of treatment is palliative relief of biliary obstruction. This aim is achieved when the patient is free of pruritus, cholangitis and the effects of liver failure. The primary goals of palliative management are therefore to increase both the length and quality of survival.

Various non-operative and operative options are available for patients with unresectable perihilar cholangiocarcinoma. Non-operative alternatives include easily changeable percutaneous transhepatic stents, indwelling plastic endoprostheses and self-expanding metallic stents. These latter two options involve insertion of the stent by either percutaneous or endoscopic techniques. However, most authorities prefer the percutaneous approach for perihilar malignancies and use metallic stents in patients whose life expectancy is less than 6 months. Nevertheless, debate continues as to whether (1) partially external or totally indwelling stents are best, (2) percutaneous or endoscopic placement is preferred, and (3) plastic or metallic stents provide the best results. A further discussion of this topic can be found in the chapter on pp. 417–419.

In most series less than half of the patients who are explored with curative intent actually undergo resection. Approximately 10–15% of patients will be found at laparotomy to have peritoneal and/or liver metastases that were not detected by preoperative studies. If percutaneous stents have been placed preoperatively through the tumour into the duodenum, these stents will usually be adequate for palliation of this subset of patients with their relatively short life expectancy. However, these patients are prone to develop acute cholecystitis, and the gallbladder should therefore be removed at the time of the laparotomy. If resection is not possible because of local involvement of the hepatic artery, portal vein, liver or duodenum, palliative options include segment III hepaticojejunostomy (*see* chapter on pp. 430–436) and placement of large-bore Silastic stents through the tumour into a Roux-en-Y limb of jejunum. The use of large-bore Silastic stents for palliation will be reviewed in this chapter.

Preoperative

Both patient and tumour factors must be considered when assessing patients with perihilar cholangiocarcinoma. As with all major operations, the patient's general medical condition must be evaluated before exploration. Factors such as obesity, diabetes and hypertension should be considered but, by themselves, are rarely contraindications to surgery. Cardiopulmonary factors such as a recent myocardial infarction or severe pulmonary insufficiency may be more important contraindications. However, the mere existence of coronary artery or chronic pulmonary disease does not preclude an aggressive surgical approach. On the other hand, pre-existing cirrhosis may dramatically increase the risk of surgery, especially if the patient also has portal hypertension.

A major consideration in operating on patients with perihilar cholangiocarcinoma is the multiple physiological abnormalities posed by obstructive jaundice[1]. These factors are particularly important if liver resection is being contemplated. Obstructive jaundice alters many aspects of hepatic metabolism such as hepatic mitochondrial respiratory function, hepatic protein synthesis and hepatic reticuloendothelial function. In addition, these patients often have endotoxaemia which, in turn, may contribute to renal, cardiac and pulmonary insufficiency. Altered cell-mediated immunity further increases the risk of infection, and coagulation disorders make these patients prone to bleeding problems. At first glance, the degree of jaundice might seem to be a good predictor of outcome in patients with obstructive jaundice. However, altered renal function, poor nutritional status and biliary sepsis have been shown to be the best prognostic indicators in these patients[3]. A more complete discussion of this is presented in the chapter on pp. 262–274.

In addition to patient-related factors, specific characteristics of the tumour need to be considered before making a decision to explore the patient. For many years, ultrasonography and computed tomographic (CT) scanning were used to assess these patients. However, neither of these studies has proved to be particularly useful for demonstration of the full parenchymal extent of the tumour or vascular involvement.

1a,b As a result, most authorities have used a combination of cholangiography and angiography to stage these patients The efficacy of these two studies in determining resectability in 97 patients with pathologically proven perihilar cholangiocarcinoma was recently evaluated at The Johns Hopkins Hospital[1]. The predictive value of cholangiography was only 60%, but the addition of angiography increased the predictive value to 79%.

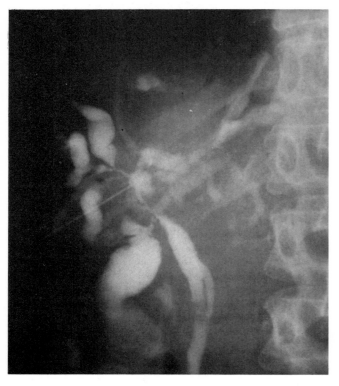

1a

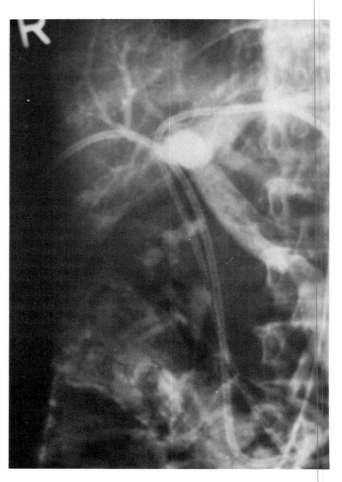

1b

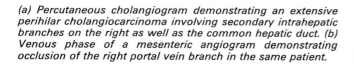

(a) Percutaneous cholangiogram demonstrating an extensive perihilar cholangiocarcinoma involving secondary intrahepatic branches on the right as well as the common hepatic duct. (b) Venous phase of a mesenteric angiogram demonstrating occlusion of the right portal vein branch in the same patient.

2a,b

The recent introduction of spiral or helical CT scanning has improved the detection of tumour involvement of both the adjacent liver parenchyma and the portal venous system. Magnetic resonance imaging (MRI) has also been shown to be particularly good at demonstrating the extent of the tumour, venous encasement and, sometimes, hepatic arterial involvement[1]. With MRI these tumours appear dark on T1 images and white on T2 images. In addition, venous anatomy is clearly demonstrated as a white image on the gradient-recalled acquisition in the steady state (GRASS) image which does not require a contrast agent.

Most recently, magnetic resonance cholangiography has been introduced which may further advance the ability to stage these patients without an invasive study. Thus, an MRI scan may currently be the study of choice for evaluating these patients.

Findings on spiral CT or MRI scanning such as bilobar peripheral metastases or extrahepatic disease preclude curative resection. Extensive bilobar hepatic parenchymal involvement also usually indicates unresectability. Atrophy of the lobe containing the tumour with hypertrophy of the other lobe is also a sign that resection may not be possible. Tumour encasement of the common hepatic artery or main portal vein has also been a contraindication to resection for most surgeons. Thus, this initial examination, even before cholangiography is performed, should provide some insight into whether a non-operative or an operative approach is in order.

The role of preoperative biliary decompression remains controversial. Most authorities agree that endoscopic stents, while often useful for periampullary lesions, are frequently harmful for patients with perihilar lesions. The introduction of bacteria into an obstructed biliary system without adequately relieving the obstruction leads to biliary sepsis that may be life-threatening. As a result, some experts recommend exploration without preoperative biliary drainage. However, many authorities believe that preoperative biliary decompression is essential if hepatic resection is contemplated. Thus, the placement of bilateral percutaneous transhepatic biliary stents is considered to be an important first step by many groups who frequently manage these patients. A more complete discussion of this topic, as well as the use of antibiotics, the management of fluids and the treatment of coagulopathies, is given in the chapter on pp. 262–274.

Anaesthesia

Placement of percutaneous transhepatic biliary drainage catheters can usually be performed with intravenous sedation and narcotics. Surgery for perihilar cholangiocarcinoma requires general endotracheal anaesthesia. Agents with potential for cholestasis or hepatotoxicity

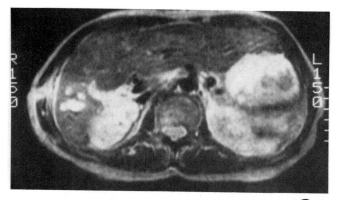

2a

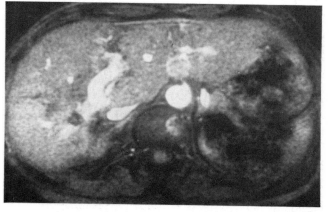

2b

(a) An MR scan T2 image in the same patient as in Illustration 1 demonstrating the tumour (white) in an atrophied right and hypertrophied left lobe. (b) The MR scan GRASS image, showing occlusion of the right and hypertrophy of the left portal vein.

should be avoided. These patients should be carefully monitored, both during and after the operation. Whether hepatic resection is contemplated or a palliative procedure is undertaken, severe cholangitis and renal insufficiency are major concerns. Thus, as a minimum, a Foley catheter and a central venous catheter should be inserted. If ongoing biliary sepsis or underlying cardiac disease are additional concerns, a Swan–Ganz catheter and an arterial line may also be in order. Repeat dosing of prophylactic antibiotics during a long procedure and intraoperative monitoring of coagulation studies are additional precautionary measures which may ensure a good outcome.

Operation

Incision

$3a,b$ If bilateral percutaneous transhepatic stents have been placed before the operation, the right stent will usually enter between the ribs while the left stent is usually placed in the upper epigastrium just to the left of the midline. These stents are prepared so that portions of them may be brought into the field during the procedure. If a right hepatic lobectomy is contemplated, a right subcostal incision will provide adequate exposure for exploration. If resection is possible, this incision may be extended to the xiphoid in the midline and laterally beneath the rib cage to provide adequate exposure. If a left hepatic lobectomy is a possibility, a midline incision is preferable. In addition, the midline incision does not interfere with the placement of the large-bore Silastic stents.

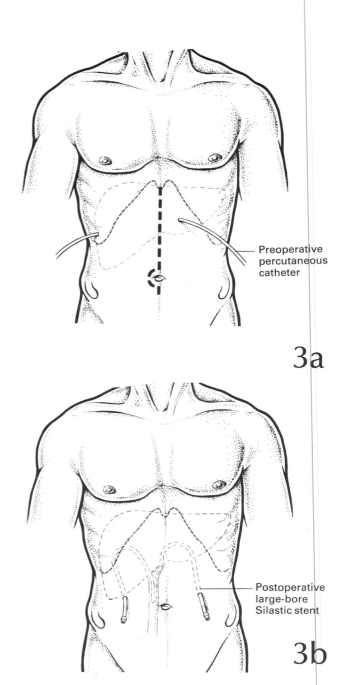

Preoperative percutaneous catheter

3a

Postoperative large-bore Silastic stent

3b

Tumour assessment

A full exploration of the entire abdomen should be the first step in this procedure. Any suspicious spots on the liver or in the peritoneal cavity should be biopsied. Tiny peritoneal metastases are frequently found on the peritoneum overlying the right kidney and along the right paracolic gutter. Lymph nodes around the coeliac axis, the hepatic artery and the portal vein are then examined. Although lymph node involvement does not preclude resection, the prognosis is adversely affected if the tumour has metastasized to the lymph nodes. Establishing a tissue diagnosis is important so that subsequent management is appropriate.

4a,b The hepatic ducts are then exposed and an attempt is made to palpate the transhepatic stents. Removal of the gallbladder will aid in this assessment on the right. If the stents cannot be palpated because the tumour has extended into secondary intrahepatic ducts on both the right and left, the lesion is usually unresectable.

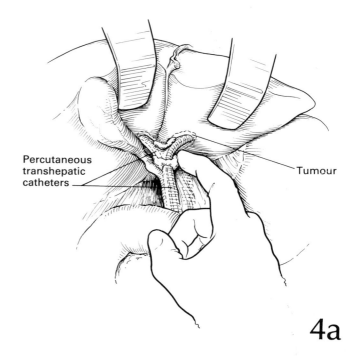

Percutaneous transhepatic catheters

Tumour

4a

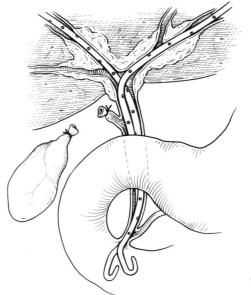

4b

Division of the bile duct

5 In some cases a decision as to resectability cannot be made without further dissection so the bile duct must be freed from the hepatic artery on the patient's left and from the portal vein (behind). The common hepatic duct is encircled with a vessel loop and a transverse choledochotomy is performed. Proximal dissection may be required to determine whether the tumour can be separated from the portal vein or hepatic artery.

Involvement of a portal vein or hepatic artery branch on the side that will require hepatic resection does not preclude resection if a negative margin can be achieved on the side of the liver that is to remain. However, resection is usually not performed if the tumour encases the main portal vein, the common hepatic artery or a branch of either vessel that goes to the liver that is to remain. If the tumour is not resectable, the distal bile duct is oversewn and large-bore Silastic stents are passed through the tumour.

Stent placement

6a,b The curved ends of the 8.3-Fr Ring catheters that were placed preoperatively are cut off. In addition, portions of the catheters that were external are retrieved into the abdomen. Guidewires are passed through these catheters, and progressively larger Coudé catheters are passed through the tumour, the bile ducts and the liver. An empty sponge forceps may be used at the liver surface to prevent tearing the parenchyma. Usually, 14 or 16-Fr Silastic biliary stents can be placed through each hepatic lobe and still fit within the common hepatic duct below the tumour. Heavy chromic mattress sutures are placed around the exit sites of the tubes from the liver to prevent bile leakage.

These large-bore stents do not become occluded as rapidly as the smaller diameter percutaneous stents and are therefore associated with fewer episodes of cholangitis in the ensuing months. In addition, placement of these stents into a Roux-en-Y limb of jejunum prevents reflux of food from the duodenum. Moreover, these stents are usually too large to fit through the normal sized distal duct and sphincter.

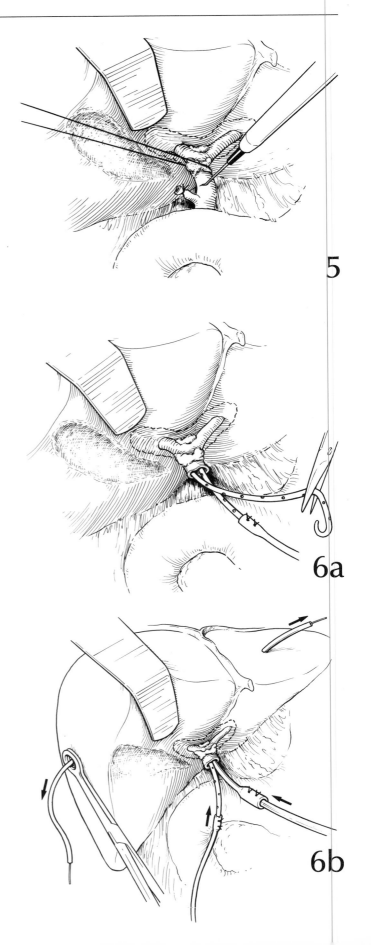

Division of jejunum

The creation of the Roux-en-Y limb of jejunum for this operation is identical to that described in the chapter on pp. 370–381. Briefly, the jejunum is divided approximately 30 cm from the ligament of Treitz at a point where there is a relatively large opening in the arcade of mesenteric vessels. The right colon is mobilized and a defect is made to the right of the middle colic vessels just above the duodenum. The distal end of the jejunum is oversewn and brought through the mesocolon in a retrocolic fashion. The retrocolic placement avoids tension on the Roux-en-Y and allows dependent drainage when the patient is in the supine position.

Choledochojejunostomy

7a–c The choledochojejunostomy is performed in an end-to-side fashion. The anastomosis may be made in one or two layers. In the case illustrated a two-layer anastomosis is being performed. An initial outer posterior row of interrupted 4/0 non-absorbable sutures is inserted, followed by an inner posterior row of interrupted 4/0 absorbable sutures. The stents are passed through the anastomosis prior to completion. The anterior portion of the anastomosis can also be performed in two layers with an inner layer of interrupted absorbable and an outer layer of interrupted non-absorbable sutures. Tube fluorocholangiography is performed to check the position of the catheters as well as to detect any leakage at their exit sites from the liver or at the anastomosis.

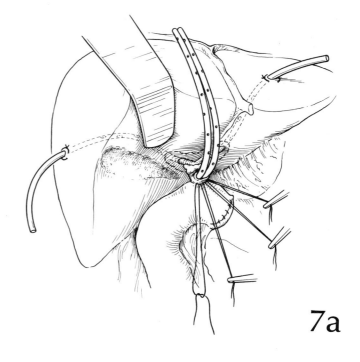

7a

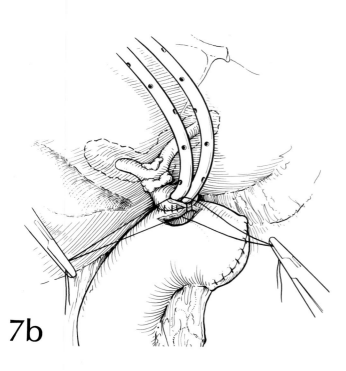

7b

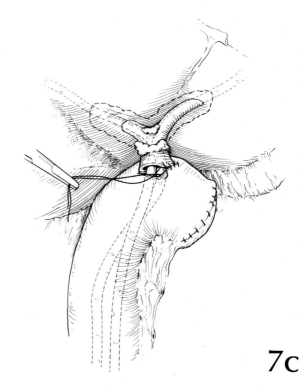

7c

Completion of Roux-en-Y

8 The procedure is completed with an end-to-side jejunojejunostomy performed 50–60 cm distal to the choledochojejunostomy. This anastomosis is usually done in two layers with an inner layer of running 3/0 absorbable sutures and an outer layer of interrupted 3/0 non-absorbable sutures. The mesenteric defects are closed with 3/0 non-absorbable sutures to prevent internal herniation. Three closed suction drains are placed to the exit sites of the two transhepatic stents from the liver and to the anastomosis. These drains and the two Silastic stents are secured to the skin. The transhepatic stents should be placed in positions in the right and left upper abdomen, respectively, that are both comfortable for the patient and easy for the interventional radiologist to change. The abdominal wall is closed in a standard fashion.

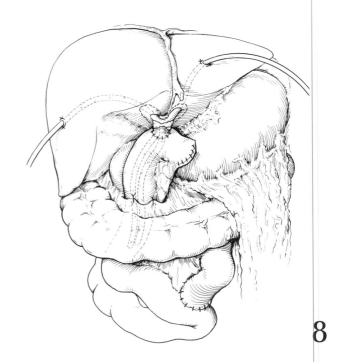

8

Postoperative care

The Silastic stents are connected to bile bags and placed on gravity drainage. Perioperative prophylactic antibiotics are continued for a minimum of 48 h postoperatively because the incidence of cholangitis is quite high after placement of large-bore Silastic stents. The nasogastric tube is left in place until bowel function has returned. On the fifth or sixth postoperative day, tube cholangiography is again performed to recheck the tube position and to be sure that no leakage has occurred at the liver edge or the anastomosis. Again, prophylactic antibiotics directed at the organisms that have been cultured from the patient's bile are begun before and continued for 24 h after cholangiography to prevent cholangitis. If no leakage has been found and no cholangitis has occurred, the biliary stents are closed the next day. If no bile is seen in the drains after an additional 12 h the drains are removed.

The patient is taught to flush both stents with 10 or 20 ml of saline twice a day to prevent the build-up of biliary 'sludge'. Nevertheless, a 16-Fr stent will become occluded with 'sludge' in approximately 4 months so these stents should be changed electively after 3 months to prevent problems with cholangitis or obstructive jaundice. This procedure can be performed on an outpatient basis by the interventional radiologist. Simply, a guidewire is passed through the old stent which is then removed. A new stent is passed over the guidewire, and its position is checked with cholangiography before the guidewire is removed. Prophylactic antibiotics should be given prior to the procedure, and the patient should be observed for signs of sepsis before discharge. In general, these stents are left in place for the remainder of the patient's life. However, when life expectancy is considered to be less than 6 months, the internal/external stents may be replaced with indwelling self-expanding metallic stents.

Outcome

Both the length and quality of survival are better if the tumour can be resected[4]. However, even when preoperative studies suggest that resection may be possible, operative findings often preclude resection. During a 17-year period at The Johns Hopkins Hospital, 53 patients were resected, 44 underwent operative palliation with large-bore Silastic stents and 21 were managed non-operatively with percutaneous stents[5]. In the 44 patients who underwent surgical exploration and palliative stenting, the actuarial survival at 1 and 2 years was 32% and 6%, respectively, with a median survival of 8 months. In contrast, in the 21 patients who had non-operative stenting the 1 and 2 year actuarial survival rates were 25% and 5%, respectively, with a median survival of 5 months.

These two groups were comparable by multiple objective criteria, but hospital mortality was, in fact, lower for the patients who underwent palliative surgery (7% versus 14%). In addition, survival for the first 6 months ($p < 0.01$) and median survival ($p < 0.05$) were also better in the patients who underwent palliative surgery. Patients who had operative palliation with large-bore Silastic stents placed into a Roux-en-Y limb of jejunum also required fewer stent changes per month of survival; however, they were more likely to undergo re-exploration for duodenal or small bowel obstruction. Since duodenal obstruction was almost always due to tumour extension, a palliative gastrojejunostomy should be considered whenever palliative surgery is being performed.

No data are available from the same institution to compare palliative surgery with large-bore stents and segment III bypass. However, the 7% hospital mortality reported in the Johns Hopkins series[5] was somewhat lower than that reported with the segment III bypass at other institutions during the same time period. In addition, in the Johns Hopkins report jaundice and pruritus were relieved in all but one patient (98%), which is also better than in most reports with the segment III bypass. The segment III bypass is more likely to relieve jaundice completely if the right and left ducts still communicate. However, the two ductal systems are separated by the majority of perihilar cholangiocarcinomas, many of which also extend into secondary branches on the left. Finally, the 8 month median survival in the patients at The Johns Hopkins Hospital who had palliative surgery with large-bore Silastic stents is also slightly longer than with other methods of palliation. However, many factors may explain these differences and randomized studies are needed.

Relatively few reports have compared the results of operative and non-operative palliation at the same institution. In addition to the report from The Johns Hopkins Hospital, Lai and colleagues from Hong Kong have compared the segment III bypass with endoscopic stenting[6]. In this and other reports, initial morbidity and mortality were similar; however, patients undergoing palliative surgery generally lived longer. In addition, if indwelling plastic endoprostheses were used, the patients managed non-operatively tended to have more late problems with recurrent jaundice and cholangitis. Thus, the additional costs of the operation were offset by the greater number of readmissions and stent changes in the patients managed non-operatively.

A final issue is whether adjuvant therapy improves survival in these patients. The use of chemotherapy alone, using 5-fluorouracil and multiple other drugs, has not been shown to improve survival in patients with either resected or unresected cholangiocarcinoma[1]. Cholecystokinin and somatostatin receptors have been identified on tumours of the biliary tract. However, whether hormonal manipulations will be helpful in these patients is unknown. Multiple retrospective analyses have suggested that radiation therapy augments survival in patients with perihilar cholangiocarcinoma. However, in these reports patients receiving radiotherapy tend to have more favourable tumours and to be relatively fit compared with those not receiving radiotherapy. By contrast, in a prospective controlled, but not randomized, analysis from The Johns Hopkins Hospital radiation without concomitant chemotherapy had no effect on survival[4]. Thus, new agents or strategies to deliver adjuvant therapy are needed to improve survival in these patients.

References

1. Pitt HA, Dooley WC, Yeo CJ, Cameron JL. Malignancies of the biliary tree. *Curr Probl Surg* 1995; 32: 1–90.

2. Klatskin G. Adenocarcinoma of the hepatic duct at its bifurcation within the porta hepatis. An unusual tumor with distinctive clinical and pathological features. *Am J Med* 1965; 38: 241–56.

3. Little JM. A prospective evaluation of computerized estimates of risk in the management of obstructive jaundice. *Surgery* 1987; 102: 473–6.

4. Pitt HA, Nakeeb A, Abrams RA *et al.* Perihilar cholangiocarcinoma. Postoperative radiotherapy does not improve survival. *Ann Surg* 1995; 221: 788–98.

5. Nordback IH, Pitt HA, Coleman J *et al.* Unresectable hilar cholangiocarcinoma: percutaneous versus operative palliation. *Surgery* 1994; 115: 597–603.

6. Lai EC, Chu KM, Lo CY, Fan ST, Wong J. Choice of palliation for malignant hilar biliary obstruction. *Am J Surg* 1992; 163: 208–12.

Bile duct cancer: palliative surgery (segment III hepaticojejunostomy)

O. James Garden BSc, MD, FRCS(Ed), FRCS(Glas)
Senior Lecturer and Honorary Consultant Hepatobiliary Surgeon, University Department of Surgery and Scottish Liver Transplantation Unit, Royal Infirmary, Edinburgh, UK

History

In 1957 Soupault and Couinaud[1] described bypass of malignant hilar obstruction by anastomosis of a jejunal limb to the segment III duct to the left hemiliver. Palliation of cancer of the hepatic duct confluence and gallbladder was effective, despite achieving only unilateral drainage of the left duct, since the biliary anastomosis was undertaken at some distance from the tumour. The technique was further refined by Bismuth and Corlette[2] who described an intrahepatic approach within the plane of the falciform ligament. Recent experience with this technique has shown that it has a place in the management of obstructive jaundice and carries an acceptable morbidity and mortality[3-5].

Principles and justification

This technique is principally employed in patients found at operation to have irresectable hilar cholangiocarcinoma but can be used for gallbladder carcinoma, lymphomatous strictures or selected cases of benign stricture. Although improved imaging techniques have enabled better selection of patients for biliary-enteric bypass, percutaneous and endoscopic methods have been used increasingly to achieve biliary drainage and this has reduced the number of potential candidates for hepaticojejunostomy. Contraindications to hepatico-jejunostomy include infection of the right duct system in patients who have previously undergone attempts at non-surgical biliary drainage. Involvement of the left hemiliver by tumour or atrophy of the left hemiliver from tumour infiltration of its vascular supply or longstanding ductal obstruction renders patients unsuitable for segment III hepaticojejunostomy.

Preoperative

It is the author's practice to rely upon Doppler ultrasonography and computed tomographic (CT) scanning to evaluate hilar tumours and to avoid percutaneous transhepatic cholangiography since this risks contaminating a right duct system isolated from the left hemiliver by tumour involvement of the ductal confluence.

Preoperative preparation is standard for all patients with obstructive jaundice, paying particular attention to renal function, adequate intravenous hydration and antibiotic prophylaxis with a broad-spectrum cephalosporin. Any coagulopathy is corrected by administration of vitamin K and blood products as necessary. A nasogastric tube is passed following induction of general anaesthesia. The patient is carefully monitored peroperatively and arterial and central venous catheters are inserted in addition to a urinary catheter.

Operation

1 Access to the peritoneal cavity can be achieved by an upper midline incision but the author prefers to use a bilateral subcostal incision, extended to the xiphisternum if required.

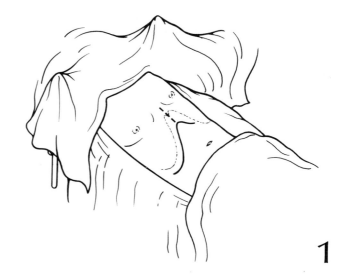

1

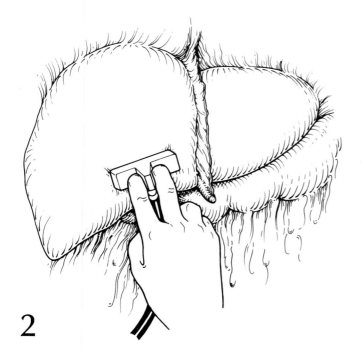

2

2 At laparotomy the hilar tumour is carefully evaluated. A thorough search is made of the abdominal cavity for peritoneal deposits and involved regional lymph nodes. The liver is carefully palpated to exclude metastatic deposits. Intraoperative ultrasonography is undertaken to confirm the absence of hepatic metastases and assess the precise level of obstruction of the biliary tree. Local invasion by tumour can be assessed and it is important to confirm that there is no involvement of the left branch of the portal vein or of the segmental biliary confluence in the left hemiliver. The segment III duct can be located precisely and the intended plane of dissection planned. Intraoperative ultrasonography can be employed during subsequent dissection to confirm the position of the segment III duct.

3 The ligamentum teres is divided between ties, one of which is secured with a haemostat to facilitate traction on the ligamentum teres and falciform ligament. The falciform ligament is divided using diathermy to maintain haemostasis. A pack is placed beneath the left lobe of the liver to protect the underlying stomach and spleen as the diathermy is used to incise the left triangular ligament which is held taut by the surgeon's retracting hand placed on the left lobe of the liver. This mobilization improves access to the icteric distended left liver.

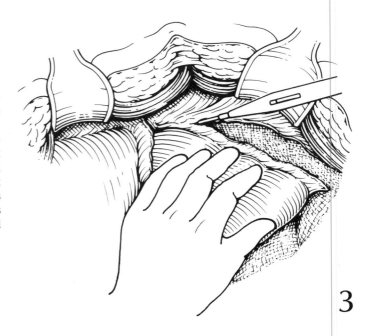

3

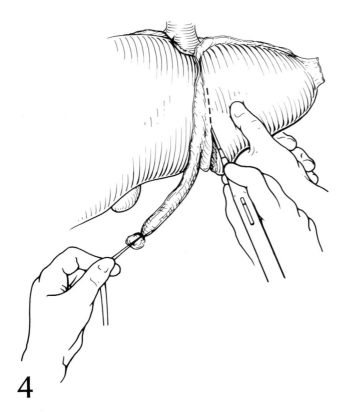

4

4 Any bridge of tissue between the quadrate (segment IV) and left lobes is divided to expose the base of the ligamentum teres. Any attempt to access the segment III duct by this approach risks injury and compromise to the blood supply to segment IV. The assistant grasps the left lobe of the liver with a loose pack and the surgeon or second assistant retracts the round ligament towards the patient's right. The capsule of the liver is incised with diathermy for a length of approximately 8 cm on its diaphragmatic surface, the incision running approximately 1 cm to the left of the falciform ligament.

5 The Cavitron ultrasonic surgical aspirator is employed to skeletonize any small vessels which can be divided following diathermy. Small dilated intrahepatic ductules are best ligated or clipped to avoid decompression of the ductal system. The dissection usually proceeds rapidly through the liver which, in the icteric patient, has a soft consistency. A subsegmental pedicle is often identified as the dissection proceeds down to the hilar plate and this generally requires division between ligatures. Dissection in this relatively avascular plane rarely results in substantial devascularization of the left lobe.

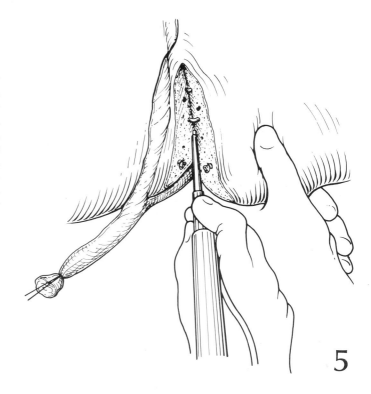

5

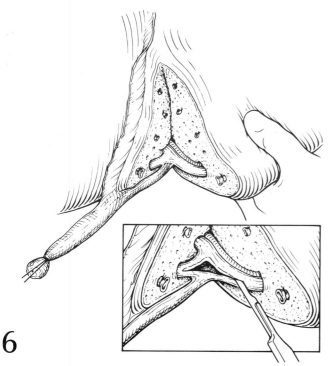

6

6 Once the hilar plate is reached, the distended segment III duct will be visible lying alongside the accompanying artery and above the segmental branch of the portal vein. A length of approximately 2–3 cm of duct can easily be exposed using the Cavitron aspirator which will trace out the confluence of the segmental ducts with the left hepatic duct.

A longitudinal incision is made in the segment III duct using a no. 15 blade (*see* inset) and a sample of bile is sent for culture. The duct can be explored with a fine malleable probe to confirm its position relative to the other segmental and left hepatic ducts. In this way, the incision can be safely extended.

7 A 70-cm Roux-en-Y limb of jejunum is then fashioned, restoring intestinal continuity with two layers of 4/0 polydioxanone (PDS) sutures. The limb of jejunum is generally passed through the transverse mesocolon to which it is secured with several interrupted 4/0 polydioxanone sutures. The limb of jejunum should reach the ducts without undue tension. The divided end of the jejunal limb is oversewn with 4/0 polydioxanone sutures.

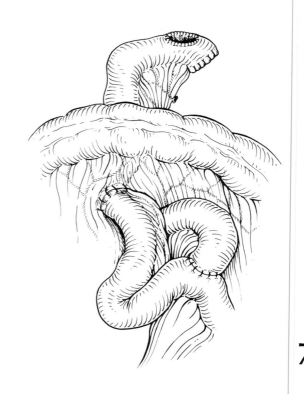

7

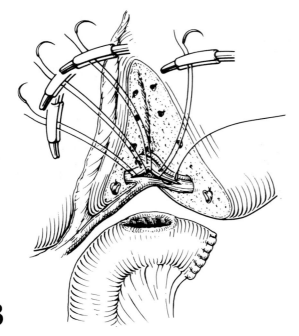

8

8 Avoiding the use of clamps, the jejunum is opened along its antimesenteric border for approximately 1 cm. A conventional biliary anastomosis is fashioned by placing 4/0 or 5/0 polydioxanone sutures in the anterior wall of the bile duct, holding these with shod clamps. The sutures are placed from left to right with the needles being passed from outside inwards to allow subsequent tying of knots outside the lumen.

9 Interrupted 4/0 polydioxanone sutures are now placed through the full thickness of the jejunum and the inferior wall of the opened bile duct and, once all are secured by shod clamps, the jejunal limb is railroaded into approximation with the liver and the duct. This posterior row of sutures is then tied with the knots on the mucosal side.

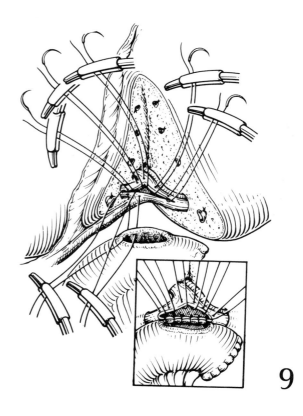

9

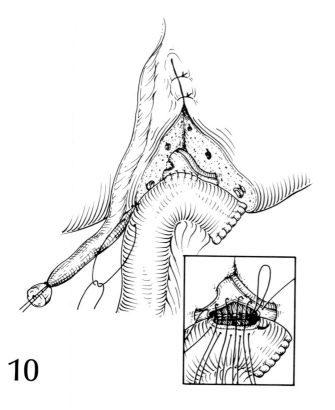

10

10 The anterior wall of jejunum is now picked up by the remaining sutures in the anterior wall of the bile duct. These sutures are then tied with the knots secured on the serosa. A stenting drain is not employed, although the author secures the jejunum to the liver capsule and/or falciform ligament with several interrupted sutures. The hepatotomy can be partially closed with several interrupted capsular sutures.

11 A single tube drain is placed down to the anastomosis and brought out through a separate stab incision before closure of the wound in layers using loop polydioxanone to muscle and staples to the skin.

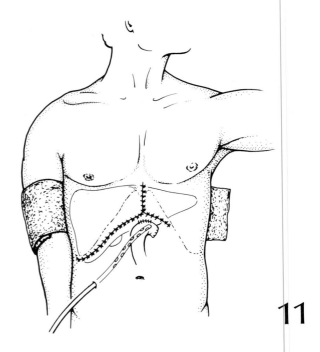

11

Postoperative care

The patient is nursed in a high dependency unit with regular haemodynamic monitoring and assessment of urinary output. Prophylactic antibiotics are generally not continued beyond 24 h, but all patients are commenced on an H_2 receptor antagonist to minimize the risk of stress ulceration in the postoperative period. The nasogastric tube is removed within 48 h and fluids and diet are introduced gradually thereafter.

Complications

Hepatorenal failure is the main cause of operative mortality and resolution of jaundice will normally occur within 3 weeks of surgery, despite involvement of the hepatic duct confluence. Recurrent biliary sepsis without jaundice may complicate this procedure when previous percutaneous or endoscopic intubation of the right duct system has been attempted or undertaken.

Outcome

In the author's institution less than 20% of patients presenting with malignant obstruction at the liver hilum are suitable candidates for segment III bypass. However, jaundice resolves in 90% of patients and the quality of palliation is excellent.

References

1. Soupault R, Couinaud C. Sur un procédé nouveau de dérivation biliare intra-hépatique: les cholangio-jéjunostomies gauches sans sacrifice héatique. *Presse Med* 1957; 65: 1157–9.

2. Bismuth H, Corlette MB. Intrahepatic cholangioenteric anastomosis in carcinoma of the hilus of the liver. *Surg Gynecol Obstet* 1975; 140: 170–8.

3. Bismuth H, Castaing D, Traynor O. Resection or palliation: priority of surgery in the treatment of hilar cancer. *World J Surg* 1988; 12: 39–47.

4. Guthrie CM, Haddock G, de Beaux AC, Garden OJ, Carter DC. Changing trends in the management of extrahepatic cholangiocarcinoma. *Br J Surg* 1993; 80: 1434–9.

5. Guthrie CM, Banting SW, Garden OJ, Carter DC. Segment III cholangiojejunostomy for palliation of malignant hilar obstruction. *Br J Surg* 1994; 81: 1639–41.

Bile duct cancer: resection

O. James Garden BSc, MD, FRCS(Ed), FRCS(Glas)
Senior Lecturer and Honorary Consultant Hepatobiliary Surgeon, University Department of Surgery and Scottish Liver Transplantation Unit, Royal Infirmary, Edinburgh, UK

Henri Bismuth MD, FACS, FRCS(Ed)
Professor of Surgery and Chairman of the Hepatobiliary Centre, Paul Brousse Hospital, Villejuif, France

Tumours involving the bile ducts pose a considerable challenge in biliary surgery. They may involve the ducts primarily or by extension from the liver, gallbladder, pancreas, the ampulla, duodenum or adjacent lymph nodes. Primary tumours of the biliary tract involving the gallbladder, ampulla and pancreas are dealt with elsewhere in this volume and this chapter is concerned only with cholangiocarcinoma involving the supraduodenal portion of the biliary tree up to and involving the confluence of the hepatic ducts. Early descriptions of bile duct tumours highlighted the difficulties of diagnosis and management given that these tumours characteristically invade locally with vascular, perineural and lymphatic involvement[1-3]. Subepithelial spread of tumour cells is of special importance in their management, and multiple lesions may arise from field change[4]. Although an increasingly aggressive approach to management has been advocated, only a minority of patients have potentially resectable disease at the time of presentation and 5-year survival following resection rarely exceeds 25%[5-7].

Principles and justification

Resection of the bile duct tumour has been shown to be the most effective way of achieving satisfactory long-term decompression of the biliary tree and clearly offers the only prospect of long-term survival. The pathological characteristics of this tumour and the absence of satisfactory imaging modalities to determine resectability may frustrate the surgeon, but mounting evidence now exists suggesting that resection can be undertaken with relatively low morbidity and mortality rates. Several studies have reported improved quality of life in patients who undergo tumour resection compared with those who have a biliary-enteric anastomosis[5,7]. The potential for improved quality of life and the long-term survival advantage require that patients who might benefit from resection be carefully identified.

The type of resection depends on the extent of the tumour within the biliary tree and its vascular involvement. For tumours that extend behind the duodenum to the pancreas, excision of the biliary tree with pancreaticoduodenectomy will be required. For lesions that extend into either the right or left duct, hepatic resection will be necessary. For the remaining tumours, wide excision of the entire supraduodenal biliary tree, cystic duct, gallbladder and related lymph nodes should be undertaken.

Preoperative

Confirmation of obstruction of the biliary tree will normally be achieved by abdominal ultrasonography. This investigation may localize accurately the level of obstruction, or this information can be inferred from the presence or absence of gallbladder distension. Advances in Doppler ultrasound imaging have enabled more accurate assessment of bile duct tumours, including the degree of vascular invasion. In many centres, endoscopic retrograde cholangiography will be undertaken to determine the nature of the obstruction, but this procedure rarely provides sufficient information about ductal involvement above the tumour. Percutaneous transhepatic cholangiography will overcome these deficiencies but, by introducing infection into the obstructed biliary tree, may compromise subsequent management if resection is not feasible.

1a–c Contrast enhanced computed tomographic (CT) scanning and nuclear magnetic resonance (NMR) imaging may allow detailed assessment of the biliary tree and tumour by non-invasive means. The CT scan shown in *Illustration 1a* demonstrates dilatation of the intrahepatic biliary tree which is more pronounced in the left hemiliver. A mass lesion is evident, predominantly involving the left hepatic duct and clearly obstructing the caudate ducts (arrowed). Long-standing obstruction above the confluence of the left and right hepatic ducts or associated vascular invasion may result in atrophy of one side of the liver. Selective hepatic arteriography with portal venous phase imaging is helpful in detecting vascular anomalies and tumour invasion. The mesenteric angiogram shown in *Illustration 1b* demonstrates an aberrant proper hepatic artery arising from the superior mesenteric artery. There is poor filling of the left hepatic artery, thought to be due to infiltration from a hilar cholangiocarcinoma which has been previously stented. The portovenous phase radiograph shown in *Illustration 1c* demonstrates tumour invasion of the left branch of the portal vein (arrowed).

These investigations indicate irresectability if there is: (1) multifocal or bilateral intrahepatic bile duct spread of tumour, (2) involvement of the portal vein, (3) bilateral invasion of the hepatic arterial and/or portal venous branches, or (4) evidence of unilateral vascular involvement with extensive contralateral invasion.

Although these criteria provide a useful guide to the radiologist and surgeon, it may be difficult to establish whether there is peritoneal dissemination of tumour, lymph node invasion or local extension into hepatic segment I. Laparoscopy and laparoscopic ultrasonography may be helpful in detecting such occult spread, but in the otherwise fit patient it may be more appropriate to contemplate operative decompression of the biliary tree rather than rely on endoscopic or percutaneous stent insertion. Furthermore, it should be borne in mind that submucosal, perineural and lymphatic spread of tumour may not be apparent before resection is attempted. Although frozen section biopsy of the bile duct may be used at the time of resection, it is unlikely that the surgeon would be able to undertake a more radical resection than that already being proposed.

Immediate preoperative assessment and preparation includes attention to the jaundiced patient's hydration and renal function, control of infection and assessment of coagulation status. The authors' practice is to undertake surgery under general anaesthesia with epidural blockade. Continuous monitoring is undertaken following placement of arterial, central venous pressure and urinary catheters.

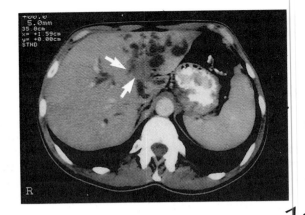

1a

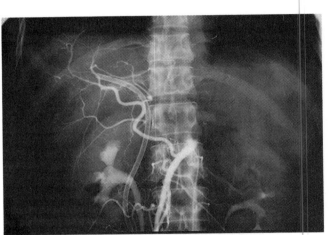

1b

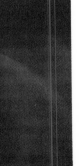

1c

Operation

2 The patient is positioned on the operating table with the right arm held beside the body by a folded towel and with the left arm extended. The abdomen is explored through a bilateral subcostal incision extended to the xiphisternum if necessary. Retraction of the costal margins is achieved by means of two large subcostal retractors secured by tapes to draped posts.

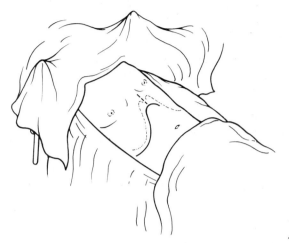

2

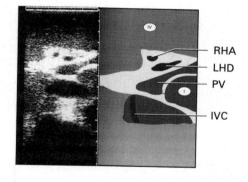

3a

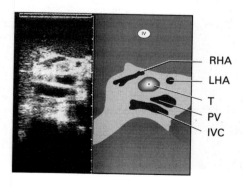

3b

3a,b The peritoneal cavity is examined to exclude peritoneal tumour deposits and hepatic and nodal metastases. Intraoperative ultrasonography is undertaken to confirm the absence of hepatic dissemination of tumour and to assess the precise level of obstruction. Vascular anomalies and invasion can also be assessed in this way. The scan depicted shows the right hepatic artery (RHA) arching over a tumour involving the common hepatic duct just below the confluence of the right and left hepatic ducts (LHD). The left hepatic artery (LHA) is visible and the portal vein (PV) and inferior vena cava (IVC) are shown posteriorly. No evidence of vascular invasion is present.

Tumours at or below the hepatic confluence

Skeletonization of the biliary tree and lymphatics from the vessels is best achieved by commencing the dissection at the level of the first part of the duodenum. When preoperative investigations and operative assessment have confirmed that it is not necessary to sacrifice liver tissue, it is necessary to free the tumour above by taking down the gallbladder, lowering the hilar plate and freeing the base of the umbilical fissure.

The ligamentum teres is divided between ties, one of which is retained on the ligament to aid exposure of the hilus of the liver. The falciform ligament is divided with diathermy towards the vena cava, but the liver is not freed from its remaining peritoneal attachments.

4 With the liver retracted upwards and with the antrum of the stomach and first part of the duodenum displaced downwards, the peritoneum at the level of the first part of the duodenum is incised towards the free edge of the lesser omentum. In some patients it may be necessary to mobilize the second part of the duodenum and to free the hepatic flexure of the colon to gain adequate exposure behind the first part of the duodenum. Lymphatic and other vessels are divided (between ties or following diathermy) down to the common bile duct as it passes through or behind the head of the pancreas. A careful search is made for an accessory hepatic artery in the free edge of the lesser omentum as the dissection is carried posteroinferiorly to the exposed portal vein. Care should be taken to avoid damage to the pancreas at this level. The dissection is continued medially towards the gastroduodenal vessel which is skeletonized of its lymphatics as one moves towards the proper hepatic artery.

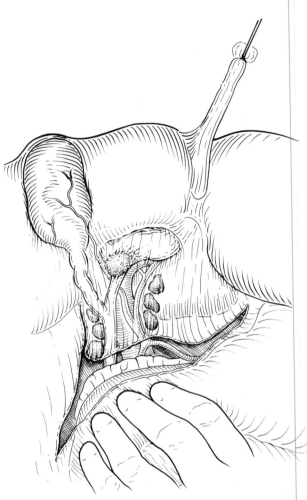

4

5 The common bile duct is freed from the underlying structures and secured above with a stout ligature, before being divided just above the pancreas. Bleeding from the two marginal arteries is controlled by suture ligation. The divided end of the bile duct is oversewn with continuous 4/0 polydioxanone (PDS). If the patient has previously been stented, to avoid delivering the intact stent through the divided duct it is transected with a pair of heavy scissors, delivering the lower end through the divided bile duct and displacing the upper end into the common bile duct, the lower end of which is ligated. In this way, contamination of the operating field by tumour cells is minimized.

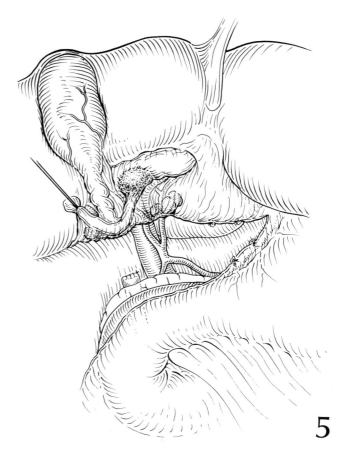

5

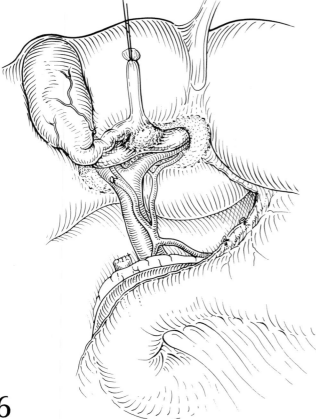

6

6 With the portal vein now exposed, the lymphatics can be cleared upwards and medially. The common and proper hepatic arteries are cleared of their associated lymph nodes as these are swept from the lesser omentum and upwards to the hilus of the liver.

7   The gallbladder is then dissected free from the liver using diathermy and retracted downwards to expose the cystic artery and the right branch of the portal vein behind. The cystic artery is divided between ties and this allows the lymphatics on the free edge of the lesser omentum to be swept from the right hepatic duct and right hepatic artery. The resected duct should now be entirely free of the skeletonized vessels posteriorly.

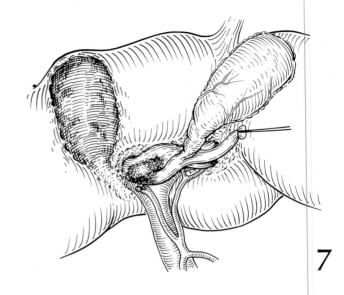

7

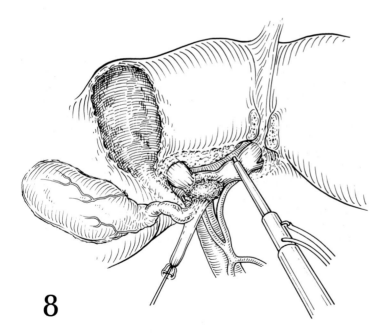

8

8   If a bridge of liver tissue is present between the quadrate and left lobes of the liver, its capsule is opened using diathermy coagulation. The Cavitron ultrasonic dissector can be used to skeletonize any intrahepatic vessels before they are coagulated and divided. By retracting the ligamentum teres upwards, the undersurface of the quadrate lobe of the liver is exposed. The peritoneum above the hepatic duct confluence is incised with diathermy and the hilar plate is lowered using the Cavitron dissector. In this way, the entire extrahepatic biliary tree and its associated lymphatics are freed from the portal vein and hepatic artery.

9 The left hepatic duct is divided as far proximally as possible, and the tumour and ductal confluence are displaced to the right to ascertain whether the main right hepatic duct can be divided or whether these should be divided at the level of the right sectoral ducts. A separate duct invariably drains the caudate lobe, and this and other adjacent ducts can be sutured together to create one or two separate orifices for anastomosis. The ducts should only be opposed without tension, and three or four interrupted 4/0 polydioxanone sutures will usually suffice.

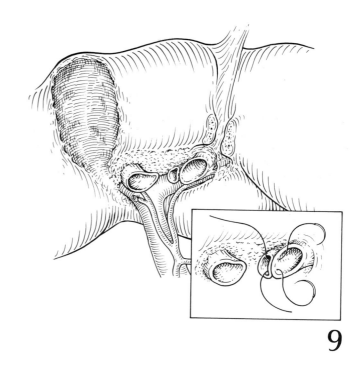

9

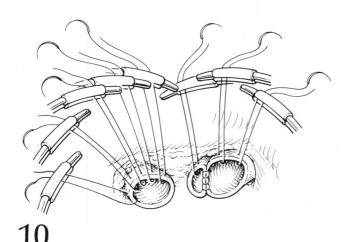

10

10 A 70-cm Roux-en-Y limb of jejunum is prepared, intestinal continuity being restored in two layers of continuous 3/0 polydioxanone sutures. The Roux-en-Y limb is delivered through the transverse mesocolon to which it is secured with several interrupted sutures. There should be no tension in the limb as it is drawn up to the hilus of the liver.

A hepaticojejunal anastomosis is undertaken in an end-to-side fashion between the ducts and the anti-mesenteric border of the jejunal limb. A conventional biliary anastomosis is undertaken, placing a single layer of 3/0 or 4/0 interrupted polydioxanone sutures into the anterior wall of the bile duct, passing the sutures from outside in. The needles are retained on shod clamps.

11   Although more than one biliary orifice may be present, it is preferable to undertake the anastomosis as if there was only one orifice. The anterior row of sutures is placed under tension and this enables precise placement of the posterior layer of sutures which are introduced from inside to outside on the jejunum and from outside to inside on the bile duct. The sutures are placed approximately 3 mm apart and secured with clamps. The jejunal limb is then 'railroaded' to the bile duct and the posterior layer of sutures is tied on the inside. The two corner sutures are retained on shod clamps while the others are cut.

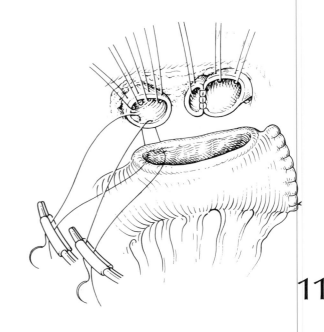

11

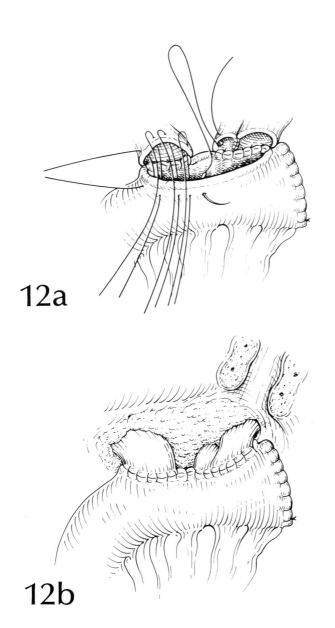

12a

12b

12a,b   The anterior layer of anastomosis is now completed by passing the needles through the jejunal wall from the mucosal side outwards. Once the sutures have been placed, the stay sutures are cut and the anterior layer of sutures tied with the knots lying anteriorly. A transanastomotic stenting tube is not normally necessary.

Once haemostasis has been confirmed, a 24-Fr silicone tube drain is passed through a separate stab incision down to the anastomosis. The wound is closed in layers using looped polydioxanone to muscle and skin staples.

Excision of bile duct tumour and hepatic resection

For tumours which unilaterally invade the secondary biliary confluence or the vessels supplying one side of the liver, it is necessary to undertake a hepatic resection employing the techniques described above and in the chapter on pp. 30–45.

13 The initial dissection of the bile duct and tumour proceeds as described above. For a tumour predominantly affecting the left hepatic duct or vessels supplying the left liver, the left hepatic artery is divided between silk ligatures at its origin and swept upwards along with the adventitial and lymphatic tissue. In this way, the portal vein and its right and left branches are identified as they enter the liver. The left branch of the portal vein is secured between clamps at its origin. Care must be taken not to traumatize any caudate branches passing posteriorly, although the left hepatectomy will normally include excision of the caudate lobe.

The falciform and the left triangular ligaments are divided and the lesser omentum is freed from the lesser curve of the stomach. As the caudate lobe is freed from the vena cava, the line of demarcation between the left and right hemilivers will be evident.

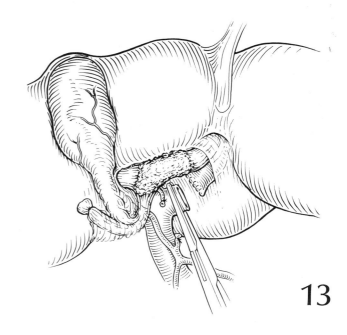

13

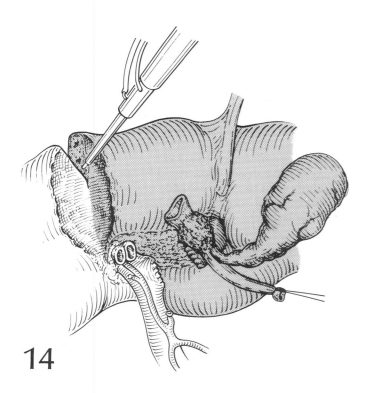

14

14 The right hepatic duct or sectoral ducts are divided well clear of the tumour, and the capsule of the liver is incised approximately 5 mm to the patient's left of the line of demarcation. The dissection into the liver is undertaken with the Cavitron dissector, skeletonizing small vessels and dividing these between ligatures. The middle hepatic vein is preserved on the right hemiliver as the dissection proceeds posteriorly and upwards. The vena cava is reached to the right of the caudate lobe.

The left hepatic vein is cleared and secured with a vascular clamp before being divided. Once the specimen is delivered from the wound, the left hepatic vein and left branch of the portal vein are oversewn using continuous 5/0 polypropylene (Prolene).

Haemostatis is secured and, if necessary, the anterior and posterior sectoral ducts are opposed with several interrupted polydioxanone sutures. The biliary anastomosis is fashioned to a 70-cm Roux-en-Y limb of jejunum as previously described.

Postoperative care and outcome

The principal source of morbidity following surgery in the jaundiced patient is the result of the development of hepatorenal failure and sepsis. A better understanding and use of prophylactic measures in the preoperative period have greatly reduced these risks. Preoperative biliary drainage remains a contentious issue and is addressed elsewhere. Peptic ulceration can develop in up to 5% of patients following Roux-en-Y hepatico-jejunostomy but, again, this risk is greatly minimized by the prophylactic administration of H_2 receptor antagonists. Most recent series report operative mortality rates of less than 5% with a 5-year survival of 5–20%.

References

1. Klatskin G. Adenocarcinoma of the hepatic duct at its bifurcation within the porta hepatis: an unusual tumour with distinctive clinical and pathological features. *Am J Med* 1965; 38: 241–56.

2. Altemeier WA, Gall EA, Culbertson WR, Inge WW Sclerosing carcinoma of the intrahepatic (hilar) bile ducts. *Surgery* 1966; 60: 191–200.

3. Longmire WP Jr, MacArthur MS, Bastounis EA, Hiatt J. Carcinoma of the extrahepatic biliary tract. *Ann Surg* 1973; 178: 333–45.

4. Gertsch P, Thomas P, Baer H, Lerut J, Zimmerman A, Blumgart LH. Multiple tumours of the biliary tract. *Am J Surg* 1990; 158: 386–8.

5. Baer HU, Stain SC, Dennison AR, Eggers B, Blumgart LH. Improvements in survival by aggressive resection of hilar cholangiocarcinoma. *Ann Surg* 1993; 217: 20–7.

6. Cameron JL, Pitt HA, Zinner MJ, Kaufman SL, Coleman J. Management of proximal cholangiocarcinomas by surgical resection and radiotherapy. *Am J Surg* 1990; 159: 91–8.

7. Guthrie CM, Haddock G, de Beaux AC, Garden OJ, Carter DC. Changing trends in the management of extrahepatic cholangiocarcinoma. *Br J Surg* 1993; 80: 1434–9.

Surgical anatomy of the pancreas

David C. Carter MD, FRCS(Ed), FRCS(Glas), FRCS, FRSE
Regius Professor of Clinical Surgery, Royal Infirmary, Edinburgh, UK

R. C. G. Russell MS, FRCS
Consultant Surgeon, The Middlesex Hospital, London, UK

Development of the pancreas

1 The pancreas forms from a dorsal and ventral anlage. Rotation of the ventral pancreas brings it into contact with the dorsal anlage early in embryonic life, the ventral pancreas coming to lie behind the primitive superior mesenteric vessels. The two anlagen and their respective draining duct systems merge as the right leaf of the dorsal mesentery of the pancreas fuses with the posterior abdominal wall, and the pancreas and duodenum take up their definitive retroperitoneal position. The avascular plane (fascia of Treitz) interposed between the posterior surface of the pancreas and the posterior abdominal wall is the plane entered during the Kocher manoeuvre used to mobilize the duodenum and head of pancreas.

The dorsal anlage forms the cranial part of the head of the gland, the body and the tail, while the ventral anlage forms the rest of the head and the uncinate process. The duct running in the dorsal pancreas normally passes downwards to fuse with the duct draining the ventral anlage (duct of Wirsung) and drain into the second part of the duodenum at the papilla of Vater. The proximal portion of the duct draining the dorsal pancreas (duct of Santorini) normally drains into the duodenum via the minor papilla but it may drain retrogradely into the duct of Wirsung or degenerate completely. If a minor papilla is present it is usually located some 2 cm proximal to the major papilla. Smaller unnamed pancreatic ducts may enter the duodenum or bile duct directly and are a potential cause of biliary or duodenal leakage after duodenum-preserving pancreatectomy.

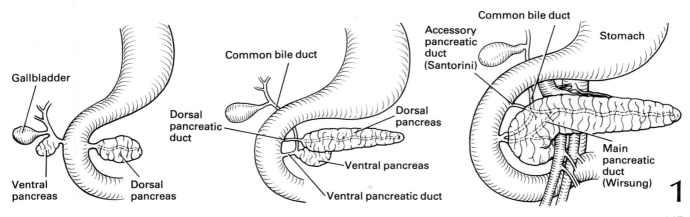

Uncommon congenital abnormalities of development of the pancreas include aplasia, annular pancreas (in which pancreatic tissue may encircle the second part of the duodenum or invade its wall), and pancreatic heterotopia (in which ectopic pancreatic tissue is found in the duodenal wall, or in less common locations such as the mesentery, omentum, colon or appendix). Failure of fusion of the duct systems of the dorsal and ventral pancreas affects approximately 10% of individuals, and although known as pancreas divisum, it is important to appreciate that there is no division of the pancreatic parenchyma. It is debatable whether pancreas divisum gives rise to pancreatitis; the anomaly is common and in the great majority of affected individuals it is discovered as an incidental finding at ERCP. In a few cases it is conceivable that problems arise because the pancreatic juice produced by the larger dorsal pancreas has to drain through the small minor papilla.

The common bile duct may be partially covered by pancreatic tissue posteriorly, or less commonly it is completely embedded in the pancreas or runs outwith and behind the pancreas on its way to enter the duodenum. In 85% of individuals the bile duct and main pancreatic duct form a common channel before emptying into the duodenum on the tip of the papilla of Vater. It is unusual for there to be ampullary dilatation at the junction of the ducts despite the frequent use of the term 'ampulla of Vater'. In a minority of subjects the two ducts have separate openings. The terminations of the common bile duct and main pancreatic duct are encircled by sphincters of smooth muscle which fuse to form the sphincter of Oddi. This sphincter varies in length between 5 and 30 mm and so may extend outwith the wall of the duodenum. When dividing the sphincter (endoscopically or surgically), division is commenced anterolaterally and the sphincterotomy should not extend in length beyond 10 mm so as to avoid injury to the pancreas.

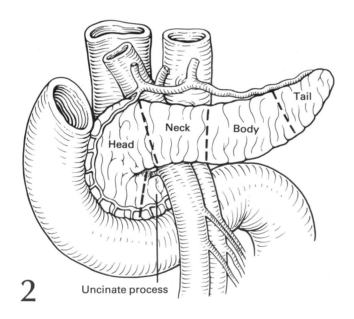

2

Uncinate process

Tail

Neck   Body

Head

Surgical anatomy of the pancreas

2   The head of the pancreas lies within the curve of the first three parts of the duodenum and the gland extends transversely and upwards from the right of the second lumbar vertebra to the splenic hilum at the level of the 12th thoracic vertebra. The gland has no distinct capsule although parts of its anterior surface are covered by the posterior layer of the peritoneum of the lesser sac. The lack of a capsule makes the normal pancreas friable and difficult to suture whereas a chronically inflamed pancreas contains large amounts of fibrous tissue and holds sutures well.

The head of the pancreas is firmly adherent to the second and third parts of the duodenum, with which it shares a blood supply, and merges with the neck of the gland along an arbitrary line marked by the gastro-duodenal artery above and anteriorly, and by the superior mesenteric vein/portal vein behind. The uncinate process extends downwards and backwards from the inferior margin of the head and passes behind the superior mesenteric vein (and in some cases behind the superior mesenteric artery as well). There are usually small veins which run directly from the anterior aspect of the uncinate process into the right side of the superior mesenteric vein; although small, these veins can give rise to troublesome haemorrhage during pancreatectomy and must be individually ligated and divided.

3 The proximal duodenum and head of pancreas are mobilized by division of the lateral leaf of the peritoneum which binds them to the retroperitoneum, the Kocher manoeuvre. Access is improved greatly if the hepatic flexure of the colon is mobilized downwards after extending the incision in the peritoneum down the lateral aspect of the ascending colon. Vessels running within the peritoneal leaf are dealt with by diathermy coagulation or individual ligation. Mobilization of the head of the pancreas exposes the hilum of the right kidney, the right renal vessels, the right gonadal vein and the inferior vena cava, and the mobilization is normally extended to expose the right anterior aspect of the aorta.

The neck of the pancreas is that part of the gland which lies in front of the superior mesenteric vein/portal vein and the superior mesenteric artery. The coeliac axis lies above it and the common hepatic artery and splenic artery run along the upper border of the neck from their origins. The splenic vein and superior mesenteric vein normally join behind the neck of the pancreas to form the portal vein, and the pancreas does not normally send venous tributaries to the anterior aspect of the superior mesenteric vein or portal vein as they pass in the tunnel behind the neck of the pancreas.

The body of the pancreas commences to the left of the superior mesenteric artery. It is triangular in cross section and has broad anterior and posterior surfaces and a narrow inferior surface. The splenic vein is embedded in the body of the pancreas posteriorly and receives tributaries directly from it, while the splenic artery runs a tortuous course along its upper border. The body of the gland terminates in the short tail which is more mobile and passes forwards to end in the splenic hilum. The essentially avascular plane behind the body and tail of the pancreas enables this part of the gland to be lifted forwards (with the splenic vessels) from the aorta, diaphragm, left adrenal gland, left renal vessels and upper part of the left kidney. When performing this manoeuvre, care must be taken not to injure the friable left adrenal gland.

The anterior surface of the head of the pancreas is normally overlain by the first part of the duodenum and pylorus above, and by the transverse colon below. The transverse mesocolon is very short or almost non-existent in front of the head of the gland, but is much longer in front of the neck and body. As one passes to the left, the transverse mesocolon is attached to the

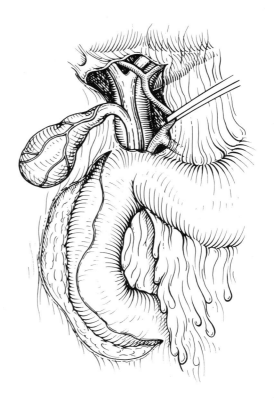

3

inferior border of the pancreas, and provided care is taken not to damage the middle colic artery (which runs within the leaves of the mesocolon), the body of the pancreas can be approached from below by opening an avascular window in the mesocolon. This approach may be useful when performing a blunt necrosectomy in patients with necrotizing pancreatitis, but access to the neck, body and tail is more usually provided by wide division of the gastrocolic omentum with ligation and division of its contained vessels. Numerous avascular adhesions bind the front of the pancreas to the back of the stomach, and must be divided to give full access to the gland.

Blood supply to the pancreas

The blood supply to the pancreas is derived from both the coeliac axis and the superior mesenteric artery. There are plentiful collateral pathways so that, during pancreatic resection, the incised gland bleeds profusely until the last arterial source of supply has been divided.

4 The head and uncinate process are supplied from above by the gastroduodenal artery which divides into anterior and posterior superior pancreaticoduodenal arteries before reaching the gland. These vessels pass downwards with the curve of the second and third parts of the duodenum, and anastomose with the anterior and posterior branches of the inferior pancreaticoduodenal branch of the superior mesenteric artery. This last vessel is often short and, in the final stages of the Whipple operation, undue lateral tension on the resection specimen can pull the superior mesenteric artery out from behind the superior mesenteric vein and into jeopardy. The pancreaticoduodenal arcades formed on the anterior and posterior aspects of the head of the pancreas also provide a plentiful supply of blood to the duodenum. Despite this shared blood supply, it is now recognized that the duodenum can be preserved after division of the pancreaticoduodenal arteries in the operation of duodenum-preserving total pancreatectomy (*see* pp. 551–556).

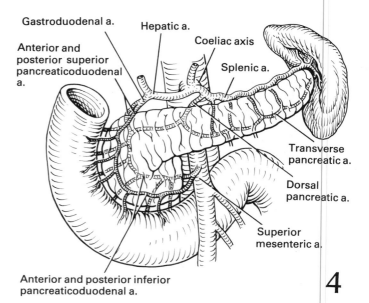

Gastroduodenal a.
Hepatic a.
Coeliac axis
Anterior and posterior superior pancreaticoduodenal a.
Splenic a.
Transverse pancreatic a.
Dorsal pancreatic a.
Superior mesenteric a.
Anterior and posterior inferior pancreaticoduodenal a.

4

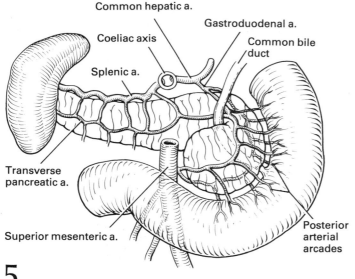

Common hepatic a.
Coeliac axis
Gastroduodenal a.
Splenic a.
Common bile duct
Transverse pancreatic a.
Superior mesenteric a.
Posterior arterial arcades

5

5 The body and tail of the pancreas are supplied by the splenic artery as it courses along their upper border. The dorsal pancreatic artery is a significant named branch which arises close to the origin of the splenic artery and, in addition to supplying the body and tail of the pancreas from behind, it gives branches to the back of the head and uncinate process.

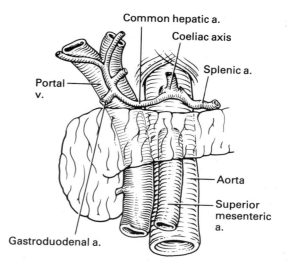

Common hepatic a.
Coeliac axis
Splenic a.
Portal v.
Aorta
Superior mesenteric a.
Gastroduodenal a.

6a

6a–c

Arterial anomalies which affect pancreatic surgery are present in about one in three individuals. The most common significant variant consists of an anomalous hepatic arterial supply in which the right hepatic artery (25% of subjects) or common hepatic artery (5% of subjects) arises from the superior mesenteric artery and courses upwards behind the head or neck of the pancreas. This anomaly should be suspected whenever arterial pulsation is felt behind or to the right of the common bile duct and common hepatic duct and, once recognized, seldom poses undue problems during pancreatic resection. In exceptional cases, the aberrant vessel passes through the head of the pancreas and can cause problems during resection. Variations in the anatomy of the pancreaticoduodenal arcades are also relatively common; the arcades may be doubled or even tripled, the superior pancreaticoduodenal artery may arise from the right gastric artery, or the superior and inferior pancreaticoduodenal vessels may both arise from an aberrant right hepatic artery.

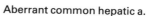

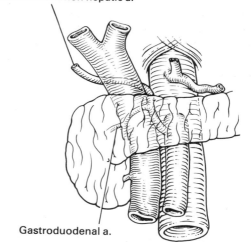

Aberrant common hepatic a.

Gastroduodenal a.

6b

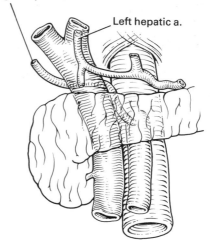

Aberrant right hepatic a.
Left hepatic a.

6c

7 The veins draining the pancreas generally run in parallel to the arteries but drain into the splenic, superior mesenteric and portal veins. The anterior superior pancreaticoduodenal vein requires careful division early in the course of a Whipple resection as it runs down to join the superior mesenteric vein just below the neck of the pancreas. This vessel is often joined to the right gastroepiploic vein. The posterior superior pancreaticoduodenal vein is usually a substantial vein which leaves the upper border of the head of the pancreas to run directly into the portal vein. The inferior pancreaticoduodenal veins often merge to form a single substantial short trunk which drains to the superior mesenteric vein behind the uncinate process, and this can give rise to troublesome bleeding in the later stages of pancreatic resection. As mentioned earlier, a number of small veins running directly from the front of the uncinate process to the superior mesenteric vein require careful ligation during pancreatic resection.

The inferior mesenteric vein is usually described as entering the splenic vein near its termination, but in up to one-third of cases it enters the confluence of the splenic and superior mesenteric veins, and in a further one-third it enters the superior mesenteric vein. The left gastric or coronary vein also enters the splenic vein near its junction with the superior mesenteric vein and should be preserved during pancreaticoduodenectomy as the major venous effluent from the gastric remnant.

Uncommon anomalies of the portal vein include drainage into the superior vena cava, involvement of the portal venous system in total anomalous pulmonary venous drainage, and a portal vein which runs anterior to the duodenum. Congenital stricture, cavernous transformation and acquired thrombosis of the portal vein and its major tributaries may result in troublesome development of venous collaterals.

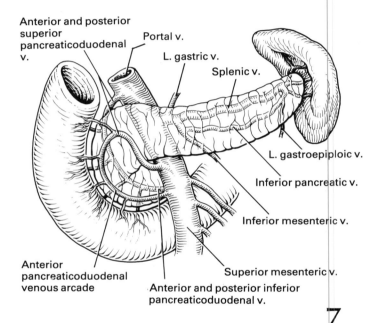

7

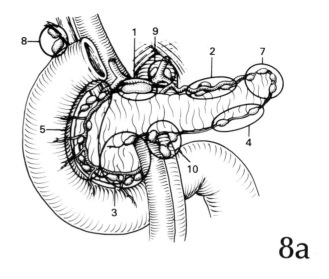

8a

Lymphatic drainage of the pancreas

8a–c The pancreas has a profuse network of lymphatics which drain to a large number of peripancreatic and retroperitoneal lymph nodes. There may be as many as 150 nodes and these have been classified into 11 groups – namely: (1) superior head, (2) superior body, (3) inferior head, (4) inferior body, (5) anterior pancreaticoduodenal, (6) posterior pancreaticoduodenal, (7) splenic, (8) portal, (9) coeliac, (10) mesenteric and (11) para-aortic. Japanese workers have attached particular significance recently to para-aortic nodes lying between the aorta and inferior vena cava, and there is ongoing debate about whether extending the radicality of resection for pancreatic cancer to include removal of such peripancreatic nodes can improve prospects for survival.

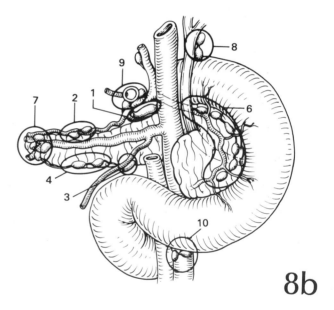

8b

Nerve supply to the pancreas

Painful stimuli are transmitted from the pancreas by sympathetic nerve fibres which travel alongside the arteries supplying the pancreas (common hepatic, splenic and superior mesenteric) to reach the coeliac ganglion. Thereafter, impulses travel in the greater and lesser splanchnic nerves to reach segments T5–10 of the thoracic spinal cord.

Further reading

Deki H, Sato T. An anatomic study of the peripancreatic lymphatics. *Surg Radiol Anat* 1988; 10: 121–35.

Michels NA. *Blood Supply and Anatomy of the Upper Abdominal Organs with a Descriptive Atlas*. Philadelphia: JB Lippincott, 1955.

Skandalakis JE, Gray SW, Skandalakis LJ. Surgical anatomy of the pancreas. In: Howard JM, Jordan GL Jr, Reber HA, eds. *Surgical Diseases of the Pancreas*. Philadelphia: Lea and Febiger, 1987: 11–36.

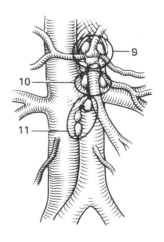

8c

Acute pancreatitis: gallstone pancreatitis

David C. Carter MD, FRCS(Ed), FRCS(Glas), FRCS, FRSE
Regius Professor of Clinical Surgery, Royal Infirmary, Edinburgh, UK

Principles and justification

Gallstones are the commonest cause of acute pancreatitis in the majority of reported series and currently account for at least 50% of cases. The incidence in some countries appears to be increasing[1], due largely to an increased number of cases of gallstone pancreatitis in older women, and it is now appreciated that particulate matter (granules of calcium bilirubinate and cholesterol crystals) in 'biliary sludge' may also trigger pancreatitis[2]. It is probable that many patients once labelled as having had idiopathic pancreatitis in fact had pancreatitis due to gallstones which had passed or which were too small to be detected readily.

Not every patient with gallstones will develop acute pancreatitis; the stones must pass into the common bile duct and impact, usually transiently, at the papilla of Vater. Indeed only 6–8% of patients with symptomatic stones develop pancreatitis, although the proportion may be as high as 20–30% in those with microlithiasis and cholesterosis[3].

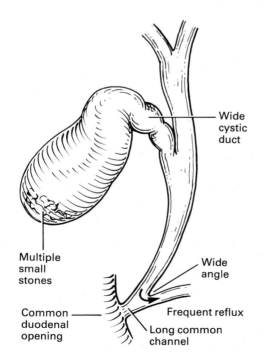

Wide cystic duct

Multiple small stones

Common duodenal opening

Wide angle

Frequent reflux

Long common channel

1 Factors known to be associated with an increased risk of developing acute pancreatitis are a gallbladder containing multiple small stones, a relatively wide cystic duct, a wide angle between the common bile duct and the main pancreatic duct, and a long common channel between the bile duct and pancreatic duct with a common opening into the duodenum.

When cholangiography is performed, patients who have had gallstone pancreatitis show reflux of contrast medium from the bile duct into the pancreatic duct in 50–67% of cases, whereas patients with gallstones who have not had pancreatitis only show reflux in 10–20% of cases.

1

Management of gallstone pancreatitis

There is general agreement that the prognosis in terms of recurrent attacks of pancreatitis is excellent if the gallbladder is removed once the acute attack of pancreatitis has settled and the biliary duct system has been cleared or shown to be free from stones. The urgent problems following admission to hospital are the need to establish that gallstones are indeed responsible for the attack, and then to deal appropriately with the minority of patients (about 20%) who do not settle promptly on conservative management and who may go on to develop potentially lethal necrotizing pancreatitis and its complications. Prognostic factor scoring systems such as those first proposed by Ranson in New York and Imrie in Glasgow are a useful means of identifying patients with severe disease who are more likely to develop complications, require surgical intervention, and succumb; as a general rule, one in four patients will have severe disease using these criteria and, of these, one in four will die.

Detection of gallstones

An algorithm for the investigation of patients with gallstone pancreatitis is shown in *Figure 1*.

Clinical and biochemical factors

If a patient is known to have gallstones, these should be assumed to be responsible for the attack of pancreatitis until proved otherwise. A history of biliary colic, acute cholecystitis or obstructive jaundice strengthens the suspicion that gallstones are responsible. Further pointers are female gender, age over 50, particularly high serum amylase levels (> 4000 u/l), and raised levels of serum bilirubin, alkaline phosphatase, and alanine aminotransferase[4].

Ultrasonography

Transcutaneous ultrasonography is the mainstay of diagnosis in the early period after admission with acute pancreatitis, and is best performed on the day of admission or on the following morning. The investigation is non-invasive, relatively inexpensive and easily repeatable, and does not depend on excretion of contrast medium by the liver and biliary system. It detects gallstones in the gallbladder and biliary tree (although it is less reliable in detecting stones at the lower end of the common bile duct), measures bile duct diameter, detects gallbladder inflammation, and provides useful information about the degree of inflammation in the pancreas. Unfortunately, ileus and gaseous

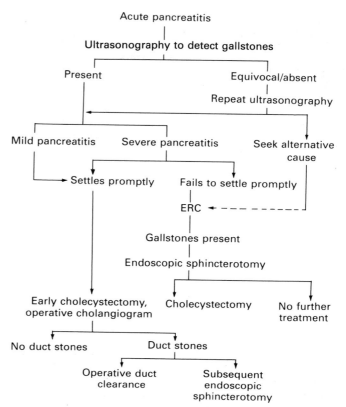

Figure 1 Algorithm for the investigation of patients with gallstone pancreatitis

distension are common features of acute pancreatitis and the gallbladder is visualized in only 70% of patients in this critical early period. When the gallbladder is seen, ultrasonography has an accuracy of 90–95% in gallstone detection; false positives are exceptional and the difficulty lies in the detection of small stones. With clinical improvement of the patient, the accuracy of ultrasonography rises progressively to about 90% but never reaches 100%, reflecting the problem of detecting small stones and microlithiasis capable of causing further attacks of pancreatitis.

Endoscopic retrograde cholangiography (ERC)

ERC offers an excellent means of displaying the biliary tree and may be considered in patients with severe pancreatitis potentially due to gallstones when the attack fails to settle promptly on conservative management. Given that endoscopic retrograde pancreatography (ERP) can trigger an attack of acute pancreatitis in patients who do not have pancreatitis, there has been reluctance to use the investigation in patients who already have active pancreatic inflammation. However, in the present context it should be stressed that the objective is to detect gallstones in the bile duct and not to fill the pancreatic duct system and so exacerbate the pancreatitis. ERC is partly used to resolve diagnostic doubt (are gallstones present?) and partly as a means of aborting the attack of pancreatitis by proceeding to endoscopic sphincterotomy if stones are found in the biliary tree (*see* below).

In patients with pancreatitis which is classified as mild on prognostic factor grading and in those with severe disease which settles promptly, *urgent* ERC is probably meddlesome and potentially dangerous. However *non-urgent* ERCP may be useful when an aetiological cause for the pancreatitis has not been identified and should be carried out after an arbitrary interval of some 2–4 weeks.

Surgical management

The management of necrotizing pancreatitis and its complications is discussed elsewhere (*see* chapter on pp. 458–462), and this chapter is concerned only with the management of the biliary tree in patients with gallstone pancreatitis. When gallstones have been detected and the acute attack of pancreatitis has settled, there is general agreement that the gallbladder should be removed at the earliest appropriate opportunity. Opinion has hardened against *urgent* biliary surgery undertaken within 24–48 h of admission[5]; operating conditions may be suboptimal, inflammation may be exacerbated, and exploration of the biliary system may be needed for stones which would have passed spontaneously into the duodenum over the next few days. Similarly, opinion has hardened against *deferred* biliary surgery because sending the patients home for 4–8 weeks exposes them needlessly to the dangers of recurrent attacks of pancreatitis, cholangitis and cholecystitis while awaiting readmission and incurs the social and financial consequences of two admissions to hospital. There is good evidence that *early* biliary surgery is safe when carried out on the next convenient elective operating list, and there is growing evidence that it can be carried out just as safely by laparoscopic means as by open operation. This is not to say that technical difficulty is not encountered during early laparoscopic cholecystectomy for gallstone pancreatitis, and dilatation of the cystic duct may require large ligating clips or an externally tied Roder slip knot if leakage is to be avoided[6].

2 Opinions vary as to the need for operative cholangiography, but in the author's unit this is carried out routinely, regardless of whether cholecyst-ectomy is being undertaken laparoscopically and whether or not the patient has had pancreatitis. The need for cholangiography may be greater in patients who have had gallstone pancreatitis, given the import-ance of duct stones as a cause of further acute pancreatic inflammation. However, such stones will be present in less than 20% of cases and failure of contrast medium to flow readily into the duodenum or duct dilatation must not be misinterpreted as evidence of residual duct stones. Oedema at the lower end of the bile tree and sphincter spasm may merely reflect the fact a stone has been present at the lower end of the common bile duct, impacting transiently before passing onwards into the duodenum. If duct stones are revealed unequivocally they should be removed, but the operator will have to decide whether it is safer to explore the duct at the time of cholecystectomy or to rely on subsequent endoscopic sphincterotomy to remove residual duct stones.

If surgery is being performed laparoscopically then particular expertise is needed for duct exploration (*see* chapter on pp. 324–336). There is a good argument for preferring endoscopic sphincterotomy to potentially difficult operative exploration in patients with small calibre bile ducts. In deciding between endoscopic and operative duct clearance it must also be borne in mind that endoscopic sphincterotomy does not always succeed, and much will depend on the balance between the operative and endoscopic skills available in the institution concerned.

Endoscopic management

As indicated earlier, ERC may be invaluable in confirming that gallstones are responsible for an attack of acute pancreatitis which does not settle promptly on conservative management. If duct stones are detected in such patients there is accumulating evidence that endoscopic sphincterotomy offers a better prospect of avoiding major complications and mortality than urgent biliary surgery. In over 1100 reported cases of endoscopic sphincterotomy in acute pancreatitis, the overall mortality rate is less than 2% and there have been very few deaths related to the procedure[3]. The major objective is to remove stones impacted at the lower end of the common bile duct, to avoid the possiblity of further stone impaction, and to relieve (and avoid) cholangitis due to biliary tract obstruction. Experimental and clinical evidence suggests that the 'window of opportunity' for the relief of obstruction of the biliary and pancreatic ductal systems may extend for 3–4 days, but even if this window has passed there may still be an argument for relieving obstruction when the disease has progressed to necrotizing pancreatitis.

The technique of endoscopic sphincterotomy is described in the chapter on pp. 282–289 but it is worth stressing that much depends on the skill of the endoscopist, avoidance of pancreatic duct filling, and avoidance of excessive manipulation in the region of the sphincter of Oddi.

If endoscopic sphincterotomy has been used to relieve biliary and pancreatic duct obstruction in gallstone pancreatitis, consideration will then have to be given to the need for surgical management of the gallbladder and its contained stones. In general, early cholecystectomy is advisable but it may be reasonable to avoid surgical intervention in frail elderly patients where the risks of abdominal surgery may outweigh those of restricting management to endoscopic sphincterotomy alone. A similar case may be argued for those ill from intercurrent disease and patients in whom there are major contraindications to abdominal surgery.

References

1. Carter DC. Special aspects of gallstone pancreatitis. In: Trede M, Carter DC, eds. *Surgery of the Pancreas*. Edinburgh: Churchill Livingstone, 1993.

2. Lee SP, Nicholls JF, Park HZ. Biliary sludge as a cause of acute pancreatitis. *N Engl J Med* 1992; 326: 589–93.

3. Neoptolemos JP. Endoscopic sphincterotomy in acute gallstone pancreatitis. *Br J Surg* 1993; 80: 547–9.

4. Blamey SL, Osborne DH, Gilmour WH *et al*. The early identification of patients with gallstone associated pancreatitis using clinical and biochemical factors only. *Ann Surg* 1983; 198: 574–8.

5. Kelly TR, Wagner DS. Gallstone pancreatitis: a prospective randomized trial of the timing of surgery. *Surgery* 1988; 104: 600–5.

6. Tate JJT, Lau WY, Li AKC. Laparoscopic cholecystectomy for biliary pancreatitis. *Br J Surg* 1994; 81: 720–2.

Necrotizing pancreatitis

Hans G. Beger MD, FACS
Professor of Surgery, Chairman and Head of the Department of General Surgery, University of Ulm, Ulm, Germany

Michael H. Schoenberg MD
Department of General Surgery, University of Ulm, Ulm, Germany

Principles and justification

Natural course of acute pancreatitis

In most patients acute pancreatitis takes the course of an oedematous interstitial inflammation, characterized by periacinar and interstitial oedema. Mild acute pancreatitis generally causes low morbidity and conservative treatment results in a rapid improvement of symptoms with a complete cure in a matter of weeks (*Table 1*). In 10–20% of patients a necrotizing acute pancreatitis develops, identified morphologically by acute inflammation of the tissue with necrosis of the exocrine and endocrine pancreatic parenchyma and fatty tissue in and around the pancreas; moderate to severe clinical symptoms develop as a result of local and systemic complications. Bacterial contamination of the pancreatic and retroperitoneal necrotic tissue occurs in about 40% of patients with necrotizing pancreatitis. The subgroup of patients with infected necrosis may develop multisystem organ failure caused by vasoactive and toxic substances released from the pancreatic, peripancreatic and retroperitoneal inflammatory tissue. After the acute phase of the disease, a pancreatic abscess may develop in the third to sixth week as a result of bacteria within the inflamed, often necrotic, tissue. This abscess is liquified and surrounded by a fibrous wall which then forms a pseudocapsule. Pancreatic abscess and infected pancreatic necrosis are two different entities according to morphological, clinical, and laboratory criteria because, in patients with a pancreatic abscess, signs and symptoms of acute pancreatitis have generally subsided when pain, fever and leucocytosis reappear. Pseudocyst after acute pancreatitis represents either collections of peripancreatic fluid with or without connection to the pancreatic duct system. These fluid collections are surrounded by a capsule of fibrous tissue. An infected pseudocyst leads to clinical symptoms that are identical to those of a pancreatic abscess (*Table 2*).

Table 1 Classification of acute pancreatitis based on clinical, morphological, radiological and bacteriological criteria

	Frequency (%)
Interstitial oedematous pancreatitis	75
Necrotizing pancreatitis	10–20
Sterile necrosis (60%)	
Infected necrosis (40%)	
Pancreatic abscess	3
Pseudocyst after acute pancreatitis	5–7

Table 2 Incidence of infection in acute pancreatitis

	Necrotizing pancreatitis (%)	Acute pancreatitis (%)
Infected necrosis	30–40	5–8
Pancreatic abscess	~ 5	2
Infected pseudocyst	< 2	< 0.5
Total	35–45	7–10

Preoperative staging of the severity of the disease

Clinical management of patients with necrotizing pancreatitis should be based on clinical and radiological criteria and on bacteriological investigations. To evaluate the prognosis of patients with acute pancreatitis within 48 h after admission the Ranson criteria are the most widely accepted. However, the important clinical decision during the course of acute pancreatitis is related to the identification of patients suffering from interstitial oedematous or necrotizing pancreatitis; accurate identification is achieved by the use of biochemical data and computed tomographic (CT) scans. C reactive protein, lactate dehydrogenase and phospholipase A$_2$ are highly sensitive biochemical markers of occurrence of a necrotizing process during the course of acute pancreatitis (*Table 3*). Ultrasonography is much less useful in the staging of the severity of acute pancreatitis because of a low sensitivity for pancreatic and retroperitoneal necrosis.

Table 3   Criteria for diagnosis of a necrotizing pancreatitis

	Cut-off point	Detection rate (%)
C reactive protein	> 150 mg/l	93
Lactate dehydrogenase	> 5 U/l	87
Phospholipase A$_2$	> 5 U/l	84
Dynamic contrast CT scans	Non-perfused area	88

Medical management of necrotizing pancreatitis

The primary treatment for all patients with necrotizing pancreatitis ought to be conservative. Medical treatment follows the generally accepted guidelines of analgesia, maintenance of parenteral volume, energy supply and interruption of pancreatic secretion. Decompression of the stomach with a tube is important as is bladder drainage. Medical treatment with atropine, glucagon, calcitonin, somatostatin and the enzyme inhibitor aprotinin has not found general approval after controlled clinical studies failed to confirm their value. The use of albumin is essential in most patients for adequate volume replacement. An arterial oxygen pressure below 60 mmHg indicates the need for supplemental nasal oxygen or mechanical ventilation. Antibiotics should be used in patients with necrotizing pancreatitis, with imipenem or mezlocillin being the most effective drugs against the Gram-positive and Gram-negative bacteria found in pancreatic necrotic tissue. Intensive medical therapy is mandatory for patients with necrotizing pancreatitis.

Surgical treatment of necrotizing pancreatitis

Surgical treatment of necrotizing pancreatitis is based on the experience that patients who do not undergo surgery have a mortality rate exceeding 60% despite maximum intensive care treatment. The surgical treatment of necrotizing pancreatitis is indicated in patients who develop signs of an acute surgical abdomen, suffer from shock, sepsis or organ failure (*Table 4*). Persisting organ failure, such as pulmonary insufficiency, renal insufficiency and gastrointestinal bleeding, or severe metabolic insufficiency are criteria for surgical treatment if these complications persist or deteriorate in spite of maximum intensive care treatment. Patients who develop infected necrosis, based on ultrasound or CT-guided fine-needle puncture, are candidates for surgical treatment.

In patients suffering from a sterile pancreatic necrosis, surgical management has not been proved by controlled trials to be superior to non-surgical management. Sterile pancreatic necroses are therefore not an indication for surgical management.

Surgical treatment of necrotizing pancreatitis involves removal of devitalized tissue from the pancreas and retroperitoneal fatty tissue spaces and evacuation of fluid collections containing vasoactive and toxic substances and bacteria. Careful surgical treatment of pancreatic necrosis preserves functional pancreatic tissue between or below areas of devitalized tissue to minimize late functional impairment.

Table 4   Criteria for surgical treatment of necrotizing pancreatitis

Surgical acute abdomen
Sepsis persisting > 48 h
Shock
Severe local and/or persisting systemic complications:
    in spite of maximum intensive care treatment
    increasing pulmonary insufficiency
    persisting renal insufficiency
    infected necrosis
Severe local bleeding
Increasing adynamic ileus
Stenosis of gastrointestinal tract segments causing ileus

An algorithm which may be used to decide the best method of treatment is shown in *Figure 1*.

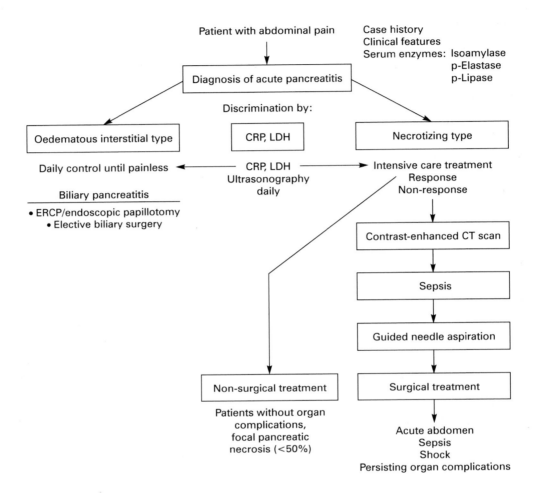

Figure 1   Algorithm defining pathways in acute pancreatitis. CRP, C-reactive protein; LDH, lactate dehydrogenase; ERCP, endoscopic retrograde cholangiopancreatography.

Operations

Surgical debridement and local lavage

An upper abdominal midline incision is used; in cases with body and tail necrosis and retroperitoneal necrosis, an upper abdominal transverse incision might be advantageous. After entering the lesser sac, devitalized haemorrhagic tissue is easily identified. Necrosectomy or debridement means dissection without a knife. A combination of necrosis debridement with the finger and intraoperative and postoperative local lavage of the lesser sac provides an atraumatic and continuous evacuation of devitalized tissue as well as removal of bacterially contaminated dead tissue and biologically active substances.

In order to preserve macroscopically normal tissue any *en bloc* resection should be avoided. Surgical haemostasis of bleeding vessels is of major importance for the patient's survival.

1 For postoperative continuous local lavage of the area of necrotic cavities, at least two large double lumen silicon rubber tubes are inserted (28–34 Fr). In cases of large extrapancreatic retroperitoneal necrosis, additional tubes are placed as required for complete evacuation of devitalized tissue and exudate. The gastrocolic and duodenocolic ligaments are used to create a closed retroperitoneal lesser sac lavage cavity.

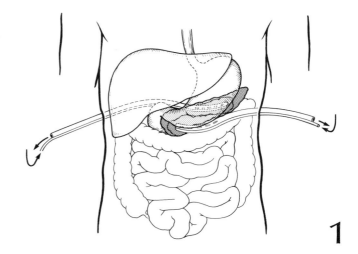

1

The advantage of local lavage of the lesser sac and the cavities containing necrotic tissue is the atraumatic continuous removal of devitalized tissue in the weeks after the operation with removal of bacteria. The rate of flow of the lavage fluid in the first 48 h is 1–2 l/h of a continuous ambulatory peritoneal dialysis solution through the lesser sac to cleanse mechanically the inflamed areas and provide an antipyretic effect.

It is generally found that the inflammatory process after debridement continues to be active up to the second or third week of the disease. Short-term continuous local lavage for the first five postoperative days has many advantages. The criteria for discontinuing lavage are absence of any sign of acute pancreatitis and complete cleansing of the cavity confirmed by measuring endotoxins and enzymes and assessing the amount of bacteria in the lavage fluid.

It is well documented that surgical debridement and local lavage, even in the first 2–5 postoperative days, reduces the severity of the disease immediately in terms of an improvement of pulmonary function and of the Apache II scoring system.

The frequency of reoperation is 25–35%, mainly due to persistent sepsis; other causes of reoperation are massive diffuse local bleeding and appearance of progressive necrosis or development of a colonic fistula leading to an intra-abdominal abscess. Pancreatic fistulas are observed in about 10% of patients after surgical debridement, but usually close spontaneously. The occurrence of local complications is proportional to the extent of intraperitoneal and retroperitoneal parenchymal necrosis. The overall time spent in hospital by surviving patients is about 60 days; this length of stay is almost always related to uncontrollable local and systemic sepsis. Hospital mortality after surgical debridement and local lavage is between 10% and 20%.

Open packing

The use of open packing with multiple redressing reduces the risk of life-threatening complications caused by prolonged inflammation, even after surgery. An open abdomen with multiple redressing tends to remove the necrosis and can be carried out in combination with intraoperative lavage. However, multiple redressing entails many reoperations and a prolonged phase of intensive care; intestinal fistula, stomach outlet syndrome, mechanical ileus and incisional hernias as well as severe local bleeding into cavities are not infrequent complications of the technique. Hospital mortality after open packing is similar to that following debridement and local lavage.

Surgical treatment of pancreatic abscess

Pus collection in the area of the pancreas or in peripancreatic retroperitoneal spaces may occur after acute pancreatitis. Treatment with interventional ultrasound-guided drainage is the first choice. Drainage in connection with local lavage of the abscess cavity interrupts the septic reaction. A transabdominal surgical procedure is indicated if ultrasound-guided drainage of pancreatic abscess fails to interrupt the sepsis syndrome. A small incision in the upper abdomen is

Table 5   Principles of surgical management of acute pancreatitis

	Treatment
Interstitial oedematous pancreatitis	Non-surgical*
Necrotizing pancreatitis	Non-surgical; surgery if no response to
Sterile necrosis	ICU treatment
Infected necrosis	Surgical debridement
Pancreatic abscess	Interventional drainage; surgical drainage in cases of persisting sepsis
Postacute pseudocyst	Interventional drainage; surgical drainage is second choice

*Except biliary tract surgery in biliary pancreatitis.

mandatory to maintain direct access to the abscess cavity.

The principles of the surgical management of acute pancreatitis are shown in *Table 5*.

Further reading

Beger HG, Bittner R, Block S, Büchler M. Bacterial contamination of pancreatic necrosis: a prospective clinical study. *Gastroenterology* 1986; 91: 433–8.

Beger HG, Bittner R, Büchler M, Hess W, Schmitz JE. Hemodynamic data pattern in patients with acute pancreatitis. *Gastroenterology* 1986; 90: 74–9.

Beger HG, Krautzberger W, Bittner R, Block S, Büchler M. Results of surgical treatment of necrotizing pancreatitis. *World J Surg* 1985; 9: 972–9.

Beger HG, Büchler M, Bittner R, Block S, Nevalainen T, Roscher R. Necrosectomy and postoperative local lavage in necrotizing pancreatitis. *Br J Surg* 1988; 75: 207–12.

Beger HG, Büchler M, Bittner R, Oettinger W, Block S, Nevalainen T. Necrosectomy and postoperative local lavage in patients with necrotizing pancreatitis: results of a prospective clinical trial. *World J Surg* 1988; 12: 255–62.

Bittner R, Block S, Büchler M, Beger H. Pancreatic abscess and infected pancreatic necrosis: different local septic complications in acute pancreatitis. *Dig Dis Sci* 1987; 32: 1082–7.

Ranson JH, Rifkind KM, Roses DF, Fink SD, Eng K, Localio SA. Objective early identification of severe acute pancreatitis. *Am J Gastroenterol* 1974; 61: 443–51.

Warshaw AL, Richter JM. A practical guide to pancreatitis. *Curr Probl Surg* 1984; 21: 1–79.

Acute pancreatitis: operations for complications

R. C. N. Williamson MA, MD, MChir, FRCS
Professor and Head, Department of Surgery, Royal Postgraduate Medical School, Hammersmith Hospital, London, UK

Definitions

Roughly 20% of patients with acute pancreatitis develop pancreatic necrosis, but less than half of these will require operative treatment. Sterile pancreatic necrosis may resolve spontaneously or progress to form a pseudocyst, which is defined as a loculated effusion of fluid with a high amylase content; a small proportion of pseudocysts develop secondary infection. Infected pancreatic necrosis implies bacterial contamination of the necrotic tissue leading to a peripancreatic abscess. Necrosis may involve part or most of the pancreas, but frequently the gland itself remains viable and the necrotic process is confined to the peripancreatic fat (retroperitoneal, mesenteric, mesocolic). The septic process may ramify widely within the retroperitoneal space causing severe toxicity with the risk of multiple organ failure and death. The other 'surgical' complications of acute pancreatitis – haemorrhage, intestinal obstruction or necrosis, pancreatic fistula – are virtually confined to patients with infected pancreatic necrosis. Those who survive may develop residual collections of pus within the abdominal cavity.

Operations for necrotising pancreatitis may be divided into those for pseudocyst and those for infected pancreatic necrosis (and associated complications), the salient difference being the absence or presence of systemic sepsis.

Pancreatic pseudocyst

Indications for operation

All inflammatory cysts of the pancreas are technically pseudocysts, since they have no epithelial lining. The cysts that follow an attack of acute pancreatitis are generally extrapancreatic, being contained within the lesser sac, and they seldom communicate with the main pancreatic duct. By contrast, cysts can develop insidiously in chronic pancreatitis, in which case they are mostly intrapancreatic in site and will often communicate with the duct; these cysts are considered in the chapter on pp. 497–505. Some degree of peripancreatic fluid extravasation is common in acute pancreatitis, but most of these fluid collections resolve spontaneously. Thus, operation is reserved for large and persistent cysts and especially those that cause symptoms.

A developing pseudocyst is best managed conservatively unless it causes troublesome pain or obstructive symptoms (jaundice, vomiting) and unless it becomes infected, as evidenced by pyrexia and leucocytosis. Operation should be deferred until 5–6 weeks after the onset of the attack of acute pancreatitis to allow the development of a mature fibrous wall that can be sutured to a hollow viscus to permit internal drainage.

Symptomatic cysts that demand decompression during this waiting period are best managed by percutaneous catheter drainage, the initial needle puncture being carried out under guidance with ultrasound or computed tomographic (CT) scanning. If percutaneous drainage is unavailable or unsuccessful, early laparotomy may occasionally be required, but the immature cyst wall is generally too thin to hold sutures so that external tube drainage becomes the best procedure.

The choice between radiological (percutaneous) drainage and operative internal drainage is a matter of individual judgement. The percutaneous technique may avoid a major operation in a patient with a small acute pseudocyst, and this is especially desirable in the elderly or frail. On the other hand, it is less suitable for managing large cysts which can be difficult to obliterate completely without the need for prolonged external drainage and/or repeat interventions. Moreover, percutaneous drainage is much less satisfactory for chronic pancreatic pseudocysts that communicate with the main duct and can therefore lead to an external pancreatic fistula.

Preoperative

Clinical and radiological diagnosis

A pancreatic pseudocyst typically presents 1–2 weeks after the onset of an attack of acute pancreatitis with abdominal pain, renewed elevation of serum amylase and an enlarging mass in the epigastrium. There may be mild jaundice from compression of the common bile duct and vomiting from distortion of the gastric outlet. Ultrasonography and/or CT scanning should be used to diagnose the cyst, identify its exact position and monitor its progress. Such imaging is a crucial part of interventional radiological procedures (*see above*), and an up-to-date scan should be available in any patient undergoing operative treatment for pseudocyst.

If there is suspicion of underlying chronic pancreatitis, endoscopic retrograde cholangiopancreatography (ERCP) may be indicated to look for dilatation of the pancreatic duct and communication with the pseudocyst. Other potential indications for ERCP are a search for gallstones as the cause of acute pancreatitis (if these were not seen on ultrasound scan) and the investigation of pronounced jaundice. Antibiotics should be given to 'cover' the ERCP and prevent the introduction of infection into the cyst cavity. In patients with chronic

pancreatic pseudocyst, visceral angiography or angio CT scanning should be considered to look for arterial pseudoaneurysms or compression and occlusion of the portal vein and its tributaries, but these complications are rare in the pseudocysts that develop after acute inflammation of an organ that was previously healthy.

Choice of internal drainage procedure

For practical purposes the choice of drainage procedure for mature pseudocyst lies between cystgastrostomy and cystjejunostomy Roux-en-Y. As already stated, percutaneous drainage is a better option than surgical external drainage for immature cysts that require decompression. Cystduodenostomy is appropriate for the occasional small cyst localized in the pancreatic head and abutting against the medial wall of the duodenum, but this is an unusual development in acute pancreatitis.

Cystgastrostomy is a well established method for dealing with an acute pseudocyst that has collected in the lesser sac of the peritoneum. Before selecting this approach, it is important to ensure from the scans that the cyst is closely applied to the back of the stomach. There are theoretical disadvantages to the procedure: gastric acid entering the cyst cavity might provoke haemorrhage, dehiscence of the 'anastomosis' can lead to an awkward gastric fistula, and it is difficult to achieve dependent drainage if the cyst is large and extends well below the stomach. In practice, these drawbacks do not emerge as major problems. Follow-up studies show that the gastric communication generally closes over once the cyst cavity has been obliterated.

Cystjejunostomy is a more versatile procedure, since a Roux loop can be joined to the cyst or cysts wherever they develop. It does involve an additional anastomosis, however. It is the author's preference to use a Roux loop to drain almost all pseudocysts, irrespective of site and chronicity.

In recent years it has become possible to carry out either cystgastrostomy or cystduodenostomy by means of endoscopy, using a diathermy wire to burn a hole through the posterior wall of the stomach or the medial wall of the duodenum; often an indwelling stent is placed. Experience with this type of endoscopic internal drainage remains limited, and there is a certain incidence of troublesome bleeding. The technique should only be undertaken by an experienced endoscopist and probably only for cysts that can be seen to bulge into the lumen of the stomach or duodenum.

Operations

LAPAROTOMY

Incision

1 The abdomen is explored through a generous transverse upper abdominal incision that is convex on its superior aspect. Alternatively, a vertical midline incision can be used. Appropriate single shot antibiotic prophylaxis should be given as for any pancreatobiliary operation.

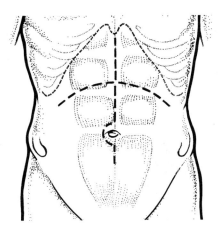

1

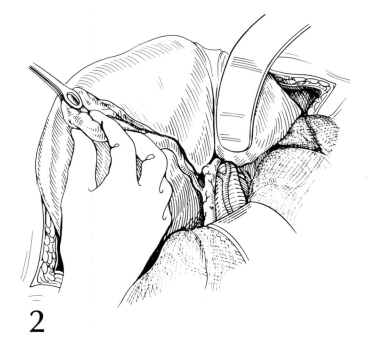

2

Examination of the biliary tree

2 The gallbladder is thoroughly examined for calculous disease and is removed in standard fashion if gallstones are felt or the wall is inflamed. On-table cholangiography is undertaken if gallstones are confirmed, and the surgeon must be prepared to proceed to exploration of the bile duct if there are obvious filling defects in the bile duct (*see* chapter on pp. 337–350).

External tube drainage

3 Attention now turns to the pseudocyst, which is often adherent to adjacent loops of small bowel. Sometimes on freeing the intestine one or more thin-walled collections of turbid fluid are drained. If the main fluid collection is disturbed during this procedure and it becomes clear that it does not have a well defined wall, it is best to abandon any attempt at anastomosis to the stomach or bowel and to proceed to external tube drainage. All communicating cavities are gently de-roofed by digital dissection, fluid contents are sucked out after obtaining a bacteriological culture and solid debris is detached (again with the finger) and removed. At least two drains are left in the cyst cavity before closing the abdomen.

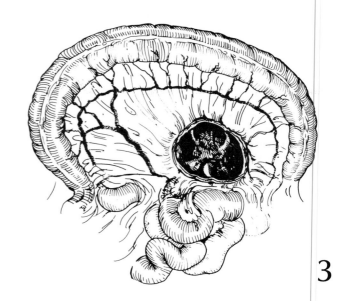

3

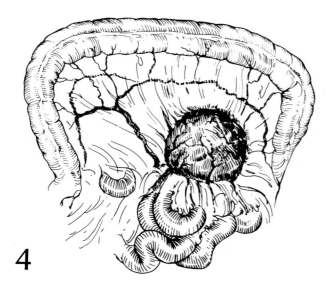

4

Formal internal drainage

4 If a month of more has elapsed since the onset of acute pancreatitis, laparotomy will generally confirm the preoperative scan appearances of a mature pseudocyst. It may be possible to palpate the cyst behind the stomach. Frequently the cyst will be 'presenting' through the transverse mesocolon to the left of the middle colic vessels, and such a cyst is particularly suitable for cystjejunostomy. Depending upon the operative findings and the surgeon's preference (*see above*), a choice is now made between cystgastrostomy and cystjejunostomy.

CYSTGASTROSTOMY

Anterior gastrostomy

5 The body of the stomach is opened obliquely using diathermy. The gastric wall is held up with a pair of Babcock's forceps or stay sutures on either side of the line of incision. Bleeding vessels are secured with diathermy or polyglactin (Vicryl) sutures.

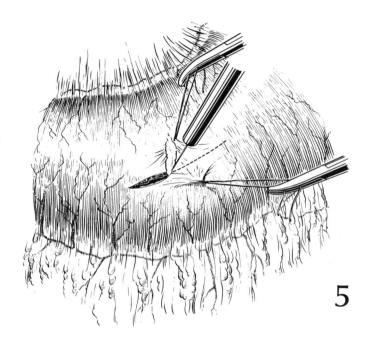

5

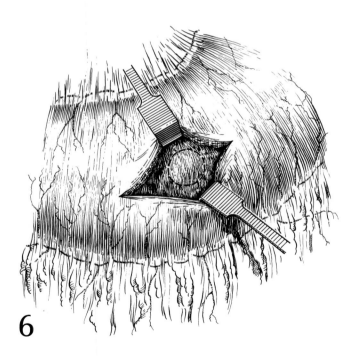

6

Exposure of posterior gastric wall

6 The anterior gastrostomy is retracted to expose the posterior wall of the stomach. The cyst may bulge into the stomach from behind, but otherwise it can be localized by palpation, by inserting a needle and syringe or by the use of an intraoperative ultrasound probe.

Opening the cyst

7 A full-thickness disc of posterior gastric wall is excised with diathermy, and the cyst cavity is entered. Fluid contents are sucked out (after bacteriological culture), and necrotic debris is gently removed by suction, insertion of a finger or sponge holders. Adherent slough is best left undisturbed as severe haemorrhage can ensue.

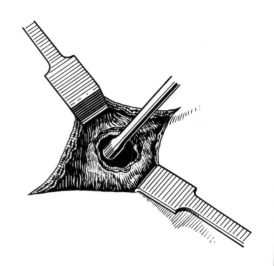

7

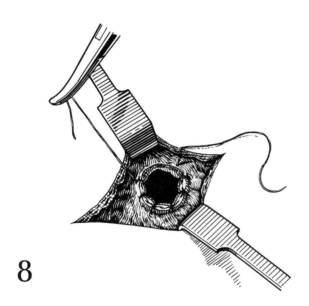

8

Closure of posterior gastrotomy

8 A circumferential suture is used to secure haemostasis and anastomose the cyst to the back of the stomach. Either a continuous suture or interrupted sutures of 2/0 polyglactin are employed. The anterior cyst wall is not seen as a separate layer, having blended with the gastric serosa.

Closure of anterior gastrotomy

9 The anterior wall of the stomach is closed either in two layers of sutures or with a GIA stapler; the staple line is oversewn with sutures. A drain may be left to this area.

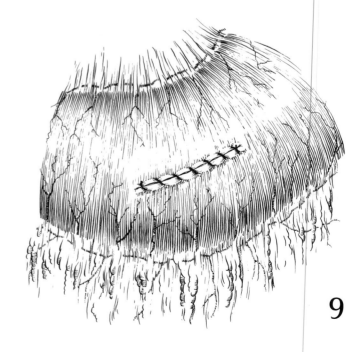

9

CYSTJEJUNOSTOMY

Approach to the pseudocyst

10 After elevating the transverse colon, a bulge can be seen and felt near the root of the mesocolon. Adherent loops of small bowel may need to be dissected off the mesocolon at this point. The cyst is entered to the left of the middle colic vessels using scissors or a haemostat. Any bleeding vessels in the mesocolon are under-run with sutures.

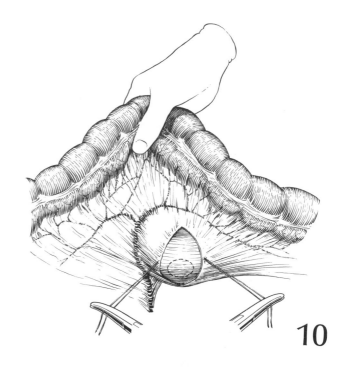

10

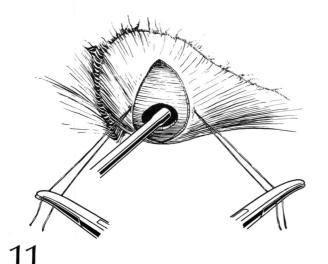

11

Evacuation of cyst contents

11 A sucker is inserted into the cyst cavity after sampling the fluid for bacteriological culture. Following evacuation of the fluid contents, a finger is inserted to explore the cavity. Loculi are broken down, necrotic tissue is gently dissected free and any communicating cysts are entered. Care is taken during this manoeuvre not to create too large or ragged an orifice into the cyst, since this subsequently needs to be used for anastomosis.

Creation of the Roux loop

12 A Roux loop of jejunum is fashioned, approximately 40 cm in length, using standard technique. The upper end of the loop is closed and invaginated.

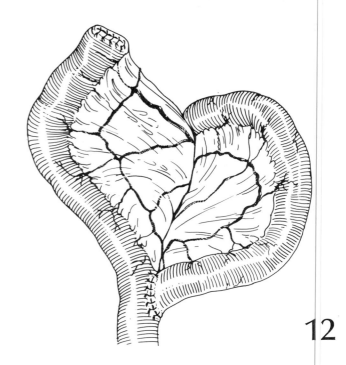

12

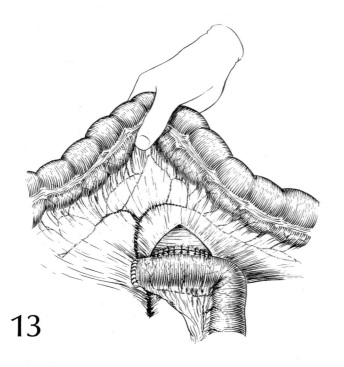

13

Cyst–jejunal anastomosis

13 The seromuscular layer of jejunum is approximated posteriorly to the mesocolon using a few interrupted sutures of 3/0 silk or polyglactin. The bowel is then opened longitudinally to match the orifice of the cyst, and an anastomosis is created using 2/0 polyglactin sutures, either interrupted or continuous. Finally, an anterior seromuscular layer is completed, and a tube drain is placed to the region of the anastomosis.

Infected pancreatic necrosis

Indications for operation

This complication carries a high mortality rate and demands prompt surgical debridement and drainage. In most patients the severity of the attack will have been apparent from the outset. Although the fluid deficit has been corrected and the general condition has stabilized at first, there is subsequent deterioration with evidence of toxicity (fever, leucocytosis, peritonism) and incipient failure of one or more organ system (cardiac, respiratory, renal, hepatic, cerebral). The crucial indication for laparotomy is failure to improve after maximal supportive treatment in an intensive therapy unit for 2–3 days.

Preoperative

Clinical and radiological diagnosis

It can be difficult to determine the severity of an attack of acute pancreatitis at the time of admission to hospital; many patients who appear very ill will rapidly improve with standard supportive care. Several tests or combinations of tests have been advocated to identify those with necrotizing pancreatitis who are at particular risk of complications and death. The scoring system introduced by Ranson is based upon age, fluid deficit, white cell count and another eight laboratory parameters of metabolic upset and organ damage. The acute phase protein, C reactive protein (CRP), can also be used to indicate the extent of toxicity and to monitor its progress. Thus the initial presence of three or more Ranson criteria with subsequent persistence (or increase) of leucocytosis and raised CRP suggests the development of infected pancreatic necrosis.

Contrast-enhanced CT scanning may have shown early swelling of the pancreas and surrounding tissues; a repeat scan will now reveal an enlarging phlegmon with patchy or subtotal ischaemia of the pancreas (failure to enhance with intravenous contrast material), collections of fluid and evidence of abscess formation (pockets of gas). Fine-needle aspiration of non-enhancing areas allows bacteriological confirmation of the presence of infecting organisms and is a further guide to the need to operate. Percutaneous aspiration can be an appropriate means to deal with residual infected collections at a later stage, but the initial management requires surgical debridement of the necrotic material. Although CT scanning delineates the presence and extent of this necrosis, the timing of laparotomy should be dictated by clinical progress and not by radiological appearances.

Choice of drainage procedure

Following debridement and lavage for necrotizing pancreatitis, the surgeon is faced with the following choice of procedures: (1) to close the abdomen leaving 2–4 wide-bore drains within the infected cavities for postoperative lavage – the *closed* drainage technique; or (2) to make no attempt at closure but to leave the abdomen widely open using moist packs to cover the exposed organs and prevent evisceration – the *open* technique or laparostomy.

The chief advantage of laparostomy is that it permits inspection of the abdominal cavity on a daily basis, with drainage of any further collections and digital removal of further necrotic tissue once demarcation becomes apparent. Since these patients are already ventilated, such re-explorations can be carried out under intravenous sedation and, if necessary, in the intensive therapy unit itself. The disadvantages of laparostomy are the difficulty in nursing these patients with an open abdomen and the increased potential for haemorrhage and intestinal fistula. By contrast, the closed drainage technique facilitates nursing at the expense of the need for repeat laparotomy in at least one-third of cases. The timing of such reinterventions is a matter of difficult clinical judgement.

The author adopts a flexible policy. If there is a widespread necrotic process involving both the supracolic and infracolic compartments, the abdomen is left open because of the probable need for one or more subsequent laparotomies. If contamination is less severe and confined to the vicinity of the pancreas, then an attempt is made to reconstitute the lesser sac for postoperative lavage (i.e. the closed technique). Should future laparotomy then be required, laparostomy would be considered. Alternatively, should a patient improve rapidly following primary laparostomy, secondary suture of the abdominal wall would be considered. Lastly, the development of troublesome haemorrhage during the initial laparotomy may tip the scales towards an open packing technique.

Preoperative preparation

A patient who is suspected of developing infected pancreatic necrosis requires admission to an intensive therapy unit for aggressive resuscitation and vigilant monitoring. Fluid and electrolyte deficiencies and acid/base balance must be corrected. Broad-spectrum antibiotics are given intravenously to counter sepsis, the choice of drug being modified by the results of bacteriological culture of blood, sputum or needle aspirate. Ventilatory and inotropic support may be required, together with standard measures for acute renal failure. Central venous access is obtained for total parenteral nutrition. Coagulopathy should be reversed with parenteral vitamin K or transfusion of fresh frozen plasma, as appropriate. Several units of blood should be cross-matched for laparotomy, and an experienced anaesthetist is required to manage a patient who is septic and at risk of operative haemorrhage and multiple organ failure.

Operations

LAPAROTOMY

Access

Thorough exposure of the abdominal viscera and retroperitoneum is required. The incision of choice is transverse, as described for a pseudocyst (*see Illustration 1* on page 465). Within the abdomen, small bowel adhesions are broken down and the transverse colon is elevated to display the peritoneum.

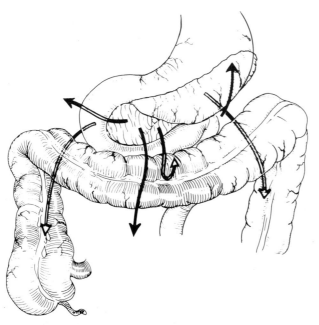

14

Assessment

Concomitant gallstones should be sought and removed by means of cholecystectomy, with exploration and T tube drainage of the bile duct (if indicated). Transduodenal sphincteroplasty is best avoided in the presence of infected pancreatic necrosis because of the risk of leakage from the duodenotomy incision. Liver biopsy should be considered in a jaundiced patient. An attempt is now made to define the extent of the necrotizing pancreatitis, correlating the operative findings with the appearances on a recent CT scan. Since the lesser sac has often been obliterated, it may be best to commence the exploration by incising the peritoneum at the root of the small bowel mesentery rather than dividing the gastrocolic omentum.

The principles of the operation are: (1) to drain all infected collections of fluid; (2) to remove all necrotic material, this mostly being peripancreatic fat; and (3) to avoid formal pancreatic resection unless a portion of the gland has clearly undergone infarction. In these adverse circumstances pancreatectomy risks uncontrollable haemorrhage from the portal vein and its tributaries. Moreover, since diabetes and steatorrhoea are rare among those who survive, total pancreatic necrosis is uncommon and perfusion defects on the contrast-enhanced CT scan may simply represent areas of recoverable ischaemia.

Debridement

14 The debridement process needs to be radical, following all pathways of spread of the infective process. Turbid fluid and necrotic debris may extend upwards from the pancreas towards the diaphragm, laterally into either flank, downwards in one or other paracolic gutter as far as the pelvis, and forwards into the root of the small bowel mesentery and the transverse mesocolon. Sharp dissection should be avoided because of the ever-present risk of bleeding from retroperitoneal or mesenteric vessels (there may be some element of portal vein compression from a swollen neck of pancreas). The best 'instrument' for exploration is the surgeon's finger, which is used gently to break down loculations and to detach and scoop out the dead fat. A thorough technique is required to enter and debride all collections of infected or necrotic material; this procedure is sometimes termed 'digital necrosectomy'. Sometimes a portion of necrotic pancreas itself can be removed with sponge-holding forceps.

Control of haemorrhage from cavity

15 Some bleeding from the large raw cavity is almost inevitable, but it can usually be controlled by temporary packing followed by suture-ligation of the relevant vessel. Persistent haemorrhage, for example from the splenic vein, should if possible be managed along similar lines without recourse to splenectomy and distal pancreatectomy, which escalate the procedure and may exacerbate the bleeding. Diffuse or uncontrollable bleeding may occasionally necessitate tight packing of the abdominal cavity and termination of the operation. The patient is returned to the intensive therapy unit, transfusion is given to restore haemoglobin and clotting factors, and the packs are removed after 24–48 h.

Lavage

Following the debridement, the ramifying cavities are washed out using copious quantities of warm saline. Some authorities recommend the addition of an antibiotic such as tetracycline to the lavage fluid.

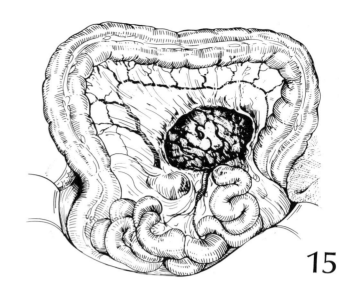

15

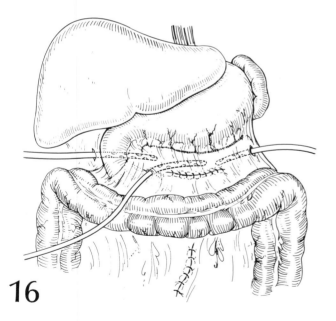

16

CLOSED DRAINAGE

16 Several silicone tube drains are placed within the lesser sac cavity. Two wide-bore drains are brought out, one in each flank. One or two drains are then brought out anteriorly to allow entry of lavage fluid. If double-lumen sump tubes are available, each can be used for inflow and egress of fluid and two may suffice. For necrosis limited to the upper abdomen, an attempt should be made to 'compartmentalize' the abdomen by suturing the 'exploratory' defects made in the transverse mesocolon and gastrocolic omentum and/or by tacking the transverse colon to the parietal peritoneum along the lower margin of the abdominal incision. It may then be possible to irrigate the infected cavity without disturbing the infracolic compartment of the abdominal cavity. A feeding jejunostomy (14 Fr latex T tube) may be placed to permit enteral nutrition. Particular care must be taken during closure of the abdominal wall because of the risk of dehiscence.

The abdominal cavity is left to seal off overnight, and lavage is then commenced down one of the tubes using 500–1000 ml of normal saline per hour (with added potassium if indicated by serum estimations). Lavage with diminishing volumes is continued for several days or even weeks, depending upon the nature of the effluent and the clinical condition of the patient.

LAPAROSTOMY

17 One or more tube drains are placed into deep cavities and brought out through stab incisions. Several gauze rolls are thoroughly moistened in saline and then spread out to cover the exposed viscera (liver, stomach, omentum, colon, small bowel). No attempt is made to suture the abdominal wall. The packs are covered by a sheet of transparent plastic film which adheres to the surrounding skin. The first change of packs is carried out after 24–48 h. Removal of the packs may reveal obvious areas of superficial slough to be cleansed, and the small bowel loops can be manually separated to permit exploration of the depths of the abdominal cavity and the release of further infected collections. Paraffin gauze can be used to cover the viscera before new moist packs are placed. It is a simple matter to biopsy the liver, suture a bleeding vessel, close a small bowel defect or insert a feeding jejunostomy, as appropriate. Once healing progresses, rapid epithelial ingrowth may obviate the need for secondary suture.

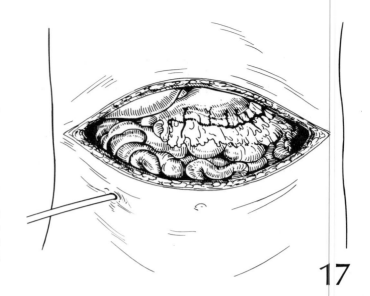

17

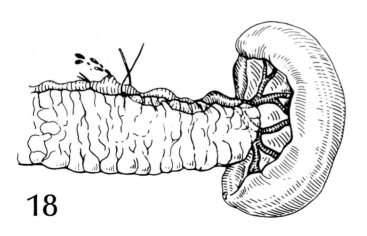

18

Other complications

Haemorrhage

18 Necrotizing pancreatitis may be complicated by stress ulceration in the stomach and duodenum or, more specifically, by haemorrhage from arteries or veins in the wall of an abscess cavity or pseudocyst. Arterial pseudoaneurysms are more often associated with the cysts of chronic pancreatitis; typically they bleed into the gut a few days after internal cyst drainage. In acute pancreatitis the bleeding is generally secondary and takes place into the abdominal cavity and then down any drains that have been inserted. Endoscopy may reveal the cause of haematemesis or melaena and allow rational treatment, including ranitidine or omeprazole and local haemostatic measures. A brisk bleed down the drains following a debridement operation requires urgent angiography and an attempt at transcatheter embolization of any arterial blush. Failure to control the bleeding demands immediate laparotomy. The cavities are explored, all clot is removed, and a search is made for the bleeding source. Arterial blood will usually be coming from the splenic artery, but alternatively from the gastroduodenal, middle colic or mesenteric arteries. Venous blood will usually be coming from the splenic or main portal vein. Precise suture of the offending vessel is the best option, but diffuse venous bleeding may require packing.

Colonic necrosis

19 Ischaemia, necrosis and perforation may develop in the region of the hepatic flexure of the colon as a consequence of thrombosis of the mesocolic vessels in fulminating pancreatitis. The patient may present with peritonitis or a faecal fistula. Alternatively, the ascending colon and/or transverse colon appear discoloured or frankly gangrenous at laparotomy for infected pancreatic necrosis. Right hemicolectomy should be performed if there is serious concern about the viability of the bowel. The terminal ileum is brought out as a spout ileostomy, and the left transverse colon is oversewn within the abdomen as a blind end. Reconnection of the bowel is delayed until complete healing and recovery have occurred.

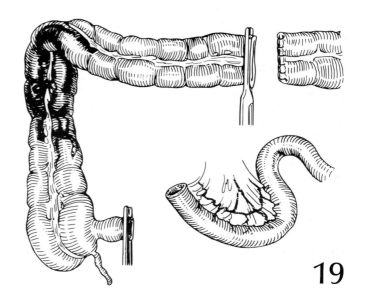

19

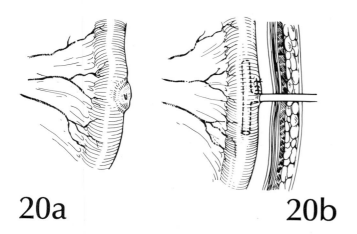

20a   **20b**

Small bowel fistula

20a,b Necrosis of the small intestine is rare, but should be dealt with by local resection with either anastomosis or exteriorization of either end of the bowel according to the patient's local and general condition. Small bowel fistulae may result from inadvertent injury to an adherent loop of gut during laparotomy for infected necrosis or from erosion of bowel exposed at laparostomy. The fistula may be controlled by suture of the defect or catheterization or just local drainage depending upon the particular circumstances. Nutrition is maintained by the parenteral route until the patient improves, when formal closure of the defect may be undertaken.

Duodenal obstruction

21 Occasionally ongoing inflammation in the pancreatic head leads to duodenal oedema and compression and gastric outlet obstruction. The condition may resolve spontaneously with nasogastric suction. Sometimes a fine-bore feeding tube can be negotiated through the narrowed segment of duodenum under endoscopic or radiological control. Occasionally, gastroenterostomy is required to circumvent persisting obstruction at this site.

Residual abdominal abscess

Some patients survive an attack of severe pancreatitis and debridement operations only to develop renewed fever and leucocytosis from residual collections of pus deep in the abdominal cavity. Ultrasound and CT scanning should be used to localize these collections and permit percutaneous insertion of a fine tube drain. Operative drainage should be reserved for the occasional case in which the contents are too viscous to be evacuated by this means.

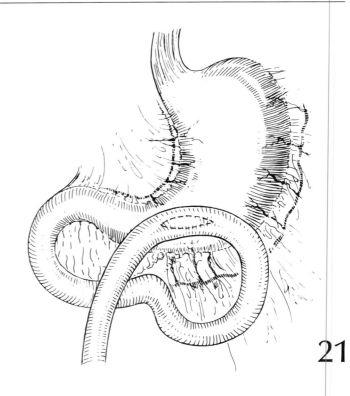

21

22

Pancreatic fistula

22 Some patients who survive one or more debridement procedures may develop a persistent pancreatic fistula through the wound itself or a drain site. The initial treatment is conservative since most pure pancreatic fistulae will dry up spontaneously; the greyish effluent can be collected in a colostomy bag and will generally not damage the skin. A mixed fistula that contains bile or small bowel contents in addition to pancreatic juice is more of a problem because of the risk of infection and skin excoriation by activated pancreatic enzymes; it should be managed along the lines of a small bowel fistula. The author has twice had to operate for a chronic pancreatic fistula that persisted for months. In each case the mature fistulous track was dissected out and anastomosed to the bowel.

Illustrations by Patrick Elliott

Accessory papilla sphincteroplasty for pancreas divisum

Andrew L. Warshaw MD

Harold and Ellen Danser Professor of Surgery, Chief of General Surgery and Associate Chief of the Surgical Services, Massachusetts General Hospital, Harvard Medical School, Boston, Massachusetts, USA

Principles and justification

The pancreas is the product of the fusion of dorsal and ventral precursors during the fifth and sixth weeks of embryological development. The duct systems of the two segments usually fuse as well, producing alternative outflow tracts for the pancreatic duct system at either the major papilla (of Vater) or the minor (accessory) papilla. The duct leading to the major papilla is commonly called the duct of Wirsung, and that to the minor papilla is the duct of Santorini.

1a–e

In nearly 10% of western populations there are significant anomalies of pancreatic duct development. The most widely recognized is pancreas divisum, in which the dorsal and ventral ducts fail to fuse and empty separately into the minor or major papilla, respectively (*Illustration 1c*). In other cases the ventral duct may regress or never form, and all pancreatic secretions egress via the minor papilla (*Illustration 1d*). In an additional 10% the communicating duct between the dorsal and ventral systems is too fine to provide a functional channel, and the resistance to flow dictates that the secretory pathways will remain separate (*Illustration 1e*). These variations may be grouped under the rubric of 'dominant dorsal duct', which indicates that the dorsal duct system emptying via the minor papilla is the principal secretory pathway of the pancreas.

In most persons with a dominant dorsal duct, the anatomical variant is of no clinical significance. In a few, however, the orifice of the minor papilla may be too small to transmit the large volume of pancreatic secretions, especially during the times of maximum flow. It is believed that the pressure in the pancreatic duct may rise inordinately in such persons and cause either recurrent acute pancreatitis or perhaps recurrent pain ('obstructive pancreatopathy'). This complex of illnesses has been called the 'dominant dorsal duct syndrome'. The combination of relative accessory papilla stenosis and dominant dorsal duct anatomy is required to cause a dominant dorsal duct syndrome. Neither condition suffices alone. While the anatomical configuration of the ducts is congenital, it is not known whether accessory papilla stenosis is congenital or acquired. Three-quarters of the reported cases have been in women, and the typical age at diagnosis is in the thirties.

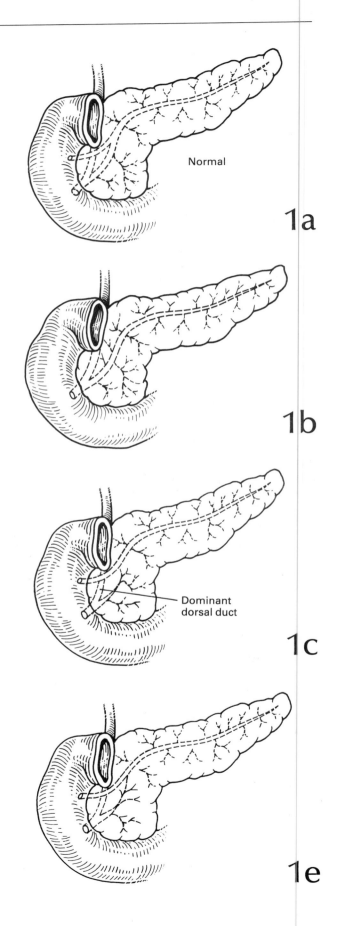

Normal

1a

1b

Dominant
dorsal duct

1c

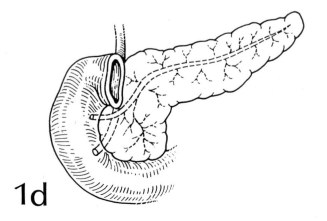

1d

1e

Diagnosis

2a,b The diagnosis of dominant dorsal duct syndrome (pancreas divisum) is initiated by endoscopic pancreatography (ERP) which delineates the anatomy of the pancreas. The ventral duct is typically foreshortened to 2–3 cm and ends in fine terminal secondary branches (*Illustration 2a*). If the ventral duct cannot be found, it may be absent. The definitive diagnosis requires opacification of the dorsal duct through the minor papilla (*Illustration 2b*).

The dorsal duct usually has a normal size and morphology, and does not appear dilated or obstructed at rest. Changes of chronic pancreatitis in the dorsal duct are quite exceptional and should raise the question of an alternative aetiology of pancreatitis. Changes in the ventral duct similarly imply a different form of chronic pancreatitis. Neither calcification nor pseudocysts are found in the majority of patients with dominant dorsal duct syndrome.

Differentiation of pancreas divisum – a congenital anomaly – must be made from acquired pancreatic duct obstruction at the junction of the dorsal and ventral ducts. The latter may occur as a consequence of cancer or injury to the duct system from pancreatitis, pseudocyst, surgical debridement or trauma. In such cases, there is a blunt termination of the ventral duct, rather than progressive arborization.

There is no universally agreed method for ascertaining whether the accessory papilla is stenotic. Endoscopic assessment including calibration and manometry has been unreliable. A trial of dorsal duct stenting has been suggested to see if the symptoms are ameliorated but no decision has been made. The authors have used ultrasound to monitor the size of the pancreatic duct under conditions of secretin stimulation (the ultrasound secretin test); prolonged duct dilatation implies restricted emptying.

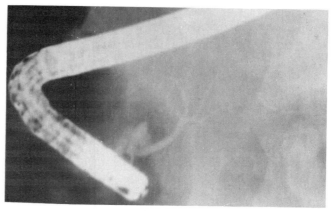

2a

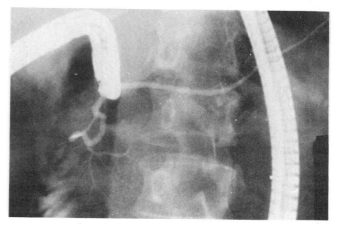

2b

Operation

The abdomen is opened by a right subcostal or midline incision. The gallbladder is removed if it is still present. Cholecystectomy not only excludes the possibility of overlooked small stones as a cause of recurrent pancreatitis, but also obviates any possibility that the gallbladder will be a cause of recurrent pain.

3 A small catheter or paediatric feeding tube can be passed down through the cystic duct into the duodenum to aid in identifying the major papilla and to determine the optimal location for the duodenotomy. It is not necessary to open the common duct to pass a catheter when the gallbladder has previously been removed. After the duodenum and head of the pancreas have been mobilized by an extensive Kocher manoeuvre, the major papilla is usually palpable along the medial wall of the duodenum. A transverse duodenotomy is made just above the major papilla.

The accessory papilla lies proximal and anterior to the papilla of Vater, usually at a distance of 2–3 cm, occasionally up to 4 cm. It is most often a 2-mm nodule on the surface of the duodenal mucosa and may be difficult to identify within the folds of the duodenum. It may be more easily palpated than visualized. Bruising and trauma to the duodenal mucosa should be minimized as the duodenal mucosa rapidly swells and becomes distorted, thereby increasing the difficulty in

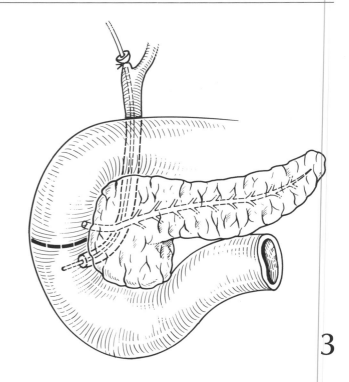

3

locating the papilla. Administration of intravenous secretin (1 unit/kg) is helpful in locating the accessory papilla. Not only does secretin induce an immediate visible flow of pancreatic juice, but also the papilla often balloons out and enlarges during secretin infusion because of the partial obstruction to flow.

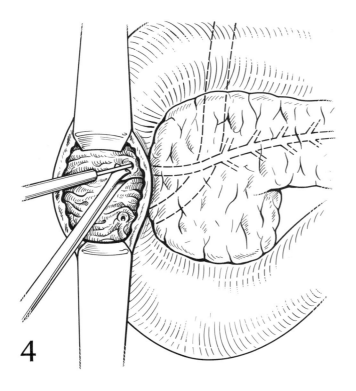

4

4 When the accessory papilla is located, the mucosa just distal to it is grasped with an Allis' clamp. This manoeuvre puts the papilla on stretch, fixes its position, and maximizes its visualization. A fine lacrimal duct probe is then inserted into the papillary orifice. If the orifice is stenotic, it will be difficult to insert even the finest (0.75 mm) lacrimal duct probe. It may occasionally be necessary to penetrate a membranous obstruction or to amputate the tip of the papilla.

5 Traction sutures of fine (4/0) absorbable synthetic material are placed on either side of the inferior margin of the papilla. With a probe in the pancreatic duct, an incision is made in the papilla on its cephaloanterior side. The probe is crucial to guiding the incision accurately into the lumen. The stenosis is almost always short and caused by the mucous membrane of the papilla. It does not extend far along the duct or involve the pancreatic substance. Therefore the incision almost immediately lays open a vestibule behind the papilla. If secretin has been given, the release of secretions is obvious.

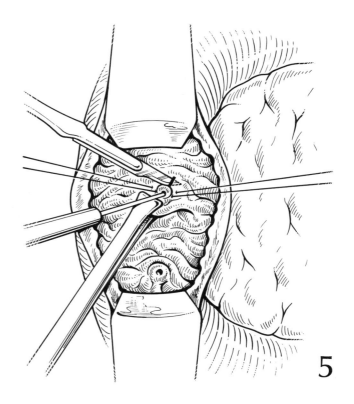

5

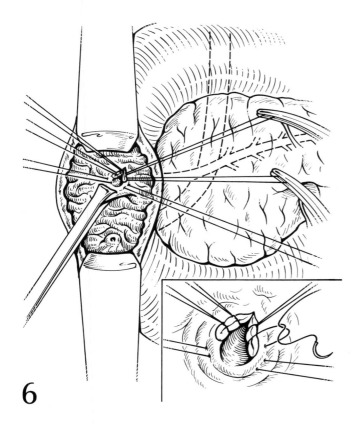

6

6 4/0 sutures are carefully placed to approximate the duodenal and pancreatic duct mucosa without narrowing the duct lumen. These sutures provide haemostasis and improve the exposure by leaving them long and holding them gently on traction with haemostats.

7 Fine clamps, either individually or in pairs, are then
   progressively placed on the septal tissue in order to
include the duodenal and pancreatic duct mucosa. The
incision is extended along these clamps, and in each bite
of tissue an additional suture is placed. In this fashion,
the sphincteroplasty is progressively extended for about
1 cm, or as far as practicable, and the mucosa is rolled
back on itself to open a tunnel. It is completed with a
final suture at the apex of the incision. The duct of
Santorini is orientated straight into the pancreatic
substance. There appears to be little or no actual
sphincter muscle in the accessory papilla. For these
reasons, the length of the sphincteroplasty is much
shorter than that usually performed on the major
papilla.

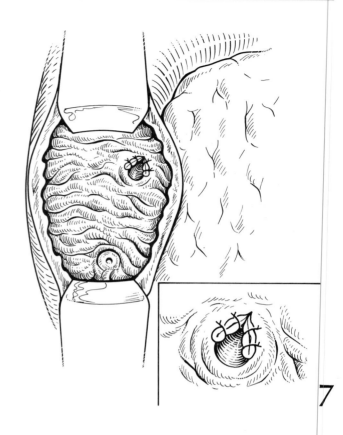

7

8 A 5-Fr catheter is threaded into the dorsal duct to
   verify that there is no obstruction along its length.
A pancreatogram may be obtained if desired and if the
dorsal duct has not been visualized preoperatively.
Leaving the catheter in the dorsal duct for postoperative
drainage will assure that the pancreas is decompressed
and may contribute to a reduced risk of postoperative
pancreatitis. The catheter can be introduced through
the duodenal wall distal to the duodenotomy through a
14 gauge needle.

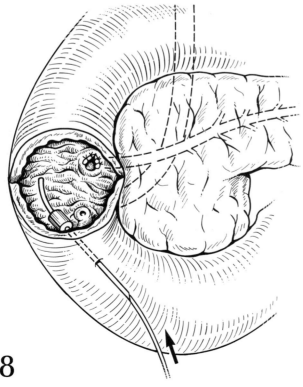

8

9 The catheter is threaded into the pancreatic duct and positioned to assure free flow. The catheter is fixed to the duodenal wall in an inverted tunnel created with double purse-string sutures and is brought out through the abdominal wall where it is connected to gravity drainage.

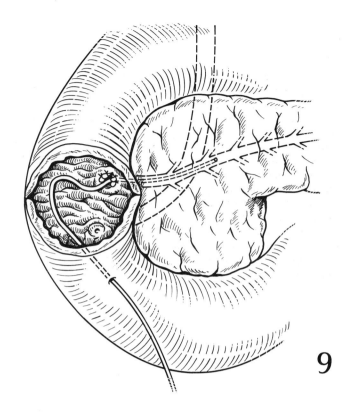

9

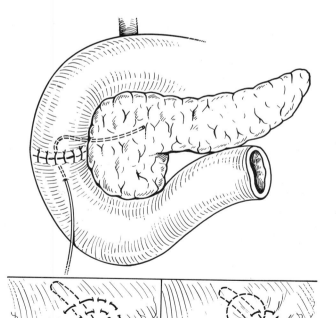

10

10 The duodenum is closed transversely with a running absorbable suture and a second layer of interrupted inverting non-absorbable sutures. Subhepatic drainage is not necessary.

It is the author's practice to place a gastrostomy tube at the time of the transduodenal sphincteroplasty. Patients appreciate this in lieu of a nasogastric tube, especially if the required period of gastric decompression is longer than anticipated.

Postoperative care

Meticulous gentle intraoperative techniques and postoperative catheter drainage of the pancreatic duct will minimize the possibility of the occurrence of postoperative pancreatitis. Pancreatography at any time should be performed with a minimal volume of dye injected at low pressure. Minimizing instrumentation near the papilla will prevent distortion of tissues and the creation of false passages.

Duodenal obstruction at the duodenotomy site is not likely to occur if a transverse duodenotomy with transverse closure has been performed and the amount of tissue inverted during the duodenal closure is minimal. With proper surgical technique, a duodenal fistula should not occur. Gastric drainage and decompression should be continued for 3–5 days after the operation. The pancreatic duct catheter and gastrostomy tube are left in place for a minimum of 10 days until a secure tract has formed around them to allow safe removal. A pancreatogram can be obtained, if desired, before catheter removal.

Several other operations aimed at reducing the volume of pancreatic secretion and the strain on the abnormally small drainage system have been proposed. Distal pancreatectomy has had little success and is not often used. Distal drainage by pancreaticojejunostomy is usually not feasible because the pancreatic duct is small and the pancreas is so soft and friable that it will not easily hold sutures. Conversely, patients with significant pancreatic duct dilatation clearly have a form of chronic pancreatitis rather than simple recurrent acute pancreatitis and do not respond well to treatment by sphincteroplasty. Such patients are best treated by other procedures that are more appropriate to their duct anatomy such as a Puestow-type pancreaticojejunostomy.

There is no effective medical treatment for recurrent pancreatitis associated with pancreas divisum. Patients with intermittent bouts of pancreatitis due to pancreas divisum should have an accessory papilla sphincteroplasty once the diagnosis is made.

Further reading

Bernard JP, Sahel J, Giovannini M, Sarles H. Pancreas divisum is a probable cause of acute pancreatitis: a report of 137 cases. *Pancreas* 1990; 5: 248–54.

Lans JI, Geenen JE, Johanson JF, Hogan WJ. Endoscopic therapy in patients with pancreas divisum and acute pancreatitis: a prospective, randomized, controlled clinical trial. *Gastrointest Endosc* 1992; 38: 430–4.

Lehman GA, Sherman S. Pancreas divisum: diagnosis, clinical significance and management alternatives. *Gastrointest Endosc Clin North Am* 1995; 5: 145–70.

Lehman GA, Sherman S, Nisi R, Hawes RH. Pancreas divisum: results of minor papilla sphincterotomy. *Gastrointest Endosc* 1993; 39: 1–8.

Warshaw AL, Simeone JF, Schapiro RH, Flavin-Warshaw B. Evaluation and treatment of the dominant dorsal duct syndrome (pancreas divisum redefined). *Am J Surg* 1990; 159: 59–66.

Warshaw AL, Simeone J, Schapiro RH, Hedberg SE, Mueller PE, Ferrucci JT Jr. Objective evaluation of ampullary stenosis with ultrasonography and pancreatic stimulation. *Am J Surg* 1985; 149: 65–72.

Illustrations by Gillian Lee Illustrations

Drainage procedures in chronic pancreatitis

David C. Carter MD, FRCS(Ed), FRCS(Glas), FRCS, FRSE
Regius Professor of Clinical Surgery, Royal Infirmary, Edinburgh, UK

Kelvin R. Palmer MD, FRCP(Ed)
Consultant Physician, Western General Hospital, Edinburgh, UK

Principles and justification

Drainage operations in chronic pancreatitis have been based on the premise that relief of ductal obstruction and distension would relieve pain and might at least arrest the decline in pancreatic endocrine and exocrine function associated with the disease. However, there is an extremely variable relationship between duct size, histological evidence of pancreatitis, ductal pressure and pain, and the explanation for the relief afforded to the majority of patients by pancreaticojejunostomy remains uncertain.

1 Early attempts at pancreatic drainage such as the DuVal procedure involved retrograde drainage of the gland into a Roux loop of jejunum after amputation of the tail of the pancreas and splenectomy. It was soon appreciated that pain relief was short-lived and that more extensive pancreatic drainage was needed to deal with multiple duct strictures and ensure long-term patency of the pancreaticojejunal anastomosis.

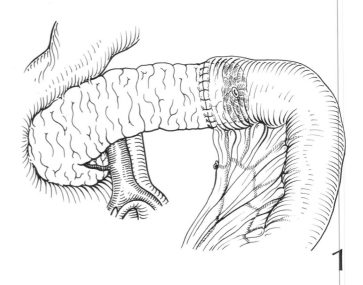

1

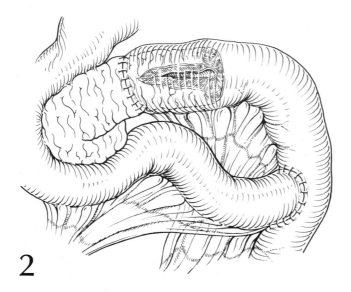

2

2 In the Puestow and Gillespie operation, the pancreatic duct was deroofed from the tail to the neck of the pancreas, and the body and tail were then implanted into a Roux loop.

In the modern operation developed by Partington and Rochelle, a side-to-side anastomosis is created between the opened pancreatic duct and the side of a Roux loop of jejunum, the tip of the pancreas is not amputated, and the spleen is not removed. In the Partington–Rochelle operation the opened jejunum was simply sutured to the pancreatic capsule, whereas emphasis is now often placed on creating a mucosa-to-mucosa anastomosis between the duct and the jejunum. Alternative methods of duct drainage include the endoscopic insertion of stents to overcome obstruction of the pancreatic duct in the head of the gland (*see* page 495) and surgical drainage of the pancreatic duct into the back of the stomach (pancreaticogastrostomy) rather than the jejunum. Although pancreaticogastrostomy has advocates, the window created is small and most surgeons still regard pancreaticojejunostomy as the drainage operation of choice.

Preoperative

The diagnosis of chronic pancreatitis is not in itself an indication for operation as many patients can be managed conservatively. Pain which cannot be controlled by medical means is usually the cardinal indication for elective surgery and, as will be discussed, additional factors favouring surgical intervention are the presence of a pseudocyst (common), biliary tract obstruction (less common) and duodenal obstruction (rare). Most surgeons consider that pancreaticojejunostomy should only be performed if the pancreatic duct system is distended to a diameter of more than 7–8 mm (normal 2–4 mm), and the operation is easiest in patients with greatly distended ducts. On the other hand, there have been recent suggestions that duct distention is not the crucial determinant and that incising the chronically inflamed pancreas down to a non-distended duct may still allow pain relief, possibly by serving as a permanent 'fasciotomy' when the opened gland is anastomosed to the jejunum.

Ultrasonography and/or computed tomography can provide useful information about the pancreas and its duct system, the liver and biliary tree, and neighbouring vascular structures such as the splenic vein. It is now appreciated that splenic vein thrombosis is a not infrequent complication of chronic pancreatitis and the surgeon is best to be forewarned about the presence of large varices and splenomegaly.

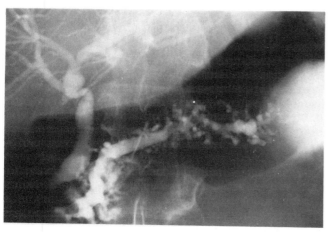

3

3 Endoscopic retrograde cholangiopancreatography (ERCP) provides the most valuable information about pancreatic duct size, presence of strictures and calculi, communicating pseudocysts, and biliary tract morphology. If a pancreatogram cannot be obtained endoscopically, percutaneous antegrade pancreatography is possible in skilled hands under ultrasound guidance or a pancreatogram can be obtained by direct puncture of the duct at operation. Intraoperative ultrasonography now offers an alternative means of defining pancreatic morphology, including duct morphology, if a pancreatogram has not been obtained before operation.

It must always be borne in mind that pancreatic cancer may be difficult clinically and at operation to distinguish from chronic pancreatitis, and operative biopsy may not always detect underlying malignancy. Calcification does not exclude cancer, the two conditions frequently coexist, and there is now some evidence that chronic pancreatitis is potentially a premalignant condition. Particular suspicion should be aroused if there is an isolated stricture of the pancreatic duct or a 'double duct sign' at ERCP with neighbouring strictures of the common bile duct and main pancreatic duct. Anxieties about malignancy are particularly important when pancreaticojejunostomy is being contemplated for chronic pancreatitis, given that the gland is left *in situ*, and most large series of patients treated by pancreaticojejunostomy include individuals in whom pancreatic cancer was overlooked at the time of surgery or developed subsequently. At the same time, the fact that pancreaticojejunostomy conserves the gland may avoid or defer the critical deterioration in pancreatic exocrine and endocrine function which is commonly precipitated by pancreatic resection in this disease.

Operations

PANCREATICOJEJUNOSTOMY

Pancreaticojejunostomy is carried out under general anaesthesia with the patient positioned supine and flat on the operating table. The availability of intraoperative ultrasonography means that intraoperative radiography can now be avoided. Although the operation can be performed through a vertical incision, a transverse or bilateral subcostal incision gives optimal exposure and can be reused if pancreatic resection is required subsequently.

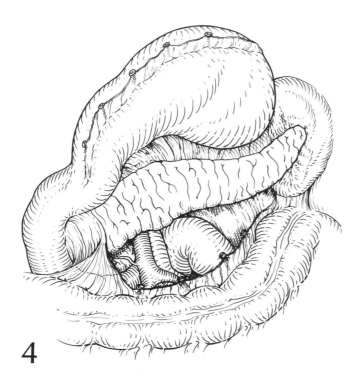

4

4 The lesser sac is opened widely by dividing the gastrocolic ligament between ligatures. The entire anterior surface of the pancreas must be exposed so that a large window is created which extends from the short gastric vessels on the left to divide the origin of the gastroepiploic vein on the right as it passes down to join the superior mesenteric vein just beneath the neck of the pancreas. It is also important to expose the front of the head of the pancreas and uncinate process by dividing the connective tissue which tethers the transverse mesocolon to the gland. It is safer and easier to begin this part of the dissection by dividing the tissue between the transverse mesocolon and the third part of the duodenum so that the superior mesenteric vein can be seen and safeguarded during the rest of the dissection. Avascular adhesions between the posterior aspect of the stomach and the front of the pancreas are divided fully with dissecting scissors to expose the front of the body and tail of the pancreas.

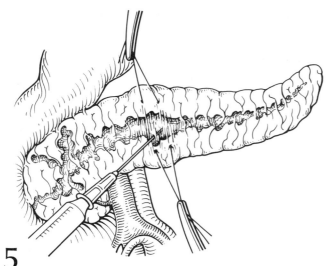

5

5 The pancreatic duct may be palpable when it is grossly distended and it is then a simple undertaking to enter it by a small longitudinal incision in the anterior aspect of the body of the gland. It is often helpful to locate the duct by needle puncture and a pair of stay sutures are then inserted above and below it at a convenient point in the body of the gland. The parenchyma is incised longitudinally between the stay sutures.

In patients with smaller ducts it is easy to pass above or below the duct and care must be taken not to cut through the entire thickness of the pancreas and enter the underlying splenic vein. Further needle puncture may be helpful in such cases and, if entry is still not achieved, a small transverse incision will locate the duct.

Once the duct has been opened a specimen of fluid is sent for cytological examination and a piece of parenchymal tissue is incised from the edge of the opened pancreas for histological examination. Some surgeons routinely measure intraduct pressure by inserting a needle attached to a manometer before incising the duct, while others insert a fine needle into the parenchyma to measure interstitial pressure.

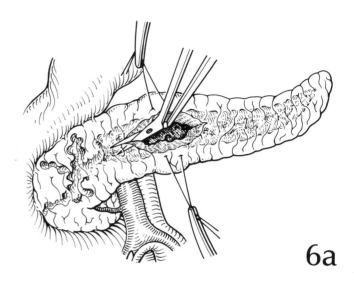

6a, b The pancreatic duct system is then incised widely along its entire length and any calculi are picked out. The length of this incision is critical to the long-term success of the operation, and it must extend from just within the anterior pancreatico-duodenal arcade on the right to the tail of the pancreas on the left. Extensions may be necessary to deroof the accessory pancreatic duct and significant branches of the duct system in the uncinate process must be opened.

6a

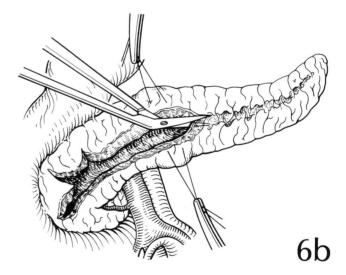

6b

7 In the operation described by Frey, the conventional operation of pancreaticojejunostomy is augmented by excising pancreatic tissue from the front of the head of the pancreas and uncinate process so that the entire duct system is laid fully open.

Dissecting scissors may be suitable for opening the duct but if there is calcification it is better to tent its anterior wall between stay sutures or the jaws of artery forceps and incise the pancreas with a scalpel.

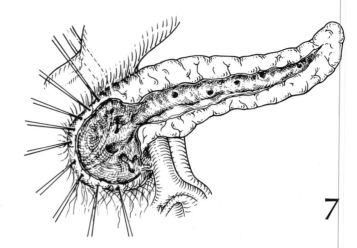

7

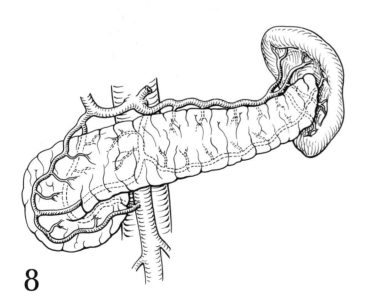

8

8 The arterial circulation is normally so disposed that there are no major vessels running on the anterior surface of the pancreas until the pancreaticoduodenal arcade is reached.

Occasionally the gastroduodenal artery gives off a significant branch to the transverse colon but this can usually be sacrificed with impunity given the collateral supply. If there is any doubt, the vessel can be occluded temporarily with a bulldog clamp while the mesocolon and greater omentum are inspected for pulsation. Bleeding points encountered while the duct system is being opened are best dealt with by suture-ligation and excessive diathermy should be avoided.

9a, b A Roux loop of jejunum is now prepared, dividing the arterial arcade, mesentery and jejunum at a convenient point in the proximal small bowel. A linear stapler allows the jejunum to be divided quickly, but the staple line is not haemostatic and it is advisable to oversew the transected distal staple line with a continuous 3/0 resorbable suture of polydioxanone (PDS). A window is now created in the transverse mesocolon and the distal end of the jejunum is passed through into the lesser sac.

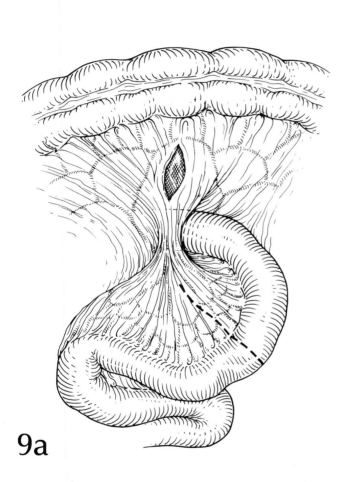

9a

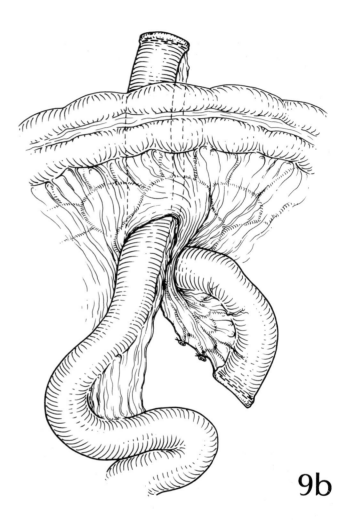

9b

10 The Roux loop is orientated so that its blind end is placed on the tail of the pancreas. This is usually the most 'comfortable' way for the jejunum to lie, and has the added advantage that more jejunum can be brought through the window in the mesocolon if biliary bypass is also needed.

Some surgeons have used 'triple bypass' in which the jejunal loop is used for anastomosis to the pancreas, biliary system and stomach. In the authors' view, patients who might be considered for triple bypass usually have such severe disease in the head of the pancreas that they are better served by resection of the head of the pancreas with formal restoration of pancreatico-enteric, biliary-enteric and gastro-enteric continuity. In patients with a communicating pseudo-cyst, the Roux loop can be used to drain the pseudocyst as well as the pancreatic duct.

Classical descriptions of longitudinal side-to-side pancreaticojejunostomy usually employed two layers of sutures for the anastomosis, but one layer of interrupted 2/0 or 3/0 delayed resorbable sutures is sufficient.

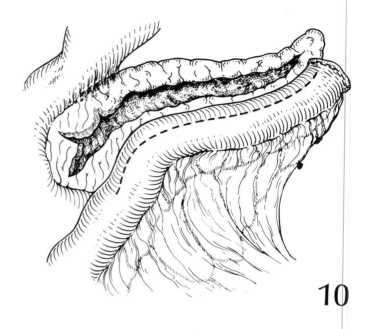

10

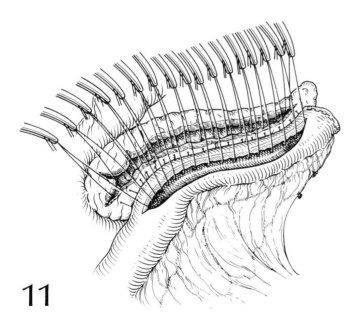

11

11 The jejunum is incised longitudinally along its antimesenteric border over a length equal to that of the pancreatic incision. The interrupted sutures are first inserted to create the inferior border of the anastomosis and it is often simpler to insert the entire layer before beginning to tie them. The sutures pick up the entire thickness of the jejunum and are inserted so that the knots will be on the inside of the anastomosis.

One school of thought holds that the pancreatic sutures should not be inserted so that they pass into the lumen in case they occlude side branches of the pancreatic duct system. However, the authors' usual practice is to create a mucosa-to-mucosa anastomosis, taking care not to occlude obvious side branches of the duct during suture insertion. The pancreatic tissue in chronic pancreatitis is usually much more fibrous than normal and is not friable. Once the sutures forming the inferior margin of the anastomosis have all been inserted and tied, they are cut short, retaining the two end sutures as stays.

12 The superior margin of the anastomosis is then performed, the sutures being inserted so that the knots are on the outside of this part of the anastomosis. It is good practice to insert the corner sutures first and to tie and retain them so that the stay sutures retained at the ends of the inferior margin can be cut. Once again it is usually easiest to insert all of the sutures and then to tie them, rather than tie each suture once it has been inserted.

Access is usually good but, on occasions, it is simpler to insert the superior row of sutures into the upper margin of the pancreatic incision, retaining their needles before commencing the inferior margin of the anastomosis. If this manoeuvre is adopted, the superior margin of the anastomosis is completed by picking up the jejunum as the final step.

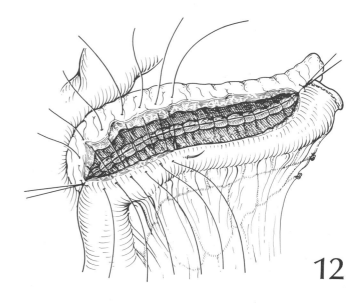

12

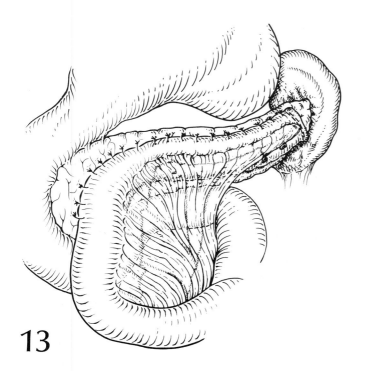

13

13 Whichever technique is adopted, the completed anastomosis should lie without tension in the lesser sac, and there should be no kinks in the Roux loop. One or two 'tacking' sutures can be inserted between the Roux loop and anterior surface of the pancreas to ensure that there are no kinks.

14 Intestinal continuity is now restored beneath the mesocolon by an end-to-side anastomosis between the cut proximal end of the jejunum and the side of the Roux loop. A twin occlusion clamp such as a Lane's clamp is ideal for the purpose and the anastomosis is created using two layers of continuous 2/0 resorbable material such as polydioxanone (PDS). Whereas the length of Roux loop used in gastric and biliary surgery is critical to avoid biliary reflux into the stomach or reflux of intestinal content into the biliary system respectively, the length of Roux loop in pancreaticojejunostomy does not appear to be vital. In general, the entero-enteric anastomosis is created at the most convenient point after the Roux loop emerges from the mesocolon into the infracolic compartment. Once the anastomosis is complete, defects in the mesocolon and small bowel mesentery are closed with interrupted sutures inserted carefully to avoid damaging blood vessels. If biliary enteric bypass is also to be performed, the anastomosis is created at this stage using one layer of interrupted 3/0 resorbable sutures to anastomose the side of the opened bile duct or the cut end of the transected bile duct to the side of the jejunum as it bends inferiorly from the pancreatico-jejunal anastomosis.

Haemostasis is checked and the abdomen is normally closed without drainage.

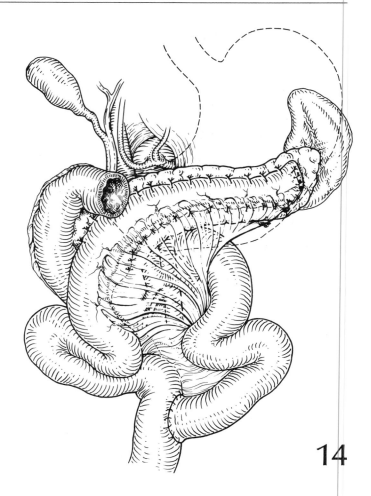

14

Outcome

Longitudinal pancreaticojejunostomy is a safe procedure which should carry no operative mortality and minimal morbidity. Patients must not be encouraged to believe that the operation will banish all of the problems associated with chronic pancreatitis, and a reasonable guideline is that about 70% of patients are pain-free or significantly improved when assessed 5 years after the operation. The procedure may prevent or defer the onset of troublesome exocrine pancreatic insufficiency and insulin-dependent diabetes, but cannot be expected to reverse existing insufficiencies. Much depends on the adequacy of drainage of the pancreatic duct system, on continuing wide patency of the anastomosis, and in the case of patients with alcoholic chronic pancreatitis, whether they abstain from alcohol consumption. Recurrence of pain is an indication to carry out ERCP and computed tomographic scanning to reassess the pancreas. In some cases it may be worthwhile attempting to provide more effective pancreatic drainage if the original pancreaticojejunostomy has been inadequate, and consideration should also be given to the Frey procedure as a means of eradicating ongoing inflammation in the head of the pancreas without exposing the patient to the risks and consequences of formal resection. However, many patients who experience major difficulties with pain after pancreatico-jejunostomy become candidates for some form of partial, subtotal or total pancreatectomy.

ENDOSCOPIC DRAINAGE OF THE PANCREATIC DUCT

Endoscopic retrograde cholangiopancreatography (ERCP) and endoscopic ultrasonography now have a defined role in the investigation of pancreatic disease. Endoscopic sphincterotomy and stone retrieval are used widely to deal with choledocholithiasis, and endoscopic biliary stenting has an established place in the management of malignant low bile duct obstruction. However, the role of therapeutic endoscopic techniques in the management of chronic pancreatitis and its complications is much less clear. While it is technically possible to perform a wide range of procedures endoscopically, the results are often imperfect and these approaches should only be undertaken after full consideration of other options, and in centres with a full range of facilities and experience in imaging and pancreatic surgery.

Indications

(1) Patients with painful chronic pancreatitis with calculi or a stricture obstructing the main duct can be considered for endoscopic therapy with pancreatic sphincterotomy, stone extraction (with or without extracorporeal lithotripsy) and stent insertion (see below). A chronic pancreatic fistula or pseudocyst which persists because of a distal duct stricture can often be dealt with by endoscopic stenting of the stricture, although the procedure is often technically demanding, particularly if the duct system is disrupted and a guidewire cannot be passed readily through the narrowed area.

(2) Pseudocysts complicating chronic pancreatitis can be dealt with endoscopically, but only after the relative merits of the approach have been compared with those of conventional surgery or percutaneous drainage techniques. Large pseudocysts indenting the stomach or duodenum can be drained directly into the lumen of the gastrointestinal tract using a diathermy 'needle knife' followed by insertion of a double pigtail stent.

(3) Gastric varices which develop following splenic vein thrombosis can be dealt with endoscopically by injection of thrombin to stop bleeding or prevent rebleeding, although splenectomy and interruption of the short gastric vessels is often still needed for definitive treatment of this problem.

(4) Obstruction of the bile duct from chronic pancreatitis may be dealt with by endoscopic stenting as a temporary expedient but surgery is usually needed for definitive management.

(5) Pancreas divisum has been dealt with on occasions by endoscopic stenting or sphincterotomy of the accessory ampulla in patients troubled by persistent pain and recurrent attacks of pancreatic inflammation. The results of treatment are unpredictable and are often poor; patients with dilatation and slow emptying of the dorsal pancreatic duct are most likely to derive benefit from this approach. Even if long-term relief of symptoms is not afforded, the endoscopic approach at least allows rational decisions to be made regarding the likelihood of success following surgical attempts to improve duct drainage.

Technique

If therapeutic intervention is considered likely in patients undergoing diagnostic ERCP, the patient should receive prophylactic antibiotics, blood clotting is checked and blood is taken for grouping and cross-matching. ERP is first performed using standard technique and if endoscopic stenting of the pancreatic duct is indicated, pancreatic sphincterotomy is undertaken using a sphincterotome with a guidewire and following deep cannulation of the duct. The technique is identical to that used for biliary sphincterotomy, but the size of the opening created is more modest. It is sometimes difficult to insert the sphincterotome into the pancreas, and 'needle knife' sphincterotomy can be undertaken to facilitate its introduction (or, in some cases, to serve as a definitive procedure).

Balloon dilatation can be used as an alternative to minimize the risk of bleeding, to allow extraction of small calculi and to facilitate stent insertion. A Gruntzig type low profile balloon is inserted over a guidewire placed across the sphincter and dilated for 1–2 min to the pressures defined by the manufacturers. Overdilatation must be avoided as it can cause undue trauma and the development of severe pancreatitis.

If a sphincterotomy has been performed, calculi can be extracted using a conventional Dormia basket or occlusion balloons. In some cases, the small size of the pancreatic duct prevents these instruments passing beyond or capturing stones, and extracorporeal lithotripsy has been used in some centres to overcome this problem.

15 A hydrophilic catheter is next inserted deeply across the stricture. To achieve this it is first necessary to pass the guidewire through a stiff Teflon overtube and the assembly is then passed through the biopsy channel of the duodenoscope. The overtube is necessary to prevent kinking of the catheter in the duodenum. The stricture is intubated using a combination of guidewire insertion followed by forward movement of the overtube as the guidewire is slowly withdrawn. Once the guidewire is appropriately positioned the overtube is removed and a double barbed 3-Fr or 4-Fr plastic stent is railroaded across the stricture using the overtube as a 'pusher'. The objective is to leave the distal end of the stent protruding into the duodenum so that it can be removed easily if this becomes necessary.

Further reading

Carter DC. Surgical drainage procedures. In: Trede M, Carter DC, eds. *Surgery of the Pancreas*. Edinburgh: Churchill Livingstone, 1993; 309–19.

Ebbehoj N, Klaaborg KE, Kronberg O, Madsen P. Pancreaticogastrostomy for chronic pancreatitis. *Am J Surg* 1989; 157: 315–7.

Frey CF, Smith GJ. Description and rationale for a new operation for chronic pancreatitis. *Pancreas* 1987; 2: 701–5.

Prinz RA, Greenlee HB. Pancreatic duct drainage in 100 patients with chronic pancreatitis. *Ann Surg* 1981; 194: 313–20.

Prinz RA, Aranha GV, Greenlee HB. Redrainage of the pancreatic duct in chronic pancreatitis. *Am J Surg* 1986; 151: 150–6.

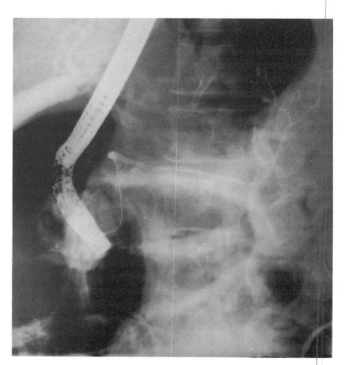

15

Chronic pancreatitis: Frey operation

Charles F. Frey MD, FACS
Professor, Department of Surgery, University of California, Davis Medical Center, Sacramento, California, USA

Hung S. Ho MD
Assistant Professor, Department of Surgery, University of California, Davis Medical Center, Sacramento, California, USA

History

It is believed that pain associated with chronic pancreatitis is caused by pancreatic ductal hypertension with activation of the stretch fibres in the duct wall as a result of obstruction, or neural and perineural inflammation. Some patients may have more than one cause of pain. Obstruction of the pancreatic ductal system may result from calcium carbonate calculi, single or multiple fibrotic strictures, or discontinuity of the main pancreatic duct. Attempts to decompress the pancreatic ductal system were initiated in 1883 and consisted of removal of calculi from the obstructed main pancreatic duct. The concept of enteric drainage of the main pancreatic duct was first advanced by DuVal and Zollinger who, in the mid 1950s, employed a technique of retrograde drainage of the main pancreatic duct, but this technique was only effective if the obstruction was at a single site between the pancreatic tail and the ampulla of Vater. Recognizing the fact that multiple sites of obstruction are the rule in chronic alcoholic pancreatitis, the longitudinal or side-to-side pancreaticojejunostomy was proposed by Puestow and Gillesby. This procedure was further refined to avoid distal pancreatectomy and splenectomy by Partington and Rochelle. Recently, evidence has been reported that decompression of ductal hypertension may prevent further loss in pancreatic endocrine and exocrine function[1].

Principles and justification

The ideal surgical procedure for chronic pancreatitis and its complications is still to be defined. It should be simple to perform, have low mortality and morbidity, provide long-lasting pain relief and resolve complications caused by pancreatitis, and yet preserve both pancreatic endocrine and exocrine reserve.

While longitudinal pancreaticojejunostomy does provide good immediate pain relief in 80% of patients, the long-term result is poor with only 54% still free of pain at 5 years. Failure of longitudinal pancreaticojejunostomy to provide long-lasting pain relief may result from technical failure to perform the operation as designed (i.e. carrying the opening of the duct of Wirsung to the duodenum) or from failure of the design of the operation. Longitudinal pancreaticojejunostomy does not provide adequate drainage of the duct of Wirsung if the pancreatic head is markedly enlarged. Under these circumstances, simply opening the duct from the anterior surface of the pancreas will not adequately decompress the proximal duct. For example, if the head is 5 cm thick and the distance from the duodenum to the main pancreatic duct where the duct courses posteriorly and inferiorly is 3 cm, then there is at least a 6-cm segment of proximal duct in a deep narrow crevice (see Illustration 2c). An even more serious deficiency of longitudinal pancreaticojejunostomy is the absence of any provision to decompress the duct of Santorini, the duct to the uncinate process, or the obstructed tributary ducts associated with the ducts of Wirsung and Santorini or the duct to the uncinate process.

Radical distal pancreatectomy (85–90% resection) does provide long-term pain relief but is associated with a high incidence of exocrine and endocrine insufficiency. The incidence of diabetes mellitus increases from 28% preoperatively to 72% postoperatively[2].

Pancreaticoduodenectomy provides excellent pain relief, especially when the disease is concentrated in the head of the pancreas and the main pancreatic duct is small. It is technically challenging, however, with a higher mortality and morbidity rate than drainage procedures[3].

More recent operations proposed by Beger and Buchler[4], Warren et al.[5] and Frey and Amikura[6] aim at treating the large bulky pancreatic head where multiple cysts and impacted calculi may be present. Long-term results from the Beger and Frey operations are still awaited, but results at 3 and 4 years indicate marked improvement in pain relief in about 75% of patients. Follow-up data on the five patients originally reported by Warren et al. are not available.

Rationale of local resection of the head of the pancreas combined with longitudinal pancreaticojejunostomy

Local resection of the head of the pancreas combined with longitudinal pancreaticojejunostomy[6] was proposed to treat the patient with chronic pancreatitis and severe pain who has a multiply strictured main pancreatic duct, a markedly enlarged fibrotic pancreatic head and uncinate process impacted with calculi and small pseudocysts along the ducts of Santorini, Wirsung and their tributary ducts, as well as a dilated duct in the body and tail of the pancreas. However, any patient who is a candidate for longitudinal pancreaticojejunostomy may benefit from local resection of the head of the pancreas combined with longitudinal pancreaticojejunostomy due to the advantages associated with decompressing the duct of Santorini, the duct to the uncinate process and their tributary ducts. It is also useful for the treatment of patients with common bile duct or duodenal obstruction, or small pseudocysts unconnected to the main pancreatic duct. With the coring out of the head of the pancreas, diseased tissue is removed and the drainage of the pancreatic head improved. Removal of calculi is also facilitated and occult areas of necrosis debrided.

Preoperative

The status of the pancreas should be studied by abdominal computed tomographic scanning and endoscopic retrograde cholangiopancreaticography to define ductal and structural abnormalities. Selective mesenteric and coeliac angiographies with both arterial and venous phases are helpful in identifying abnormal vascular anatomy and conditions such as pseudoaneurysms and mesenteric, portal and splenic vein thrombosis which could alter the operative plan.

Total parenteral nutrition may be indicated in patients with weight loss of more than 20% of ideal weight. Biliary tract disease should be ruled out or addressed before any direct operative intervention on the pancreas itself. Elevated serum alkaline phosphatase and total bilirubin levels are indications of common bile duct stricture or obstruction.

In order to assess whether the patient has benefited from the operation when it is performed to relieve pain it is essential that pain is assessed both before and after surgery. The authors recommend the use of a pain scale in which 0 = no pain and 10 = the worst pain imaginable, assessed by the patient. Minimal pain is defined as < 2 on the pain scale. Narcotic intake is categorized as follows: minimal, 500 mg paracetamol (acetaminophen) equivalent required 1–2 days/month; moderate, paracetamol weekly/daily; and major, pethidine equivalent weekly/daily. Endocrine insufficiency is categorized as either requiring control by diet, oral hypoglycaemic agents or insulin.

Anaesthesia

A combination of general endotracheal and high epidural anaesthesia is ideal with the patient supine.

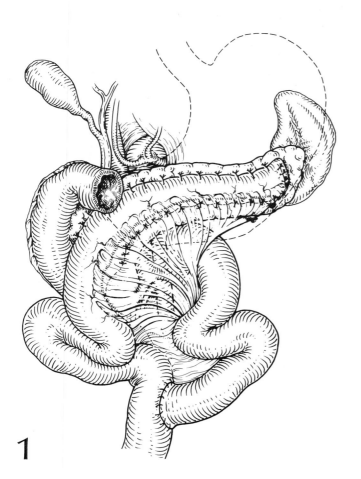

1

Operation

Incision and exploration

1 A bilateral subcostal incision is used to open the abdomen. Systematic exploration of the abdomen is carried out. The gallbladder is palpated for stones and the common bile duct palpated and inspected for choledocholithiasis and dilatation. The procedure consists of local resection of the head of the pancreas combined with a longitudinal pancreaticojejunostomy in the body and tail of the pancreas. An overview of the completed procedure is depicted.

Exposure of the head of the pancreas

2a–c An extended Kocher manoeuvre is performed. The hepatic flexure and right transverse colon are mobilized and retracted medially and downward. The duodenum and head of the pancreas are exposed. The peritoneum and areolar tissue lateral to the second and third portions of the duodenum are divided, allowing manual palpation on both sides of the head of the pancreas. This step is important in determining the extent of the local resection later. The gastroduodenal artery should also be identified at this time, as it may need to be ligated for haemostasis. At this stage the rationale for the procedure is appreciated as the extent of fibrosis within the head of the pancreas is palpated.

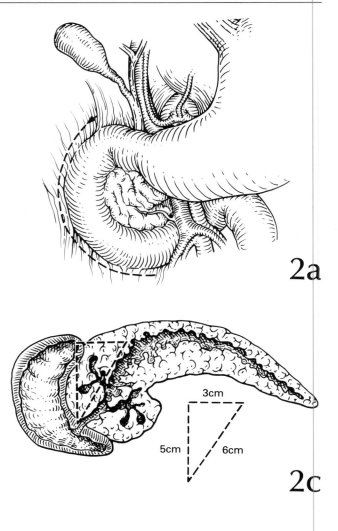

2a

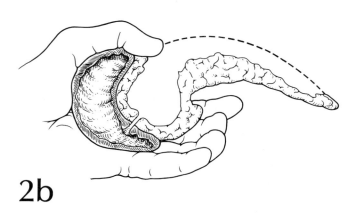

2b

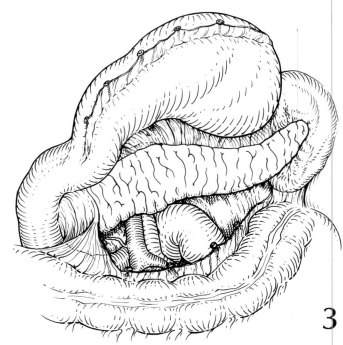

2c

Exposure of the body and tail of the pancreas

3 The gastrocolic ligament is divided, allowing entrance to the lesser sac. Lysis of adhesions may be required to separate the posterior aspect of the stomach from the anterior surface of the pancreas. With the stomach retracted superiorly and the transverse colon retracted downward, the body and tail of the pancreas are clearly exposed. The portal vein above and the superior mesenteric vein below the pancreas are identified and kept under direct vision. This is a very important step in preparation for local resection (coring out) of the head of the pancreas in order to avoid injury to these structures.

3

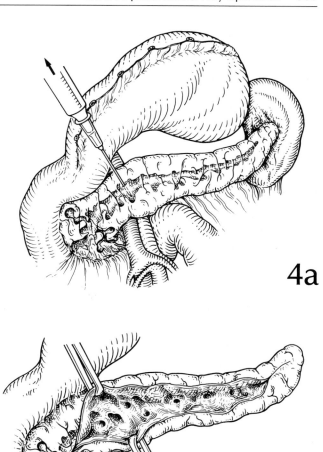

4a

Palpation, measurement of ductal pressure and opening of the main pancreatic duct

4a, b The body and tail are palpated and the dilated pancreatic duct is located. Ductal pressure is recorded using a 21-gauge guide needle and a manometer. Normal pressure is 8–12 cmH$_2$O. In the authors' experience the average pressure in patients with chronic pancreatitis is 32 cmH$_2$O with a range of 20–47 cmH$_2$O. The capsule of the pancreas is incised directly over the guide needle. Haemostasis is achieved with electrocoagulation or fine suture. The entire distal duct is opened and impacted calculi are removed.

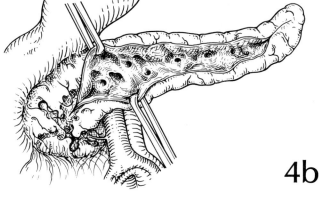

4b

Coring out the pancreatic head and uncinate process

5 Absorbable 3/0 or 2/0 sutures are placed along the inner aspect of the duodenum, on the pancreas and 3–4 mm from the border between the pancreas and duodenum for haemostasis. Attempts should be made to preserve the anterior pancreaticoduodenal arcade. The head of the pancreas is cored out with electrocoagulation and sharp dissection. A rim of pancreatic tissue is preserved along the inner aspect of the duodenum laterally. Medially, a margin of at least 5 mm of pancreatic tissue to the right of the portal vein and superior mesenteric vein is preserved to avoid vascular injury. Care is taken not to injure the common bile duct. A short segment of pancreatic duct extending to the ampulla of Vater will remain. This should be inspected and impacted calculi should be removed. A probe should pass freely into the duodenum. In patients with biochemical and anatomical evidence of intrapancreatic common bile duct obstruction, it is necessary to free the intrapancreatic portion of the common bile duct from the overlying fibrotic pancreas. In order to do this safely without injury to the bile duct, a choledochotomy should be performed and a Bake's dilator passed toward the ampulla of Vater so that the position of the common bile duct can be ascertained. The coring out process then proceeds and the fibrotic tissue around the common bile duct is completely released.

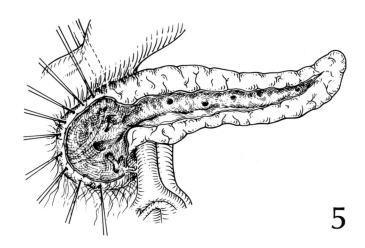

5

Preparation of the Roux loop

6a, b The Roux loop is fashioned based on the jejunal primary, secondary and tertiary vascular arcades. The site should be selected distal (about 15 cm) to the ligament of Treitz, and care must be taken to assure good blood supply and no tension after the loop is placed in the lesser sac through an opening in the transverse mesocolon, to the left of the middle colic vessels.

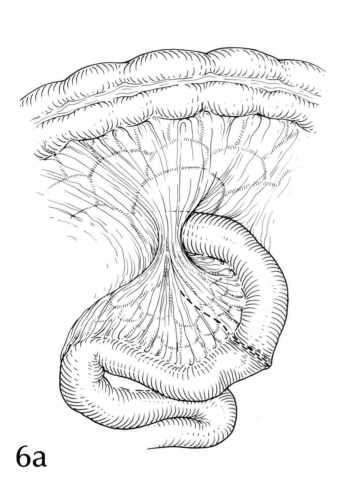

6a

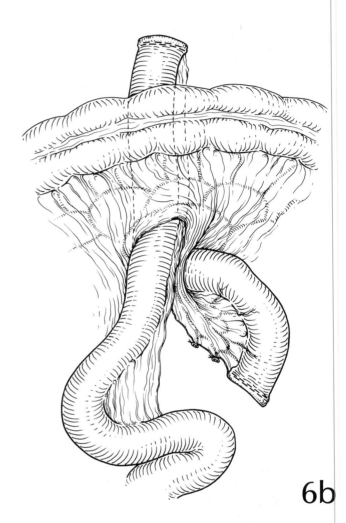

6b

Pancreaticojejunostomy

7 The jejunum is attached along the opened pancreatic duct with interrupted 3/0 silk sutures, fixing the serosa of the jejunum to the lower edge of the pancreas. The jejunum is then opened along the dotted line. An inner layer of running 4/0 polydioxanone (PDS) sutures attaches the cut edges of the open pancreatic duct to the jejunum, extending all the way around the cored out head of the pancreas. A mucosa-to-mucosa anastomosis is not necessary. It is important to have adequate purchase of the pancreatic capsule.

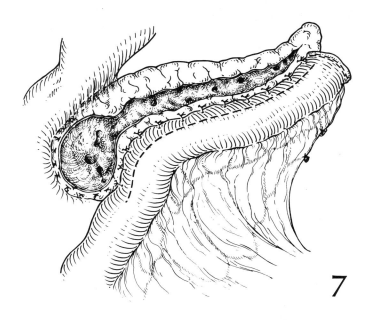

7

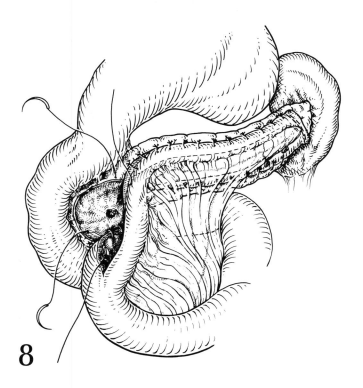

8

Completion of pancreaticojejunostomy

8 The upper edges of the open pancreatic duct and jejunum are attached in a similar two-layer closure.

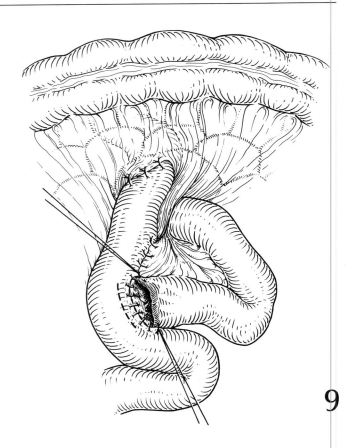

Restoration of gastrointestinal continuity

9 The jejunojejunostomy is completed in an end-to-side fashion with an inner layer of absorbable 4/0 polydioxanone sutures and an outer layer of silk.

Postoperative care

Patients are routinely managed in the intensive care unit for the first 2–3 days after surgery, where haemodynamics, fluid balance, serum glucose levels and drain amylase output and volume are closely monitored. High levels of drain amylase are an indication of a leak at the site of the pancreaticojejunostomy. Should sepsis develop, early re-exploration is indicated to provide additional drainage. Intraoperative and postoperative use of octreotide has been shown to reduce these complications. Drains are removed once there is no evidence of pancreatic leakage or fistula. In the authors' experience the average postoperative length of stay in hospital is 14 days (range 7–40 days)[6].

Outcome

The operation has been performed on 60 patients by Frey and results of pain relief have been reported for the first 50 patients[6]. The perioperative mortality was zero. There was a 10% late death rate from 6 to 91 months, most of which were related to alcoholic hepatopathy. Pain relief was excellent in 75% of patients and improved in 13%. Worsening of diabetes was experienced by 10% of patients. There were no gross changes in exocrine function; 64% of patients gained weight. Although only 32% returned to work, most of them had not been working for 4–5 years before their operation.

References

1. Nealon WH, Thompson JS. Progressive loss of pancreatic function in chronic pancreatitis is delayed by main duct decompression. A longitudinal prospective analysis of the modified Puestow procedure. *Ann Surg* 1993; 217: 458–68

2. Prinz RA, Greenlee HB. Pancreatic duct drainage in chronic pancreatitis. *Hepatogastroenterology* 1990; 37: 295–300.

3. Gall FP, Zirngibl H, Gebhardt C, Schneider MV. Duodenal pancreatectomy with occlusion of the pancreatic duct. *Hepatogastroenterology* 1990; 37: 290–4.

4. Beger HG, Buchler M. Duodenum-preserving resection of the head of the pancreas in chronic pancreatitis with inflammatory mass in the head. *World J Surg* 1990; 14: 83–7.

5. Warren WD, Milliken WJ Jr, Henderson JM, Hersh T. A denervated pancreatic flap for control of chronic pain in pancreatitis. *Surg Gynecol Obstet* 1984; 159: 581–3.

6. Frey CF, Amikura K. Local resection of the head of the pancreas combined with longitudinal pancreaticojejunostomy in the management of patients with chronic pancreatitis. *Ann Surg* 1994; 220: 492–507.

Illustrations by Gillian Oliver

Chronic pancreatitis: distal pancreatectomy

R. C. G. Russell MS, FRCS
Consultant Surgeon, The Middlesex Hospital, London, UK

Principles and justification

All who undertake a distal pancreatectomy for benign disease must ask themselves if they are undertaking the right operation. So often the manifestations of the disease may be most obvious in the body and tail of the pancreas, but the cause of these manifestations lies in the head of the pancreas. In other words, much of the problem in the body of the pancreas is related to obstruction of the duct and, if that obstruction lies in the head or ampulla, a distal pancreatectomy will not resolve the situation. The common indication for resection of the body and tail of the pancreas is disruption of the duct at the neck of the pancreas due to trauma or an episode of severe acute pancreatitis with or without cyst formation. Occasionally, it is associated with duct strictures secondary to chronic pancreatitis, but this is rare and more usually the whole of the pancreas is involved.

Preoperative

Preoperative investigation

The essential investigation is contrast enhanced computed tomographic scanning using a spiral scanner to obtain good views of the arterial and venous phases. It is appropriate to undertake endoscopic retrograde cholangiopancreatography (ERCP) to ensure that the papilla is normal and the head of the pancreas has a normal duct system. The objective is to select patients who have a normal head of pancreas with disease confined to the body and tail of the pancreas. A Puestow-type procedure is not appropriate in these patients as the duct in the head of the gland is normal.

1a, b The ERCP shows a normal duct system in the head of the pancreas with complete obstruction at the level of the neck of the pancreas. There is no calcification in the head of the pancreas.

The computed tomographic scan confirms the presence of a normal pancreatic head with disease in the body and tail of the pancreas. In the scan shown in *Illustration 1b* there is complete transection at the level of the neck giving rise to a cyst and a dilated duct in the tail of the pancreas.

Preoperative preparation

Distal pancreatectomy for chronic pancreatitis is a major operation and, indeed, the procedure can be technically more demanding than a pancreato-duodenectomy because of the increased number of adhesions encountered which may result in a much greater blood loss. It is therefore appropriate to approach this operation circumspectly and, if there is much inflammation and the patient is in pain from that inflammation, a period of pancreatic rest with parenteral nutrition and nil orally can enable the inflammation to resolve and ease the operative procedure.

The immediate concern is to ensure that the patient is fit for surgery with a stable cardiovascular system, and is well hydrated with an infusion commenced the evening before the operation. The patient is catheterized and given preoperative antibiotics and thromboembolic prophylaxis with subcutaneous heparin and TED stockings. Because infection is a problem in these patients, invasive monitoring is avoided apart from an arterial line.

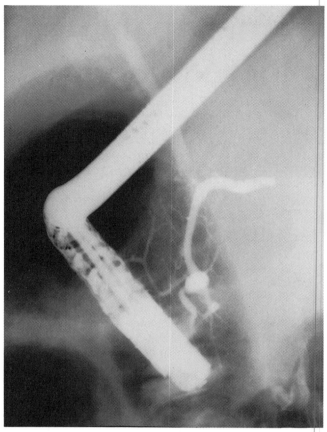

1a

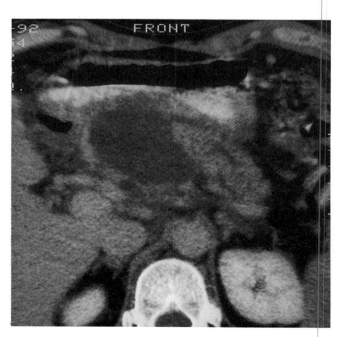

1b

Operation

There is a series of defined steps in this procedure which do much to ease the performance of the operation. First, the lesser sac is opened, then the splenic artery is tied near the coeliac axis, the short gastric arteries are tied, the colon is separated from the spleen and the mesocolon from the body of the pancreas, and finally the spleen is mobilized with the tail of the pancreas. There is a vogue for splenic-preserving pancreatectomy but this is more suited to resection of benign tumours because the spleen is often intimately involved in the inflammatory process in chronic pancreatitis.

Incision

A straight transverse incision is suitable, starting at the tip of the 12th rib and extending to the right as far as is required. A bilateral subcostal or midline incision can be used, but the advantages of one over the other are minimal. After opening the abdomen a full laparotomy is performed to assess the extent of the disease.

Exposure of the pancreas

2   The body of the pancreas is best exposed by mobilizing the omentum from the greater curve of the stomach within the epiploic arch, and displacing the omentum and the colon with its mesocolon inferiorly away from the front of the pancreas.

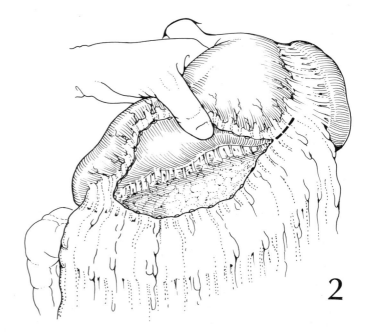

2

Divison of the gastrosplenic ligament

3 The dissection is continued up the greater curve, dividing the short gastric vessels near the stomach up to the uppermost short gastric artery level with the upper pole of the spleen, which should then fall away from the stomach with division of adhesions between the posterior wall of the stomach and pancreas.

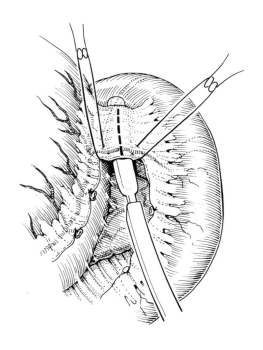

3

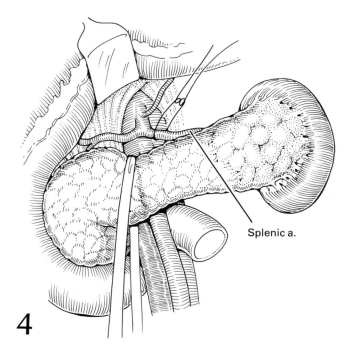

Splenic a.

4

Ligation of the splenic artery

4 Using a stabilized ring retractor (Buchwalter) the stomach is retracted superiorly and the colon displaced downwards. The borders of the pancreas are defined from tail to neck above and below the pancreas. Attention is next turned to the trifurcation of the coeliac axis at the upper border of the neck of the pancreas. The hepatic artery is identified and freed from the superior margin of the pancreas. This artery is then followed towards the left until it merges with the splenic artery at its origin from the coeliac axis. The splenic artery is now tied to reduce the vascularity of the organs to be removed. As this dissection proceeds the upper border of the neck of the pancreas is displayed with the portal vein beneath. A little time spent dissecting the portal vein from the neck of the pancreas will be advantageous later in the operation. A tape is passed around the neck of the pancreas.

Mobilization of the splenic flexure

5 The left gastroepiploic artery is traced down to the hilum of the spleen and there ligated. The remaining part of the omentum between the splenic hilum and the colon is divided, and the peritoneum which tethers the splenic flexure to the splenic hilum, the front of the kidney and the paracolic gutter is divided to enable the splenic flexure and its mesentery to be mobilized inferiorly. This enables the inferior border of the pancreas to be further exposed.

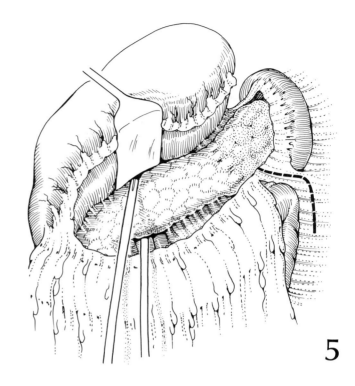

5

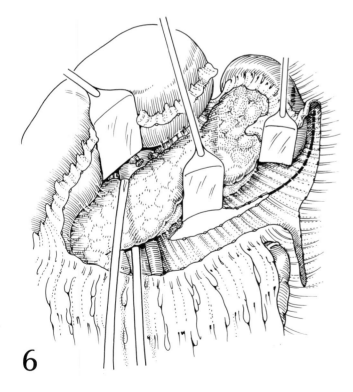

6

Mobilization of the spleen

6 The dissection of the inferior border of the pancreas is continued and extended beneath the pancreas where there is often an avascular plane, uninvolved by the inflammation of the pancreatitis. The plane is developed and extended laterally beneath the spleen where the lienorenal and lienophrenic ligaments are divided, so mobilizing the spleen upwards and anteriorly away from the posterior abdominal wall.

Dislocation of the spleen

7 In chronic pancreatitis there is often severe inflammatory change around the spleen. Careless hand mobilization of the spleen can cause much blood loss. This can be avoided by carefully dissecting the spleen away from the diaphragm with meticulous attention to haemostasis. The spleen so mobilized is now free from the diaphragm and can be dislocated to the right, enabling the plane of dissection developed posteriorly to be extended to the upper border of the pancreas. At the upper border of the pancreas care should be taken to avoid the adrenal gland which can be involved in the inflammatory process.

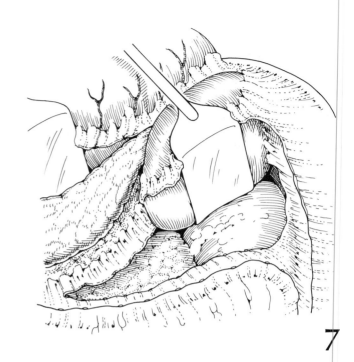

7

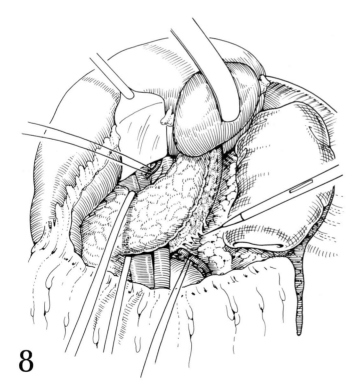

8

Dissection of the body of the pancreas

8 With the spleen and tail of the pancreas mobilized, care is required to dissect the body of the pancreas away from the posterior abdominal wall, avoiding deep dissection with damage to the renal vein and adhering closely to the posterior surface of the pancreas. Inferiorly, the inferior mesenteric vein should be avoided or tied if it joins the splenic vein, and superiorly the left gastric vein is tied and the coeliac axis avoided. As the dissection extends to the right, the position of the tape on the neck of the pancreas should be watched. To aid haemostasis, packing of the large exposed raw area reduces blood loss.

Control of the splenic vein

9 With the pancreas and spleen fully mobilized and brought over to the right side of the patient, the splenic vein is dissected onto the portal vein. With the tape around the neck of the pancreas as a guide, the splenic vein can be dissected, clamped and oversewn with 4/0 polypropylene (Prolene) on the portal vein.

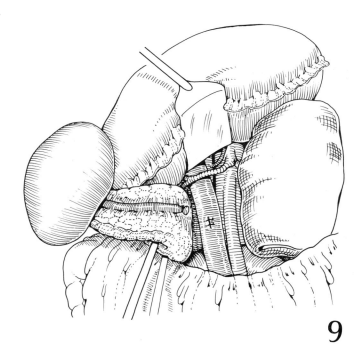

9

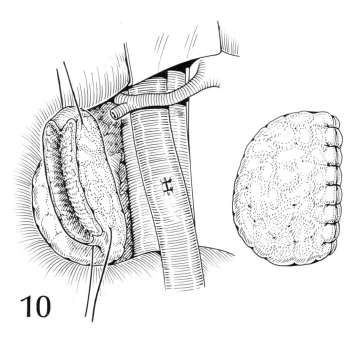

10

Division of the pancreas

10 The pancreas is now attached to the head by a narrow neck of tissue, which is divided cleanly with a knife with the head side controlled with stay sutures. Bleeding is controlled by sutures. The duct is carefully identified and closed with 4/0 polypropylene sutures. There is no advantage in draining the duct into a Roux loop. The pancreas is carefully closed with interrupted 2/0 sutures. Occasionally this closure is made easier by cutting with a 'fish mouth', but this can make the duct more difficult to find.

Closure

Careful haemostasis is essential before closure. A single closed tube drain is passed down to the bed of the pancreas and the wound is closed by the preferred method.

Postoperative care

The patient is maintained on intravenous infusion and nasogastric drainage until gastric emptying resumes a normal pattern. Occasionally gastric stasis may be prolonged, but it always resolves and patience is all that is required. The main complication of this operation is sepsis, either in the pancreatic bed or a left lower lobe atelectasis with secondary infection. Both resolve with conservative management. A fistula from the pancreatic duct is uncommon.

Approximately 70% of the pancreas has been removed, and as a consequence diabetes mellitus will occur in one-third of patients. Similarly, enzyme deficiency may be present requiring treatment by enzyme replacement therapy.

The overall mortality of this procedure should be 1–2%, and the morbidity 30% at most. Approximately 80% of patients have a good long-term result. The outcome in the remainder depends to a large degree on the success of the removal of the underlying cause of the chronic pancreatitis.

Further reading

Aldridge MC, Williamson RC. Distal pancreatectomy with and without splenectomy. *Br J Surg* 1991; 78: 976–9.

Geghardt C. Left resection in chronic pancreatitis. In: Beger H, Büchler M, Malfertheiner P, eds. *Standards in Pancreatic Surgery*. Berlin: Springer-Verlag, 1993: 392–5.

Konishi T, Hiraishi M, Kubota K, Bandai Y, Makuuchi M, Idezuki Y. Segmental occlusion of the pancreatic duct with prolamine to prevent fistula formation after distal pancreatectomy. *Ann Surg* 1995; 221: 165–70.

Sawyer R, Frey CF. Is there still a role for distal pancreatectomy in surgery for chronic pancreatitis? *Am J Surg* 1994; 168: 6–9.

Shankar S, Theis B, Russell RC. Management of the stump of the pancreas after distal pancreatic resection. *Br J Surg* 1990; 77: 541–4.

Warshaw AL. Conservation of the spleen with distal pancreatectomy. *Arch Surg* 1988; 123: 550–3.

Chronic pancreatitis: pancreaticoduodenectomy – conventional operation

David C. Carter MD, FRCS(Ed), FRCS(Glas), FRCS, FRSE
Regius Professor of Clinical Surgery, Royal Infirmary, Edinburgh, UK

History

Originally used in the treatment of pancreatic and periampullary neoplasia, the Whipple operation of pancreaticoduodenectomy has been used extensively as one form of surgical treatment of chronic pancreatitis. The Italian surgeon, Alessandro Codivilla, is credited with having performed the first pancreatico-duodenectomy in 1898 for a patient with a lesion in the head of the pancreas. Codivilla resected the duodenum, pylorus and head of pancreas, closed the duodenal stump and performed a gastrojejunostomy-en-Y, and then carried out a cholecystojejunostomy after ligating the divided bile duct. His patient survived for only 24 days. In 1909, Kausch in Berlin performed a successful staged pancreaticoduodenectomy in a patient with periampullary tumour who survived for 9 months. Whereas Kausch had attempted to restore pancreatico-intestinal continuity, Whipple and colleagues in New York ligated the main pancreatic duct as part of their two-stage pancreaticoduodenectomy for cancer of the periampullary region, an operation described in 1935. Brunschwig was probably the first to use the operation successfully for carcinoma of the head of the pancreas in 1937, but it was not until 1940 that the operation was accomplished as a one-stage procedure. Although normally known as the Whipple operation, it is clear that pancreaticoduodenectomy was performed many years earlier than the description published by Whipple and colleagues.

Principles and justification

Indications

Pancreaticoduodenectomy may be employed in patients with chronic pancreatitis when the disease is maximal in the head of the gland and the pancreatic duct system is not sufficiently dilated for pancreaticojejunostomy (*see* page 488). Pain which cannot be controlled by other means is the major indication for the operation, but other factors include the inability to exclude cancer in the head of the pancreas, biliary tract obstruction, duodenal obstruction and the presence of cysts or vascular complications such as pseudoaneurysm formation and haemorrhage. The Whipple operation entails *en bloc* resection of the head and neck of the pancreas, duodenum, pylorus and distal half of the stomach, gallbladder and common bile duct. Variants include pylorus-preserving pancreaticoduodenectomy (page 528), duodenum-preserving resection of the pancreatic head (page 544) and the Frey operation (page 497).

As in all areas of surgery, operative morbidity and mortality are influenced by patient selection, patient preparation, standards of perioperative care, and the skill and experience of the surgeon. Whereas Whipple's operation once carried an overall operative mortality rate of over 20%, a number of specialist centres now report large series of patients with operative mortality rates ranging between zero and low single figures. As a rough guide, approximately 70% of patients are pain-free or significantly relieved of pain when assessed 5 years after the operation, but the patient must understand that freedom from pain is by no means guaranteed. The risk of developing insulin-dependent diabetes mellitus and significant exocrine insufficiency is increased by any form of pancreatic resection, and in patients with alcohol-associated disease the long-term outlook depends greatly on whether the patient is able to abstain from alcohol.

Preoperative

It is assumed that appropriate investigations such as ultrasonography, elective retrograde cholangiopancreatography (ERCP), and computed tomographic (CT) scanning will have been undertaken to define the nature and extent of the patient's disease and to help to determine the choice of surgical procedure. While percutaneous fine needle aspiration or Tru-Cut biopsy can provide cytological or histological confirmation of the nature of a mass in the pancreatic head before surgery is undertaken, there is a growing tendency to use percutaneous sampling only in patients with presumed pancreatic cancer in whom surgery appears inappropriate and who will be treated by non-surgical means such as endoscopic stenting. When dealing with chronic pancreatitis, it is frequently difficult to exclude pancreatic cancer by radiological means, and it is often impossible to be confident that a tissue sample obtained percutaneously is truly representative. In other words, a negative biopsy or aspirate does not exclude cancer and resection of the head of the pancreas may both resolve the diagnostic dilemma and effectively treat the patient's problems.

Angiography was once regarded as a valuable means of detecting vascular anomalies likely to affect the course of resection. While significant vascular anomalies such as origin of the right hepatic or common hepatic artery from the superior mesenteric artery are present in up to one-third of patients (*see* page 450), such lesions are usually apparent at operation and appropriate care can be taken not to interrupt the arterial supply to the liver. For example, an anomalous right hepatic artery originating from the superior mesenteric artery usually courses behind or to the right of the common bile duct and arterial pulsation in these areas should immediately arouse suspicion. Furthermore, intraoperative ultrasonography now allows vascular anatomy to be defined at operation.

In all patients being considered for major pancreatic surgery, routine haematological and biochemical investigations are necessary to detect anaemia, coagulation abnormalities, and to monitor hepatic and renal function. Obstructive jaundice may complicate inflammation in the pancreatic head and can cause malabsorption of fats and fat-soluble vitamins. Lack of absorption of vitamin K is a potential cause of coagulopathy due to inadequate production of prothrombin by the liver. This abnormality is usually readily correctable by daily intramuscular injection of vitamin K_1 (10 mg), but more complex clotting abnormalities occasionally require fresh frozen plasma or provision of specific clotting factors and platelets. Jaundiced patients may benefit from a period of preoperative biliary drainage following endoscopic stenting of the obstructed biliary tree. Any diabetes mellitus must be stabilized by appropriate means including prescription of insulin if necessary before surgery.

Prophylactic antibiotics are commenced just before operation and the importance of adequate hydration before, during and after operation cannot be over-emphasized in jaundiced patients (*see* page 262).

Anaesthesia

A combination of light general anaesthesia and high epidural anaesthesia allows optimal operating conditions with profound muscle relaxation, minimal blood loss and effective postoperative analgesia.

Operation

Incision

1 The patient is placed supine on the operating table. A bilateral subcostal (roof top) or transverse incision provides ideal access but the right half of the incision is opened in the first instance to determine the need for further exposure. A vertical midline incision can also give adequate access in tall thin patients but, in general, transverse incisions are preferred both for access and ease of healing. The incision is extended laterally well beyond the lateral edge of the rectus sheath and the lower skin flap is retracted by suturing it to the anterior abdominal wall beneath the umbilicus. A fixed retraction system such as the Omnitract greatly eases the task of the assistant(s); alternatively, the costal margin(s) can be retracted by taping a broad-bladed Doyen's retractor to a vertical pole attached to the operating table so that the costal margin is drawn upwards and slightly forwards.

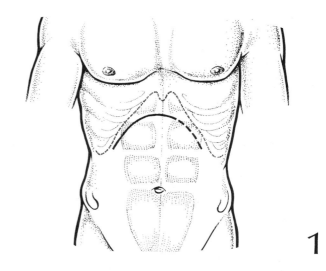

1

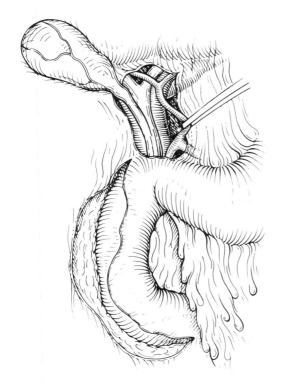

2

Mobilization of the head of the pancreas

2 Following systematic examination of the abdominal contents, any adhesions involving the gallbladder are divided. The peritoneum lateral to the descending duodenum, hepatic flexure and ascending colon is then incised with dissecting scissors so that the colon can be packed downwards out of the operative field. Small vessels running across the incision line are dealt with by diathermy. The right kidney, inferior vena cava and right gonadal vein are identified in the operating field and their integrity is carefully respected. The incision in the peritoneum can then be extended superiorly so that it runs on to the peritoneum covering the right side of the common bile duct. The opening into the lesser sac is often obliterated in chronic pancreatitis and care is exercised when developing the plane between the inferior vena cava and the common bile duct. Chronic pancreatitis typically produces peripancreatic inflammation and fibrosis which at every stage may make for greater difficulty in defining and opening tissue planes than is encountered when carrying out the Whipple resection for neoplasia.

3 The duodenum is then mobilized forwards and to the left (Kocher manoeuvre) and the dissection proceeds behind the pancreatic head and uncinate process until the aorta comes into view. This dissection plane is normally avascular and major vessels are not encountered. At this stage the fingers of the left hand can be passed behind the head of the pancreas so that it can be palpated between fingers and thumb.

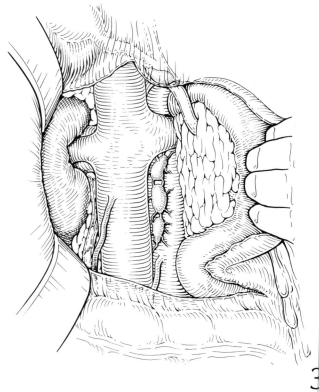

3

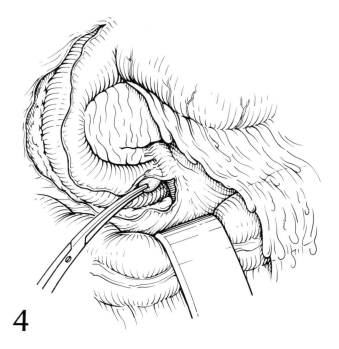

4

4 Attention is next turned to developing the plane between the front of the third part of the duodenum and transverse colon. A combination of sharp dissection (dissecting scissors) and blunt dissection (peanut swabs held in a pair of Mayo's forceps) is used to sweep the colon downwards, exposing first the front of the duodenum and then the right side of the superior mesenteric vein. If the planes are developing easily, the line of dissection can then continue upwards alongside the superior mesenteric vein as it passes upwards alongside the uncinate process. In some cases it is easier to leave this area for the moment and to open the lesser sac by dividing the gastrocolic omentum at a point near the junction of the antrum and body of the stomach.

5 Vessels within the omentum are divided between ligatures as one moves towards the pylorus; access to the lesser sac and front of the pancreas is improved if avascular adhesions between the pancreas and back of the stomach are divided with dissecting scissors. The back of the first part of the duodenum is also carefully cleared and at this point the gastroduodenal artery (or at least its anterior pancreaticoduodenal branch) comes into view. The right gastroepiploic vein is mobilized and divided as it courses downwards and backwards to join the superior mesenteric vein immediately before it disappears behind the neck of the pancreas. Veins in this region are friable and are best dealt with by using a Lahey forceps to pass fine ligatures around the vein, tying the ligatures and then cutting the vein with dissecting scissors. Ligaclips are best avoided as they may be dislodged during the subsequent dissection leading to troublesome venous bleeding which can soon emanate from the superior mesenteric vein or portal vein. Venous anatomy is also variable and the middle colic vein may be found passing to the gastroepiploic vein rather than entering the superior mesenteric vein directly.

Attention returns at this stage to clearing the bridge of tissue between the uncinate process and the superior mesenteric vein. This bridge contains a variable number of veins passing directly from the uncinate process into the vein and, once again, scrupulous care is needed to divide the veins between ligatures and to avoid major venous bleeding. As in all forms of pancreatic resection, it is sensible to have a vascular tray of instruments open and available at the start of the operation and to have a needle holder loaded with a 5/0 polypropylene (Prolene) suture so that any troublesome venous bleeding can be dealt with promptly by direct suture. Once these tributaries of the superior mesenteric vein have been dealt with, the anterior surface of the vein can be cleared as it passes behind the neck of the pancreas to become the portal vein. At this stage the temptation to develop the plane between the portal

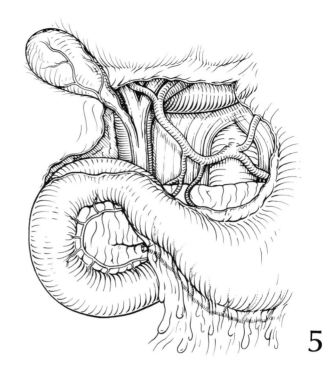

5

vein and neck of the pancreas should be resisted. Although the plane is normally avascular and older textbooks stressed the importance of defining it in cancer patients so as to be certain that the lesion was resectable, development of the plane serves little purpose at this point and it is much safer to leave the manoeuvre to a much later stage when it can be developed from above as well as from below. In some patients with chronic pancreatitis the plane is far from avascular or easy to develop, and major bleeding may only be controllable after the neck of pancreas has been divided.

Mobilization of the stomach

6 A window is now opened in the gastrohepatic omentum and the right gastric artery is doubly ligated and divided at the point where it leaves the common hepatic artery and passes to the upper border of the pylorus and antrum. The descending branches of the left gastric artery are next divided between ligatures at the level of the gastric incisura on the lesser curvature, and it is advisable to take this block of tissue in two sets of ligatures rather than to attempt to encircle too much tissue in one ligature which may slip. This manoeuvre clears a section of the lesser curve serosa at the anticipated point of division of the stomach.

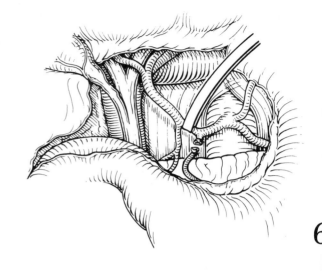

6

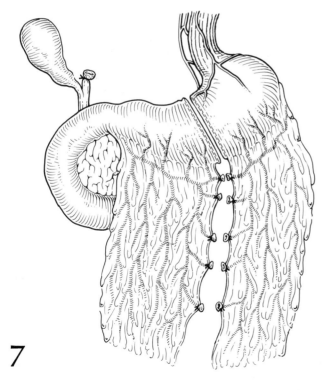

7

7 The point of division of the greater curvature is now also cleared by doubly ligating and dividing the gastroepiploic vessels at the junction of gastric corpus and antrum. The stomach is then divided using a linear stapler such as the TLC 75.

8 Division of the stomach allows the antrum and pylorus to be retracted to the right so that the gastroduodenal artery is brought into view. This vessel is cleared by a combination of sharp and blunt dissection so that it can be encircled by a ligature and divided as it descends from the common hepatic artery but before it reaches the pancreas. Attempts to divide this vessel on the front of the pancreas are inadvisable as, by this stage, the gastroduodenal artery has usually divided into its anterior and posterior superior pancreaticoduodenal arteries, and the vessel being divided may prove to be the anterior branch rather than the parent vessel. If there is any doubt about vascular anatomy, the common hepatic artery can be dissected for a short distance and the pulsation within the hepatic artery can be palpated while the gastroduodenal artery is temporarily occluded.

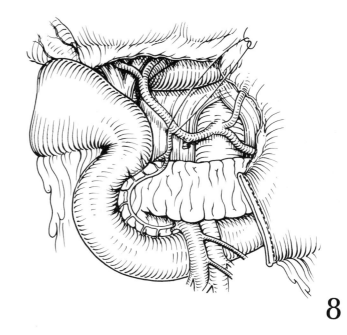

8

Mobilization of the gallbladder and bile ducts

9 The peritoneum between the common bile duct and hepatic artery is now cleared so that a plane can be developed around the common bile duct. Small vessels running to the common bile duct can usually be dealt with by diathermy but care is taken not to devascularize the common hepatic duct which will remain after the resection is complete. Vessels which appear too large to be dealt with by diathermy should be treated with respect as they are much more likely to represent anomalous branches of the hepatic artery and be destined to supply the liver rather than the bile ducts. Lahey forceps are useful when developing the plane around the bile duct and care must be taken not to injure the portal vein which normally lies behind the dissection plane. Small repeated manoeuvres are better than single forceful movements when developing this plane and it is often advisable to work alternately from the right and left side of the duct. In patients with a large bile duct and significant periductal inflammation, it may be easier and safer to open the duct formally and to dissect the opened duct from the tissues which surround it. If the bile duct is not opened during its mobilization, it is encircled by a loop which can then be used for retraction. Retraction of the common bile duct to the right exposes the front of the portal vein but a further fine fascial layer usually remains in front of the vein and has to be cleared at this stage or once the bile duct has been formally divided. Careful blunt dissection in front of the portal vein now begins to develop the plane between the vein and the back of the neck of pancreas. Once again, the temptation to fully develop the plane is best resisted at this stage in patients with

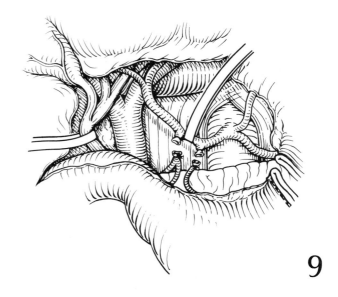

9

chronic pancreatitis. The gallbladder is now mobilized from its bed and removed after ligation and division of the cystic duct and artery. Some surgeons retain the gallbladder but, in the author's view, it is better removed given its potential for subsequent disease. Furthermore, the bilioenteric anastomosis is better created using a fully vascularized common hepatic duct than a common bile duct of marginal viability.

Mobilization of the duodenojejunal flexure

10 The proximal jejunum is now mobilized by dividing the peritoneal attachments on its lateral aspect as it leaves the duodenojejunal flexure. The inferior mesenteric vein is identified in the field of dissection and preserved. The fascial attachments which constitute the ligament of Treitz are next divided and, although largely avascular, they often contain a vessel or vessels which need to be divided between ligatures.

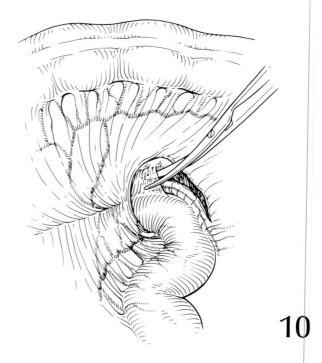

10

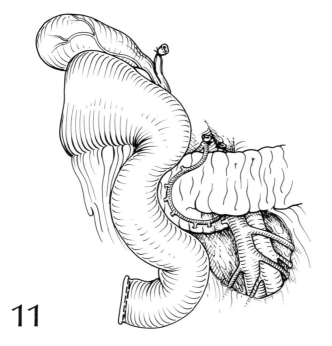

11

11 The short mesenteric vessels which supply the proximal 5 cm of jejunum are then divided between ligatures and it is safer to ligate them individually rather than run the risk of ties slipping following attempts to ligate too much tissue. Undue traction on the jejunum must also be avoided as it can cause ligatures to slip. It is not necessary to clear more than 5 cm of proximal jejunum before dividing the bowel with a linear stapler (TLC 55). Provided that the duodenojejunal flexure has been mobilized fully, it can then be drawn to the right behind the superior mesenteric vessels and into the main operating field.

Some surgeons do not mobilize the proximal jejunum at this stage, preferring to do this as the final stage in the resection. The author prefers to divide the jejunum early so that the dissection is complete before beginning to separate the pancreas from its retroperitoneal attachments.

Division of the bile duct, neck of pancreas and retroperitoneal attachments

12 The common hepatic duct is now occluded temporarily with a bulldog clamp and divided just above the normal point of entry of the cystic duct. Bleeding from the distal bile duct is controlled if significant. Any remaining dissection of the front of the portal vein above the neck of the pancreas is completed at this point. The plane between the back of the neck of the pancreas and the front of the portal vein is then developed by careful blunt dissection from above and below, and a loop is passed through the tunnel so that the pancreatic neck can be retracted.

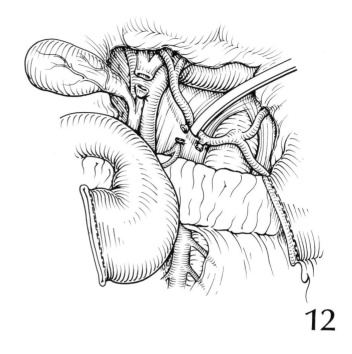

12

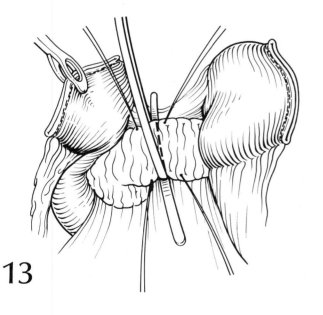

13

13 Four sutures are now placed in the neck of the pancreas and tied, partly to avoid excessive bleeding when the neck of the gland is divided and partly to serve as retractors. Two of these sutures are inserted in the upper border of the neck of the pancreas on either side of the proposed line of division, and two are inserted in the lower border of the neck of the pancreas on either side of the line of division.

14 A grooved dissector is placed behind the neck of the pancreas to protect the portal vein, and the pancreatic neck is divided with a scalpel. Major bleeding points on either side of the divided pancreas are controlled by suture ligation. Some surgeons use a linear stapler to divide the pancreas or use occlusion clamps to control bleeding.

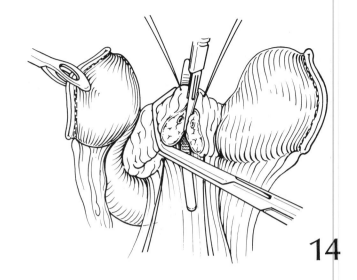

14

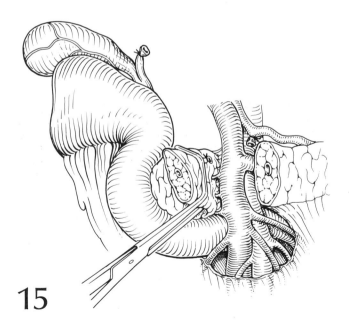

15

15 The superior pancreaticoduodenal vein is then cleared, doubly ligated and divided as it passes from the back of the upper part of the head of the pancreas to enter the right side of the portal vein as it emerges from behind the neck of the gland. All other remaining venous tributaries passing to the portal vein from the head and uncinate process of the pancreas are now divided between ligatures. The inferior pancreaticoduodenal vessels are identified if possible as they pass into the back of the inferior pole of the head and uncinate process. The inferior pancreaticoduodenal artery continues to supply the gland with a substantial amount of arterial blood until late in the operation, but it is often difficult to dissect out these vessels given their relatively short course to the pancreas from the posterior aspect of the superior mesenteric vessels. As stressed earlier, the dissection in chronic pancreatitis is frequently very difficult, given the inflammation, fibrosis and loss of tissue planes, and it may be safer to leave a small cuff of uncinate process rather than encounter even more difficulty by dissecting close to the major superior mesenteric vessels.

16 Undue retraction of the resection specimen to the right runs the very real risk of pulling the superior mesenteric artery behind the superior mesenteric vein and into the operating field where it may be damaged with devastating consequences. If a cuff of uncinate process is to be left behind, pairs of small artery forceps are used to clamp small portions of uncinate process which are then sequentially divided with careful ligation of the stump of tissue that remains. The technique is analogous to that used in partial thyroidectomy.

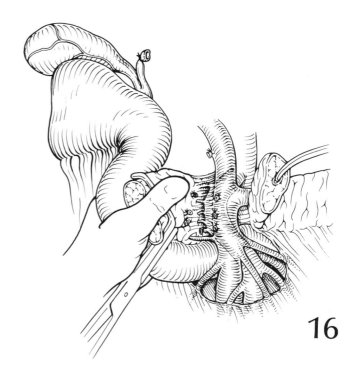

16

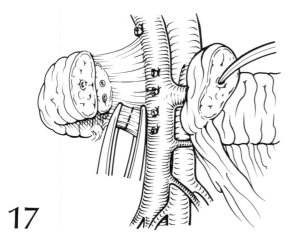

17

17 Even if it is not necessary to leave a small cuff of uncinate process, a thick layer of fascial tissue still attaches the back of the pancreas to the retroperitoneum. Some surgeons have advocated the use of a linear stapler to divide this fascial layer but in the author's experience this is rarely sensible, particularly in patients with chronic pancreatitis. The layer is best dealt with by using pairs of artery forceps in the manner just described. Once the specimen has been removed, the tissue enclosed within each pair of forceps is ligated. Absolute haemostasis must then be obtained as subsequent access to the area is difficult if not impossible once the reconstruction has been undertaken.

Reconstruction

18 The stapled end of the jejunum is brought through a convenient window in the mesocolon and is first anastomosed to the pancreatic remnant. One good feature of resection in chronic pancreatitis is the fact that the pancreatic remnant is more fibrous than normal and that sutures are less likely to cut out. There are many ways of dealing with the pancreatic remnant and much depends on personal preference. It is the author's practice to oversew the stapled end of the jejunum and create an end-to-side anastomosis between the cut end of the pancreas and the side of the jejunal loop. A single layer of interrupted 3/0 delayed absorbable material such as polypropylene or polydioxanone (PDS) is used for this purpose and it is imperative to mobilize the pancreatic remnant so that it can be rotated forwards to allow deep bites to be taken when inserting sutures into the posterior aspect of the gland. The entire posterior layer of sutures is inserted into the pancreas and jejunum before being tied and cut, leaving the two end sutures as temporary stays.

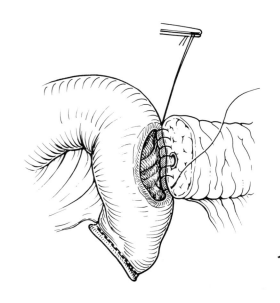

18

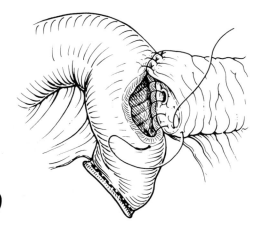

19

19 The anterior layer is commenced by burying these two stay sutures at either end of the suture line, and the entire anterior layer of sutures is then inserted before being tied and cut.

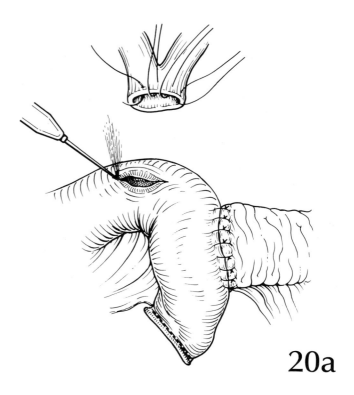

20a

20a,b An end-to-side hepaticojejunostomy is created downstream of the pancreaticojejunal anastomosis at the most distal point which does not produce kinking of the jejunum. The technique is similar to that described for the pancreaticojejunal anastomosis. The entire posterior row of sutures is inserted before they are tied and cut with the knots on the inside of the anastomosis. The two end sutures are left long and the anterior layer of the anastomosis begins with a corner stitch at either end so that the two stays can be buried and cut.

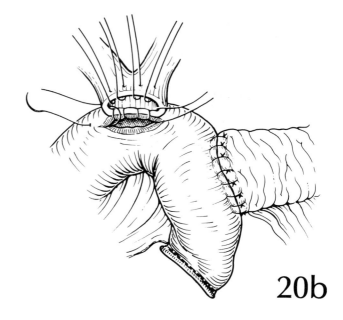

20b

21 The entire anterior layer of sutures is then inserted so that the knots will be on the outside. The sutures are then tied and the ends are cut. If access is difficult and the bile duct small, it may be easier to insert the anterior layer of sutures into the bile duct (leaving the needles on each suture) before commencing the posterior layer of the anastomosis.

Opinions vary regarding the need to stent the pancreaticojejunal and hepaticojejunal anastomoses. The author does not employ a stent for the pancreaticojejunal anastomosis but leaves a tube which provides access to the jejunal loop. This acts as a 'safety valve', preventing leakage from the two anastomoses if pressure builds within an obstructed jejunal loop, and also allows access for radiology if this is needed in the postoperative period. This access can be provided by inserting a T tube into the bile duct so that it splints the hepaticojejunal anastomosis. Alternatively, a Silastic tube (3–5 mm diameter) can be placed in the jejunal loop through a stab incision distal to the hepaticojejunal anastomosis and left so that its end passes into the hepatic duct. If this latter technique is adopted it is advisable to use a 3/0 catgut suture to fix the end of the stent temporarily within the hepatic duct.

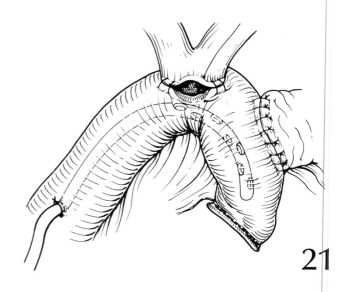

21

22a, b Finally, a gastrojejunal anastomosis is performed some 50 cm distal to the hepaticojejunal anastomosis. The anastomosis can be created by bringing the gastric remnant through a window in the mesocolon but it is the author's practice to perform an antecolic anastomosis. The upper half of the cut end of stomach is first closed using two layers of continuous suture (2/0 polyglactin (Vicryl)) and the remaining half is then anastomosed to the side of the jejunum, once again employing two layers of continuous 2/0 polyglactin. The inner layer is an all coats haemostatic layer while the outer layer is a seromuscular layer of sutures.

Once the anastomoses have been completed and haemostasis confirmed, the peritoneal cavity is lavaged and the abdominal wound is closed leaving two large Redivac drains in place. One of these drains is placed in front of the right kidney and the other is placed so that it lies above the pancreaticojejunal anastomosis.

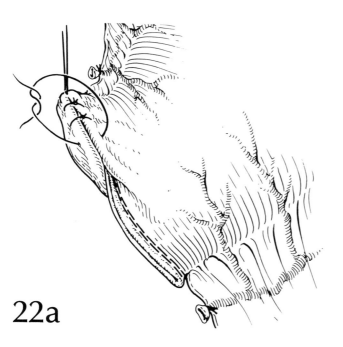

22a

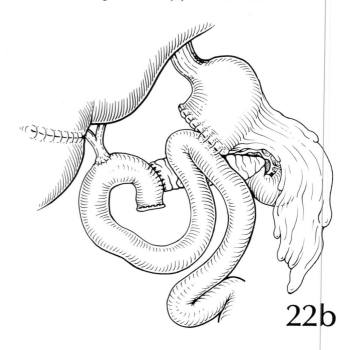

22b

Postoperative care

The patient is usually extubated on the operating table and nursed in a high dependency unit unless intensive care is advisable because of particular risk factors. The nasogastric tube is removed on the first or second postoperative day unless there is copious gastric aspirate, and the patient is encouraged to keep the chest clear by deep breathing and coughing. The epidural anaesthesia is usually maintained for 48 h to minimize pain and assist the physiotherapist in avoiding respiratory complications. The urinary catheter can normally be removed within 24–48 h. Blood glucose levels should be checked frequently as many patients develop insulin-dependent diabetes mellitus after pancreatic resection or need adjustment of their normal insulin requirements.

Antibiotic prophylaxis is continued for 24 h, low dose subcutaneous heparin is maintained for 7–10 days, and H$_2$ receptor antagonists are prescribed for 3 months as a safeguard against stress ulceration. In some centres the somatostatin analogue, octreotide, is used to reduce the risk of leakage from the pancreaticojejunal anastomosis. However, after resection for chronic pancreatitis there is a relatively low risk of leakage from the pancreatic remnant and octreotide is not used routinely by the author. The abdominal drains can usually be removed within 5 days but the T tube or splinting jejunal tube is retained for at least 14 days. Contrast medium can be used to check the integrity of the various anastomoses before removing the tube if there is any cause for concern.

Further reading

Trede M, Carter DC. *Surgery of the Pancreas*. Edinburgh: Churchill Livingstone, 1993.

Illustrations by Peter Cox and Gillian Lee Illustrations

Pancreaticoduodenectomy: pylorus preservation

Henry A. Pitt MD

Professor and Vice Chairman, Department of Surgery, The Johns Hopkins Medical Institutions, Baltimore, Maryland, USA

History

Pancreaticoduodenectomy was popularized by Whipple and his colleagues in the 1930s[1]. Numerous modifications of the original two-stage operation were introduced in the 1940s and 1950s and, by the 1960s, the 'standard Whipple procedure' was a one-stage operation that included a partial pancreatic resection and an antrectomy. During the 1970s, a trend evolved towards more radical operations including total pancreatectomy, portal vein resection and extensive retroperitoneal lymph node dissection. However, concerns about increased postoperative morbidity and mortality as well as a poorer quality of life with these more radical operations led Traverso and Longmire[2] to introduce the pylorus-preserving pancreaticoduodenectomy in 1978.

Principles and justification

Pylorus-preserving pancreaticoduodenectomy was originally described by Traverso and Longmire for the management of patients with chronic pancreatitis. Many pancreatic surgeons believe that it is the procedure of choice when the pancreatitis is most severe in the head and uncinate process and the pancreatic duct is not dilated. In this situation a Puestow procedure cannot be performed, and a distal pancreatectomy is less likely to relieve the pain that is usually the primary indication for surgery. In addition, many of these patients also have relative or significant narrowing of the distal bile duct which is also easily dealt with by pylorus-preserving pancreaticoduodenectomy.

The operation may also be indicated for a variety of other benign as well as malignant diseases. At present the most common indication for pylorus-preserving pancreaticoduodenectomy is a tumour arising in the periampullary region[3-5]. These tumours include adenocarcinomas that arise in the head of the pancreas, the ampulla of Vater, the distal bile duct and the duodenum. Pylorus-preserving pancreaticoduodenectomy is also indicated for the other less common neoplasms that may arise in the head of the pancreas. These tumours include the cystic neoplasms, both cystadenomas and cystadenocarcinomas, the islet cell tumours which may be either benign or malignant, and cystic and papillary (Hamoudi) tumours as well as a variety of very rare lesions.

Some surgeons have expressed concern that pylorus-preserving pancreaticoduodenectomy may not be an adequate operation for pancreatic cancer. However, at The Johns Hopkins Hospital and at several other institutions it is performed in more than 80% of these patients[4, 5]. For those who express concern about the pylorus-preserving procedure, recurrence at the duodenal margin and the adequacy of the lymph node dissection are the major issues. On the other hand, those who are advocates of pylorus-preserving pancreaticoduodenectomy point out that frozen section of the duodenal margin prevents local recurrence, and they also report excellent survival data[3-5]. In addition, the quality of survival has been reported to be better with pylorus preservation than with either the standard Whipple procedure (which includes an antrectomy) or with more radical operations including total pancreatectomy and extensive retroperitoneal lymph node resection[6].

Preoperative

Regardless of the underlying pathology, the most likely presenting symptoms for patients who will require pancreaticoduodenectomy are pain and jaundice. A history of excess alcohol intake and chronic pain in middle-aged patients are most suggestive of chronic pancreatitis. On the other hand, the onset of relatively painless jaundice in an elderly patient makes an obstructing carcinoma the most likely diagnosis. In these jaundiced patients, the presence on physical examination of a non-tender, palpable gallbladder almost confirms the diagnosis of a malignancy. By the time these patients present, they may be severely jaundiced and may have lost considerable weight. Thus, the decision of whether or when to operate cannot be taken lightly.

In deciding whether to perform surgery, several patient and disease characteristics must be considered. The patient's age in itself should not be a factor in this decision. Most carefully selected elderly patients will tolerate pancreaticoduodenectomy without difficulty[3], while a younger patient with severe cardiac, pulmonary or renal disease may not fare so well. Similarly, underlying cirrhosis, especially if the patient also has portal hypertension, may significantly increase the risk of surgery. Patients who present with obstructive jaundice experience a myriad of physiological abnormalities which alter cardiac, pulmonary, hepatic, renal and immune function. In addition, these patients frequently have coagulation defects, impaired wound healing and a moderate degree of malnutrition.

As a result, a number of experts have recommended preoperative biliary drainage. However, the routine use of preoperative drainage remains controversial, but most authorities agree that jaundice should be relieved and surgery should be delayed in patients who are severely malnourished, have underlying renal disease and/or biliary sepsis. Abnormal laboratory data will provide information about sepsis, nutrition, renal function, the degree of biliary obstruction and coagulation.

1a,b In addition to deciding whether the patient can withstand surgery, in those with a malignancy it is necessary to determine whether the tumour is resectable. Percutaneous ultrasonography will demonstrate dilated bile ducts, a distended gallbladder and larger liver metastases. However, ultrasonography is not the best way to evaluate the pancreas or mesenteric vasculature and does not usually detect small liver metastases. Computed tomographic (CT) scanning is better at visualizing the pancreas, and newer spiral or helical techniques provide good information about the mesenteric vessels as well as detecting small liver metastases (*Illustration 1a*). Magnetic resonance imaging has not proved to be better than current CT techniques in staging these patients. Some experts have recommended the routine use of mesenteric angiography to assess vascular involvement by a pancreatic tumour (*Illustration 1b*), but the newer CT techniques may obviate the need for routine angiography.

Having information about the anatomy of the biliary tree prior to surgery is also usually helpful. An ultrasonogram or CT scan normally determines the level of obstruction. However, a cholangiogram will define the exact anatomy and is also very accurate in determining the specific diagnosis. The cholangiogram can be obtained by either the percutaneous transhepatic or the endoscopic retrograde (ERCP) technique. In patients with disease in the periampullary area, ERCP is usually preferred because the duodenum and ampulla can be visualized. In addition, biopsies can be taken and, if the diagnosis is in doubt, a pancreatogram can also be obtained. Moreover, in some patients who have not developed jaundice, the pancreatogram may detect a malignant stricture in the pancreatic neck or uncinate process or may suggest chronic pancreatitis.

A newer technique that may also be helpful in staging these patients is endoscopic ultrasonography. This investigation will usually detect obstruction of the bile and pancreatic ducts and visualize the tumour. Vascular involvement and lymph node metastases may also be detected with this technique. However, its accuracy in comparison with CT scanning and angiography or spiral CT scanning in determining resectability has yet to be determined. Another approach for staging these patients is laparoscopy. Laparoscopic examination will usually detect metastases on the surface of the liver and on the peritoneum. The addition of ultrasonography to laparoscopy increases its ability to determine resectability. However, laparoscopy is considered to be unnecessary by those who believe that operative palliation has advantages over non-operative palliation and that the decision with respect to resectability can only be made by the operating surgeon.

Another issue that must be considered is the need for a tissue diagnosis. In patients with obvious liver metastasis whose jaundice can be relieved with an endoprosthesis, needle biopsy of a liver lesion will

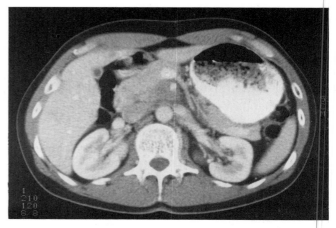

1a

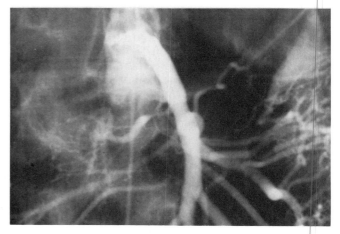

1b

usually provide the diagnosis. Similarly, in patients with large, unresectable lesions of the body or tail of the pancreas who do not require palliation of jaundice or duodenal obstruction, needle biopsy will avoid the need for a laparoscopy or laparotomy. However, if the CT scan demonstrates a potentially resectable mass in the periampullary area in a fit patient, preoperative biopsy is not indicated because the results of the biopsy will not alter the decision to operate. Moreover, some concern exists that the biopsy may spread tumour cells and adversely affect outcome. Additional issues to consider in preoperative preparation such as the perioperative use of prophylactic antibiotics and fluid management in these jaundiced patients are discussed in the chapter on pp. 262–274.

Anaesthesia

ERCP, endoscopic ultrasonography, percutaneous or endoscopic placement of biliary stents and angiography can usually be performed with intravenous sedation and analgesia. On the other hand, laparoscopy usually requires a general anaesthetic. Similarly, laparotomy to determine resectability and undertake a pancreatico-duodenectomy is also performed under a general endotracheal anaesthesia. In choosing an anaesthetic regimen, agents which can cause cholestasis or hepato-toxicity should be avoided in these jaundiced patients.

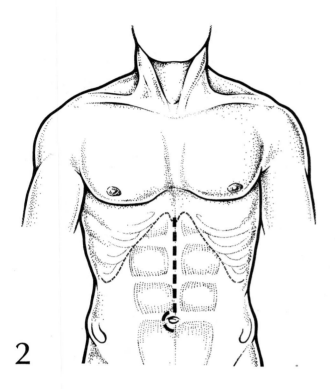

Operation

Incision and exploration

2   A pylorus-preserving pancreaticoduodenectomy may be performed through either a midline or a right and partial left subcostal incision. However, the midline incision allows more flexibility in tube and drain placement and avoids wound problems that commonly occur in the right flank.

Once the abdomen is open, a thorough exploration is undertaken. The liver and all peritoneal surfaces are carefully inspected for any sign of metastatic disease. Any suspicious lesions are biopsied, and the presence of liver or peritoneal metastases is generally taken as a contraindication to resection. On the other hand, tumour involvement of lymph nodes within the boundary of resection is not a contraindication to resection. However, spread of tumour to lymph nodes outside the usual areas of resection may be a reason to forgo resection. Most tumours that require pancreatico-duodenectomy are localized to the head, uncinate and/or neck of the pancreas. Spread throughout the body and tail of the gland is present in some cases, and the decision to undertake resection in such cases requires considerable judgement.

Kocher manoeuvre

3a,b If tumour spread has been excluded, an extensive Kocher manoeuvre is performed. The incision along the lateral border of the duodenum should also be carried to the right to free some of the attachments of the hepatic flexure of the colon from the retroperitoneum. The duodenum, head of the pancreas and the tumour can usually be easily separated from the inferior vena cava and aorta. However, extension of tumour into these structures occasionally precludes resection. Extensive mobilization of the head of the pancreas is also important to determine the extent of tumour spread into the uncinate process. The tumour may extend behind the superior mesenteric or portal vein and still be resectable. However, encasement of the superior mesenteric artery is usually regarded as a contraindication to resection.

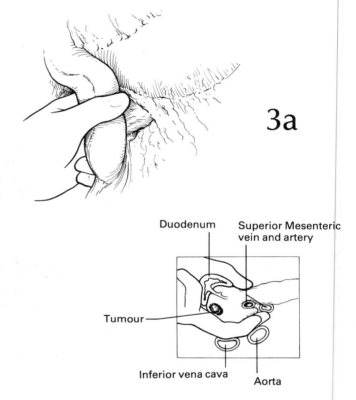

3a

Duodenum

Superior Mesenteric vein and artery

Tumour

Inferior vena cava

Aorta

3b

Cholecystectomy and division of the bile duct

4a,b The next step in deciding on resectability is to expose the portal and superior mesenteric veins. Detachment of the gallbladder from the liver and division of the bile duct facilitates determination of the relationship between the portal vein and the tumour.

Before undertaking this step, a decision needs to be made as to whether the gallbladder would be used for bypass if the tumour is not resected. However, the long-term results of choledochojejunostomy are better than those of cholecystojejunostomy. On the other hand, if the portal vein is occluded by the tumour and multiple venous collaterals have developed around the bile duct, the gallbladder may be the best option for the biliary bypass as long as the cystic duct is still patent and not too close to the tumour. Assuming that this rare situation does not exist, the gallbladder is removed in a standard fashion, and the bile duct is transected just above or below the cystic duct entrance but at least 2 cm from the tumour. This manoeuvre will expose the portal vein more fully.

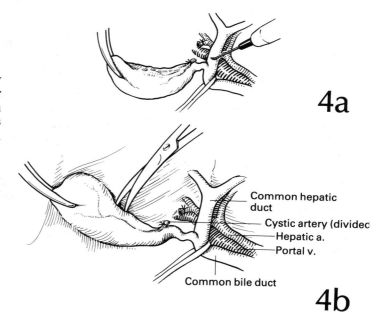

4a

Common hepatic duct
Cystic artery (divided
Hepatic a.
Portal v.
Common bile duct

4b

Exposure of the superior mesenteric vein

5a–c To determine whether a tumour in the head, uncinate or neck of the pancreas is resectable, the superior mesenteric vein must also be exposed. To facilitate this manoeuvre, the transverse mesocolon is freed from the head and uncinate process, and the Kocher manoeuvre is extended to the third portion of the duodenum, thus exposing the right lateral edge of the superior mesenteric vein. Dissection of this vein is then carried up to the neck of the pancreas (*Illustration 5a*). Venous branches draining the transverse mesocolon and the head of the pancreas may need to be divided to continue tracing the superior mesenteric vein beneath the pancreatic neck. Dissection can then be continued between the superior mesenteric vein (below) and portal vein (above) and the neck of the pancreas. When this dissection is completed, fingers may be passed in this plane (*Illustrations 5b* and *5c*) to assess further the extent of the tumour. A judgement must be made at this point as to whether the tumour extends into the superior mesenteric or portal veins or into the superior mesenteric artery which lies to the left and somewhat behind (dorsal) the veins.

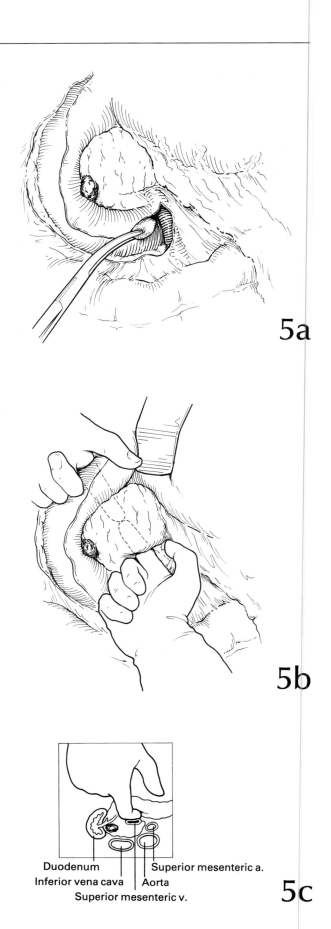

5a

5b

Duodenum | Superior mesenteric a.
Inferior vena cava | Aorta
Superior mesenteric v.

5c

Division of the duodenum

6 If the lesion is resectable, the next step is to divide the first portion of the duodenum. Multiple small vessels communicating between the first portion of the duodenum and the head of the pancreas have to be ligated before the duodenum can be divided. However, the right gastric artery, which usually extends from the common hepatic artery to the pyloric region, and associated nerves should be preserved. In addition, the first 2–3 cm of duodenum should be preserved, along with the pylorus. The pacemaker of the small intestine lies in this proximal segment of the duodenum, and preservation of the neurovascular supply should help with postoperative motility. Once adequate mobilization of the proximal duodenum has been completed, division with a GIA stapler is performed.

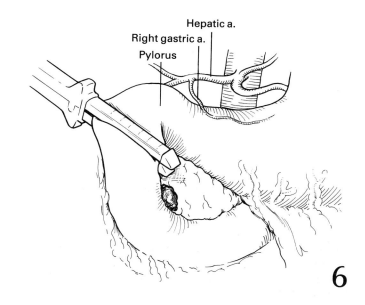

6

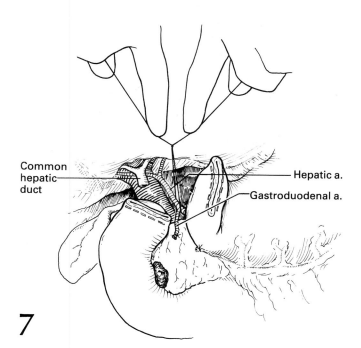

7

Division of the gastroduodenal artery

7 After the proximal duodenum has been divided, the gastroduodenal artery can be exposed more easily. A sufficient length of artery should be dissected to allow room for both ligation and suture ligation on the side leading from the hepatic artery. Care should be taken in this process not to interrupt flow through the hepatic artery. The gastroduodenal artery runs along the ventral surface of the neck of the pancreas and becomes the right gastroepiploic artery. This artery also needs to be ligated and divided to separate fully the pylorus from the specimen. If the patient has a replaced right hepatic artery extending from the superior mesenteric artery, this vessel usually runs ventral to the portal vein along its right side and dorsal to the common duct, also along its right side. Care should be taken to identify and preserve a replaced right hepatic artery which occurs in 15% of the population.

Division of the pancreatic neck

8 Despite division of the gastroduodenal and gastro-epiploic arteries, a considerable amount of blood continues to flow into the pancreatic neck through branches from the superior mesenteric artery. Larger vessels usually run along the cephalad and caudal borders of the pancreas at the neck, and placement of stay sutures along these borders of the pancreas reduces blood loss during division of the pancreatic neck. A vascular clamp applied to the specimen side will also minimize blood loss during this process. Protection of the portal vein with a finger or forceps is another wise move during the division of the pancreatic neck. Use of the cautery for the division also minimizes blood loss. If the tumour extends close to this margin, frozen section of the pancreatic neck should be performed at this point rather than when the entire specimen has been excised.

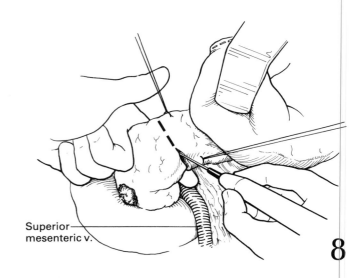

Superior mesenteric v.

8

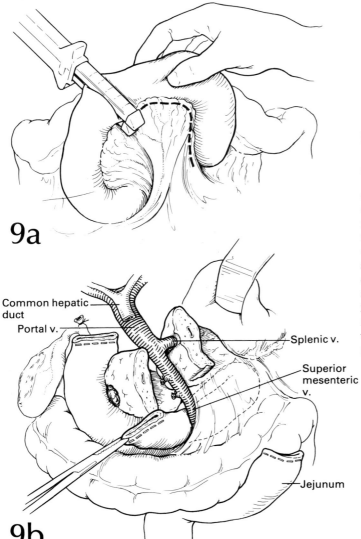

9a

Common hepatic duct
Portal v.
Splenic v.
Superior mesenteric v.
Jejunum

9b

Division of the jejunum

9a,b The ligament of Treitz is mobilized and the jejunum is then divided with a GIA stapler about 8–10 cm distal to the ligament. The mesentery is divided relatively close to the jejunum to avoid any injury to the superior mesenteric artery or vein. Usually, a double row of short vessels attaches the fourth portion of the duodenum to the uncinate process. Once these short vessels have been divided, the proximal jejunum can be passed behind the superior mesenteric artery and vein to the patient's right. This manoeuvre facilitates dissection of the uncinate process from the right and dorsal sides of the superior mesenteric vein, as well as from the right side of the superior mesenteric artery.

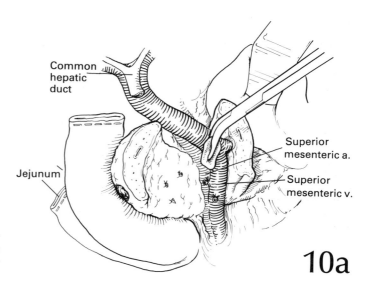

Dissection of the uncinate process

10a,b At this point the only remaining attachments of the specimen are between the uncinate process and the mesenteric vessels. Relatively few venous branches drain from the uncinate process into the superior mesenteric and portal veins. However, these branches are relatively short and need to be carefully ligated and suture ligated to avoid bleeding from or narrowing of the superior mesenteric or portal vein. In addition to these venous attachments, multiple arterial branches extend from the superior mesenteric artery into the uncinate process and these vessels should be ligated close to the superior mesenteric artery, especially if the tumour extends into the uncinate process. During this dissection, care should be taken to avoid injury to the superior mesenteric artery. The chance of injuring the artery may actually be less if it is identified and exposed in the process of dissection.

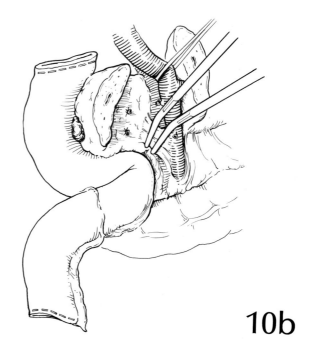

Resected specimen

11a,b The resected specimen consists of the gallbladder, the distal bile duct, the second, third and fourth portions of the duodenum, the proximal jejunum, and the head, neck and uncinate portions of the pancreas. When the resection has been performed for malignancy, frozen sections of the bile duct, duodenum and pancreatic neck and uncinate process are performed. If any of these margins, except the uncinate, are positive, further tissue may be removed in an effort to achieve a negative margin. In selected cases, however, resection of a segment of the portal or superior mesenteric vein may also be performed to achieve a negative margin. A primary anastomosis of the vein will normally suffice, but autologous vein is occasionally required to bridge the gap. Rarely, the coeliac axis is stenotic so that a significant proportion of the blood flow to the liver comes through collaterals in the pancreatic head. In this rare situation, an arterial bypass from the aorta or right renal artery to the hepatic artery or division of the arcuate ligament may need to be performed.

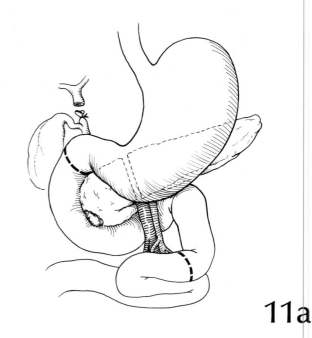

11a

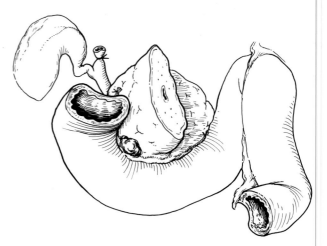

11b

Pancreatic anastomosis

12a–d A variety of methods exist to reanastomose the pancreas to the intestinal tract. Common options that are performed include an end-to-end (dunking) pancreaticojejunostomy (*Illustration 12a*), an end-to-side (mucosa-to-mucosa) pancreaticojejunostomy (*Illustration 12b*) or an end-to-side pancreaticogastrostomy (*Illustration 12c*). Any of these anastomoses may be stented with a short internal stent or with a longer stent which exits the jejunum and abdominal wall. If an end-to-side (mucosa-to-mucosa)

pancreaticojejunostomy is carried out, the outer layer is performed with 3/0 non-absorbable sutures which extend from the pancreatic capsule to the jejunal serosa (*Illustration 12d*). A 2–3 mm opening is made in the jejunum adjacent to the pancreatic duct, and an anastomosis is performed with 4/0 absorbable sutures. This anastomosis is usually stented with a short segment of paediatric feeding tube which is attached to the jejunum with a single 4/0 absorbable suture.

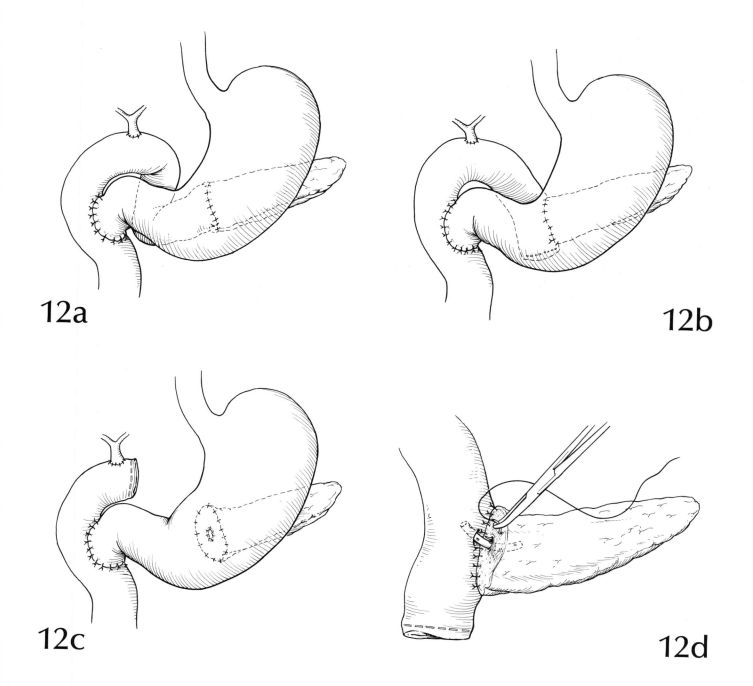

12a

12b

12c

12d

Hepaticojejunostomy

13a–d The hepaticojejunostomy usually lies only 6–8 cm distal to the pancreatico-jejunostomy. The hepaticojejunostomy is performed in an end-to-side fashion and may be done in one or two layers. The anastomosis which is illustrated is two-layered with an outer layer of interrupted 4/0 non-absorbable sutures (*Illustration 13a*) and an inner layer of running 4/0 absorbable sutures (*Illustration 13b*). A T tube is placed through a separate stab incision in the common hepatic duct (*Illustration 13c*). The anterior row of sutures is also completed in two layers, and the jejunum is tacked to periportal tissues to take tension off the anastomosis (*Illustration 13d*). Fluorocholangiography is performed to assess proper positioning of the T tube and to check for leaks. The use of an operatively placed T tube or a preoperatively placed transhepatic stent is controversial. However, if a leak occurs at the biliary or the pancreatic anastomosis, external drainage may facilitate closure of the leak.

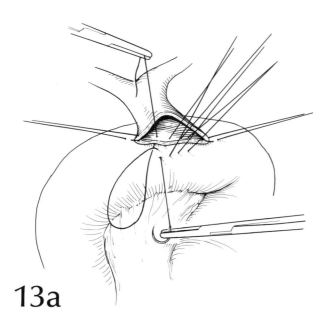

13a

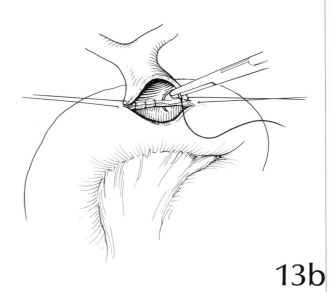

13b

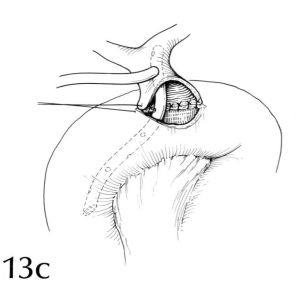

13c

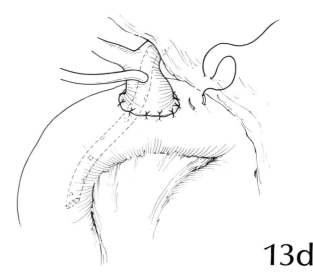

13d

Duodenojejunostomy

14a–d The third anastomosis is an end-to side duodenojejunostomy. This anastomosis is performed 15–20 cm distal to the hepaticojejunostomy. The duodenojejunostomy is performed in two layers. First, an outer layer of interrupted 3/0 non-absorbable sutures is placed (*Illustration 14a*). The staple line is removed from the duodenum, the blood supply is checked and an enterotomy is made in the jejunum (*Illustration 14b*). An inner layer of running 3/0 absorbable sutures is inserted (*Illustration 14c*) and the anastomosis is completed with an outer layer of interrupted 3/0 non-absorbable sutures (*Illustration 14d*).

This anastomosis is left just above the transverse mesocolon. However, the jejunum just below the anastomosis is tacked to the mesocolon to prevent internal herniation as well as obstruction. Two closed suction drains are inserted, one via the right flank and the other via the left upper quadrant. The right drain extends dorsal to the hepaticojejunostomy and ventral to the pancreaticojejunostomy. The left drain goes through the old ligament of Treitz area and lies behind (dorsal) the pancreaticojejunostomy. The T tube is brought out through a stab incision in the right upper quadrant. Both drains and the T tube are sutured to the skin, and the abdominal wall is closed in a standard fashion.

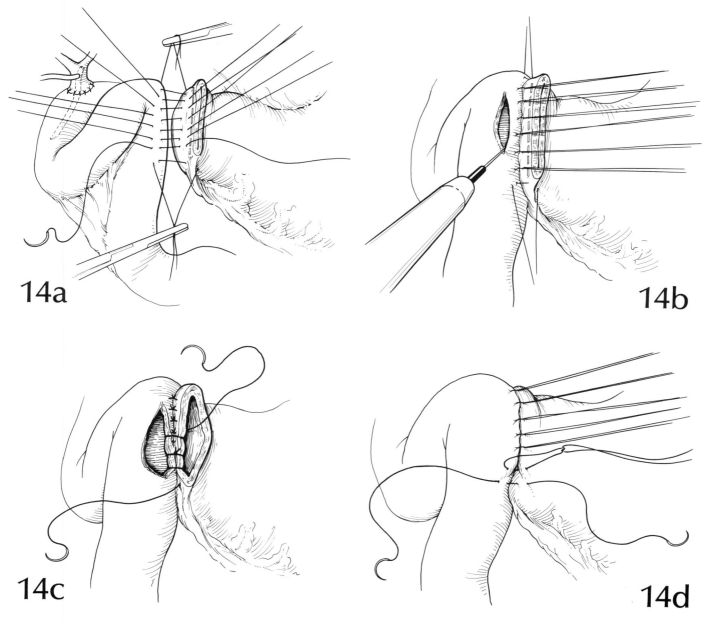

14a

14b

14c

14d

Postoperative care

Prophylactic antibiotics are normally stopped after 24 h. The routine use of octreotide to prevent a pancreatic anastomosis that remains controversial. The nasogastric tube is left in until bowel function returns and drainage has diminished to less than 500 ml in 24 h. The incidence of delayed gastric emptying in the early postoperative period may be as high as 30–40% so the routine use of an intravenous prokinetic agent such as erythromycin has been recommended by some authorities. A pancreatic fistula may also occur in 5–15% of patients so the drainage fluid should be analysed for amylase on about the fifth postoperative day and again after oral intake has started. A T tube cholangiogram is performed on the fifth or sixth postoperative day. Prophylactic antibiotics directed at the organisms cultured from the bile are given before and for 24 h afterwards if no cholangitis occurs. If no bile or pancreatic leak is demonstrated and no cholangitis is experienced, the T tube is closed on the day after cholangiography. If a pancreatic or a bile leak is discovered, the T tube is left on drainage and a CT scan is performed. Any unusual fluid collections which do not communicate with an existing drain are percutaneously aspirated and drained.

In most circumstances in which a pancreatic leak is documented, the patient is kept on nil by mouth and total parenteral nutrition is begun. Re-exploration is usually not required unless bleeding develops. Oral intake is not begun until bowel function has returned, the stomach is properly emptying, and bile or pancreatic leaks have healed. Drains are not removed until the T tube has been closed, any fistulas are healed and the patient is eating. An unusual problem is drainage of very large amounts of ascites in the early postoperative period which requires urgent re-exploration to assess venous obstruction. On the other hand, if the ascites is chylous, an injury to a main lymphatic channel may have occurred, and this problem can usually be managed by stopping oral intake and beginnig parenteral nutrition. When the patient does begin eating, blood sugars and bowel movements are monitored. Most patients who do not have pancreatic endocrine or exocrine insufficiency before pancreaticoduodenectomy do not develop these problems after surgery, because more than half of the pancreas remains after the head of the gland has been resected.

Outcome

The mortality rate following pancreaticoduodenectomy has diminished significantly in recent years although morbidity remains high[1,3–5]. In a recent series of 145 consecutive patients who underwent pancreaticoduodenectomy at The Johns Hopkins Hospital the hospital mortality was zero[3]. However, in this series, in which 81% of patients underwent a pylorus-preserving pancreaticoduodenectomy, the postoperative morbidity was 52%. The most common complication was delayed gastric emptying which occurred in 36% of the patients. Although some authorities have suggested that this problem is more common after pylorus-preserving pancreaticoduodenectomy, comparative data have not confirmed this contention[1]. Delayed gastric emptying is often caused by other intra-abdominal problems such as pancreatitis or a pancreatic fistula. When these other complications resolve, gastric emptying usually improves so that long-term problems with gastric stasis are unusual.

The next most common complication after pancreaticoduodenectomy is development of a pancreatic fistula[3–5]. In a recent randomized trial of pancreaticojejunostomy versus pancreaticogastrostomy performed at The Johns Hopkins Hospital the overall incidence of pancreatic fistula was 11%[5]. However, the incidence was the same regardless of the type of anastomosis employed. Pancreatic fistula can lead to intra-abdominal abscess, haemorrhage and death. However, careful monitoring of amylase levels in the drainage fluid resulting in early diagnosis, percutaneous drainage of intra-abdominal collections, and parenteral nutritional support have all diminished the severity of this complication. Total pancreatectomy, of course, avoids the problem of pancreatic fistula, but the overall morbidity is actually higher with total than with partial pancreaticoduodenectomy[1]. Moreover, with total pancreatectomy the diabetes mellitus can be quite brittle, and late problems with hepatic fibrosis have been reported.

In a collected series of 339 pylorus-preserving pancreaticoduodenectomies published in 1990, the hospital mortality was 4% which compared favourably with the 3% mortality reported in a collected series of standard Whipple procedures reported during the same time period[1]. During this period, the hospital mortality in collected series of regional and total pancreatectomies was 6% and 18%, respectively[1]. Since 1990 several large series of pylorus-preserving pancreaticoduodenectomies have been published with mortality rates of 0–2%.

Thus, pylorus-preserving pancreatiocduodenectomy can usually be performed with equal or greater safety than the other alternatives. On the other hand, controversy continues as to whether it provides the best chance for long-term survival in patients with cancer. Critics argue that the area resected is reduced and suggest that pylorus-preserving pancreaticoduodenectomy should not be performed for pancreatic cancer. However, advocates point out that the bile duct, uncinate process and pancreatic neck margins are usually closer to the tumour than the duodenal margin. Moreover, survival rates after the pylorus-preserving procedure have been the same or better than those with the classic Whipple procedure or with total pancreatectomy[1,4]. Finally, the quality of survival can be better with pylorus-preserving pancreaticoduodenectomy than with either the classic Whipple procedure or with regional pancreatectomy[6].

References

1. Pitt HA. Curative treatment for pancreatic neoplasms: standard resection. *Surg Clin North Am* 1995; 75: 891–904.
2. Traverso LW, Longmire WP Jr. Preservation of the pylorus in pancreaticoduodenectomy. *Surg Gynecol Obstet* 1978; 146: 959–62.
3. Cameron JL, Pitt HA, Yeo CJ, Lillemoe KD, Kaufman HS, Coleman J. One hundred and forty-five consecutive pancreaticoduodenectomies without mortality. *Ann Surg* 1993; 217: 430–8.
4. Yeo CJ, Cameron JL, Lillemoe KD *et al*. Pancreaticoduodenectomy for cancer of the head of the pancreas: 201 patients. *Ann Surg* 1995; 221: 721–33.
5. Yeo CJ, Cameron JL, Maher MM *et al*. A prospective randomized trial of pancreaticogastrostomy versus pancreaticojejunostomy following pancreaticoduodenectomy. *Ann Surg* 1995; 222: 580–92.
6. Yasuda H, Takada T, Uchiyama K *et al*. Social function following pylorus-preserving pancreaticoduodenectomy for cancer of the head of the pancreas. *Asian J Surg* 1993; 16: 228–31.

Illustrations by Peter Cox

Duodenum-preserving resection of the head of the pancreas

Hans G. Beger MD, FACS
Professor of Surgery, Chairman and Head of the Department of General Surgery, University of Ulm, Ulm, Germany

Michael H. Schoenberg MD
Department of General Surgery, University of Ulm, Ulm, Germany

During the course of chronic pancreatitis 45–65% of patients need surgical treatment because of intractable abdominal pain or severe local complications. Abdominal pain not responding to medical and analgesic treatment is the critical symptom in severe chronic pancreatitis. About one-third of patients with chronic pancreatitis develop an inflammatory mass in the head of the pancreas. Such patients suffer severe abdominal pain and episodes of cholestasis due to stenosis of the intrapancreatic common bile duct early in the clinical course; in this subgroup of patients a stenosis of the peripapillary duodenum and obstruction of the portal vein occur frequently. Elective retrograde cholangiopancreatography (ERCP) often demonstrates a major stenosis in the prepapillary segment of the main pancreatic duct with signs of advanced duct deformity and, occasionally, a chain of lakes in the duct system.

Table 1 Imaging features and pathology of patients with chronic pancreatitis treated by duodenum-preserving resection

Imaging data:	
Pancreatic head enlargement (> 4 cm)	84%
Stenosis of the common bile duct	49%
Duodenal stenosis, severe	6%
Portal vein compression/occlusion	17%
Pancreatic main duct stenosis, single	36%
Pathology in the pancreatic head:	
Cystic lesions	54%
Tissue calcification	36%
Duct stones	31%
Necrosis	10%
Chronic pancreatitis + pancreatic cancer	2.8%

Source: 325 patients treated between November 1972 and April 1982 at the Surgical Department, FU Berlin and between May 1982 and March 1994 at the Department of General Surgery, University of Ulm

Principles and justification

Indications

Surgical treatment is mandatory in patients with severe abdominal pain not responding to analgesic treatment, as well as in patients with common bile duct stenosis, recurrent episodes of jaundice or a severe stenosis of the duodenum. Patients with clinical signs of portal hypertension due to compression of the portal vein by the enlarged head of pancreas are candidates for surgical decompression. The association of chronic pancreatitis with an inflammatory mass and cancer of the head of the pancreas is not well established; however, in about 3% of patients with a long history of chronic pancreatitis a ductal cancer is found. Therefore patients with established chronic pancreatitis are candidates for a surgical resection if there is a suspected malignancy. A decision to proceed to surgery is based on the clinical features, contrast enhanced computed tomography of the pancreas, ERCP, and the level of endocrine and exocrine dysfunction as determined by the glucose tolerance test and pancreolauryl test (PLT), respectively.

Table 1 summarizes the complications caused by an inflammatory mass in the head of the pancreas and its pathology.

Contraindications

Patients with chronic pancreatitis and dilatation of the main duct of more than 8 mm should have a Partington-Rochelle drainage procedure of the main pancreatic duct. Chronic pancreatitis and cancer of the head of the pancreas are treated by a partial duodenopancreatectomy using oncological criteria for resection.

Operation

Incision

Access to the peritoneal cavity is achieved by an upper abdominal midline incision. Sometimes a transverse upper abdominal incision provides advantages for exposure of the whole pancreas. Duodenum-preserving resection of the head is a three-step surgical procedure: (1) exposure of the head of the pancreas, (2) subtotal resection of the head of the pancreas, and (3) reconstruction using an upper jejunal loop for interposition.

Exposure of the pancreas

1   The objective of duodenum-preserving resection of the head of the pancreas is the local excision of an inflammatory tumour by subtotal excision of the head from the portal vein to the intrapancreatic common bile duct. A Kocher manoeuvre is first performed to mobilize the duodenum. The anterior surface of the pancreas is then exposed by dividing the omentum and duodenocolic ligament to reveal the head, neck and body of the pancreas. Finally the plane between the pancreas and the portal vein is developed by dissecting carefully beneath the neck of the pancreas in the fascial plane surrounding the superior mesenteric vein, starting inferiorly and dissecting superiorly in the direction of the porta hepatis. A tape is placed around the neck of the pancreas.

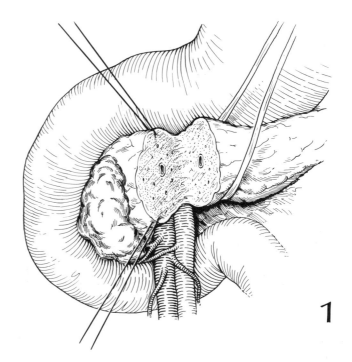

Dissection of the neck of the pancreas

2   With the tape as a guide, the neck of the pancreas is transected along the duodenal side of the portal vein, and the vessels within the pancreatic gland are ligated. Stay sutures are placed on the divided pancreas. The head of the pancreas is everted to expose the superior and inferior pancreaticoduodenal veins which are carefully tied (*see inset*). These are fragile vessels and care is required as tears in the vessel are difficult to control.

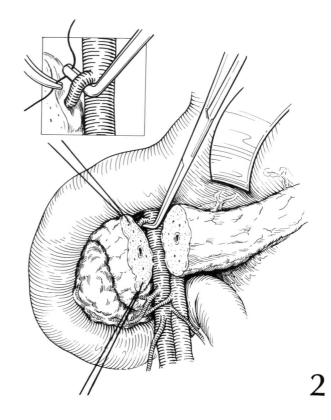

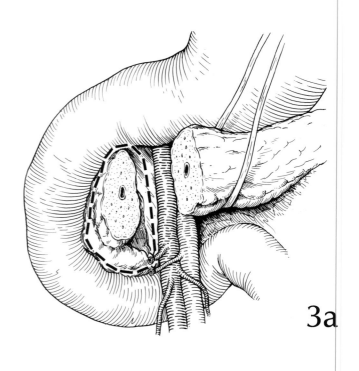

3a

Resection

$3a, b$ With the head of the pancreas completely exposed, the extent of the resection is planned and, in particular, the position of the bile duct defined. Subtotal resection entails incision of the pancreas along the common bile duct to the prepapillary area and subtotal excision of the uncinate process. In most patients it is not difficult to dissect the pancreatic tissue along the wall of the intrapancreatic segment of the common bile duct. For identification, in cases of difficulty, a sound is introduced into the common bile duct towards the papilla, and the pancreas is divided away from the bile duct down to the papilla. A 5–8-mm shell-like piece of the pancreatic head is preserved. This shell along the first and second part of the duodenum is continued round the wall of the third and fourth part of the duodenum leaving a rim of uncinate process.

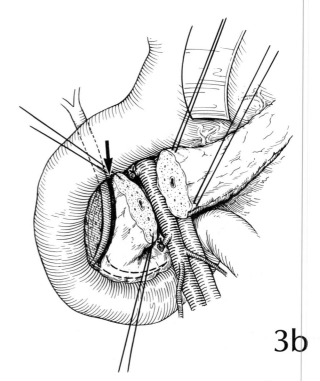

3b

The pancreatic remnant

4 The shell-like piece of preserved pancreas should be just enough to preserve the blood supply to the duodenum, by avoiding injury to the supraduodenal artery and the retropancreatic duodenal arcades. In two-thirds of patients with an inflammatory mass in the head of the pancreas causing stenosis of the intrapancreatic common bile duct, resection of the head results in decompression of the narrowed common bile duct.

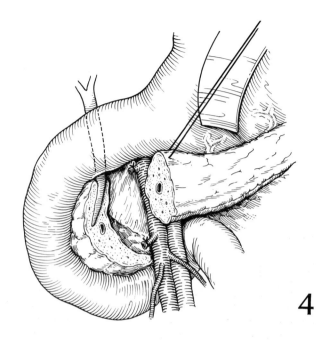

4

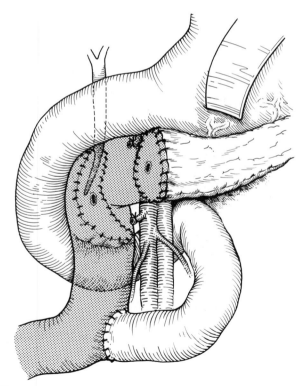

5

Reconstruction

5 A Roux-en-Y jejunal loop is constructed and brought up into the supracolic compartment by a retrocolic route. The end of the loop is anastomosed to the transected pancreas, and a side-to-side anastomosis is constructed between the pancreatic remnant and the jejunum. In 15% of cases a side-to-side choledochojejunostomy is required.

6a–d Two pancreatic anastomoses are required. The end of the jejunum is sutured with interrupted sutures to the fibrous capsule of the pancreas. No attempt is made to suture the mucosa to the duct, but a few sutures are used to tether the duct to the fibrous tissue to prevent retraction. The antimesenteric border of the Roux loop is sutured to the capsule on the posterior wall of the remaining shell of the pancreas. The jejunum is then opened and the mucosa is sutured to the cut edge of the pancreas. The two layers are completed anteriorly so that the shell of the pancreas is completely covered by jejunum.

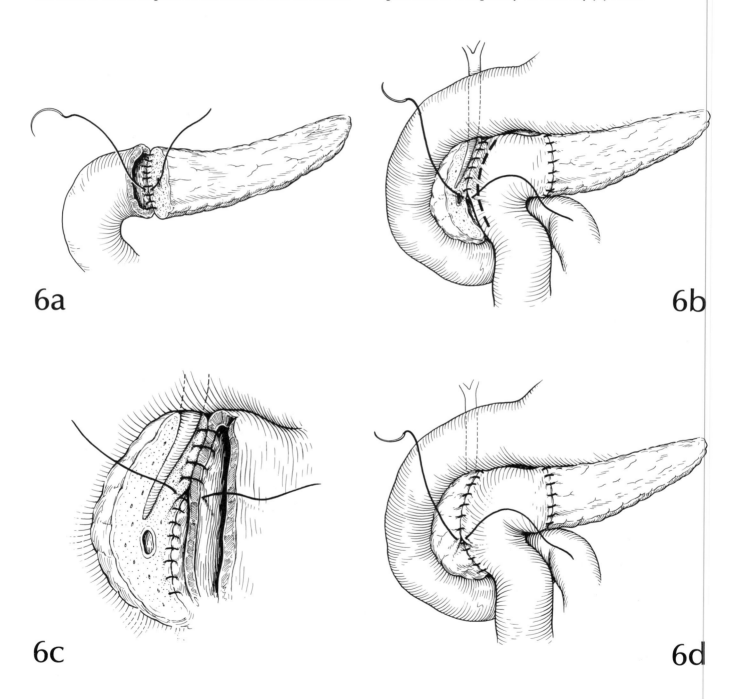

6a

6b

6c

6d

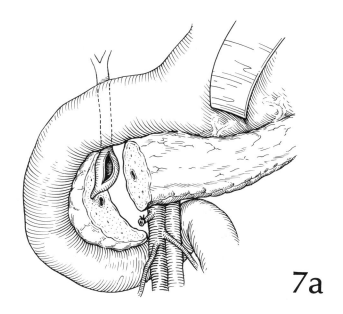

Bile duct anastomosis

7a, b In the 15% of patients with common bile duct stenosis unrelieved by the earlier dissection, an additional anastomosis is required between the prestenotic common bile duct and the jejunal loop. This anastomosis should be performed above the pancreatic duct as a separate procedure.

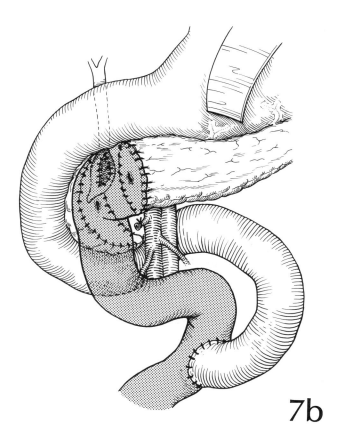

Stenosis of the pancreatic duct

8 In some patients preoperative investigation has shown that there are multiple strictures in the duct in the pancreas to the left of the portal vein. Provided that the duct is enlarged, a Puestow-type side-to-side anastomosis between the pancreatic duct and the jejunal loop has to be performed.

When the patient is first assessed it may be apparent that there is either duodenal obstruction or portal vein compression, or both, causing the vascular signs of portal hypertension. Once the inflammatory mass has been excised the obstruction and compression are seen to resolve and operative intervention is not required.

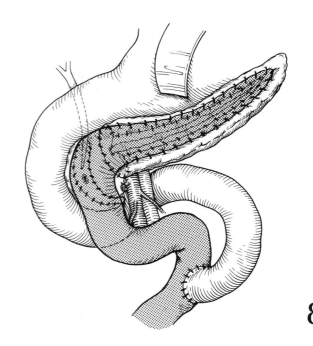

8

Postoperative care

Early postoperative complications are due to bleeding into the intestine from the pancreas, anastomotic leakage causing an intra-abdominal abscess, ileus, or persistence of the common bile duct stenosis. The rate of reoperation is about 5%, and the majority of complications resolve with conservative management. The median postoperative stay is 13 days (range 7–59), and the hospital mortality rate is 0.8%.

Outcome

Most patients increase their body weight after operation. Abdominal pain is completely relieved in 77% of patients, 11% suffer a few periods of abdominal pain per year, but 11% continue to have severe pain. About two-thirds of patients return to work. The late mortality rate is about 6% after a follow-up of up to 22 years.

Subtotal excision of the head of the pancreas with conservation of the duodenum does not result in impaired glucose metabolism in the early postoperative period because only 20–25% of the pancreatic parenchyma has been removed. In 5–10% of patients endocrine function improves in the early postoperative period due to the reduction of glucagon and pancreatic polypeptide baseline secretion originating from the head of the pancreas. An increase in the frequency of diabetes mellitus is observed later due to progressive impairment of islet cell function.

Further reading

Beger HG, Büchler M, Bittner R. The duodenum preserving resection of the head of the pancreas (DPRHP) in patients with chronic pancreatitis and an inflammatory mass in the head. An alternative surgical technique to the Whipple operation. *Acta Chir Scand* 1990; 156: 309–15.

Beger HG, Büchler M, Bittner R, Oettinger W, Roscher R. Duodenum-preserving resection of the head of the pancreas in severe chronic pancreatitis: early and late results. *Ann Surg* 1989; 209: 273–8.

Beger HG, Krautzberger W, Bittner R, Büchler M, Limmer J. Duodenum-preserving resection of the head of the pancreas in patients with severe chronic pancreatitis. *Surgery* 1985; 97: 467–73.

Beger HG, Witte C, Kraas E, Bittner R. Erfahrung mit einer das Duodenum erhaltenden Pankreaskopfresektion bei chronischer Pankreatitis. *Chirurgie* 1980; 51: 303–7.

Bittner R, Butters M, Büchler M, Nägele S, Roscher R, Beger HG. Glucose homeostasis and endocrine pancreatic secretion in patients with chronic pancreatitis before and after surgical therapy. *Biomed Res* 1988; 9(Suppl 1): 28.

Illustrations by Gillian Oliver

Duodenum-preserving total pancreatectomy

R. C. G. Russell MS, FRCS
Consultant Surgeon, The Middlesex Hospital, London, UK

Principles and justification

The importance of the pylorus and duodenum in the maintenance of intestinal function is now acknowledged, and it is accepted that major disease of an inflammatory nature can be managed by excision of the head of the pancreas with duodenal preservation. Several approaches have been made to achieve this; the first, to excise some of the head as in the Beger procedure (*see* page 544); the second, to excise all the pancreas within the duodenal loop; and the third, to decompress the head of the pancreas by excising all the tissue in front of the duct and to anastomose the raw area to a jejunal loop. The latter approach – the Frey procedure – is probably best limited to patients with a cyst in the head of the pancreas or those with a large duct and much calcification in the side branches indicating virtual destruction of the head of the pancreas.

Of the remaining two procedures, it is debatable whether all or only part of the head should be excised. For the majority of patients the Beger procedure is preferable, as there is less danger of damage to the blood supply of the duodenum and intrapancreatic bile duct. Nevertheless, the longer term outlook of these patients has to be assessed to ensure that pancreatic disease does not recur in the remaining pancreas. Thus, total excision of the head is indicated in the younger patient who has already had a previous operation, often a distal pancreatectomy, and who is left with severe pain. To ablate the pancreas in these patients ensures that any further pain is not of pancreatic origin.

Preoperative

A thorough assessment of the patient is required to ensure suitability for surgery, that the certainty of diabetes and enzyme deficiency is accepted, and that there should be no further requirement for narcotic analgesics after the procedure. Particularly in patients who have recently had severe symptoms with computed tomographic evidence of marked inflammatory changes, the management is eased by a period of pancreatic rest with parenteral nutrition only. As the pain resolves, so the analgesics can be reduced and the patient's postoperative rehabilitation will be much improved.

Intravenous fluids should be commenced the evening before surgery, and immediately before the operation a urinary catheter should be passed and limited non-invasive peroperative monitoring arranged.

Operation

For ease of description, it is assumed that the patient has had a previous distal pancreatectomy (*see* page 505) and that the transected pancreas lies on the right side of the portal vein. If only the head is removed, preserving the body and tail of the pancreas, a Roux loop is anastomosed to the neck of the pancreas as described in the Beger procedure (*see* page 547).

Incision

A right upper transverse incision is most convenient; it should not extend across the midline. After a full laparotomy and assessment of the extent of the disease in the head of the pancreas, a cholecystectomy is performed in order to avoid stasis in the gallbladder if there is malfunction of the sphincter of Oddi after the extensive dissection.

Exposure of the head of the pancreas

1 A stabilized ring retractor is ideally suited to provide exposure of the pancreas. The hepatic flexure of the colon is dissected off the front of the pancreas and duodenum. The epiploic artery and vein should be preserved. At the end of this dissection the whole of the duodenal C loop, the head of the pancreas and the portal vein should be exposed. The head of the pancreas and the duodenum are not further mobilized by the Kocher manoeuvre.

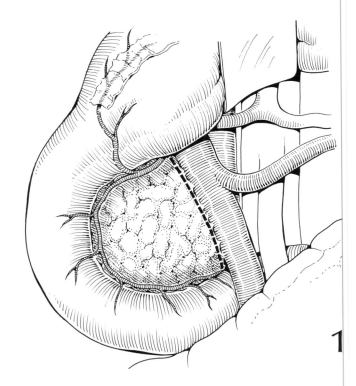

1

Mobilization of the pancreas

2 The neck of the pancreas is dissected off the portal vein, and the uncinate process is dissected away from the superior mesenteric vein. At the point where the duodenum passes under the superior mesenteric vein, the uncinate process of the pancreas is grasped and retracted in an anterosuperior direction. The vessels on the surface of the duodenum are dissected and tied to separate the pancreas from the duodenum.

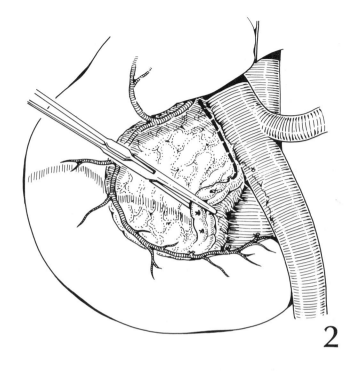

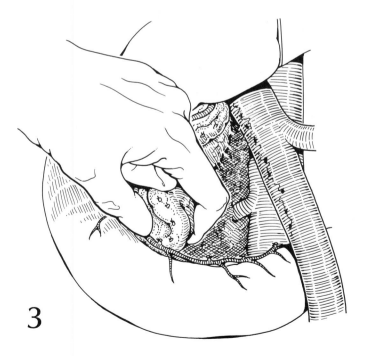

3 The dissection is continued posteriorly to ensure that the duodenum is free from the pancreatic tissue, but this posterior dissection should not be so deep as to destroy the vessels running in the floor of the C loop of the duodenum. The tip of the uncinate process is brought further forwards and a finger is inserted on the posterior surface of the uncinate process. With the finger lifting the pancreas forward and tensing the vessels, it is easier to dissect the arcade between the pancreas and duodenum, and the vessels passing from the pancreas to the mesenteric vessels. This dissection is continued along the superior mesenteric vein and the portal vein until the upper border of the pancreas is reached. The dissection is now continued along the fourth part of the duodenum.

4 As the pancreas becomes more mobile, it is possible to separate it by finger dissection from the floor of the C loop. This helps the tedious dissection of the arcade on the duodenum away from the pancreas until the ampulla of Vater is reached. At this point the pancreas is firmly adherent to the duodenum. Careful dissection is required to isolate the pancreatic duct which is divided near its junction with the bile duct.

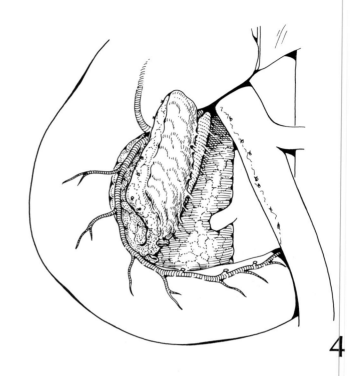

4

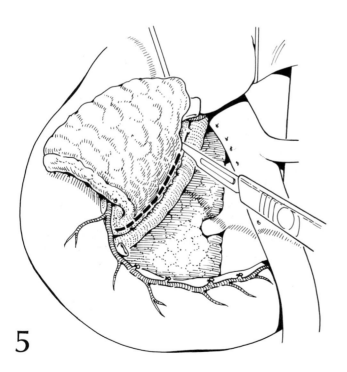

5

Dissection of the bile duct

5 The bile duct is identified either near the ampulla, on the posterior surface, or in the angle between the first part of the duodenum and the portal vein. Once identified, the duct is carefully dissected out from the pancreas by sharp dissection. Sometimes there is a well defined plane but, if not, sharp dissection is required. The pancreas can be sacrificed but the bile duct must not be damaged or devascularized.

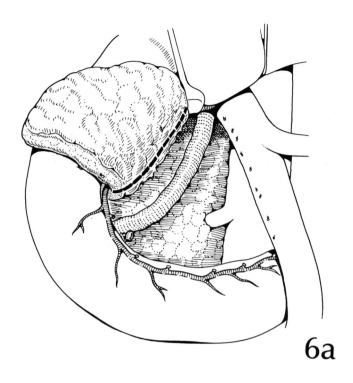

6a

Dissection of the groove

6a, b Once the bile duct is dissected away from the pancreas it remains for the groove of the pancreas between the bile duct and the first and second parts of the duodenum to be removed. This can be achieved by sharp dissection; bleeding, which is minimal at this stage, can be controlled by pressure or by use of the bipolar diathermy. The specimen is then released.

Final assessment

The duodenum is now carefully inspected to ensure that there are no perforations. Any bleeding from the duodenal wall is managed by oversewing. Similarly, the bile duct is inspected to ensure that it is not perforated; a leak can be managed by decompression using a catheter placed into the bile duct via the cystic duct stump. Any defect in the bile duct is sutured with 6/0 polypropylene (Prolene). The colour of the duodenum is carefully assessed; if left with a warm pack the bluish tinge near the ampulla will invariably resolve. When the operative site is satisfactory, a silicone drain is placed down to the duodenum.

Closure

This is performed in the routine manner.

The procedure takes 2.5–4.5 h to complete. Intra-operative blood loss should be less than 750 ml.

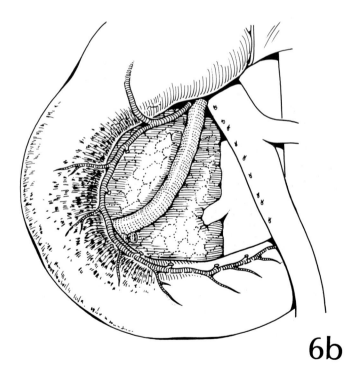

6b

Postoperative care

The patient is monitored carefully, with particular attention being paid to the oxygen saturation level. Oxygen should be given during the first 24 h. An intravenous infusion is maintained until nasogastric aspiration indicates gastric emptying is normal. The median time before normal emptying resumes is 14 days.

The most frequent complication after the operation is sepsis, with chest infection, infection of the infusion line and a urinary tract infection occurring most often. A duodenal leak has occurred in three of 30 patients, and all have resolved spontaneously.

Outcome

Long-term morbidity, mortality and quality of life have been good. A better quality of life has been achieved than in those who underwent standard total pancreatectomy.

Further reading

Büchler MW, Friess H, Muller MW, Wheatley AM, Beger HG. Randomized trial of duodenum-preserving pancreatic head resection versus pylorus-preserving Whipple in chronic pancreatitis. *Am J Surg* 1995; 169: 65–70.

Lambert MA, Lineham IP, Russell RC. Duodenum preserving total pancreatectomy for end stage chronic pancreatitis. *Br J Surg* 1987; 74: 35–9.

Lineham IP, Lambert MA, Brown DC, Kurtz AB, Cotton PB, Russell RC. Total pancreatectomy for chronic pancreatitis. *Gut* 1988; 29: 358–65.

Total pancreatectomy

R. C. G. Russell MS, FRCS
Consultant Surgeon, The Middlesex Hospital, London, UK

Principles and justification

The role of total pancreatectomy has evolved over the last decade, and now has little or no place in the management of malignant disease while, for chronic pancreatitis, it is used as a last resort when previous surgery has failed to control the symptoms. The operation should only be performed after most careful consideration as it will render the patient both endocrine-deficient and exocrine-deficient, a burden of no small magnitude.

Indications

The traditional indications include extensive maligant disease, but this is limited to the rarer duct tumour dysplasias in which there is a papillary neoplasm involving the complete duct system. Multifocal APUD tumours occasionally demand a total pancreatectomy, but blind total resection for functioning islet cell tumours is no longer acceptable. However, a near total or total resection is necessary for nesidioblastosis. The most common indication is failure of the primary operation for chronic pancreatitis; such patients are often already diabetic and enzyme-deficient, so the burdens of insulin and enzyme replacement have already been encountered. It should never be considered in the management of acute pancreatitis.

Contraindications

The operation should rarely, if ever, be performed in persons over 70 years of age or in frail patients with multisystemic disorders and a limited life expectancy. There is no therapeutic benefit in treating those addicted to alcohol or narcotics by this technique, as the postoperative management requires numerous admissions for control of unstable diabetes and steatorrhoea. Once a patient has had this operation, life-long care will be required in order to manage the diabetes and steatorrhoea. This is preferably done by a diabetologist well versed in the management of these patients; thus, the operation should not be performed as a 'one-off' procedure but as part of a long-term pancreatic programme.

Preoperative

Investigation

The decision to perform this operation is based on clinical factors brought together over a period of months. The key investigation is a contrast enhanced spiral computed tomography (CT) scan which will define the anatomy and blood supply clearly. Occasionally, endoscopic retrograde cholangiopancreatography (ERCP) is required to outline the duct anatomy, particularly if there is evidence of stenosis, but by the time the decision has been made to undertake a total pancreatectomy, the surgeon is familiar with the patient, his disease and the anatomical state of his pancreas.

Preparation

In the assessment of the patient and in the preparation for pancreatic resection, meticulous attention must be paid to the general wellbeing of the patient. Emphasis should be placed on the following aspects of preoperative care.

Nutrition and hydration

Many patients who require a total pancreatectomy for benign disease will have suffered significant weight loss. Vitamin and trace element deficiency may be present and require replacement. For inflammatory disease, a period of preoperative pancreatic rest makes the operation easier by allowing resolution of the inflammation. While waiting for this response, parenteral nutrition with vitamin and trace element supplements will be of value in aiding a more rapid recovery postoperatively. In malignant disease there is less time and less need for prolonged preoperative preparation, but in such patients it is important to ensure adequate hydration, a good urine output, and appropriate vitamin supplements.

Haematology

Anaemia and coagulopathy should be corrected.

Cardiopulmonary function

Cardiopulmonary function should be carefully assessed by pulmonary function tests, chest radiography and electrocardiography. If there is any doubt about cardiac function an echocardiogram and MUGA scan are of value.

Infection

Prophylactic systemic antibiotics are recommended for all patients with biliary tract obstruction, especially if the patient has had an endoscopy or preoperative biliary stent. There is no ideal combination and local bacteriological advice should be sought.

For the patients who are jaundiced, endoscopic stenting is advised and the operation should be postponed until liver function tests return to near normal levels.

Anaesthesia

A standard general anaesthetic is appropriate with good muscle relaxation. A nasogastric tube is necessary to decompress the stomach, and an arterial line should be inserted for convenient sampling, particularly of the blood glucose level. Two large cannulae for venous access are appropriate. Oxygen saturation and the end tidal carbon dioxide pressure should be monitored throughout the operation.

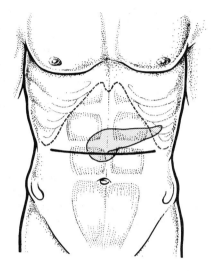

1a

Operation

Incision

1a,b In most patients an oblique or transverse muscle-cutting incision along the long axis of the pancreas is preferable to the long midline vertical incision, but preference depends on previous scars and the build of the patient.

Abdominal exploration

For both malignant and benign disease a systematic and thorough examination of the abdominal cavity is required. In malignant disease, any suspicious nodule should be excised and subjected to frozen section examination. Some advocate a laparoscopy to hasten this stage of the procedure, but there is still no substitute for careful palpation. Pancreatic cancer can occur in patients with pancreatitis and can cause obstruction of the pancreatic duct which produces changes identical to those of chronic pancreatitis. Such dilemmas are usually resolved by ultrasound or CT-guided biopsy and, if these are unhelpful, the decision to resect must be made on clinical grounds before the operation commences.

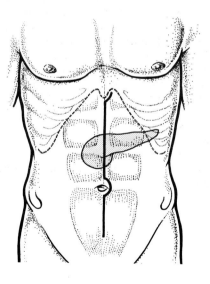

1b

Mobilization of the duodenum and head of the pancreas

2a,b A cholecystectomy can be performed initially to help expose the operative field. The peritoneal reflection lateral to the second part of the duodenum is incised in front of the right kidney, and the duodenum and pancreatic head are mobilized anteriorly and to the left by careful sharp dissection with meticulous haemostasis. Diathermy scissors aid this procedure. In benign disease the dissection is close to the duodenum and pancreas, while in malignant disease Gerota's fascia is opened on the front of the kidney and the fascia and fat are removed from the kidney, the right renal vein, the inferior vena cava, the left renal vein and the aorta.

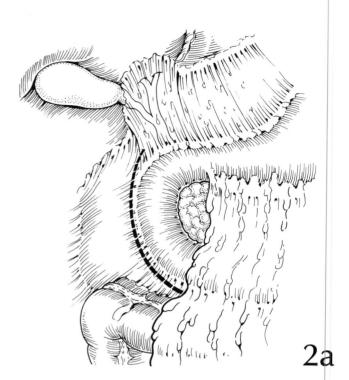

2a

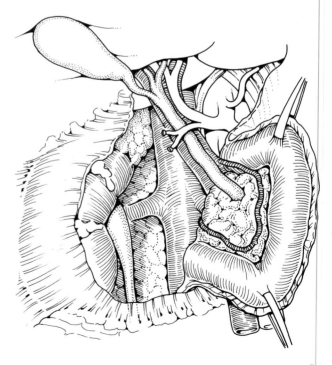

2b

Exposure of the body and tail of the pancreas

3a–c The greater curve of the stomach is mobilized by dividing the vessels within the epiploic arcade from the right epiploic artery and vein to the left epiploic artery and vein. The lesser sac exposure is completed by dividing the short gastric vessels up to the apex of the spleen (*Illustration 3a*). The spleen is exposed by dividing the left gastroepiploic vessels on the hilum of the spleen, and continuing this dissection to the splenic flexure of the colon and the left paracolic gutter to mobilize the splenic flexure of the colon and its mesentry (*Illustration 3b*). The superior mesenteric vein is identified and the neck of the pancreas mobilized from it and the portal vein; a tape is placed round the neck of the pancreas. The splenic artery is exposed at the upper border of the pancreas and tied (*Illustration 3c*).

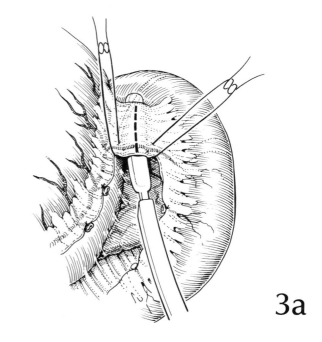

3a

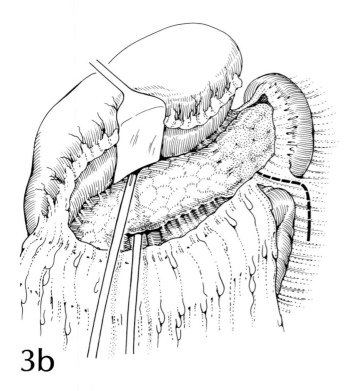

3b

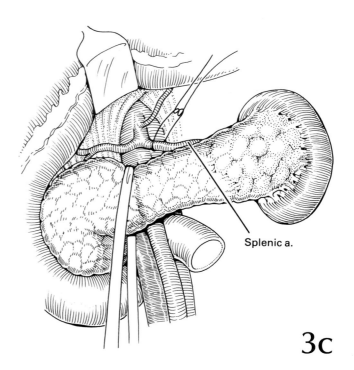

Splenic a.

3c

Dissection of the vessels

4 From the splenic artery, the hepatic artery is traced along the upper border of the pancreas and separated from it by dividing the right gastric artery and the gastroduodenal artery. In malignant disease all the lymph nodes around these vessels are removed with adjacent fat so that the porta hepatis is skeletonized.

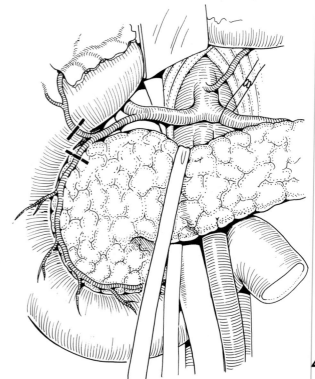

4

Mobilization of the spleen and pancreas

5a–d Attention is directed to the tail of the pancreas. The inferior border of the body and tail of the pancreas is dissected, and this plane beneath the body and tail of the pancreas is extended laterally to divide the lienorenal and lienophrenic ligament (*Illustration 5a*). The spleen, now mobile, is carefully dissected off the diaphragm, if attached by adhesions, with the diathermy scissors. The spleen and tail of the pancreas are dissected from the posterior abdominal wall, the left gastric vein is tied and dissection is continued to the neck of the pancreas (*Illustrations 5b* and *5c*). By holding up the tape around the neck of the pancreas, the junction of the splenic vein with the portal vein is defined. The proximal end is oversewn on the portal vein and the neck of the pancreas is dissected from the portal vein (*Illustration 5d*).

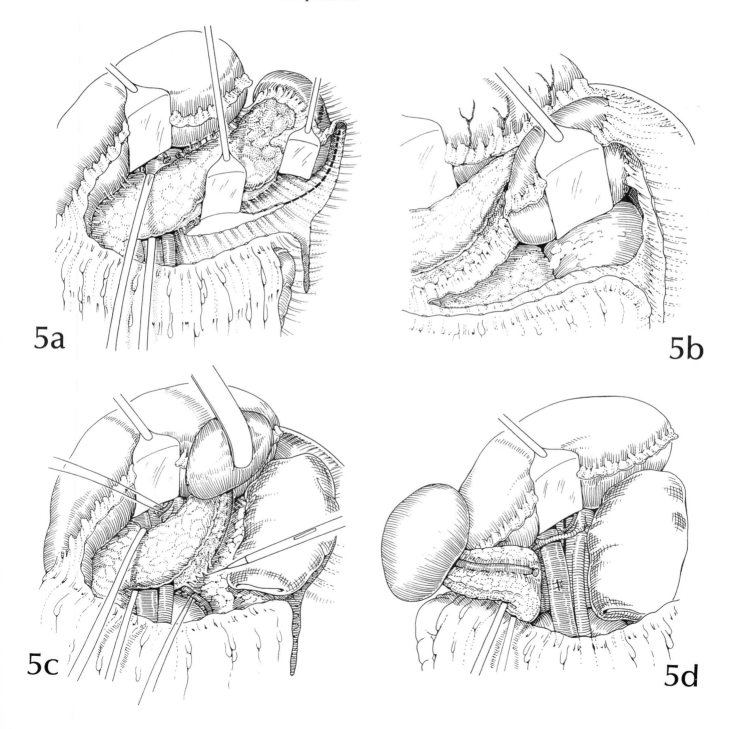

5a

5b

5c

5d

Division of the stomach

6 A limited gastrectomy or a pylorus-preserving resection may be performed. With the latter, a more conservative dissection of the vessels of the lesser curve is necessary to obtain a well vascularized duodenum. The fourth part of the duodenum is carefully dissected and the jejunum delivered into the supracolic compartment where it is transected.

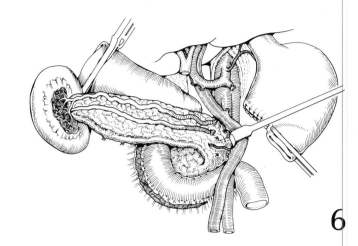

6

Resection of the head of the pancreas

7 With the stomach divided, the body of the pancreas and spleen mobile, and the jejunum divided and separated from its mesentery, only the vascular attachments of the uncinate process and the head of the pancreas maintain the viability of the specimen. Starting inferiorly at the ligament of Treitz, the pancreatic branches of the superior mesenteric artery and vein are clipped, divided and ligated. The pancreatic veins to the portal vein are divided last, leaving only the common bile duct to transect to release the specimen.

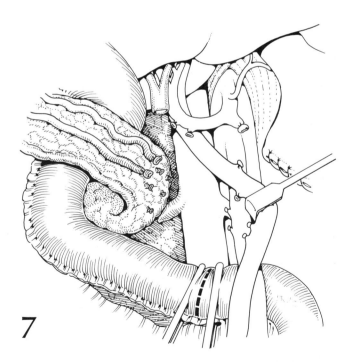

7

Reconstruction

8 The great advantage of total pancreatectomy is that there is no pancreatic anastomosis. The jejunum is brought up from the ligament of Treitz and anastomosed end-to-end with the duodenum. An end-to-side choledochojejunostomy is formed 10 cm distally. A silicone drain is inserted into the pancreatic bed and the abdomen is closed.

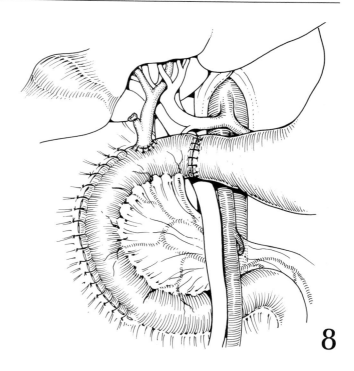

8

Postoperative care

Careful monitoring of urine output, pulse, blood pressure and oxygen saturation is required in the initial postoperative period. Ventilation should be unnecessary. Hourly blood glucose estimation is required. Insulin is given as an infusion, the most convenient technique being to infuse Actrapid insulin (50 i.u. in 50 ml normal saline) via a syringe driver. The rate of infusion is adjusted to maintain the blood glucose level at 4–8 mmol/l. In order to standardize the infusion, 2 litres of 5% dextrose are infused at a constant rate over 24 h. A separate infusion of normal saline should run concurrently, the volume delivered being dependent on the fluid and electrolyte balance.

The most common complication after a total pancreatectomy is sepsis. Fistulae and haemorrhage are unusual due to the absence of the pancreas. Despite this, the mortality rate following a total pancreatectomy is invariably higher than after a subtotal procedure, being 3–5% with a 50% morbidity due to infection. The median length of stay in hospital is 21 days, at least some of which is spent ensuring that the patient is off all narcotics and in control of their diabetes.

Long-term management

The future for the patient with no pancreas is governed by his diabetes, and the diabetic control is governed by the bowel. Much of the fragile nature of diabetes after total pancreatectomy is related to variable absorption of carbohydrate. A rapid transit due to a high fat load leads to inconsistent absorption and an unstable diabetic state. Adequate enzyme consumption is the key to health. Far higher doses of enzyme are required than are recommended in the pharmaceutical literature, many patients requiring up to 60 capsules per day of the high potency preparations. Once the patient has grasped the need to balance his intake (particularly the quantum of

fat in the diet) with the number of capsules of enzyme replacement, then a stable absorption pattern is achieved and the diabetes is managed with ease. Patients have difficulty in managing these fundamentals, and much counselling by dedicated liaison nurses is required during the early months.

Outcome

Once the patient is stable, the long-term future is good. However, because of the aetiology of their pancreatitis, these patients are prone to an increased mortality rate from drug abuse, alcohol-related and cardiovascular disease. After total pancreatectomy for cancer few patients live long enough to determine whether the same problems arise. Once a total pancreatectomy has been performed, the patient remains a patient for life.

Further reading

Cooper MJ, Williamson RC, Benjamin IS *et al*. Total pancreatectomy for chronic pancreatitis. *Br J Surg* 1987; 74: 912–15.

Linehan IP, Lambert MA, Brown DC, Kurtz AB, Cotton PB, Russell RC. Total pancreatectomy for chronic pancreatitis. *Gut* 1988; 29: 358–65.

Stone WM, Sarr MG, Nagorney DM, McIlrath DC. Chronic pancreatitis – results of Whipple's resection and total pancreatectomy. *Arch Surg* 1988; 123: 815–19.

Chronic pancreatitis: other procedures including pain relief operations

Ingemar Ihse MD, PhD
Professor and Chairman, Department of Surgery, University Hospital, Lund, Sweden

Åke Andrén-Sandberg MD, PhD
Associate Professor, Department of Surgery, University Hospital, Lund, Sweden

Masao Kobari MD
Visiting Scientist, Department of Surgery, University Hospital, Lund, Sweden

Principles and justification

Pain is the principal clinical feature of chronic pancreatitis and both its frequency and its duration vary. Only about 5% of patients will be pain-free throughout the course of their disease. Operative intervention aims to achieve pain relief by removal of inflamed pancreatic tissue and/or by decompressing the main duct of the gland. The alternative treatment options, based on our current knowledge of regulation of pancreatic secretion and of neural anatomy, are presented in this chapter.

Cause of pain in chronic pancreatitis

The opinion that pain in patients with chronic pancreatitis has many causes is supported by the clinical experience that the characteristics of pain vary, not only among patients, but also in the same patient from time to time.

The most commonly discussed cause of pain is intraductal and intraparenchymal hypertension. Increased ductal pressure has been reported in patients with chronic pancreatitis and pain compared with those without pain and those without pancreatitis as mea-sured intraoperatively or endoscopically. Similarly, pancreatic tissue fluid pressure was found to be raised in cases of painful pancreatitis, but fell to normal levels after surgical drainage procedures. Interestingly, the tissue fluid pressure was raised in those who suffered pain 1 year postoperatively while in pain-free patients it was normal[1]. There is therefore increasing evidence that hypertension of the duct and tissue is involved in pain generation in patients with chronic pancreatitis.

There also seems to be a specific pancreatitis-associated neuritis in such patients. The number of sensory nerve cells is increased in inflamed pancreatic tissue and there is infiltration of round cells and a disintegration of the perineurium, allowing influx of inflammatory mediators such as substance P and calcitonin gene-related peptide (CGRP).

Hypertension and neuritis may work together to cause pain, as the former may facilitate the influx of pain mediators through the injured perineurium. This could tentatively explain the more constant type of pancreatic pain, whereas acute attacks are associated with acute inflammation and/or autodigestion with tissue necrosis and pseudocyst formation[2].

Medical treatment

The different modalities of medical treatment of pain in chronic pancreatitis will not be fully covered; instead, attention will be focused on endeavours which have been made to relieve pain by suppressing exocrine pancreatic secretion and function. Most authors agree that in the human there is a negative feedback mechanism exerted by intraluminal proteases on the regulation of exocrine pancreatic secretion. Based on this mechanism, it has been suggested that the low levels of intraintestinal proteases in chronic pancreatitis stimulate pancreatic secretion with an ensuing tissue hypertension because of the outflow obstruction caused by ductal stenoses and stones. If this hypothesis is correct, oral enzyme replacement would be beneficial.

Several prospective studies support the hypothesis. However, there are also reports of no pain relief being achieved with this treatment[3]. Certainly, it is worthwhile to test the enzyme treatment for a couple of months before resorting to analgesics. Theoretically, somatostatin may be of value if pain is caused by hypertension of the duct tissue. This hormone has a direct inhibitory effect on pancreatic secretion, inhibits the release of cholecystokinin and secretin, and inhibits neurally-stimulated pancreatic secretion. The results of the ongoing prospective randomized studies of somatostatin in the treatment of pain in patients with chronic pancreatitis are awaited with interest.

Surgical treatment

Autonomic nerve supply of the pancreas

1 The pancreas is innervated by the sympathetic and parasympathetic nervous systems. The sympathetic nerves reach the pancreas by way of the greater and lesser splanchnic nerves. The greater splanchic nerve arises from the fifth to the ninth or tenth thoracic sympathetic ganglia and the lesser splanchnic nerve is composed of fibres from the ninth and tenth or the tenth and eleventh ganglia. These nerves pierce the diaphragmatic crura to enter the coeliac ganglia. The parasympathetic nerves reach the pancreas by way of the vagus nerves which enter the coeliac ganglia through the coeliac division of the posterior vagus trunk. Both the anterior and the posterior vagal trunks pass through the oesophageal hiatus. In the omental bursa the posterior trunk is divided into the posterior gastric and coeliac divisions. In the coeliac ganglia parasympathetic nerves form a loop with sympathetic nerves. Branches from the coeliac ganglia of both sides are connected and reach the surrounding tissues to form the coeliac plexus and superior mesenteric plexus. Thus, all nerves to the pancreas, both afferent and efferent, pass through the coeliac plexus. From the plexus the nerves accompany the vessels and enter the pancreas. The sympathetic nerve fibres are mainly distributed to the blood vessels of the gland. Parasympathetic fibres run between the pancreatic lobules to reach individual acinar, ductal or endocrine cells. Afferent pain fibres from the pancreas pass through the coeliac ganglia to enter the splanchnic nerves.

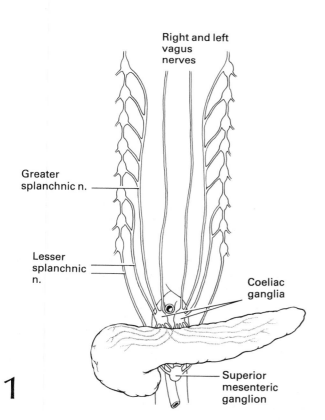

Right and left vagus nerves

Greater splanchnic n.

Lesser splanchnic n.

Coeliac ganglia

Superior mesenteric ganglion

1

COELIAC PLEXUS BLOCK

Coeliac plexus block with alcohol or phenol has been used in patients with pancreatic pain which does not have an obvious cause that might be treated by another strategy.

2 Under local anaesthesia, with the patient in the prone position, two needles are inserted 7–8 cm from the midline at the inferior edge of the 12th rib. When the needles reach the lateral body of the first lumbar vertebra (L1) they are redirected until they slide off the vertebral body. They are then advanced about 2 cm until their tips rest just anterior to the upper part of the body of the first lumbar vertebra. Ganglia are usually located 1.5 cm anterior to the front of the vertebral body, those on the left being located lower than those on the right. Aspiration through the needle is performed when the needle is in position. Injection should meet no resistance when the needle is correctly placed in the loose retroperitoneal tissue; 20–25 ml of 0.25% bupivacaine is injected through each needle. If good pain relief is achieved the procedure is repeated within 1–2 days using 25 ml 50% alcohol on each side. It is recommended that the needle is guided by fluoroscopy with injection of contrast medium. The procedure described above is called the classic approach. Modifications such as the transcrural and transaortic routes have also been tried.

There are few severe complications after coeliac plexus block, but hypotension and increased gut motility are known side effects which sometimes require treatment.

In a collective review of 18 studies comprising 432 patients with pancreatic cancer, good pain relief was achieved in 70–100% of cases by this method. In chronic pancreatitis good pain relief was reported in 0–100% (average 60%) of 77 patients reported in eight studies. The pain relief in these patients lasted for hours to a few months[2]. In a prospective randomized study the pain relief by percutaneous coeliac plexus block in patients with chronic pancreatitis was compared with that of pancreaticogastrostomy. At follow-up after 6 months the results of the surgical procedure were significantly better than those after the nerve block[4]. Most authors agree that coeliac plexus block is helpful in pancreatic pain due to cancer, but that it should be used very selectively in pancreatitis and only when a block with a local anaesthetic agent has been shown to be effective.

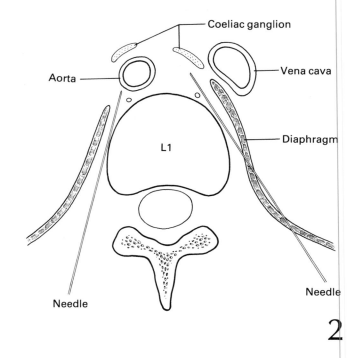

2

SURGICAL NERVE ABLATION PROCEDURES

Retroperitoneal, intraperitoneal and transhiatal splanchnicectomy have been practised in the past, especially by French surgeons[5]. Different techniques have been developed but none is widely accepted. However, long-term pain relief in 90% of patients has been reported from experienced centres[6]. Procedures such as the denervated splenopancreatic flap and complete denervation of the pancreas have not been generally accepted. The same is true for transthoracic left splanchnicectomy combined with truncal vagotomy. The results of all these operations as presented by the initial authors need confirmation.

THORACOSCOPIC SPLANCHNICECTOMY

The rapid development in the field of endoscopic surgery has led to progress in the thoracoscopic approach. For treatment of pain in patients with chronic pancreatitis, thoracoscopic splanchnicectomy has been suggested (*see also* page 592).

The procedure is performed under general anaesthesia, with the patient in the prone position, using double-lumen endotracheal intubation making single lung ventilation possible. A small trocar is introduced after local anaesthesia with adrenaline (to minimize local bleeding) through the first intercostal space encountered caudal to the inferior angle of the scapula. A pneumothorax is created by allowing air into the pleural cavity. If necessary, carbon dioxide is insufflated to improve access to the operation field. The trocar is replaced by the telescope (10 mm) and an operating cannula (5.5 mm) is inserted under direct vision in the next or subsequent intercostal space. A 30° forward oblique telescope is used. The other working instruments are a duckbill grasper and an electrosurgical hook.

The sympathetic chain lying across the neck of the ribs and overlain by the parietal pleura is easily identified and the splanchnic nerves are visualized. A small incision is made with the electrosurgical hook on each side of the nerve 10 mm from the chain. The nerve is then grasped by the hook, freed for a distance of about 6 mm, and cut so that the ends are seen to be clearly separated. The most cranial nerve is usually found on the neck of the sixth rib and is often the one which is most easily identified. The operation preferably starts at this point and the nerves are approached one by one in a caudal direction along the sympathetic chain. The number of nerves identified and divided on each side varies from four to seven.

Postoperative care

A small chest drain is inserted through the lower incision and removed after 6–8 h if there are no signs of bleeding. The operating time is about 15 minutes on each side. A chest radiograph is performed after the patient has recovered from the anaesthesia. If the postoperative course is uneventful, the patient is discharged from the hospital the day after the operation.

Outcome

The experience of the procedure is still limited but available reports show promising results. However, the follow-up time is still short. The authors' results are

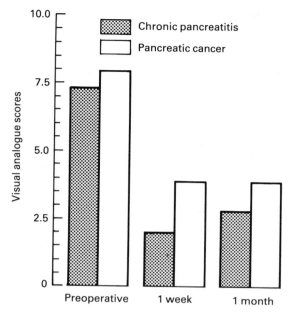

Figure 1   Results of thoracoscopic splanchnicectomy in 11 patients with chronic pancreatitis and five with pancreatic cancer. Pain relief evaluated by visual analogue scores.

summarized in *Figure 1*. The marked pain relief during the first month was accompanied by a reduced need for analgesics. Long-term follow-up will determine if thoracoscopic splanchnicectomy deserves a place in the therapeutic arsenal for patients with chronic pancreatitis and pain.

References

1. Ebbehöj N, Borley L, Bülow J, Rasmusson SG, Madsen P. Evaluation of pancreatic tissue fluid pressure and pain in chronic pancreatitis – a longitudinal study. *Scand J Gastroenterol* 1990; 25: 462–6.

2. Ihse I, ed. Pancreatic pain – causes, diagnosis and treatment. *Acta Chir Scand* 1990; 156: 257–321.

3. Ihse I. Treatment of pain in chronic pancreatitis with pancreatic enzymes. In: Lankisch PG, ed. *Pancreatic Enzymes in Health and Disease*. Berlin: Springer, 1991: 89–94.

4. Madsen P, Hansen E. Coeliac plexus block versus pancreatico-gastrostomy for pain in chronic pancreatitis – a controlled randomized trial. *Scand J Gastroenterol* 1985; 20: 1217–20.

5. Hollender LF, Laugner B. Pain-relieving procedures in chronic pancreatitis. In: Trede M, Carter DC, eds. *Surgery of the Pancreas*. Edinburgh: Churchill Livingstone, 1993: 349–57.

6. Mallet-Guy PA. Late and very late results of resections of the nervous system in the treatment of chronic relapsing pancreatitis. *Am J Surg* 1983; 145: 234–8.

Pancreatic cancer: palliation of pain

Keith D. Lillemoe MD
Associate Professor, Department of Surgery, The Johns Hopkins Medical Institutions, Baltimore, Maryland, USA

History

Significant advances have been made in the last two decades in the diagnosis and management of pancreatic cancer. Pancreaticoduodenectomy can now be performed with acceptably low perioperative morbidity and mortality, with recent reports showing improvement in overall survival. Unfortunately, at the time of diagnosis most patients with pancreatic cancer are unresectable for cure, so optimal palliation of symptoms to maximize quality of life is of primary importance in these patients. Significant improvement in the surgical palliation of pancreatic carcinoma has also been achieved in recent years. Furthermore, non-operative palliation of obstructive jaundice has been shown to relieve this symptom effectively in patients deemed to be inoperable based on either extent of disease or their general medical condition. Yet, perhaps the most disturbing and incapacitating symptom of pancreatic cancer – namely, pain – is poorly managed and can remain a significant problem for many patients until death.

The use of chemical splanchnicectomy in patients with unresectable pancreatic cancer was first described by Copping and colleagues in 1969[1]. In an update in 1978 of their series which included 41 patients, 88% of those with pain due to pancreatic cancer experienced pain relief after surgery[2]. Most of these patients underwent palliative biliary and gastrointestinal bypass at the same operation. These results were compared with a group of historical controls in which only 21% of patients experienced pain relief after similar palliative procedures. There were no reported complications of chemical splanchnicectomy. Since that time, this procedure has been advocated by a number of authors in anecdotal reports describing successful control of pain in the majority of patients. In 1993 a prospective, randomized placebo controlled study of this treatment was completed and the results suggested that chemical splanchnicectomy with 50% alcohol significantly reduced or prevented pain in patients with unresectable pancreatic cancer[3].

With the recent advances in laparoscopic and thoracoscopic surgery, technical descriptions and reports have been published of thoracoscopic pancreatic denervation performed via the left chest[4]. Preliminary results using this technique have been excellent with minimal morbidity.

Principles and justification

The pathogenesis of pain associated with pancreatic cancer can be classified into two general categories. The first mechanism is pain due to obstruction of either the biliary or pancreatic ducts. This pain will generally be located in the upper abdomen, is exacerbated by oral intake, and is associated with dilatation of the pancreatic and biliary ducts. Relief of the biliary obstruction and its associated pain can be achieved either by surgical bypass or by non-surgical endoscopic or radiological stent placement. Relief of malignant pancreatic ductal obstruction, however, is more difficult and neither pancreatic stenting nor surgical drainage procedures have provided consistent relief of pain. The second mechanism of pain due to pancreatic cancer comes from direct retroperitoneal nerve invasion. Direct nerve invasion by pancreatic cancer can be seen in most patients who undergo pancreatic resection. It is therefore likely that all patients with unresectable cancer will have progressive nerve involvement as their disease advances. Pain due to retroperitoneal nerve involvement is usually constant and is often relieved by sitting forward. This pain is often the first symptom in patients with cancers arising in the uncinate process or the body or tail of the pancreas.

Indications

The use of intraoperative chemical splanchnicectomy is limited to those patients with pancreatic cancer who, after preoperative assessment and staging, are considered surgical candidates. After determining at laparotomy that the tumour is unresectable, intraoperative chemical splanchnicectomy should be performed. The procedure is indicated whether the patient has signifi-cant pain or is pain-free at the time of surgery. The technique is applicable whether the cancer arises in the head, body or tail of the pancreas. There would appear to be no indication for chemical splanchnicectomy following pancreaticoduodenectomy or distal pancreatectomy if resection is completed with grossly clear margins. In the unusual situation where resection is completed but gross tumour is left at the margins, chemical splanchnicectomy may be performed in the hope of treating or preventing future pain due to retroperitoneal invasion of the remaining tumour.

There is no indication for laparotomy for the sole purpose of performing intraoperative chemical splanchnicectomy in patients who are otherwise not candidates for surgical resection or palliation based on either extent of disease, age or medical disability. The availability of percutaneous coeliac block with fluoroscopic or computed tomographic guidance has eliminated the need for this procedure in almost all patients. In those rare patients in whom percutaneous chemical splanchnicectomy cannot be safely performed, thoracoscopic pancreatic denervation offers an appropriate alternative. Patients requiring thoracoscopy must be suitable candidates for general anaesthesia but require no other special preparation.

Preoperative

Intraoperative chemical splanchnicectomy is simply an additional procedure performed as part of the surgical palliation of pancreatic cancer. No special preoperative assessment or preparation is therefore necessary for this technique. Patients should undergo appropriate preoperative assessment and preparation for either the planned resection or palliative procedure as discussed in the chapter on pp. 594–609.

Operations

INTRAOPERATIVE CHEMICAL SPLANCHNICECTOMY

Intraoperative chemical splanchnicectomy is performed as part of a palliative surgical procedure for pancreatic carcinoma with either an upper midline or bilateral subcostal incision providing adequate exposure. After determining that the cancer is unresectable and having completed a biliary bypass and/or gastrojejunostomy as indicated, chemical splanchnicectomy should be performed. A 50% alcohol solution should be prepared in a sterile fashion by dilution of absolute alcohol with sterile injectable saline solution. A 20-ml syringe with either a 20 or 22 gauge spinal needle is used for the injection.

1 The lesser omentum is excised and the coeliac axis can be palpated as it arises from the aorta. A palpable thrill due to the high blood flow through the coeliac axis is usually apparent.

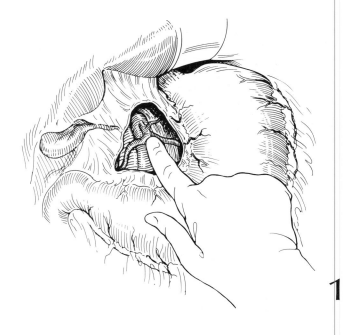

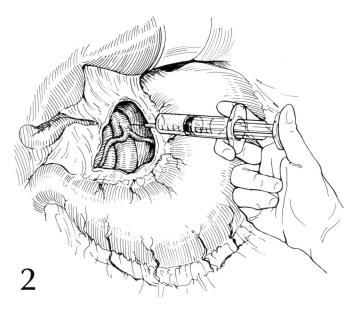

2 The 22 gauge spinal needle is then advanced on either side of the aorta at the level of the coeliac axis and 20 ml of the 50% alcohol solution is injected on each side. Both before and during the injection the syringe should be aspirated to ensure that neither the vena cava, aorta nor adjacent lumbar vessels have been cannulated.

After completion of both injections the sites are inspected for haemostasis. If minor bleeding is observed, the area is simply packed and compressed for a short period of time. At the time of injection the anaesthetist should be notified of the procedure because some degree of hypotension may occasionally be observed with an adequate sympathetic block. This situation can generally be managed by intraoperative administration of crystalloid solution.

THORACOSCOPIC PANCREATIC DENERVATION

A double-lumen endotracheal tube is inserted and the patient is placed on the operating table in the right lateral decubitus position. The arm is elevated on a sling to a 90° angle to the chest wall and the table is tilted posteriorly to about 15°.

3 A 1-cm incision is made in the fourth intercostal space in the anterior axillary line and, after single-lung (right) ventilation, an 11-mm thoracoscopic cannula is inserted and the thoracoscope is introduced. Three additional 11-mm cannulas are placed in the sixth intercostal space in the anterior axillary line and through the seventh and ninth spaces in the posterior axillary line of the left chest.

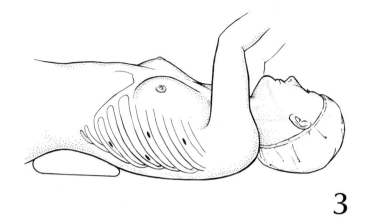

3

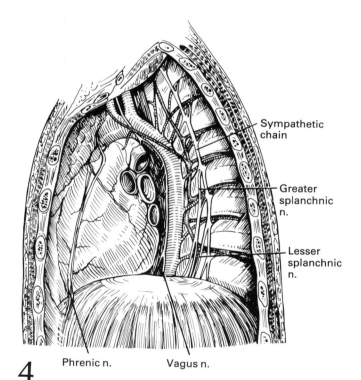

Sympathetic chain

Greater splanchnic n.

Lesser splanchnic n.

Phrenic n.   Vagus n.

4

4 The sympathetic chain is identified coursing over the ribs 2 cm posterior and lateral to the aorta. The upper end of the sympathetic chain is noted and the stellate ganglion is identified. The greater splanchnic nerve (T 5–9) and lesser splanchnic nerve (T 10–11) are identified.

5 The parietal pleura is incised and dissected superiorly and inferiorly. Each nerve should be doubly clipped and divided.

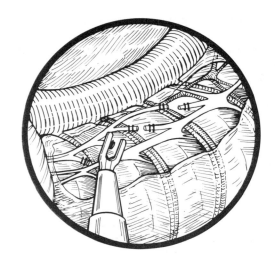

5

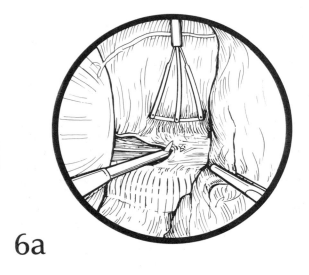

6a

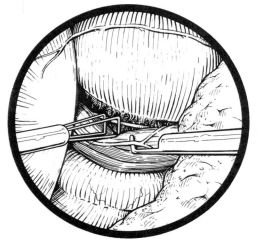

6b

6a, b In order to add a vagotomy to the procedure, a semi-flexible dilator or flexible endoscope is inserted into the distal oesophagus to facilitate identification of this structure. The left lung is retracted anteriorly and cephalad away from the oesophagus using an atraumatic fan-like instrument. It may be necessary to divide the inferior pulmonary ligament in order to retract the left lung away adequately from the distal third of the oesophagus. The pleura overlying the oesophagus is opened with either blunt or sharp dissection and the oesophagus is identified. The left vagus nerve (anterior) is easily visualized over the anterior surface of the oesophagus and is dissected free from the underlying muscle fibres. The structure is then doubly clipped and divided.

7 Access to the right (posterior) vagus nerve usually requires complete mobilization of the oesophagus, and the dilator or endoscope should be withdrawn to a point above this area. After identification of the structure it can also be doubly clipped and divided. A small (28–32 Fr) chest tube is inserted through a lower cannula incision.

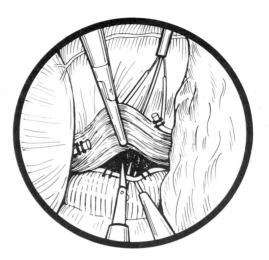

7

Postoperative care

The addition of an intraoperative chemical splanchnicectomy will require no alteration in the postoperative management of a patient undergoing laparotomy and palliative procedures for unresectable pancreatic cancer. In those patients in whom only a biopsy for tissue diagnosis and a chemical splanchnicectomy is performed, the patient can return to oral intake as tolerated and be discharged as soon as possible after the procedure. During first attempts at postoperative ambulation the patients should be observed for any evidence of orthostatic hypotension; however, this effect, if noted at all, is seldom long-lasting.

Following thoracoscopic pancreatic denervation the chest tube can be removed on the first or second postoperative day and the patient discharged shortly thereafter.

Outcome

A prospective, randomized placebo controlled trial of intraoperative chemical splanchnicectomy with 50% alcohol was recently completed at The Johns Hopkins Hospital[3]. Preoperative and postoperative pain were assessed with a questionnaire including a visual analogue scale. No significant difference was found between the patients who received chemical splanchnicectomy and the control group with respect to perioperative morbidity, mortality, length of nasogastric drainage, days until oral intake or postoperative length of stay in hospital. In the patients with pre-existing pain, a statistically significant decrease in mean postoperative pain scores was observed when compared with the control patients; 70% of those with pre-existing pain who received alcohol had a decrease in their narcotic requirement compared with none of the control group. Patients who received alcohol experienced a mean of 3.3 pain-free months compared with 0.8 pain-free months for the control patients. Unfortunately, significant pain did recur before death in 65% of the patients who received an alcohol block.

In patients with no pre-existing pain a statistically significant decrease in mean postoperative pain scores was also observed in those who received chemical splanchnicectomy compared with the placebo control group. The mean number of months without significant pain was 7.2 months in the treated group and only 3.0 months in the placebo group. Only 46% of patients receiving alcohol block ever required significant doses of narcotic pain medications compared with 60% of the placebo patients. Finally, 56% of patients who received alcohol splanchnicectomy reported no significant pain until death compared with only 34% of the patients in the placebo group.

An unexplained and surprising finding of this study was that, in those patients with significant preoperative pain who underwent chemical splanchnicectomy, a highly significant increase in survival was noted when compared with similar patients in the control group. These two subgroups were analysed with respect to age, tumour location, tumour stage, operation performed, the use of chemotherapy and radiotherapy, baseline mood and disability. No significant difference was apparent in any of these comparisons, suggesting that adequate pain control may improve survival in patients with this disease.

Although no prospective trials have been performed, a number of authors have reported significant pain control following thoracoscopic pancreatic denervation with minimal perioperative morbidity[4].

References

1. Copping J, Willix R, Kraft R. Palliative chemical splanchnicectomy. *Arch Surg* 1969; 98: 418–20.

2. Flanigan DP, Kraft RO. Continuing experience with palliative chemical splanchnicectomy. *Arch Surg* 1978; 113: 509–11.

3. Lillemoe KD, Cameron JL, Kaufman HS, Yeo CJ, Pitt HA, Sauter PK. Chemical splanchnicectomy in patients with unresectable pancreatic cancer. A prospective randomized trial. *Ann Surg* 1993; 217: 447–57.

4. Worsey J, Ferson PF, Keenan RJ, Julian TB, Landreneau RJ. Thoracoscopic pancreatic denervation for pain control in irresectable pancreatic cancer. *Br J Surg* 1993; 80: 1051–2.

Pancreatic cancer: laparoscopic staging

O. James Garden BSc, MD, FRCS(Ed), FRCS(Glas)
Senior Lecturer and Honorary Consultant Hepatobiliary Surgeon, University Department of Surgery and Scottish Liver Transplantation Unit, Royal Infirmary, Edinburgh, UK

For most patients who present with symptoms from pancreatic cancer there is already local progression of disease and metastatic spread. Conventional radiological imaging may not detect small hepatic metastases and peritoneal deposits which are readily detected by direct inspection of the peritoneal cavity at laparoscopy[1]. Laparoscopic ultrasonography is a new technique which will detect such overt dissemination of pancreatic tumour but, more importantly, it also allows assessment of local tumour invasion, regional nodal involvement and distant metastatic spread to the liver using high resolution real-time ultrasound imaging[2]. Early reports indicate that staging information additional to that obtained from laparoscopy alone is obtained in over half the patients examined, and that the technique is more specific and accurate in predicting tumour resectability than laparoscopy alone[3, 4].

Principles and justification

Any patient with suspected pancreatic malignancy in whom surgery is contemplated should be submitted to preoperative staging assessment by laparoscopy and laparoscopic ultrasonography. The examination permits sampling of ascitic fluid and suspicious lesions of the peritoneum, omentum and liver. Direct laparoscopic inspection of the pancreas through the omental bursa, lesser omentum and gastrocolic omentum or meso-colon has been described. However, access to the pancreatic head may be limited, and successful exploration of the lesser sac provides little information regarding local tumour invasion into the retroperitoneum or adjacent vascular structures. Such information can readily be obtained by laparoscopic ultrasonography without the need for laparoscopic dissection.

Laparoscopic evaluation is contraindicated in patients with obvious clinical evidence of disseminated disease, and percutaneous needle aspiration cytology of enlarged nodes or sampling of ascitic fluid may provide

sufficient confirmation. The results of transcutaneous abdominal ultrasonography, computed tomographic (CT) scanning and angiography should be interpreted with caution when assessing tumour resectability[5,6].

Preoperative

The patient will require preoperative assessment to determine fitness for general anaesthesia. When examination is undertaken in the jaundiced patient, consideration should be given to renal function and coagulation status.

The examination is performed under general anaesthesia with muscle relaxation. Passage of a nasogastric tube to decompress the stomach facilitates examination of the body and tail of the pancreas. Low-dose subcutaneous heparin (5000 IU) is administered as thromboprophylaxis in patients with normal coagulation parameters.

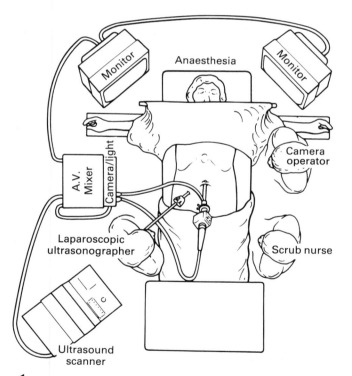

1

1 The patient is examined supine on the operating table with the laparoscopic ultrasound machine positioned nearby. The controls may be operated by the surgeon if a remote control device is available or if the control panel is covered with a sterile drape. For laparoscopic ultrasonography the author uses a probe equipped with a side-viewing 7.5 MHz linear array transducer (Aloka UST-5521-7.5, KeyMed Ltd, Southend-on-Sea, UK; TETRAD 7.5D, Englewood, Colorado, USA). Picture and picture video mixing using an audiovisual mixing desk (Panasonic WJEA5-AV, KeyMed Ltd, Southend-on-Sea, UK) allows a laparoscopic camera picture and laparoscopic sonogram to be observed simultaneously on the video monitor.

2 A 10–11-mm diameter disposable laparoscopic port is inserted via an infraumbilical incision by a direct cutdown approach. A second 10–11-mm diameter port is inserted in the right flank under direct laparoscopic vision. A probe can be introduced through this second port to elevate the liver and to displace the omentum and small bowel loops during laparoscopic inspection.

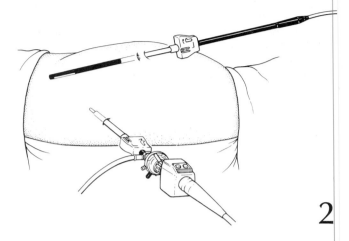

3 A search is made for serosal deposits on both the visceral and parietal peritoneum. Any suspicious peritoneal seedlings are biopsied using straight-bladed laparoscopic scissors or biopsy forceps. All lesions on the surface of the liver should be sampled as biliary ectasia is not uncommon in patients who have previously undergone endoscopic decompression of the biliary tree. The pancreatic region can be 'palpated' with the probe to assess any mass lesion. The porta hepatis, lesser omentum and the root of the mesentery should be inspected for lymphadenopathy. Mesenteric venous congestion may indicate portal vein stenosis or occlusion due to tumour invasion. The gallbladder often appears thin walled and distended in the presence of unrelieved biliary obstruction. The presence of ascitic fluid does not necessarily mean dissemination of tumour, and a sample should therefore be taken for cytological examination; 200–500 ml of warm isotonic saline may be instilled into the peritoneal cavity so that an aliquot can be retrieved and submitted to cytological examination, and to facilitate acoustic coupling of the laparoscopic ultrasound transducer with the structures to be examined. The presence of this fluid avoids the need to apply downward pressure which can produce the impression of ductal or vascular invasion.

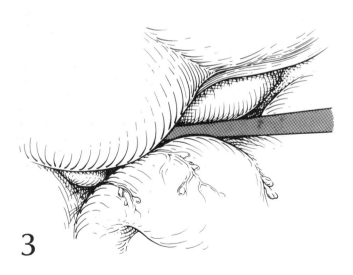

4 The liver is carefully examined with the ultrasound transducer. Metastases may appear as hyperechoic or hypoechoic lesions but are commonly circumscribed with an anechoic halo ('bullseye' lesions). Such lesions can be distinguished from haemangiomas, which are hyperechoic, by fine needle aspiration biopsy. Intra-hepatic duct dilatation may be evident in patients with unrelieved obstructive jaundice, but the previous insertion of a stent may produce considerable acoustic interference because of the presence of aerobilia.

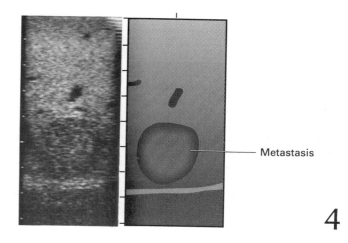

Metastasis

4

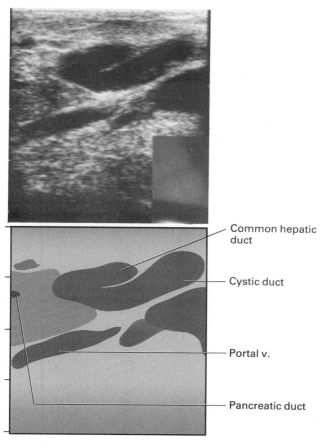

Common hepatic duct

Cystic duct

Portal v.

Pancreatic duct

5

5 With the laparoscope in the right flank port, the transducer is passed through the umbilical port and placed on the porta hepatis. The portal vein is readily identified as a landmark separated posteriorly from the inferior vena cava by the caudate lobe of the liver. The common bile duct may be dilated with a thickened wall. If a biliary stent has been inserted, its brightly hyperechoic walls may be seen, along with biliary sludge within the duct lumen. In cases of malignant biliary obstruction, the obstructing tumour in the region of the head of the pancreas or periampullary region may be identified. The confluence of the cystic duct with the common hepatic duct can be defined and its clearance from the tumour may be assessed.

6 The ultrasound transducer is gradually withdrawn to enable the portal vein to be traced from the porta hepatis to the confluence of the superior mesenteric and splenic veins. The neck of the pancreas will be seen anterior to the portal vein and measures 10–15 mm anteroposteriorly. The pancreatic duct, which normally measures less than 3 mm in diameter, will be identified in its transverse section and is normally dilated if there is a tumour in the pancreatic head. The absence of dilatation of the pancreatic duct in the presence of malignant obstruction of the common bile duct is highly suggestive of a cholangiocarcinoma rather than a pancreatic neoplasm. The position of the portal vein with respect to the tumour can be ascertained, along with any obvious invasion of the vessel by the tumour. The branches of the coeliac trunk and common hepatic artery can be traced, although arterial invasion by tumour is unusual when the lesion measures less than 3 cm in diameter. An aberrant right hepatic artery arising from the superior mesenteric artery is present in up to 20% of patients and may be identified as it runs behind the pancreatic head and portal vein.

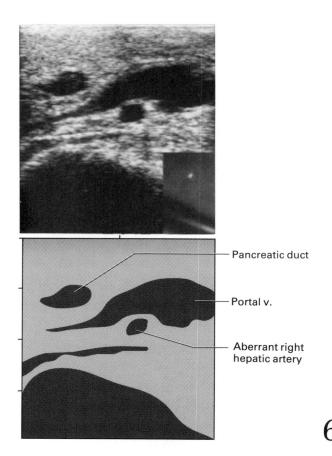

— Pancreatic duct

— Portal v.

— Aberrant right hepatic artery

6

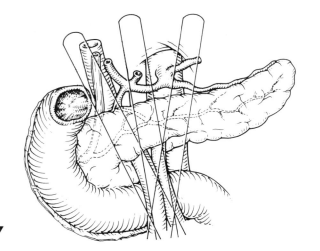

7

7 Successful examination of the pancreas is achieved by using slight rotatory probe movements, while the body and tail of the gland can be examined by gently sweeping the transducer to the left, using the stomach as an acoustic window. Gentle downward pressure with the transducer may be necessary to displace underlying gas and air in the gastric antrum and duodenum.

8 The examination is completed by transferring the transducer to the right flank port and passing the laparoscope through the umbilical port. In this way, cross-sectional images of the pancreas can be obtained as it is scanned along its longitudinal axis. Again, the portal vein and the confluence of the superior mesenteric and splenic veins are used as landmarks in the region of the neck of the pancreas.

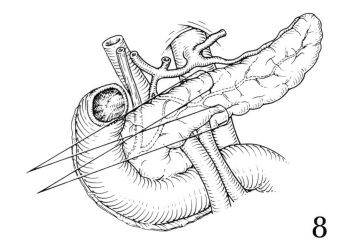

8

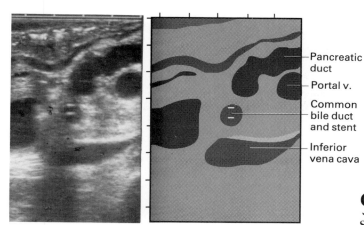

9a

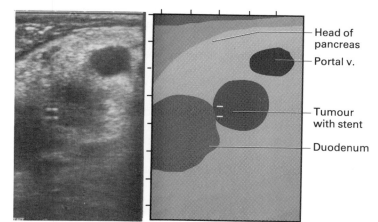

9b

9a,b A dynamic image of the tumour and the associated structures can be undertaken. Successive scans taken through the pancreatic head and neck will define the position of the tumour relative to the pancreatic duct and portal vein.

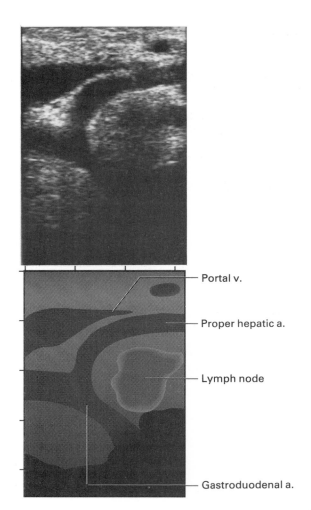

10 Pancreatic tumours tend to have a well defined hypoechoic appearance, whereas malignant nodes are said to be hyperechoic with well defined margins. Lymph node enlargement exceeding 10 mm in diameter has, in the past, been regarded as signifying malignant lymphadenopathy, but such enlarged lymph nodes frequently demonstrate reactive changes on histological examination, particularly in patients who have previously undergone biliary stent insertion.

Portal v.

Proper hepatic a.

Lymph node

Gastroduodenal a.

10

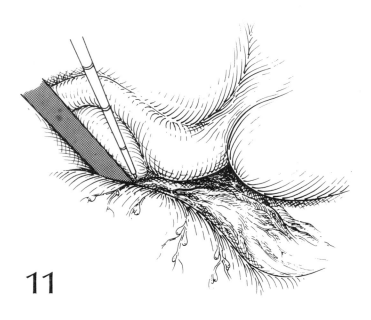

11

11 Targeted sampling of such nodes can be undertaken using fine needle aspiration. Tru-cut biopsy of the main pancreatic mass is undertaken if there is convincing laparoscopic or ultrasound evidence of irresectability. Fine needle aspiration or Tru-cut biopsy should not be performed on pancreatic lesions which are considered resectable, in order to minimize the risk of tumour dissemination before open surgery.

Once the examination is complete, the peritoneal cavity is deflated and the ports removed. The wounds are infiltrated with 0.5% bupivacaine and the linear alba at the umbilical incision is closed with interrupted 1/0 polydioxanone (PDS) sutures. The skin is opposed with interrupted subcuticular 5/0 polydioxanone sutures and the nasogastric tube is withdrawn.

Postoperative

Diclofenac suppositories are administered at the end of the procedure to minimize the need for opiate analgesia. Oral fluids are commenced when the patient has recovered from the anaesthetic.

No major complication has been observed by the author in over 100 examinations, although one patient who was found at laparoscopy to have peritoneal dissemination of tumour developed recurrence of tumour at the site of the umbilical port within 2 months of examination.

References

1. Warshaw AL, Gu ZY, Wittenberg J, Waltman AC. Pre-operative staging and assessment of resectability of pancreatic cancer. *Arch Surg* 1990; 125: 230–3.

2. Murugiah M, Paterson-Brown S, Windsor JA, Miles WFA, Garden OJ. Early experience of laparoscopic ultrasonography in the management of pancreatic carcinoma. *Surg Endosc* 1993; 7: 177–81.

3. John TG, Greig JD, Carter DC, Garden OJ. Carcinoma of the pancreatic head and periampullary region: tumour staging with laparoscopy and laparoscopic ultrasonography. *Ann Surg* 1995; 221: 156–64.

4. Bemelman WA, de Wit LT, van Delden OM *et al.* Diagnostic laparoscopy combined with laparoscopic ultrasonography in staging of cancer of the pancreatic head region. *Br J Surg* 1995; 82: 820–4.

5. Murugiah M, Windsor JA, Redhead D *et al.* The role of selective visceral angiography in the management of pancreatic and periampullary cancer. *World J Surg* 1993; 17: 796–800.

6. John TG, Garden OJ. Ultrasonography and laparoscopy. In: Brooks DC, ed. *Current Review of Laparoscopy*. 2nd edn. Philadelphia: Current Medicine, 1995: 77–95.

Further reading

Garden OJ, ed. *Intraoperative and Laparoscopic Ultrasonography*. Oxford: Blackwell Scientific, 1995.

Pancreatic cancer: laparoscopic palliation

William C. Meyers MD
Professor and Chairman, Department of Surgery, University of Massachusetts, Worcester, Massachusetts, USA

Philip R. Schauer MD
Assistant Professor, Department of Surgery, University of Pittsburg, Pittsburg, Pennsylvania, USA

Laparoscopy in the treatment of painless obstructive jaundice

Early laparoscopy is used in many patients with a suspected distal biliary malignancy. Patients are usually elderly and are admitted with painless obstructive jaundice. Ultrasonography reveals a large bile duct and there is no history or radiological imaging to suggest calculus disease. Early laparoscopy is considered appropriate without computed tomographic (CT) scanning or endoscopic retrograde cholangiopancreatography (ERCP) in otherwise healthy patients.

The initial decision is between an extensive examination and early diagnostic laparoscopy. The conventional management might include CT scanning, magnetic resonance imaging (MRI) or ERCP. Diagnostic laparoscopy is also appropriate after the conventional examination. At diagnostic laparoscopy the operation can be converted to laparotomy for possible resection. The larger operation can also be performed in a second stage after further evaluation. If the tumour is unresectable at diagnostic laparoscopy, treatment can be performed at that time or at a later stage.

A decision-making algorithm for the use of laparoscopic palliation in patients with pancreatic cancer is depicted in *Figure 1*.

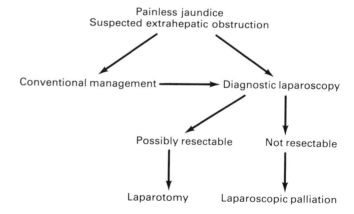

Figure 1   Decision-making algorithm for use of laparoscopic palliation in pancreatic cancer.

Diagnostic laparoscopy

Cannulation

1 The patient is placed in the reverse Trendelenburg position slightly tilted to the left. The abdomen is entered with a Hasson type cannula which enters the abdomen directly through the umbilicus with a 10–11-mm trocar. Kocher clamps are used to retract the fascia and a 0 polyglactin (Vicryl) purse-string suture is placed at the fascial level. A second purse-string is placed at the skin level with 1 nylon. The latter suture, which will be removed, is useful for maintenance of the pneumoperitoneum. Two additional trocars are placed on the right side of the abdomen, one at about the level of the umbilicus laterally and the second in the right lower quadrant. Each is a 12-mm trocar so that the ultrasound probe can be placed through either one.

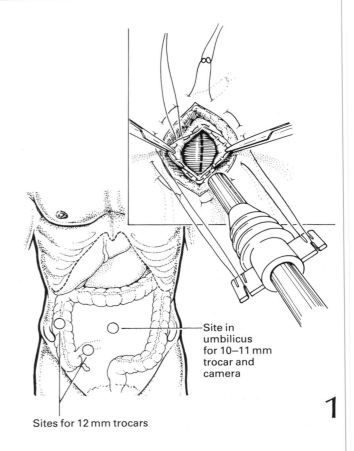

Site in umbilicus for 10–11 mm trocar and camera

Sites for 12 mm trocars

1

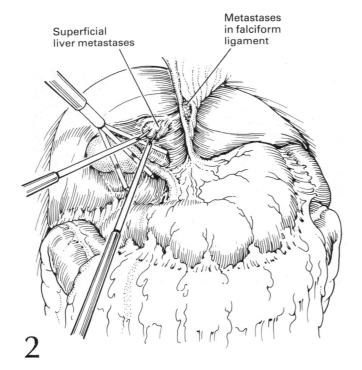

Superficial liver metastases

Metastases in falciform ligament

Biopsy of peritoneal or liver metastases

2 The superficial aspect of the entire abdomen is visualized. It is difficult to see around loops of bowel or behind organs, but the surfaces of the upper abdomen are seen and a search is undertaken for peritoneal metastases. The most likely places for peritoneal metastases are on the surfaces of the bowel, liver or falciform ligament (as shown), or other parietal peritoneal surfaces in the right upper quadrant. These are easily excised with a combination of graspers and scissors. Cautery or, rarely, clips or sutures are necessary for haemostasis.

2

Ultrasonography

Ultrasonography is routinely performed longitudinally and transversely.

Longitudinal image

3a,b The longitudinal image is obtained through the right lower quadrant port. Retraction is obtained via the other port as necessary. Under direct visualization a well lubricated ultrasound probe is placed on the superficial aspect of the duodenum in the suspected area of tumour. The portal venous anatomy is easily outlined as well as the head of the pancreas and enlarged bile duct. Colour flow Doppler scanning helps to identify the vascular structures. The primary purpose of ultrasonography here is to look for invasion of the portal structures, but occasionally other structures such as the inferior vena cava are invaded. The tumour mass is often a poorly outlined invasive mass which distorts the normal architecture. The pancreatic duct may be enlarged and a greatly enlarged bile duct is often present. Invasion of the portal vein is identified as tumour or thrombus inside the portal vein. The circumference of the portal vein may be distorted and invasion is obvious. A biopsy specimen of the tumour is taken from near the site of invasion by a transduodenal Tru-cut technique.

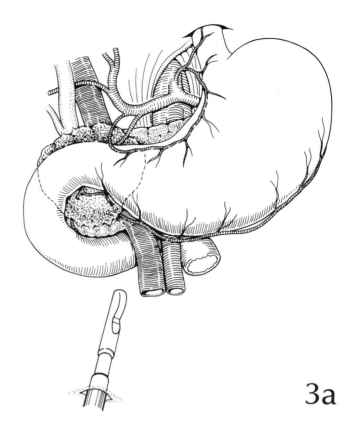

3a

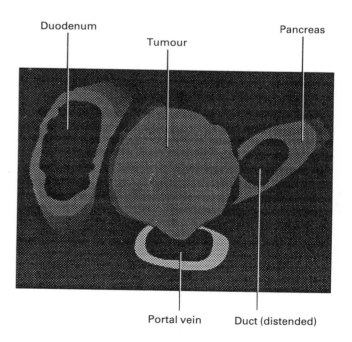

Duodenum   Tumour   Pancreas

Portal vein   Duct (distended)

3b

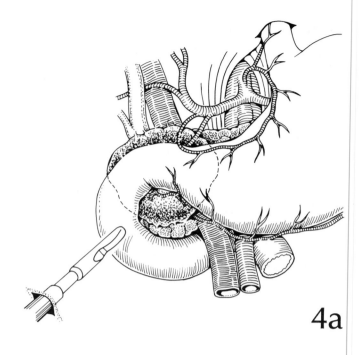

4a

Transverse image

$4a,b$ A transverse image is obtained via the right mid abdominal port. A longer length of pancreatic duct enlargement can usually be seen. Only a small section of the portal vein will be seen on each view but much of the length of splenic vein can be seen. The bile duct will be seen as a single circular luminal image. A tumour in the body of the pancreas and the junction of the tumour with the pancreas is more easily seen with a transverse than with a longitudinal image.

Closure

The trocar sites are closed with absorbable suture for both the fascia and the peritoneum.

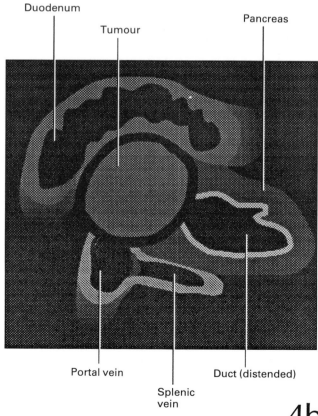

4b

Laparoscopic cholecystojejunostomy

Placement of ports

5 With the patient in the reverse Trendelenburg position a Hasson trocar is again used at the umbilical level. Two 12-mm trocar sites are chosen, one in the lateral aspect of the right upper quadrant and the other can be in the left upper quadrant. Both trocar sites may not be required. The number of sites can be determined after exploring the abdomen and visualizing the lie of the gallbladder. The Endo-GIA stapler is inserted through either site or both, as appropriate. Usually, one or two 5-mm ports are used, one in the right mid abdomen peripherally, the other in the subxiphoid region.

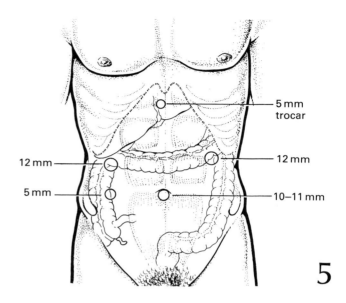

5

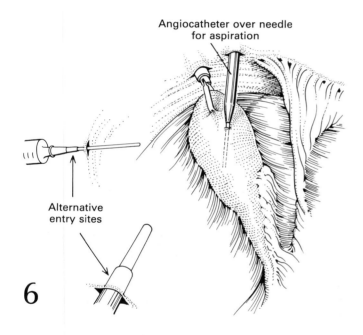

6

6 The gallbladder is aspirated and a cholangiogram is performed through a catheter in the gallbladder in order to make sure that the cystic duct communicates with the bile duct above the obstruction. It is important to make sure that the cholecystojejunostomy will drain the obstructed bile. Colourless bile is an indication that the tumour is obstructing the cystic duct. The gallbladder fundus is retracted superiorly during aspiration. Injection of contrast medium is performed under fluoroscopy.

7 The third step is identification of the proximal jejunum. The ligament of Treitz is identified easily by rotating the patient to the right while still in the reverse Trendelenburg position The proximal jejunum is identified as it exits the transverse mesocolon. A convenient portion of the proximal jejunum is then brought to the right upper quadrant. The loop is selected so that there is little tension.

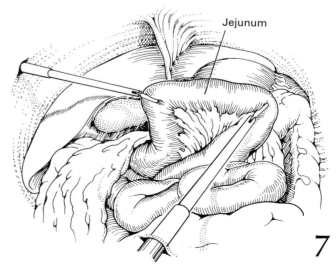

7

8 The Endo-GIA stapler is inserted through either of the 12-mm port sites. A traction suture is often useful, particularly on the right side, to hold the gallbladder, fundus and jejunum together. The Endo-GIA stapler is inserted and fired once and, following its removal, haemostasis is inspected directly. Cautery or sutures are used for haemostasis, or a well positioned clip can also be effective.

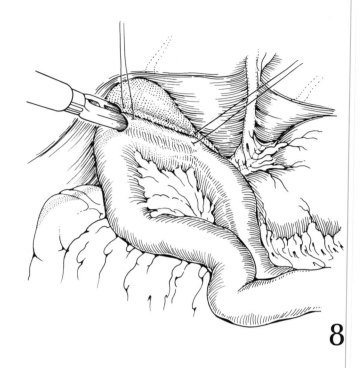

8

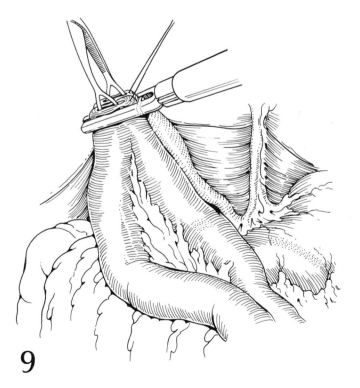

9

9 With a Babcock clamp, traction sutures or graspers for traction, the defect is closed with the Endo-GIA stapler inserted from the left upper quadrant port. Often more than one staple line is necessary to close the port. The defect can also be closed using direct suturing techniques. The Endostitch device is preferred by the authors using 4 or 5 interrupted sutures or a running suture of 3/0 silk or equivalent.

Laparoscopic gastrojejunostomy

The position of the port sites is similar to the cholecystojejunostomy, and the two operations are often performed in conjunction. Again, the patient is placed in the reverse Trendelenburg position.

10 The proximal jejunum is selected as previously and the gastrojejunostomy is performed 45 cm distal to the cholecystojejunostomy. Traction sutures on either side of the staple line are usually helpful. The Endo-GIA stapler is fired in a similar fashion to the cholecystojejunostomy, and the anastomosis is inspected for haemostasis. Usually a double suture line is necessary for an adequate sized anastomosis. The second firing is performed with a new load of staples and the same Endo-GIA device through the previous defect site. The staple line can be inspected directly with the laparoscope or with a flexible endoscope passed perorally.

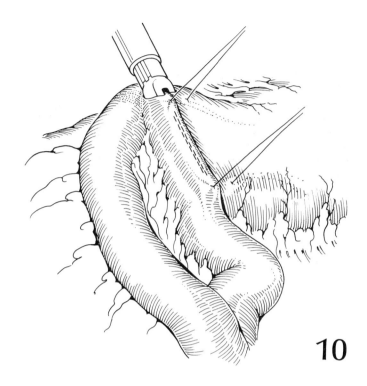

10

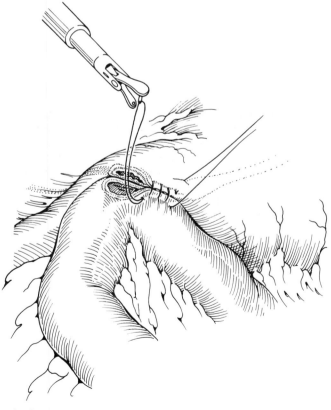

11

11 The defect is again closed with either the Endo-GIA stapler or an Endostitch device, whichever is easier.

Following the closure of the defect saline can be instilled through a nasogastric tube to check for leakage.

Additional procedures

Two additional procedures are often performed for palliation during laparoscopy for pancreatic cancer: (1) coeliac ganglion block and (2) placement of haemoclips as a reference for radiotherapy.

Coeliac ganglion block

12 This can usually be performed easily, depending on the extent of the tumour. The coeliac ganglion transmits afferent fibres from the region of the tumour and can be visualized directly via an incision in the peritoneum between the liver and lesser curvature of the stomach. The ultrasound probe is useful for identification of the anatomy. Approximately 30 ml of absolute alcohol is instilled into the region of the coeliac access after identification of the trunk. The needle is moved continuously in order to avoid injection directly into a vessel.

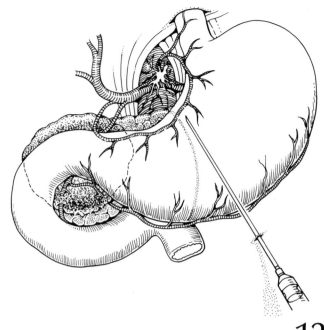

12

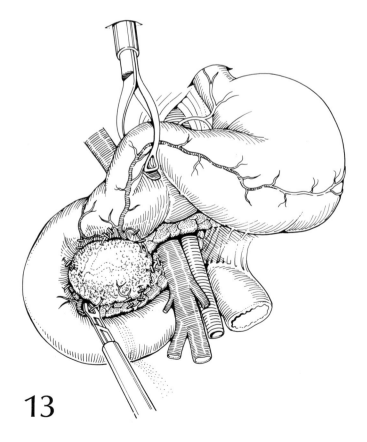

13

Placement of haemoclips

13 Haemoclips can be placed around the tumour as a reference for future radiotherapy. The mass, which may be visualized directly or via ultrasonography, is identified and clips are placed on the superior, anterior, posterior and inferior sides of it.

Thoracoscopic splanchnicectomy

Thoracoscopic splanchnicectomy is an extremely useful operation for the relief of pain from pancreatic cancer. A left thoracoscopic splanchnicectomy is usually performed as an initial procedure, and a similar procedure can be performed on the right side.

14 For the left thoracoscopic splanchnicectomy the patient is placed in a left lateral position (right side down). The surgeon faces the patient and four trocar sites are selected as depicted; 10 mm and 5 mm trocar sites are used by the operator and a 10 mm site for a fan retraction of the lung.

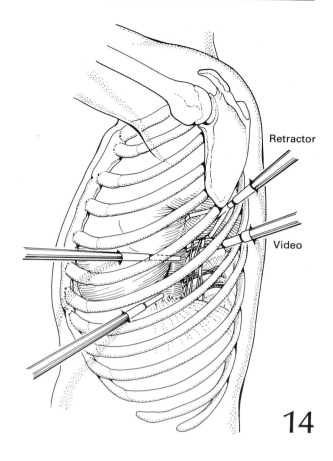

Retractor

Video

14

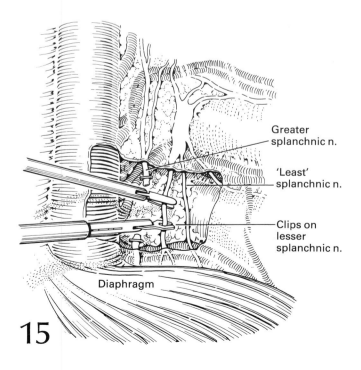

Greater splanchnic n.

'Least' splanchnic n.

Clips on lesser splanchnic n.

Diaphragm

15

15 The anatomy is visualized easily after entrance into the thorax. The greater splanchnic nerve is seen through the pleura just posterior to the aorta. The pleura is opened and the nerve identified. With appropriate retraction approximately 7.5 cm of nerve is removed. The sympathetic chain often becomes intimate with the nerve superiorly. The sympathetic chain disappears into tiny fibres at the level of the diaphragm. A portion of the sympathetic chain can be removed, even bilaterally at this level, without problems.

After division of the greater splanchnic nerve the lesser splanchnic nerve is identified as it runs obliquely about 2.5 cm peripheral to the greater nerve. The 'least' splanchnic nerve, if present, is then divided.

The trocar sites are closed with absorbable sutures.

Illustrations by Gillian Oliver

Pancreatic cancer: palliative bypass

P. C. Bornman FRCS(Ed), MMed (Surg)
Professor of Surgery and Head of Surgical Gastroenterology, University of Cape Town and Groote Schuur Hospital, Cape Town, South Africa

J. E. J. Krige FRCS, FCS(SA)
Associate Professor, Department of Surgery, University of Cape Town and Groote Schuur Hospital, Cape Town, South Africa

Principles and justification

The complexity of palliative treatment of pancreatic carcinoma is often underestimated[1]. Most patients are elderly with comorbid diseases, and additional risk factors associated with obstructive jaundice such as renal failure, coagulation disorders and sepsis further compound management strategy. Palliative treatment should aim at minimizing hospital stay while improving and maintaining quality of life. Although there are no objective criteria to validate the benefits of relieving jaundice, patient morale and performance status are generally improved, particularly when pruritus is present. Duodenal obstruction is seldom a presenting symptom, but when present is usually an indication of advanced disease. The management of pain is often difficult, particularly during the terminal stages of the disease.

Non-operative stenting has provided an alternative option for biliary bypass[2,3]. Stenting is now the treatment of choice in high-risk or frail patients and in those with obvious advanced disease without duodenal obstruction. In elderly fit patients without overt metastatic disease, the choice between palliative bypass surgery and non-operative stenting will be largely determined by ease of access to centres with endoscopic and interventional radiological facilities and expertise in stenting. Surgically fit patients with locally advanced disease (who may survive longer) should undergo surgical bypass, as the initial advantage of stenting will be eroded by the subsequent need for stent replacement and the risk of duodenal obstruction.

Choice of operation

Despite careful preoperative evaluation, the final decision determining the choice of bypass is often made during laparotomy. Selection will depend on the presence of metastases, extent of the primary tumour, proximal bile duct infiltration and the degree of duodenal involvement. Other anatomical considerations such as previous biliary surgery (e.g. cholecystectomy), obesity and mobility of the small bowel mesentery also influence the choice of bypass.

Bypass surgery should be avoided when unexpected diffuse liver or peritoneal metastases, ascites and porta hepatis involvement by tumour are encountered. These patients should rather be referred for postoperative stenting unless a gastrojejunostomy is required for overt duodenal obstruction. The morbidity and mortality in this subgroup of patients is high and the bypass procedure often proves ineffective.

Biliary bypass

For biliary drainage the options are anastomosis of either the gallbladder or the bile duct to the jejunum or duodenum. External biliary drainage via a T tube is no longer acceptable and cholecystgastrostomy is of historic interest only.

Cholecystojejunostomy using a loop of proximal jejunum is the simplest method of palliative biliary bypass and has particularr appeal in the high-risk patient. Only a small incision is required and the anastomosis is technically easy and safe. This bypass is now also performed laparoscopically (*see* page 588).

In selecting the gallbladder for biliary bypass, the surgeon must ensure that the cystic duct is patent and that entry into the bile duct is not close to the upper limit of the tumour. A tense distended gallbladder does not necessarily indicate communication with an obstructed common bile duct, but may be caused by cystic duct obstruction. Accurate assessment of cystic duct compromise may be difficult to determine at operation even with careful dissection. It is also important to ensure that there is an adequate distance between the entry of the cystic duct and the level of obstruction. Cystic duct patency is best determined preoperatively by endoscopic or percutaneous transhepatic cholangiography, or intraoperatively by cholangiography via the gallbladder. It is generally accepted that 2–3 cm of clearance is required between the obstruction and the entry of the cystic duct to safeguard against recurrent biliary obstruction[4]. The indiscriminate use of the gallbladder may have been responsible for the poor results reported in some studies. The gallbladder should not be used when chronic cholecystitis and gallstones are present.

To avoid the development of cholangitis due to reflux of the bowel contents into the biliary system, either an enteroanastomosis or a Roux-en-Y jejunal loop has been recommended. There is, however, increasing evidence that this potential complication is overemphasized when used for short-term palliation. The Roux-en-Y jejunal loop is seldom used for gallbladder drainage as it adds a further anastomosis to the procedure. The Roux loop is preferable for bile duct drainage, particularly when a simultaneous duodenal bypass is contemplated. It is useful when technical difficulties due to a shortened small bowel mesentery (caused by obesity or tumour bulk) prevent the bowel from reaching the porta hepatis without tension. A choledochoduodenostomy may also overcome this problem, but later encroachment by tumour and the development of recurrent jaundice has limited its use.

Duodenal bypass

A gastrojejunostomy is clearly indicated in patients with clinically overt gastric outlet obstruction and in the asymptomatic patient in whom there is evidence of duodenal infiltration or displacement by tumour on endoscopy, barium meal or at laparotomy. It must be emphasized that delayed gastric emptying may not only be due to a mechanical obstruction, but also occurs as a consequence of advanced disease. A gastrojejunostomy in this situation may not be effective. The role of a prophylactic gastrojejunostomy remains controversial, but a good case can be made when longer survival is anticipated as the risk of developing duodenal obstruction increases exponentially in patients who survive longer than 6 months[5].

The sequence of anastomoses when draining both the gallbladder and the stomach has never been standardized. The authors support the rationale for doing the gastric bypass first using proximal jejunum as troublesome bile reflux is thus avoided. There is no need to add a vagotomy since the risk of subsequent stomal ulceration is negligible despite the biliary diversion.

Preoperative assessment and preparation

In the selection of palliative treatment, assessment of performance status, anaesthetic risk and tumour staging are important considerations in planning preoperative preparations and surgical strategy[6].

Associated medical conditions should be identified and treated and special attention given to those risk factors related to malignant biliary obstruction. Adequate rehydration, correction of haematocrit and initiating diuresis are important measures in preventing renal failure. Mannitol (500 ml of a 10% solution infused over 1–2 h) before or during surgery remains a useful diuretic when other measures fail to establish a diuresis. The administration of one or two doses of vitamin K usually corrects the deficient coagulation factors related to reduced absorption, but additional fresh frozen plasma may be required in patients with associated liver disease.

Antibiotics are the most effective means of combating the systemic effects of endotoxaemia and the increased susceptibility to sepsis in the jaundiced patient[7]. A combination of penicillin and an aminoglycoside is commonly used, but should be avoided in elderly patients and those with renal impairment. The use of a second generation cephalosporin fulfils the same need and has the advantage of being effective against staphylococci.

Several controlled trials evaluating preoperative biliary drainage have shown no reduction in postoperative morbidity and mortality and in some studies it has been associated with life-threatening complications such as haemorrhage and cholangitis[8]. Internal stenting avoids many of the disadvantages of external biliary drainage but its use has not gained widespread acceptance. The use of preoperative biliary drainage (preferably by internal stenting) is now restricted to selected cases with cholangitis or renal failure who do not respond to medical therapy.

Operation

Incision

1 A right subcostal incision is used in most patients because it provides easy access and good exposure of the operative field. The incision can readily be extended across the midline if required. A right transverse incision is preferable in obese patients and in those with hepatomegaly. A long midline incision extending from the xiphisternum to below the umbilicus can be used in patients with a narrow subcostal angle.

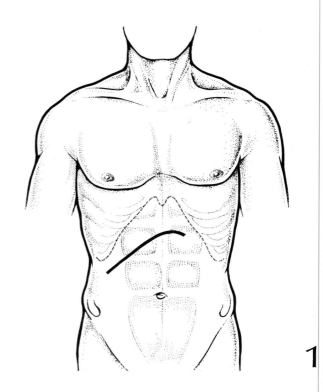

Exploration of the peritoneal cavity

2 A mechanical subcostal retractor facilitates exposure of the porta hepatis, especially if the bile duct is used for drainage. A systematic approach is used, first to exclude distant metastases, then regional nodal involvement and, finally, local tumour extension. Biopsies are taken of suspicious areas showing puckering, nodular implantation or fixation. Hepatic, omental, serosal or peritoneal seedlings are usually immediately obvious and preclude resection. Special attention is paid to examination of the liver using bimanual palpation and, if available, intraoperative ultrasonography which may detect unsuspected deep-seated liver metastases. Portal vein involvement, invasion of the hepatic artery or superior mesenteric vessels, or extension of the tumour beyond the normal limits of pancreatic resection indicate non-resectability.

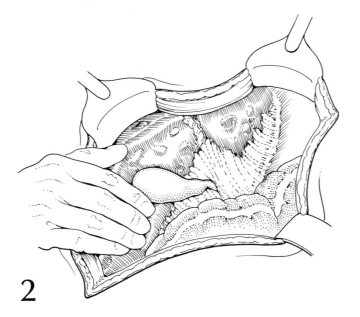

3 Extension of tumour from the neck of the pancreas or uncinate process along the superior mesenteric vessels into the base of the mesocolon is assessed by elevating the transverse colon and examining the mesocolon from below in the region of the ligament of Treitz. The base of the small bowel mesentery should also be examined for nodal involvement.

4 The gastrohepatic omentum is incised to allow inspection and palpation of the neck and body of the pancreas and to assess regional lymph nodes along the coeliac and hepatic arteries and in the porta hepatis (1). If nodal metastases or local tumour extension to surrounding structures is present, the tumour is incurable and a bypass is performed. If neither nodes nor extension are present, the lesser sac is exposed via the gastrocolic ligament which allows complete ex-amination of the body and tail of the pancreas and the nodes along the splenic vessels and the splenic hilum (2). The opening is widened and the stomach retracted upwards using a malleable retractor or a Penrose drain placed around the stomach. This allows complete visualization of the neck, body and tail of the pancreas. The duodenum is Kocherized only if no distant or regional nodes are encountered and forms part of the assessment of resectability (3). A further description of the detailed assessment of resectability is found in the chapter on pp. 610–623.

Preparation of the intestinal loop

The first loop of the jejunum is usually used to fashion the gastroenterostomy when this is necessary. The loop of jejunum distal to the stoma is next inspected either to fashion a Roux loop or, more simply, as an intact loop with or without an enteroanastomosis between afferent and efferent loops. The highest loop of the jejunum which reaches the right upper quadrant without tension is selected. An enteroanastomosis is made between the afferent and efferent loops approximately 20 cm from the apex of the loop.

The loop is next passed through an avascular window in the right transverse mesocolon so that it lies

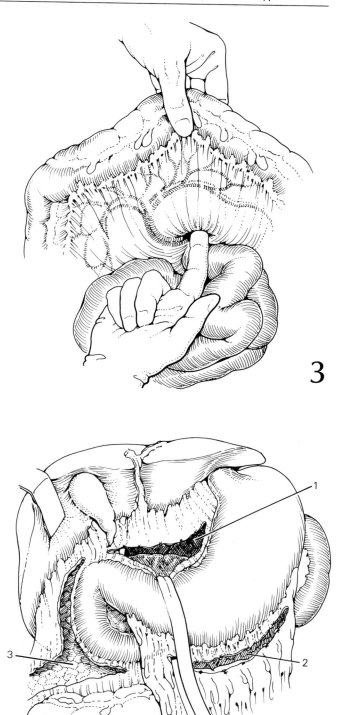

comfortably in the right subhepatic space. This retro-colic route facilitates exposure for the next phase because exposure and access is more difficult if the loop is brought in front of the colon, especially if a choledochojejunostomy is being performed.

CHOLECYSTOJEJUNOSTOMY

5 A suitable proximal jejunal loop which easily reaches the gallbladder is selected for an antecolic anastomosis. A retrocolic approach through the meso-colon of the hepatic flexure to the right of the middle colic vessels can be used if necessary. In the unusual situation where neither is possible, a Roux loop is used. A flexible approach is used when selecting the site of the gallbladder anastomosis. Either the fundus or the body of the gallbladder is suitable and the most prominent and accessible site is chosen. The gallbladder is first emptied using a trocar suction apparatus which allows it to be handled more easily than when grossly distended and avoids spillage of bile.

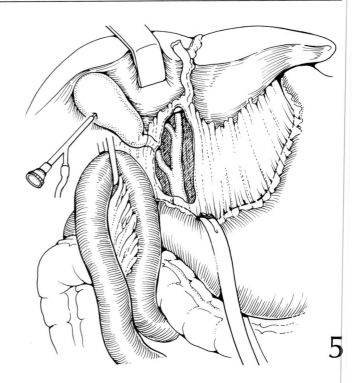

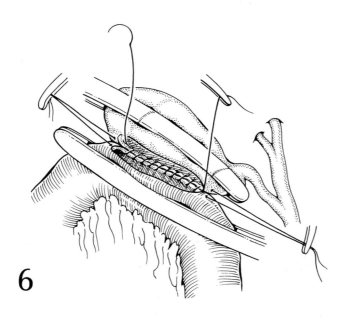

6

6 Non-crushing soft bowel clamps placed across the gallbladder and the small bowel are useful to avoid spillage. The jejunal loop and gallbladder are laid side-by-side and a continuous 3/0 monofilament suture is used to approximate the posterior walls. An incision is made in both the gallbladder and jejunum. The inner layer, incorporating the full thickness of the posterior wall of the gallbladder and the intestine, is anastomosed using a 3/0 continuous absorbable monofilament suture starting at one corner, and both the posterior and anterior inner layers are completed. A Connell stitch applied at each corner is useful to prevent mucosal pouting.

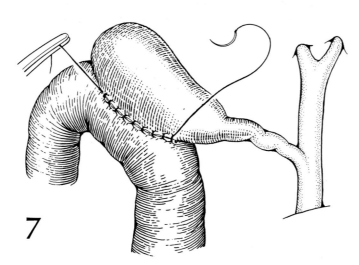

7

7 The anterior serosal surfaces are approximated using a continuous 3/0 suture. When the gallbladder wall is distended and thin, a two-layer anastomosis is preferred using 4/0 sutures and a thin needle to avoid bile leakage from the suture holes. For a thicker gallbladder wall a single-layer anastomosis is adequate.

CHOLEDOCHOJEJUNOSTOMY

8 The Roux loop is fashioned by transecting the jejunum approximately 15 cm beyond the ligament of Treitz. The proximal small bowel is held up and spread to transilluminate the mesentery and identify the vascular arcades so that the mesentery can be divided without compromising the blood supply. The authors divide only primary and secondary arcades before transecting the bowel. This usually provides sufficient length when the antimesenteric margin at the end of the loop is used for the biliary anastomosis. It is seldom necessary to divide the tertiary arcades and extend the division into the base of the mesentery. The bowel is transected between crushing clamps and the distal end of the Roux loop is secured by closure using two layers of an absorbable suture. Alternatively, staples can be used to divide the bowel and the end of the loop is closed by invagination using an absorbable suture.

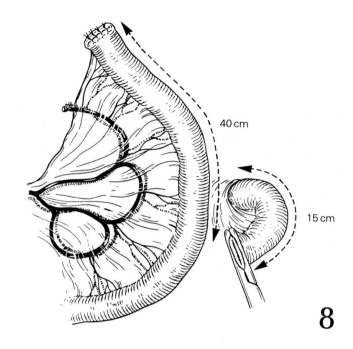

8

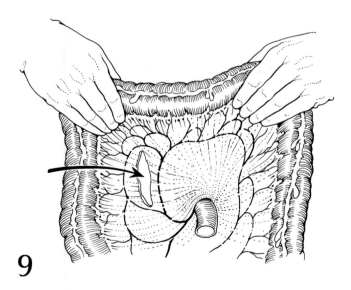

9

9 The transverse colon is retracted out of the wound and transilluminated to identify the middle colic vessels and their branches. An avascular site in the mesocolon which provides the shortest route to the porta hepatis is selected, usually to the right of the middle colic vessels. The mesocolon is opened with a scalpel or pair of scissors for a distance of about 8 cm to allow comfortable passage of the jejunal loop and accompanying mesentery.

10 The loop is manipulated through the gap in the mesocolon to a point where the end of the loop lies comfortably without tension adjacent to the porta hepatis at the site of the proposed biliary anastomosis.

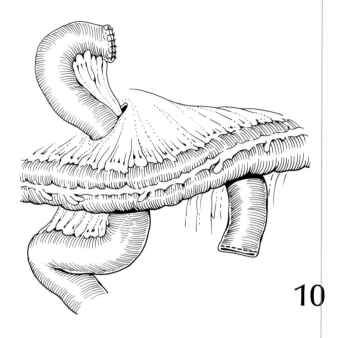

10

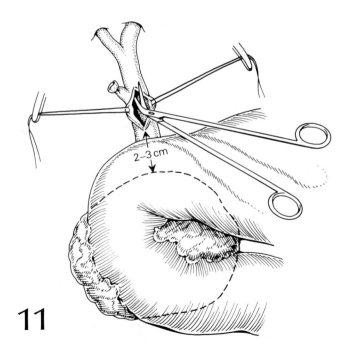

11

11 A cholecystectomy is not routinely performed. Removal of the gallbladder does, however, facilitate construction of the hepaticojejunostomy, especially if exposure is limited and a high anastomosis is required. In this situation dissection and removal of the gallbladder must be meticulous to avoid bleeding from the gallbladder bed. Emptying of the gallbladder before dissection may be useful when the gallbladder is grossly distended. The common bile duct is opened at least 2–3 cm above the macroscopic extent of the tumour. Two 5/0 stay sutures are placed at the site of the choledochotomy to support the duct and avoid injury to the posterior wall of the duct or adjacent structures during opening. The initial incision is made in the anterior wall with a no. 15 scalpel blade and the choledochotomy is enlarged to 3 cm using a pair of angled Pott's scissors. The decision whether to use interrupted or continuous sutures for the anastomosis is based on the size of the duct, the level of the anastomosis and the adequacy of exposure. A low anastomosis to a wide duct can be accomplished without difficulty using a continuous suture. For higher anastomoses, where exposure is less adequate, the technique for high bile duct reconstruction using interrupted sutures is recommended[9].

12 The selection of suture material and the size and diameter of the needle are governed by the thickness of the bile duct wall. When the wall of the bile duct is thin, 4/0 sutures, a thin needle and suture bites 2 mm apart and placed 2 mm from the edge are used. Particular care is taken to avoid undue traction on sutures placed in a thin-walled bile duct to prevent tearing of the duct wall. For ducts with thicker walls, 3/0 sutures, a larger needle and more generous bites can be used. A superior row of sutures which will constitute the anterior layer of the anastomosis is placed in the bile duct first before the posterior layer of sutures is inserted. The apex suture is placed first to mark the mid point of the anterior wall anastomosis. The sutures (absorbable monofilament) are now sequentially placed starting from the apex, working towards the two corner stay sutures. The needles are passed from the outside inwards to allow subsequent tying of the knots on the outside when the final sutures are placed through the anterior jejunal wall. This technique allows accurate and precise placement of the sutures and produces the best possible mucosa-to-mucosa approximation[9]. The needles on the anterior row of sutures are retained and each suture is clipped with a shod clamp and kept in sequential order on a clamp hanger. The row of upper sutures is lifted to elevate the anterior wall of the bile duct and facilitate exposure and placement of the posterior wall sutures. The end of the jejunal loop is positioned at a convenient distance below the inferior margin of the choledochotomy. A soft bowel clamp is applied across the jejunal loop 15 cm from the end after milking the contents back to avoid leakage and

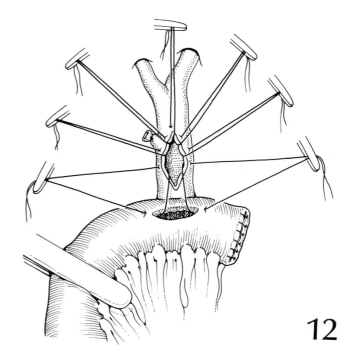

12

contamination of the operative field during the procedure. A linear incision is made into the antimesenteric margin of the jejunum near the closed end. The jejunal incision should be three-quarters the length of the biliary opening to avoid an ultimate discrepancy in size as the jejunal opening usually stretches with manipulation. Stay sutures are placed at each corner.

13 The posterior layer of sutures is placed starting from *within* the lumen of the bile duct, taking care that the full thickness of both the jejunal wall and the bile duct are incorporated in each suture to ensure accurate approximation and effective haemostasis. The needle is cut off each interrupted suture once placed. It is helpful to hold up the previously placed suture to allow close apposition of the two walls and accurate placement of the next stitch. The remainder of the posterior wall is completed with sutures placed every 3 mm. After all the sutures have been placed the jejunal limb is 'railroaded' upwards to lie in close proximity to the inferior margin of the choledochotomy. The posterior layer sutures are then tied serially. The tension applied on each knot is critical to ensure that each tie is snug and secure. The two corner stay sutures are held on shod clamps while the others are cut. The integrity of the posterior anastomosis should be assessed at this stage by inspecting the suture line from below by gently lifting and rotating the end of the loop upwards.

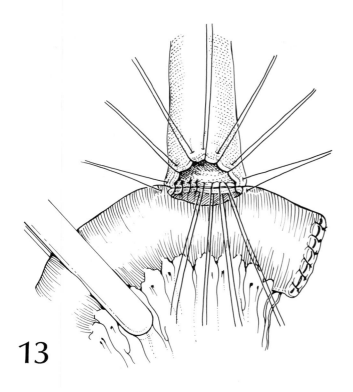

13

14 The technique of suture placement on the jejunal side is important. The needle is passed obliquely through the jejunal wall incorporating only 1 mm of mucosa from the cut edge and 3 mm of serosa. This prevents eversion and mucosal pouting and ensures a watertight closure.

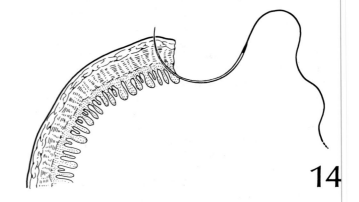

14

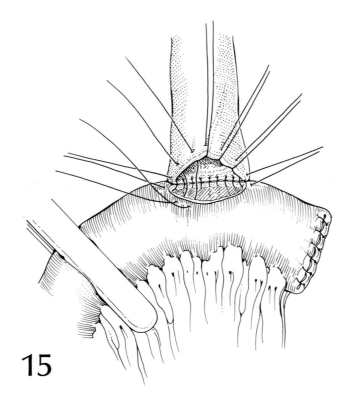

15

15 The previously placed anterior row of sutures is now used to complete the anastomosis by passing the needles from the inside outwards onto the anterior wall of the jejunum. The entire row is placed and the needles are cut from the sutures. The anterior layer of sutures is then serially tied, each knot being placed on the outside.

16 The enteroanastomosis between the end of the proximal jejunum and the side of the Roux loop 40 cm from the tip is fashioned below the transverse mesocolon. Before starting the anastomosis, particular attention is paid to ensure that the proximal small bowel mesentery is not twisted or rotated. Soft bowel clamps are applied to both the proximal jejunum and the Roux loop to avoid contamination of bowel content during the procedure. An incision is made on the antimesenteric margin of the Roux loop 40 cm from the end and a stay suture is inserted at each corner of the anastomosis. A double-armed 3/0 suture is inserted at the mid point of the posterior wall and tied. The posterior wall is completed using each of the sutures. The corner stay sutures are tied and each arm continued to fashion the anterior wall. The sutures are now tied at the point where they meet in the middle of the anterior layer.

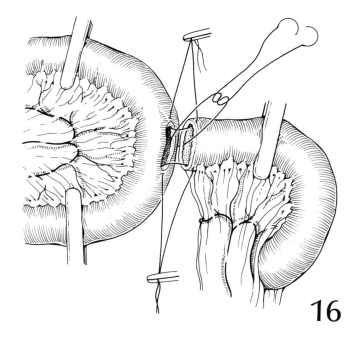

16

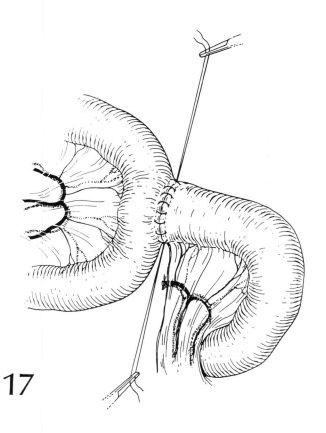

17

17 The ligated edges of the mesentery are examined to ensure that haemostasis is secure. The remaining defect in the transverse mesocolon adjacent to the jejunal loop is carefully closed using fine sutures and the divided surfaces of the mesentery are apposed to prevent internal herniation.

CHOLEDOCHODUODENOSTOMY

18 Before embarking on a choledochoduodeno-stomy, evaluation of the mobility of the duo-denum and bile duct is essential to ensure absence of tumour encroachment and tension-free approximation. A Kocher incision with freeing of the lateral margin of the duodenum may be required to achieve the necessary mobility. The gallbladder is removed and the choledochotomy performed between two 5/0 stay sutures. A longitudinal incision is made in the post-bulbar duodenum, the mid point of the incision being centred on the choledochotomy. The duodenal incision tends to stretch with manipulation and should therefore always be slightly smaller than the biliary incision. A stay suture is placed through each apex of the duodenotomy to the mid point of each wall of the choledochal incision (A). A similar stay suture is placed through the inferior apex of the choledochotomy to the mid point of the posterior wall of the duodenal incision (B). These three stay sutures are tied to fashion the posterior wall of the anastomosis. The anastomosis can be performed using either a continuous suture beginning at the mid point of the posterior wall or by using interrupted sutures.

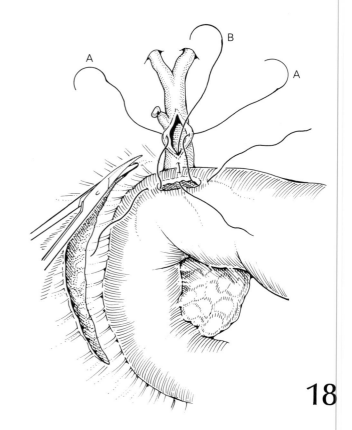

18

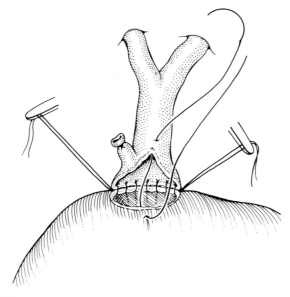

19

19 The posterior wall is completed by placing the remainder of the interrupted 3/0 absorbable monofilament sutures. The sutures are inserted so that the knots are tied on the inside of the lumen. The anterior wall is similarly constructed by placing a stay suture from the mid point of the duodenum to the superior apex of the choledochotomy.

20 Interrupted sutures are placed between the stay sutures to complete the anastomosis. The knots are tied on the outside. A 6-mm closed suction drain is placed in Morrison's pouch.

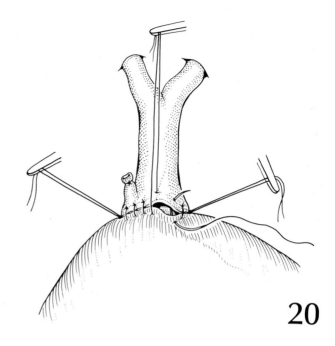

20

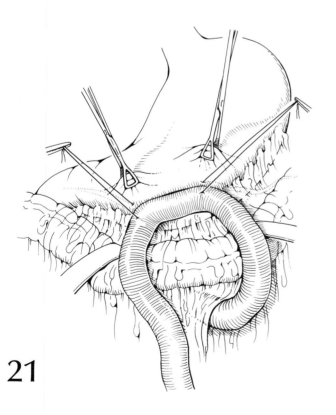

21

GASTROENTEROSTOMY

21 The gastroenterostomy can be performed by placing the jejunal loop either in an antecolic or a retrocolic position. The selection is often an arbitrary decision based on the extent of both local and regional tumour spread and anatomical factors including mobility of the small bowel mesentery and body habitus. It is important to place the gastroenterostomy in the antrum close to the greater curvature to avoid stomal malfunction. The site for the anastomosis on the anterior wall of the stomach is selected and marked by applying Babcock forceps. A loop of jejunum is then brought anterior to the colon for an isoperistaltic anastomosis. The loop is selected so that the afferent limb is short but not under any tension. An extra few centimetres of slack allows for any subsequent colonic distension without compromise behind the jejunal loop.

22 Corner sutures are first placed about 8 cm apart and the jejunum is attached to the stomach using a continuous row of 3/0 seromuscular sutures. This posterior row of sutures should be placed on the jejunum midway between the mesentery and the antimesenteric border. The opening in the stomach is made about 5 mm from the row of sutures, extending from one corner suture to the other, using cautery. If large submucosal vessels are encountered these are best secured by underrunning with 3/0 absorbable sutures. Fluid within the stomach is aspirated to avoid contamination during surgery. The opening in the jejunum is similarly made 5 mm from the previous suture line after applying a soft bowel clamp to prevent bowel content spillage. The jejunal opening should be slightly smaller than the gastric opening because the jejunal wall stretches and the opening gets larger during the performance of the anastomosis.

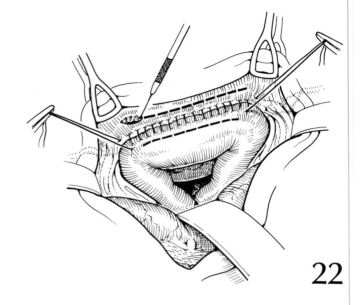

22

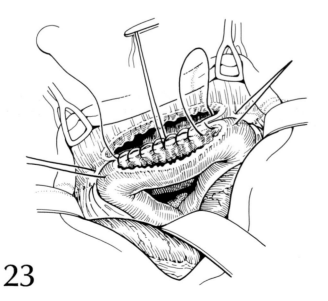

23

23 Next the posterior inner layer of sutures is placed. Continuous absorbable 3/0 sutures are used, beginning in the middle of the posterior wall and progressing laterally in both directions. These sutures are haemostatic and should encompass the full wall of both the stomach and jejunum. The suture is carried on to the anterior wall, bringing the edges of the stomach and jejunum together. This suture will form the inner layer of the anterior portion of the anastomosis. A Connell suture is useful and simplifies inversion of the mucosa when the corners of the anterior wall of the anastomosis are fashioned. Continuous 3/0 sutures are next inserted to complete the outer wall of the anterior portion of the gastroenterostomy.

24 The construction of a retrocolic gastrojejuno-stomy is similar to that of the antecolic technique. The lesser sac is entered by dividing the gastrocolic omentum and the posterior wall of the stomach is exposed. The transverse colon is retracted out of the wound and the transverse mesocolon transilluminated to visualize the middle colic vessels and its branches. An avascular portion of the mesocolon is selected, usually to the left of the middle colic vessels, and is opened for a distance of 8 cm.

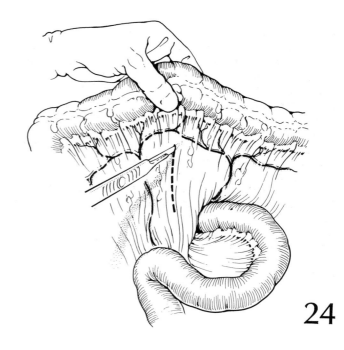

24

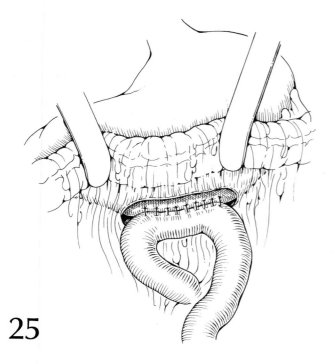

25

25 After completion of the anterior wall of the gastroenterostomy the defect in the transverse mesocolon is closed.

26 When a retrocolic Roux loop is used for biliary drainage, the same loop can be used for the gastric bypass. Passage through the transverse mesocolon should be near the hepatic flexure and to the right of the middle colic vessels. This route has the benefit of avoiding entry into the lesser sac and provides the shortest access to the porta hepatis. In addition, potential kinking of the loop is avoided by constructing the gastrojejunostomy first. The additional advantage of the gastric anastomosis above the biliary anastomosis is avoidance of troublesome bile reflux into the stomach.

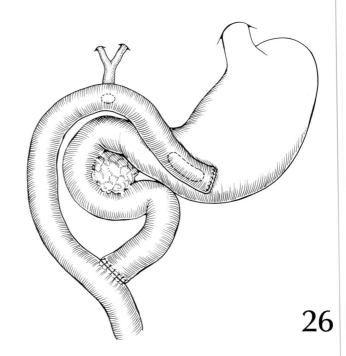

26

Postoperative care

Most patients can be managed in a general surgical ward during the postoperative period unless comorbid systemic illnesses require support in an intensive care unit. Fluid balance needs careful monitoring to avoid renal failure and perioperative antibiotic therapy should continue for 24 h unless other indications dictate longer treatment. The nasogastric tube can usually be removed after 2–3 days with return of bowel sounds, or when the nasogastric drainage is less than 500 ml over a 24 h period. Abdominal drains can be removed after 3–4 days unless the operation is complicated by a bile leak or bowel fistula.

Functional delayed gastric emptying is not infrequently encountered, particularly in patients with advanced disease who have undergone a gastroenterosotmy. Prokinetic drugs are usually unhelpful and some patients may require nasojejunal feeding or parenteral nutrition. Other complications include bleeding due to coagulopathy, renal failure as part of the hepatorenal syndrome, sepsis, and delayed healing with wound dehiscence and anastomotic leaks.

Reports on morbidity and mortality after palliative bypass operations remain distressingly high[10]. However, most complications can be avoided by careful selection of treatment options (including non-operative stenting), appropriate preoperative preparation and performance of operations by experienced surgeons.

References

1. Krige JE, Bornman PC, Terblanche J. Optimal palliation of pancreatic carcinoma. *S Afr Med J* 1992; 81: 238–40.

2. Bornman PC, Harries-Jones EP, Tobias R, Van Stiegmann G, Terblanche J. Prospective controlled trial of transhepatic biliary endoprosthesis versus bypass surgery for incurable carcinoma of head of pancreas. *Lancet* 1986; i: 69–71.

3. Smith AC, Dowsett JF, Russell RCG, Hatfield ARW, Cotton PB. Randomised trial of endoscopic stenting versus surgical bypass in malignant low bile duct obstruction. *Lancet* 1994; 344: 1655–60.

4. Singh SM, Reber HA. Surgical palliation for pancreatic cancer. *Surg Clin North Am* 1990; 63: 599–611.

5. Gudjonsson B. Cancer of the pancreas: 50 years of surgery. *Cancer* 1987; 60: 2284–303.

6. Bornman PC, Krige JEJ. Surgical palliation of pancreatic and periampullary tumours. In: Trede M, Carter DC, eds. *Surgery of the Pancreas*. Edinburgh: Churchill Livingstone, 1993: 497–513.

7. Keighley MR, Razay G, Fitzgerald MG. Influence of diabetes on mortality and morbidity following operations for obstructive jaundice. *Ann R Coll Surg Engl* 1984; 66: 49–51.

8. McPherson GA, Benjamin IS, Habib NA, Bowley NB, Blumgart LH. Percutaneous transhepatic drainage in obstructive jaundice: advantages and problems. *Br J Surg* 1982; 69: 261–4.

9. Voyles CR, Blumgart LH. A technique for the construction of high biliary-enteric anastomoses. *Surg Gynecol Obstet* 1982; 154: 885–7.

10. Schouten JT. Operative therapy for pancreatic carcinoma. *Am J Surg* 1986; 151: 626–30.

Illustrations by Gillian Lee

Resection for pancreatic cancer: Whipple's operation

Michael Trede MD, FRCS(Hon), FACS(Hon)
Professor and Chairman, Department of Surgery, Klinikum Mannheim, University of Heidelberg, Germany

History

Following an attempt by Codivilla in 1898 (in Imola), the first successful pancreatoduodenectomy was performed by Kausch in Berlin in 1908. His patient survived a two-stage resection for papillary carcinoma for some 9 months. However, it was Whipple who, in 1935, reported upon three such operations and who standardized the technique in the ensuing years in New York. By the time he retired, Whipple had personally performed some 37 pancreatoduodenectomies, an operation that carried a mortality rate of 20–30% right into the 1970s.

Principles and justification

Resection for pancreatic cancer is confined to those 25% of diagnosed cases in whom the tumour is limited to the pancreas without macroscopic evidence of spread to retroperitoneal vessels, the hepatoduodenal ligament or into the mesenteric root. Peritoneal or liver metastases are absolute contraindications to resection, whereas involvement of juxtapancreatic lymph nodes is not.

It is understood that microscopic tumour spread, e.g. along perineural lymphatics, will ultimately vitiate the results of most pancreatic resections. Nevertheless, resection at best provides the only chance for cure and at least it provides the best possible palliation as well as some prolongation of life.

The standard resection chosen – right-sided, left-sided or total pancreatectomy – depends on the localization and size of the tumour.

Preoperative

Imaging methods used to assess resectability (i.e. staging) of a pancreatic tumour include ultrasonography, angio-computed tomographic (CT) scanning endosonography, endoscopic retrograde cholangiopancreatography (ERCP), selective arteriography and portography, percutaneous fine-needle cytology and laparoscopy (including laparoscopic ultrasonography). These investigations should be performed in this sequence, but they are not all required in every patient.

Dynamic bolus angio-CT scanning is the single most informative step, and ERCP is essential only in jaundiced cases. Fine-needle sampling is confined to clearly inoperable patients who require no palliative procedure in order to confirm the diagnosis. Laparoscopy can help to avoid an unnecessary laparotomy in patients of doubtful operability who require no operative palliation.

Although old age is no longer an absolute contra-indication, routine preoperative investigations are required to assess the general operability of the patient.

Although not confirmed by controlled studies, patients with obstructive jaundice appear to have fewer postoperative complications if the obstructed bile ducts are drained preoperatively. This is best done at the time of diagnostic ERCP by means of a wide transpapillary tube. Thus bile flows once more into the gut and liver function parameters recover whilst further staging of the tumour is performed. If endoscopic transpapillary drainage fails, the patient receives daily doses of vitamin K (20 mg intramuscularly) and staging is expedited. This is preferable to attempting biliary drainage via the more invasive and complicated percutaneous transhepatic route.

Anaesthesia

General anaesthesia with adequate relaxation is always required for these pancreatic resections which usually take 4–6 h or longer.

Operation

Incision

The author prefers a transverse subcostal approach beginning on the right side for preliminary exploration, before extending the incision over to the left if no gross signs of inoperability are found. For tumours of the pancreatic tail, a left subcostal incision is made. If the patient has an acute subcostal angle or if there is already a median laparotomy scar, then a midline incision can be used.

1 The operation includes the *en bloc* resection of the pancreatic head (and varying amounts of the neck and body of the gland, depending on the size and localization of the tumour), the distal one-third of the stomach (with the right half of the greater omentum), the duodenum (and proximal 5–10 cm of jejunum), as well as the gallbladder and common bile duct.

For small periampullary tumours, some authors prefer the pylorus-preserving variant in which the stomach and first 3 cm of duodenum are left intact.

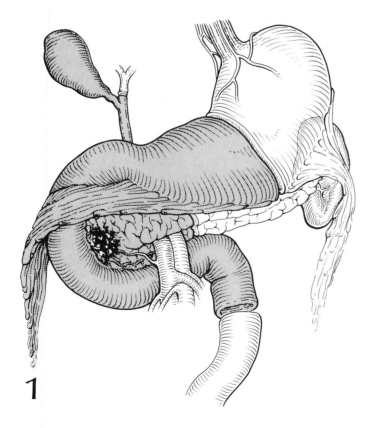

1

Exploration and mobilization

The size and mobility of the tumour are first assessed and distant metastases excluded by systematic palpation of the entire abdominal cavity. Particular attention must be paid to the liver, hepatoduodenal ligament and mesenteric root. Mobilization follows oncological principles, in that the tumour is approached centripetally from the periphery. In this way, the stepwise mobilization and *en bloc* resection of the specimen is performed without touching the tumour itself at any time. If any suspicious nodes or peritoneal nodules are encountered, they are sampled for frozen section examination. This will contribute to accurate staging of the tumour without necessarily influencing the operative strategy. Discrete tumour deposits in juxtapancreatic lymph nodes or even in those more remote (e.g. para-aortic nodes) are not a contraindication to the resection of a locally operable pancreatic tumour in a normal low-risk patient.

2a–e The duodenum and pancreatic head are mobilized from the hepatoduodenal ligament above down to the mesocolon below according to the technique of Kocher.

With the right colonic flexure freed and reflected downwards, the retropancreatic aspect of the vena cava, left renal vein and right border of the aorta are displayed. The tumour is palpated between finger and thumb and possible encasement of the superior mesenteric artery is explored. The lesser sac is entered by dividing the largely avascular adhesions between the right half of the greater omentum and the transverse colon. (If total or left-sided pancreatectomy is undertaken, the entire omentum should be taken off the colon in this fashion). Thus, adequate exposure of the ventral surface of the pancreas is obtained.

If resectability is unlikely, an easier and quicker approach to the pancreas is through the lesser omentum. Dissection between the inner curve of the ascending part of the duodenum and the uncinate process will expose the right border of the superior mesenteric vein disappearing upwards behind the pancreas (*Illustration 2e*). Infiltration of the retropancreatic segment of this vein with tumour reduces the likelihood of achieving a cure, but does not exclude resectability.

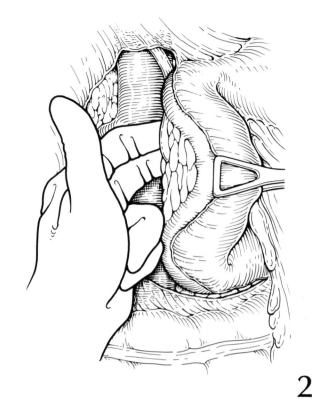

2a

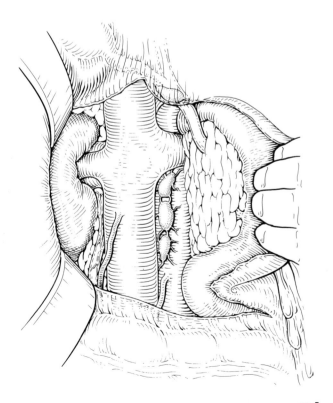

2b

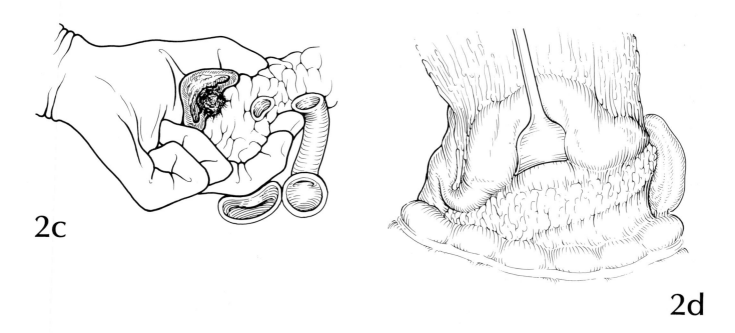

2c

2d

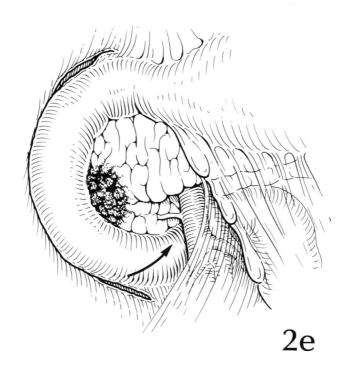

2e

Cholecystectomy and dissection of the hepatoduodenal ligament

This is routinely performed to increase the extent of the excision (particularly if the tumour extends up the common duct), to leave a shorter and well vascularized hepatic duct for subsequent anastomosis, and to obviate possible gallstone complications later.

The gallbladder is shelled out of its liver bed in an avascular plane. Any oozing is easily controlled by a pack. The cystic artery is divided and the gallbladder is left hanging from the cystic duct which serves as a guide to the hepatic duct.

3 The peritoneal covering of the hepatoduodenal ligament and the right half of the lesser omentum are incised close to the lower border of the liver. Proceeding systematically from above downward and from right to left, all lymphoid and areolar tissue is dissected until the three structures within the ligament are completely clean: the common hepatic artery with its right and left branches, the portal vein and the common bile duct. The latter is divided just proximal to the cystic duct early on in this dissection, but not before it is quite clear that there are no accessory (right) hepatic ducts draining into the common duct more distally. Similarly, the lymphoid tissue to the right of the hepatic duct (in front) and the portal vein (behind) must not be divided before the presence of an aberrant hepatic artery (emanating in 25% of cases from the superior mesenteric artery and almost invariably running in this tissue) has been excluded. The proximal stump of the bile duct is left to drain into a small pack; clamping will damage this delicate structure unnecessarily.

The distal common duct is tied and peeled off the portal vein together with more or less voluminous and haemorrhagic lymph tissue. Immediately behind the upper border of the pancreas, a small but constant tributary – the posterior superior pancreatoduodenal vein – drains into the right border of the portal vein and should be divided between clips before subsequent manoeuvres tear it off. Similarly, the delicate right gastric artery should be identified as it arises from the hepatic artery. This leaves the largest branch of the hepatic artery – the gastroduodenal – that can now be divided between ligatures. Dissection of the hepatic artery is continued along the upper border of the pancreas as far as the neck of the gland. If total pancreatectomy is planned, the dissection reaches up to the coeliac trifurcation.

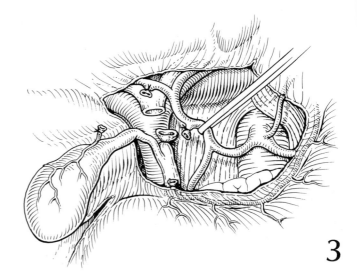

3

Mobilization of the pancreatic neck

4 This rather delicate manoeuvre is performed by a probing forefinger or Overholt clamp running along the anterior border of a portal vein from above downwards (since there usually are no tributaries here).

Downward traction of the transverse mesocolon displays the lower border of the pancreas, where the tip of the advancing finger can be met by a curved clamp in front of the superior mesenteric vein. This retropancreatic passage is then widened carefully and a tape passed through it.

If the tunnel is too narrow or obstructed by tumour infiltration of the vein, it is unwise to force a passage and it is safer to leave this step until after division of the stomach is completed. Should bleeding occur in this tunnel, it is best controlled by tamponade with narrow gauze. Any attempts at suturing should be deferred until the pancreatic neck is divided.

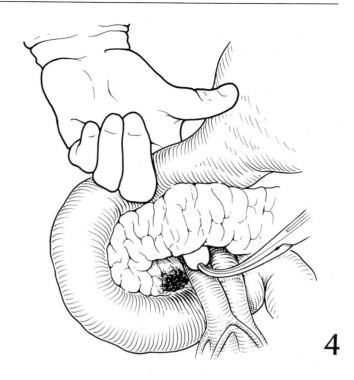

4

Partial gastrectomy

5a,b No more than the distal 40% of the stomach (including the antrum) is skeletonized and divided with the help of a stapler. Although no vagotomy is added, anastomotic ulcers have been observed in only 2.3% of the author's cases.

Another possible complication – postoperative bleeding from the blindly closed section of the stomach – is prevented by covering the right half of the staple line with two additional sutures (an over-and-over locking stitch using 3/0 chromic catgut and an outer layer of interrupted 3/0 silk sutures).

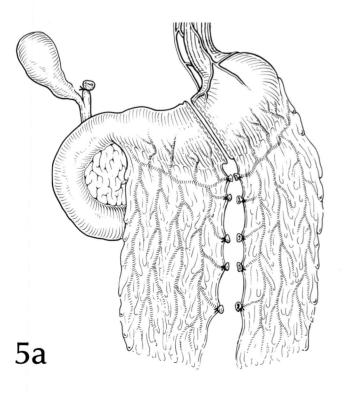

5a

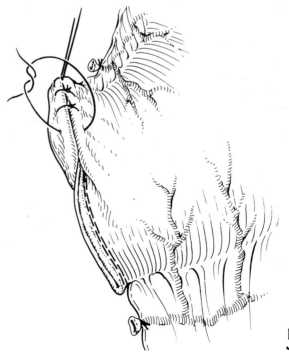

5b

Division of the pancreas

6a–c With the distal stomach retracted to the right, the pancreatic neck (already taped) is exposed. Depending on the localization of the tumour, the pancreas is divided well to the left of the taped 'tunnel' that will now easily accommodate a broad sound. To control the bleeding, the cephalad part of the pancreas is compressed by a Satinsky clamp and divided by a scalpel. Any bleeding vessels on the cut surface of the pancreatic remnant are sutured with 3/0 silk. A thin slice of the cephalad pancreatic resection surface is sent for frozen section examination. Malignant infiltration is rare in most periampullary tumours but, if found, this would logically lead on to total pancreatectomy.

The large retropancreatic veins are now freely exposed and the large superior mesenteric artery behind them is revealed.

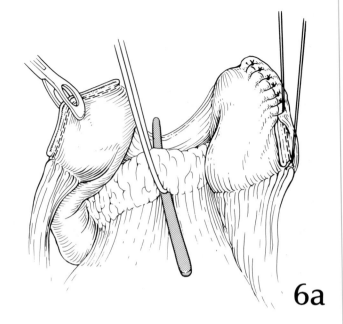

6a

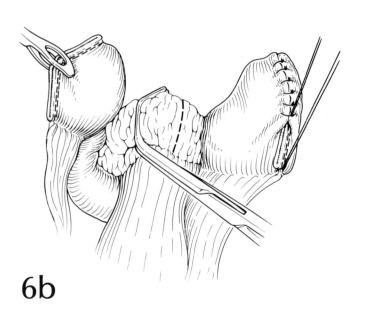

6b

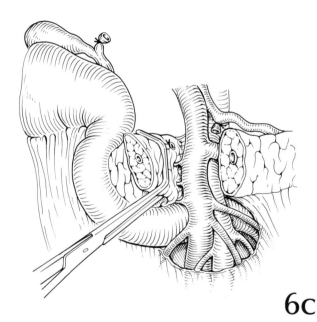

6c

Dissection of retropancreatic vessels

7a–c The mobilized specimen (including gall-bladder, distal stomach, omentum and first three parts of the duodenum) is wrapped in a pack and retracted towards the right, putting the 2–5 delicate veins draining the pancreatic head into the portal vein under tension. These veins are divided between fine metal clips whilst the large portal vein is gently 'rolled off' the pancreatic head by means of a peanut swab. Should one of the tributaries tear out, bleeding from these low pressure vessels is easily controlled by pressure with fingers behind and thumb in front of the specimen.

If damage to the large vein is to be expected (due to inflammatory or neoplastic infiltration), it is safer to obtain control of all four veins (splenic, superior and inferior mesenteric distally and portal vein proximally) by taping them with vessel loops and, if necessary, clamping all four. With such vascular control, the pancreatic head can be dissected off safely and bloodlessly, even if a segment of portal or superior mesenteric vein has to be resected (tangentially or segmentally) along with the specimen. In order to keep mesenteric congestion during portal vein occlusion to a minimum, it is good policy also to clamp the inflow, i.e. the superior mesenteric artery. Partial defects of the portal venous wall can be closed with a 6/0 suture, whereas segmental defects of up to 4 cm can usually be closed by a tension-free end-to-end anastomosis. If this is not possible, the interposition of a reinforced 10 mm polytetrafluoroethylene prosthesis will be required.

Traction of the specimen to the right will tend to pull the superior mesenteric artery into view from under its large accompanying vein. The course of this large pulsating vessel must be defined by repeated palpation to avoid injuring it. The two posterior pancreato-duodenal arteries are divided close to the superior mesenteric artery. Care must be taken not to carry skeletonization too far distally, where branches to the proximal jejunum and also the middle colic artery arise.

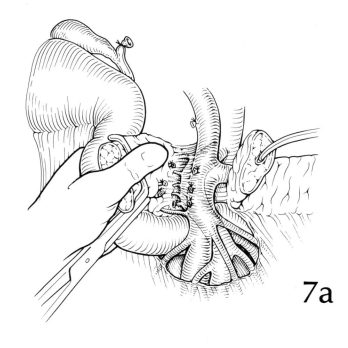

7a

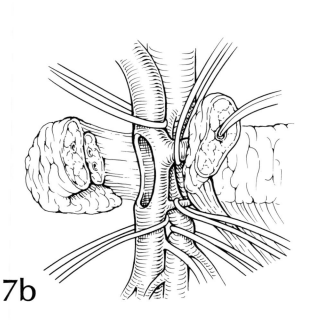

7b

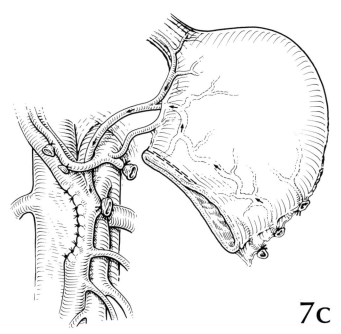

7c

Division of the jejunum

8a–c With the transverse mesocolon pulled up and the proximal jejunum downwards, the mesenteric root and the duodenojejunal flexure are put under tension. Keeping close to the antimesenteric border of the gut, the peritoneum and ligament of Treitz are divided. This creates a wide passage reaching from the lower to the upper abdomen behind the mesenteric vessels. It is through this opening that the proximal jejunum is pushed gently (from lower left to upper right) to join the rest of the specimen. A loop is passed around the most proximal jejunal segment still showing mesenteric pulsations. Keeping close to the gut, this proximal jejunal mesentery is skeletonized. The jejunum is divided by means of a stapler and the specimen can be discarded *en bloc*.

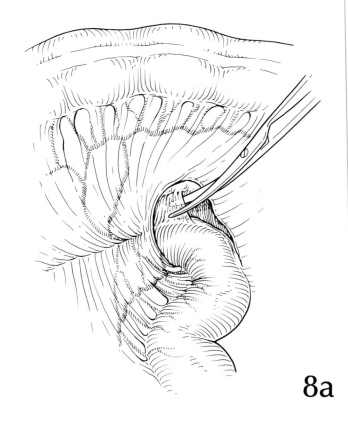

8a

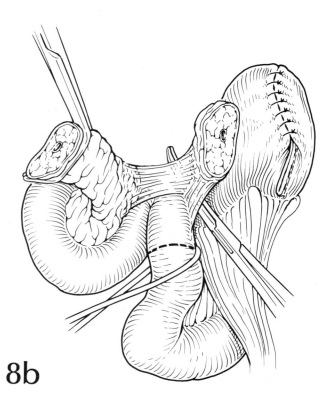

8b

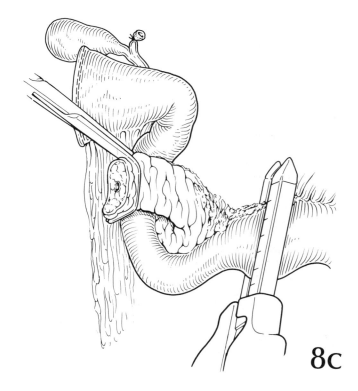

8c

Reconstruction

9 Of almost 70 variations of reconstruction after pancreatoduodenectomy, the author has largely followed the technique of Child. The pancreatic tail, hepatic duct and proximal stomach are anastomosed with the proximal jejunum in this order. The final situation is depicted here.

Pancreatojejunostomy

The stapled distal end of the jejunum is brought up behind the mesenteric vessels to lie tension-free against the cut surface of the pancreatic remnant. In cases where a local recurrence at the mesenteric root has to be considered – a recurrence that has been known to obstruct the draining jejunal loop – it is safer to pass this loop through an avascular gap in the mesocolon some distance from the mesenteric vessels.

The pancreatojejunostomy is performed as an end-to-end inverting telescope-type of anastomosis in two layers (3/0 silk outside and 3/0 chromic catgut within).

10a–d The outer posterior row of 5–7 3/0 silk sutures are placed, taking deep sero-muscular bites of jejunum and equally generous bites of the posterior pancreatic surface. The latter are facilitated by tilting the pancreatic stump to the left by means of a curved clamp placed in the pancreatic duct. When all are in position, these sutures are tied snugly and cut, leaving the two corner sutures long as markers.

The inner posterior row of 3/0 chromic catgut is placed next, catching the posterior edge of the cut pancreatic surface and a full-thickness bite of jejunal wall. If the pancreatic duct is dilated (>3 mm), 2–3 bites of its posterior edge are taken to splay it open.

Although recommended by some, the author has never placed a pancreatic ductal drainage tube; this duct is either too narrow to accommodate a useful drain or it seems too dilated to need one.

The inner anterior row is fashioned as inverting sutures placed inside-to-outside (jejunum) and outside-to-inside (anterior pancreatic edge), so that the 3/0 chromic catgut knots come to lie within the lumen (*Illustration 10c*). Again, if the duct is markedly dilated, two or three of these sutures can catch its anterior edge.

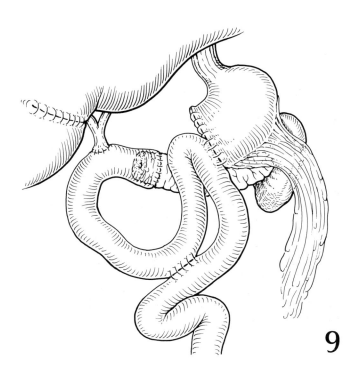

9

The final outer anterior row of 3/0 silk sutures will produce the 'telescope effect', placing the pancreatic stump deeply into the jejunum. Here big bites of anterior pancreatic surface and seromuscular layer of jejunum are taken beginning at least 2 cm away from the cut surfaces (*Illustration 10d*).

Rarely, the pancreatic remnant may be too bulky to fit into the jejunum end-to-end, in which case an end-to-side anastomosis is performed between the pancreatic stump and the antimesenteric edge of the jejunum, using exactly the same technique as that described above.

Other methods of dealing with the pancreatic remnant – the 'Achilles heel' of the whole procedure – include its removal (i.e. total pancreatectomy), its anastomosis with the posterior wall of the stomach (pancreatogastrostomy), sealing the pancreatic duct by occlusion with Ethibloc and/or ligature, or leaving the remnant open with a drain to collect the inevitable secretions.

In practised hands most of these variations produce acceptable results, but a 10% rate of leakage from the pancreatic anastomosis has to be anticipated. More important than the particular variation or suture material used is adherence to a standardized, meticulously atraumatic technique.

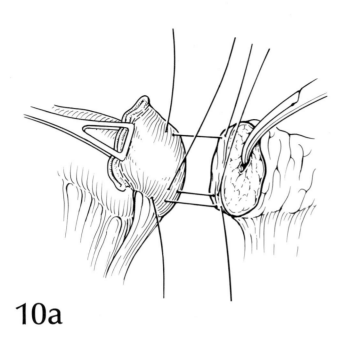

10a

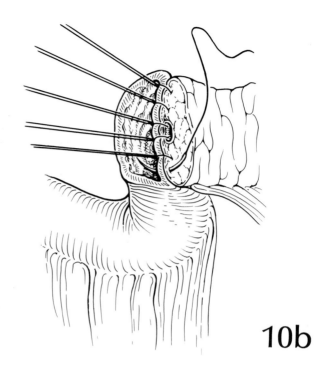

10b

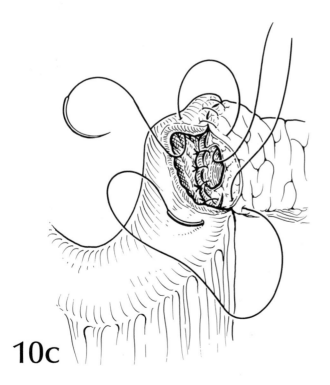

10c

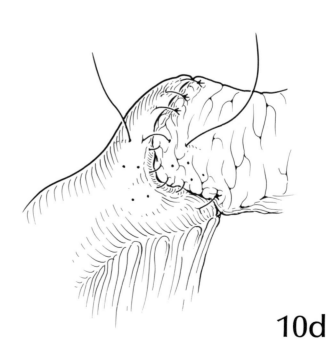

10d

Hepaticojejunostomy

End-to-side hepaticojejunostomy is performed some 10–12 cm downstream from the pancreatic anastomosis with a single row of 4/0 resorbable sutures.

11a–d The anterior sutures are placed first, taking the anterior edge of the bile duct from within to outside. An opening is then fashioned in the antimesenteric border of the jejunum using fine needle cautery. The posterior full thickness row of sutures is then placed, tied and cut. The anterior row is completed by passing the needle through the anterior jejunal edge (full-thickness) so that the resorbable knots come to lie inside (*Illustration 11c*).

Unless the bile duct is very narrow (which it hardly ever is in cases of cancer of the pancreatic head) a splinting drainage tube is not required. However, in order to drain bile away from the pancreatic anastomosis and to decompress the jejunal loop, it is advisable to place a 5 mm Silastic Völker drain into this loop. It is brought out through the jejunal wall in a Witzel-type canal and can be removed 2–3 weeks later. If there is any clinical suspicion of a leak at either of the anastomoses, this drain provides a good port for their postoperative radiographic control.

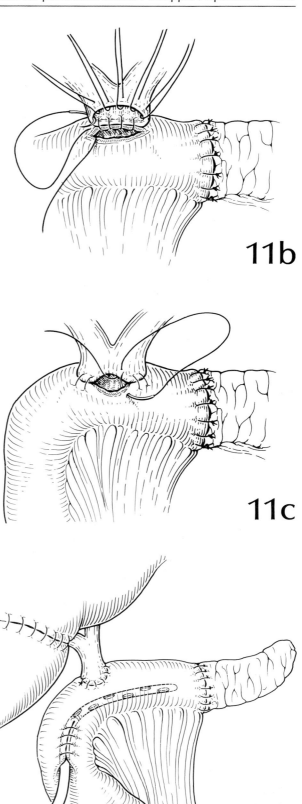

11b

11c

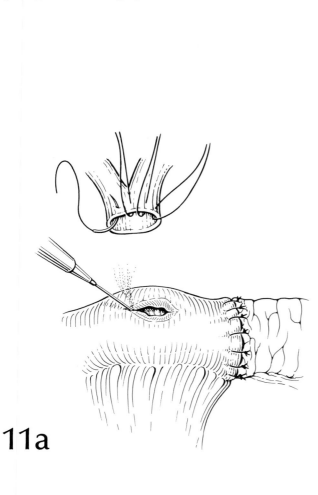

11a

11d

Gastrojejunostomy

The final anastomosis (antecolic, partial end-to-side gastrojejunostomy) lies 40–50 cm distal to the biliary anastomosis. It is performed in two layers: 2/0 silk outside and 2/0 chromic catgut within.

A Braun jejunojejunostomy is added to decompress the proximal jejunal loop and to reduce jejunal-gastric reflux to a physiological minimum. This last anastomosis is performed with a single continuous resorbable 3/0 suture.

Drainage and closure

A soft wide-bore Silastic drain is placed close to and behind the pancreatic and biliary anastomoses and is brought outside via a stab wound in the right flank some 5 cm below the Völker jejunal drain.

The abdominal wall is closed in four layers: (1) peritoneum and posterior rectus sheath with continuous 2/0 monofilament resorbable suture; (2) anterior rectus fascia with a heavy duty no. 1 monofilament resorbable suture; (3) subcutaneous interrupted 3/0 absorbable sutures; and (4) skin closure with a non-resorbable 2/0 monofilament intracutaneous pull-out suture, removable after 2 weeks.

Postoperative care

Postoperative management is kept as simple as possible and differs little from that following a partial gastrectomy. The patient is extubated on the operating table and transferred to the surgical ICU. Apart from routine input and output records and haemodynamic control, the single most important item of postoperative monitoring is the close meshed clinical observation of the patient by the same personnel and, above all, by the surgeon.

The nasogastric tube and bladder catheter are removed in the evening of the operation. As soon as peristalsis starts (48–72 h postoperatively), the patient may begin taking sips of tea. At the same time, the intravenous infusion is reduced and terminated altogether at about the fifth postoperative day.

Postoperative medication is confined to a single dose of perioperative antibiotic prophylaxis (2 g cephazoline) and adequate patient-controlled analgesia using Piritramide in 15 mg doses. Routine prophylaxis of thromboembolic, bronchopulmonary and stress ulcer problems is achieved by low molecular heparin, physiotherapy and omeprazole.

The subhepatic drain is usually shortened on the fifth day and removed completely on the seventh postoperative day. If drainage is copious, the fluid is examined for amylase or bile. Rarely, several litres of lymph fluid are drained daily, particularly after extensive retroperitoneal lymph node dissection. Such fluid loss must be restored parenterally until it subsides spontaneously in 2–3 weeks.

The average postoperative hospital stay is 16 days, by which time the Völker drain can also be removed.

Complications

The postoperative complications feared most are leaks at the pancreatic anastomosis (in up to 10% of cases) and gastrointestinal or, more rarely, retroperitoneal bleeding (in 6%). Pancreatic leaks range from a harmless fistula to disastrous peritonitis with generalized sepsis. Raised amylase values in the postoperative drain secretions may be the only sign of a pancreatic fistula that usually dries up within 2–3 weeks without any special therapy. If there is a significant anastomotic dehiscence or acute pancreatitis in the pancreatic remnant, the clinical signs (abdominal tenderness, agitation, dry tongue, tachycardia and fever) usually arouse suspicions before laboratory or radiological findings. If in doubt, early reintervention provides the best chance for averting a catastrophe. Depending on the extent of local damage and the patient's general condition, the best solution usually is a completion pancreatectomy.

Gastrointestinal bleeding is detected by melaena (more rarely haematemesis) and deterioration in haemoglobin and/or haemodynamic parameters. Localization and control of bleeding is achieved endoscopically in most cases. If bleeding recurs, laparotomy and additional suture of the bleeding site is required, usually along the gastric remnant or gastrojejunal anastomosis, and rarely at the Braun jejunojejunostomy.

Outcome

In the past 22 years, 458 consecutive Whipple pancreatoduodenectomies have been performed at the Mannheim Clinic, 328 for neoplasms and 130 for severe, complicated chronic pancreatitis afflicting mainly the head of the pancreas. The early results are shown in *Table 1*. The postoperative and in-hospital mortality rate for resections performed for neoplasms alone amounted to 2.7%.

Table 1 **Early results of pancreatoduodenectomy at the Mannheim Clinic**

Type of procedure	No. of patients	Diagnosis		Operative + hospital mortality
		Neoplasm	Pancreatitis	
Whipple's operation	458	328	130	9
Total pancreatectomy	61	44	17	4
Total	519	372 (11 deaths)	147 (2 deaths)	13 (2.5%)

Pancreatic endocrine disease

Jon A. van Heerden MS, FRCS(C), FACS, FCM(SA), FRCS(Ed), FRCS(Glas)
Fred C. Anderson Professor of Surgery, Department of Gastroenterologic and General Surgery, Mayo Clinic and Mayo Foundation, Rochester, Minnesota, USA

Chung-Yau Lo FRCS(Ed), FCS(HK)
Senior Registrar, Department of Surgery, The University of Hong Kong, Queen Mary Hospital, Hong Kong

History

The first association between islet cell tumours of the pancreas and an endocrine disorder was made by Wilder and associates at the Mayo Clinic in Rochester, Minnesota in 1927. An orthopaedic surgeon was referred for the evaluation of bizarre spells and unusual behaviour. Dr C. H. Mayo explored the patient and encountered a non-resectable, widely metastatic pancreatic islet cell tumour. Extracts of tissue excised from the tumour produced severe hypoglycaemia when injected into a rabbit. In the ensuing 50 years, aided by the refinement in immunohistochemical staining techniques, a better understanding of the amine precursor uptake and decarboxylation (APUD) cell system and the advent of electron microscopy, an increasing number of clinical syndromes secondary to the production of various peptides have been elucidated in association with functioning islet cell tumours. In addition, an increasing number of 'pancreatic incidentalomas' with no obvious endocrine function have been detected by abdominal computed tomography. With the exception of insulinoma and gastrinomas which account for at least 95% of functioning islet cell tumours, others are encountered so infrequently that they will not be considered any further in this chapter.

Principles and justification

Four important questions need to be addressed during the evaluation of these tumours:

1. *Is the tumour functioning or non-functioning?* At least 50% of islet cell tumours are non-functioning. Perhaps there is no such entity as a truly non-functional islet cell tumour. The lack of clinical hormone overproduction could be caused by the failure of these tumours to release hormones from their precursors, the failure of current biochemical detection of the hormones secreted, or the failure of the hypersecreted hormone to produce detectable clinical syndromes.
2. *Is the tumour benign or malignant?* The diagnosis of malignancy depends on the demonstration of the presence of distant metastases since the histological appearance alone is notoriously unreliable in confirming malignancy. Approximately 50–60% of gastrinomas are malignant, compared with 10% of insulinomas.
3. *Is the tumour a sporadic occurrence or is the patient a member of a family with the multiple endocrine neoplasia type I (MEN-I)?* The hallmark of pathology in the pancreas in patients with MEN-I is multiplicity of tumours and diffuse islet cell hyperplasia; these findings have important therapeutic implications in such patients. The occurrence of other endocrinopathies such as pituitary adenomas and hyperparathyroidism, usually as a result of parathyroid hyperplasia, should be sought in the patient and other family members.
4. *Is the patient a neonate or an adult?* Non-neoplastic hyperinsulinism should only be considered in newborn infants in whom a discrete adenoma is the exception. The pathology is usually that of diffuse islet cell hyperplasia (or nesidioblastosis) – a condition which is best treated by a ±95% pancreatectomy.

The goals of operative intervention are: (1) to locate and excise, if possible, all abnormally functioning tissue; (2) to differentiate between benign and malignant tumours by searching for the presence of metastatic disease; and (3) to accomplish both (1) and (2) with minimal concomitant postoperative morbidity and mortality.

Islet cell tumours, both functioning and non-functioning, benign and malignant, are indolent slow-growing tumours. Surgical resection is not only beneficial for functioning islet cell tumours of the pancreas, but also valuable for prevention or relief of symptoms arising from non-functioning malignant tumours.

However, surgery should not be performed to confirm the diagnosis. This diagnosis should be based on clinical suspicion and should ideally be secured by biochemical tests before exploration.

Choice of operation

The surgical procedure is predicated on the localization and site of the tumour, the relation/proximity of the tumour to the pancreatic duct, and the presence or absence of regional or distant metastases. The over-riding principle is that of wide exposure of the entire pancreas to allow both visual and digital examination of the gland, and the routine use of intraoperative, real-time, small-part ultrasonography, utilizing either a 7.5 or 10 MHz transducer.

Preoperative

Localization

All islet cell tumours of the pancreas should ideally be localized before exploration in order to facilitate and expedite surgical removal. Localization studies should only be entertained after the diagnosis is confirmed with biochemical tests and should not be performed to make a diagnosis. Modalities for preoperative localization vary from techniques such as ultrasonography, computed tomography, magnetic resonance imaging, octreotide radioisotope scanning and endoscopic ultrasonography to invasive and sophisticated studies including selective visceral angiography, percutaneous transhepatic portal or splenic venous sampling, and calcium or secretin-stimulated selective pancreatic and hepatic angiography with hepatic venous sampling (Imamura test). To this list should be added surgical palpation of the pancreas, intraoperative ultrasonography, intraoperative endoscopy and transillumination, and intraoperative detection of radiolabelled somatostatin analogues with a hand-held gamma-detecting probe.

The choice of localization studies before operation is controversial and each group of endocrine surgeons and endocrinologists has a favoured preoperative strategy. However, for patients with islet cell tumours of the pancreas undergoing primary operation none has yet been shown to be superior to digital palpation and inspection of the pancreas and duodenum by an experienced pancreatic surgeon. All of the other methods are of importance principally in reoperative cases in which postoperative reaction and scarring decrease the sensitivity of palpation. Extensive pre-operative localization investigation is neither indicated nor cost effective because of the high success rate of surgical exploration. Preoperative localization, in our practice, is limited to small-part ultrasonography alone which is cost effective and non-invasive and, in addition, may exclude the presence of hepatic or nodal metastases. Successful exploratory operation continues to rely on the careful surgical palpation of the entire pancreas and the routine use of intraoperative ultra-sonography[1-3].

Intraoperative glucose monitoring

Prior to exploration in patients with insulinoma all glucose intake should be stopped 3–4 h before the operation to allow for intraoperative monitoring. A glucose level should be obtained soon after induction of anaesthesia as a baseline and to prevent undue and potentially hazardous hypoglycaemia. This level is monitored at 15–20-min intervals until the tumour is removed. Following removal, glucose should be monitored at 5-min intervals. A prompt rise in glucose level (> 20 mg/dl or 1.2 mmol/l) within 15–20 min following removal of the tumour is an indication of complete tumour excision. However, since there may be a delay in rebound hyperglycaemia (>90 min) in 10% of patients, no operative decision should be made based solely on these levels.

Perioperative octreotide (somatostatin)

Octreotide acetate in a dose of 100–150 µg sub-cutaneously should be given 1 h before operation and may be continued for 3–5 days in a dose of 100–150 µg every 6 h. Sufficient data have substantiated the role of octreotide in decreasing the incidence of postoperative pancreatic fistulae in patients undergoing pancreatic surgery[4].

Anaesthesia

General anaesthesia with adequate muscle relaxation is similar to that used in other upper abdominal opera-tions. The patient is placed supine on the operating table, a nasogastric tube should be inserted for gastric decompression, and a urinary catheter inserted in the bladder.

Operation

Incision

1a, b A transverse epigastric incision (from nipple line to nipple line) is preferred for most upper abdominal operations, particularly those on the pancreas. Unless the patient is thin, midline incisions are confining and less than ideal. Exposure is greatly facilitated and enhanced by the liberal use of the mechanical third arm or upper hand retractor.

After entry into the peritoneal cavity, a careful and systematic laparotomy is performed with particular emphasis on the liver and peripancreatic areas to rule out the possibility of metastatic disease.

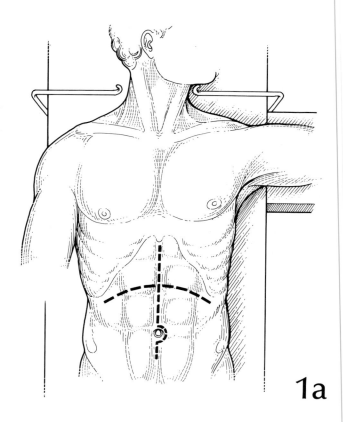

1a

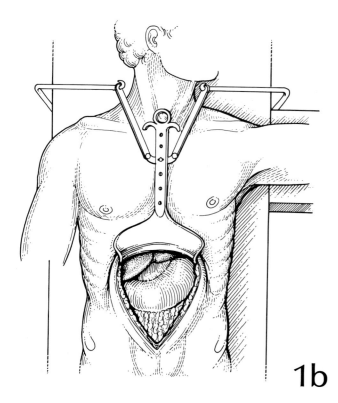

1b

Duodenum and head of the pancreas

2   If the tumour is thought to be in the head of the gland or the uncinate process of the pancreas a wide Kocher's manoeuvre of the duodenum is imperative. The peritoneum and loose areolar tissue lateral to the second part of the duodenum are incised to allow the entire duodenum (particularly the third and fourth portions) and head of the pancreas to be lifted forward off the inferior vena cava. This manoeuvre allows excellent access for palpation of the first, second and third portions of the duodenum, and the head and neck of the pancreas, as well as the uncinate process.

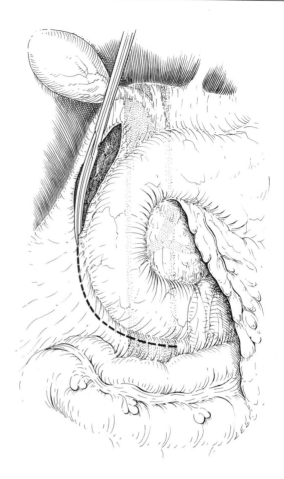

2

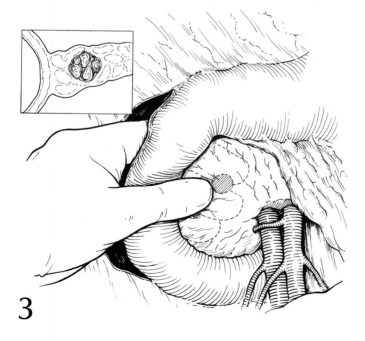

3

Patients with insulinoma

3   Bimanual or bidigital gentle palpation of the entire head of the gland and uncinate process is the key to successful localization in patients with insulinoma. Subtle difference in consistency when palpating the pancreas is the hallmark of islet cell adenomas. Insulinomas are slightly firmer than normal pancreatic tissue and this subtle difference in consistency can be readily appreciated with a gentle and soft palpation. Most of these tumours are less than 1.5 cm in size and are seldom visible to the naked eye.

Patients with the Zollinger–Ellison syndrome

4 In these patients particularly careful search by palpation of the entire duodenum is required to detect the presence of the usually small (4–6 mm) duodenal gastrin-producing carcinoid tumours. These tumours are characterized by their firmness to palpation of the duodenum after wide mobilization ('millet seed feel')[5]. Longitudinal incision of the second part of the duodenum and separate palpation of the anterior and posterior wall can be considered for patients with a suspected gastrinoma in the duodenal wall.

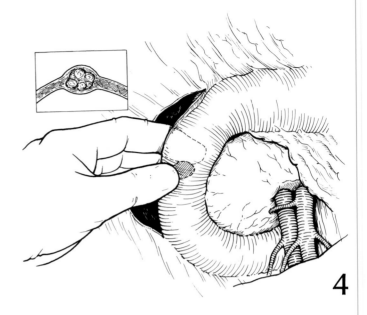

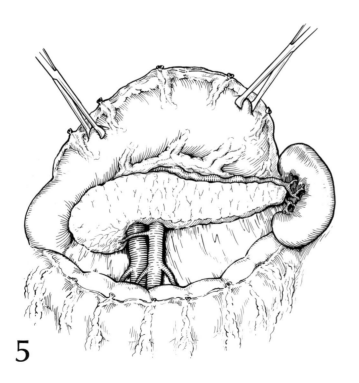

Body and tail of the pancreas

5 Exposure of the body and tail of the pancreas is obtained by wide division of the gastrocolic omentum and entry into the lesser sac. Any adhesions between the posterior wall of the stomach and the pancreas are lysed.

6 The avascular peritoneum along the inferior border of the pancreas, to the left of the superior mesenteric vessels, is incised with electrocautery which allows mobilization of the pancreas to the splenic hilus.

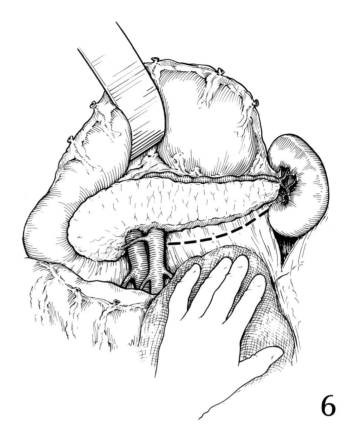

6

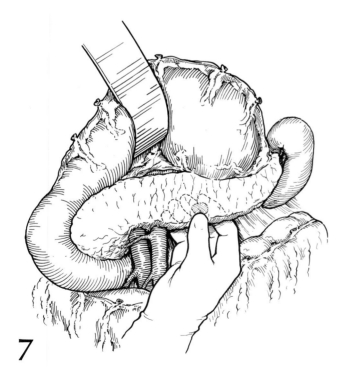

7

7 The body and tail of the pancreas is reflected upwards and can be 'stood on end' with this extensive mobilization. Once again, bimanual or bidigital palpation can be done between the thumb and the forefinger of either hand in a gentle, unhurried and systematic way.

Intraoperative ultrasonography (IOUS)

The utilization of intraoperative, small-part real-time ultrasonography should be a routine in pancreatic endocrine surgery. An enthusiastic radiologist skilled in ultrasonography should not only interpret the images obtained by the real-time ultrasonography but should be an integral part of the operating team.

8 The advantages of this technology include: (1) localization of islet cell tumours; (2) delineation of proximity of tumour to main pancreatic duct; and (3) demonstration of the presence of multiple tumours in patients with MEN-I syndrome.

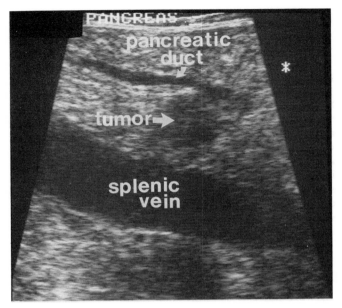

8

Enucleation versus resection

Once the tumour is localized the decision has to be made whether it can be enucleated or whether a pancreatic resection (proximal or distal) will be required. Since about 85% of islet cell adenomas are less than 1.5 cm in diameter and are located in a superficial position, simple enucleation can be safely performed in most cases and major resections such as pancreatico-duodenectomy are seldom required. This crucial decision has been facilitated by the routine use of intraoperative ultrasonography.

Enucleation

9 This is facilitated by the use of electrocautery or the cavitron ultrasonic aspirator (CUSA) in combination with small haemoclips. Initial experience has shown that enucleation with the CUSA has been particularly helpful when the tumours are located close to the pancreatic duct and may lead to a decrease in the number of postoperative pancreatic fistulae.

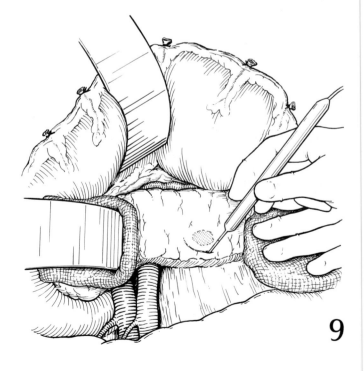

9

Repair of pancreatic bed

10 The enucleation site should be carefully inspected for haemostasis and possible major pancreatic duct injuries. If such a suspicion is present, 1 mg of secretin should be injected intravenously to affirm this suspicion. Pancreatic resection should be seriously considered for any major pancreatic duct injury. The 'pivot' in the pancreatic bed should be carefully and gently approximated or repaired with non-absorbable sutures (silk or polypropylene (Prolene)), if possible, reinforced with a plug of omentum similar to the Graham patch-type closure for perforated duodenal ulcers. Liberal peripancreatic suction drainage should always be used.

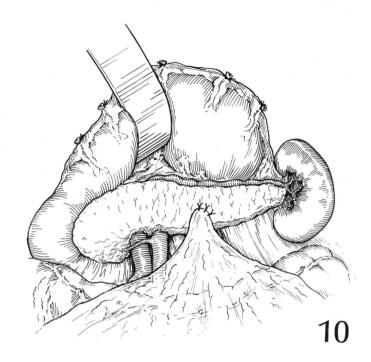

10

Distal pancreatectomy and radical pancreaticoduodenectomy

For tumours located in the tail that are deep-seated or in juxtaposition to the main pancreatic duct, distal pancreatectomy should be performed. The decision regarding enucleation may become difficult for tumours located at the head or uncinate process of the pancreas; radical pancreaticoduodenectomy is rarely necessary although there is concern with the 10% incidence of postoperative pancreatic fistulae, most of which, however, close without reoperative intervention. The technical aspects of distal pancreatectomy and radical pancreaticoduodenectomy are discussed on pp. 654–656.

'Blind' distal pancreatectomy

This is never indicated, even when no tumour is identified during operation, because: (1) islet cell tumours are evenly distributed throughout the pancreas and distal pancreatectomy will result in failure in 50% of cases; (2) the inherent morbidity and mortality associated with pancreatic resection; and (3) the increasingly effective medical management of hypergastrinaemia (H_2 blocker or omeprazole) and hyperinsulinaemia (somatostatin and/or diazoxide).

Postoperative care

For patients with insulinoma, glucose-containing solution should not be given during the first 24 h after surgery. Rebound hyperglycaemia of up to 200–300 mg/dl (11–17 mmol/l) within 12–18 h after surgery is not an uncommon phenomenon and does not require treatment. During this phase the urine is frequently tested for the presence of ketone bodies, a circumstance which is extremely rare in our practice. The nasogastric tube can be removed in the recovery room after operation unless indicated otherwise. Intravenous fluid should be continued until the return of gastrointestinal motility and the progressive resumption of oral intake. Suction drains are normally removed if drainage has ceased, but are left in position if there is a persistent drainage and suspicion of a pancreatic leakage.

Despite meticulous surgical techniques and routine pancreatic drainage, morbidity occurs in 10–15% of patients after enucleation or resection. Complications include secondary haemorrhage, pancreatitis, and pancreatic fistulae or formation of subphrenic abscess (which are secondary to a pancreatic leakage). Pancreatic fistulae are evident by excessive or persistent drainage of pancreatic juice from the suction drain. Most of the leakage is temporary from the raw surface of the pancreas, which will close spontaneously with hyperalimentation and other simple management. A second operation is rarely necessary. Other complications should be managed according to surgical principles.

Outcome

Insulinoma

Mortality rates following operation range from 0% to 6%[6]. In a recent series of 30 consecutive patients, palpation and intraoperative ultrasonography localized all tumours. The most common surgical procedure undertaken was tumour enucleation in 20 patients, followed by distal pancreatectomy in nine. One patient with MEN-I underwent an 85% distal pancreatectomy plus enucleation of an adenoma in the head of the remaining gland. Intraoperative glucose monitoring was positive in 26 out of 27 patients (96%). There was no operative mortality and significant morbidity occurred in four patients (13%), which included two with a pancreatic fistula that closed spontaneously. All patients were rendered normoglycaemic after the operation.

Gastrinoma

Since 50–60% of patients with Zollinger–Ellison syndrome have malignant tumours and at least two-thirds have metastasized when they are discovered, the surgical cure rate is at present approximately 30%[6]. However, exploration in carefully selected patients seems to be the treatment of choice with an increased cure rate in this group of patients.

References

1. Rothmund M. Localization of endocrine pancreatic tumours. *Br J Surg* 1994; 81: 164–6.

2. Grant CS, van Heerden JA, Charboneau JW, James EM, Reading CC. Insulinoma: the value of intraoperative ultrasonography. *Arch Surg* 1988; 123: 843–8.

3. van Heerden JA, Grant CS, Czako PF, Service FJ, Charboneau JW. Occult functioning insulinomas: which localizing studies are indicated? *Surgery* 1992; 112: 1010–15.

4. Buchler M, Friess H, Klempa I *et al.* Role of octreotide in the prevention of postoperative complications following pancreatic resection. *Am J Surg* 1992; 163: 125–31.

5. Thompson NW, Vinik AI, Eckhauser FE. Microgastrinomas of the duodenum: a cause of failed operations for the Zollinger-Ellison syndrome. *Ann Surg* 1989; 209: 396–404.

6. van Heerden JA, Thompson GB. Islet cell tumours of the pancreas. In: Trede M, Carter DC, eds. *Surgery of the Pancreas*. London: Churchill Livingstone, 1993: 545–61.

Pancreatic transplantation: islet transplantation

D. W. R. Gray DPhil(Oxon), MRCP, FRCS
Clinical Reader and Consultant Surgeon, Department of Surgery, John Radcliffe Hospital, Oxford, UK

Principles and justification

The technique of isolated pancreatic islet transplantation has been developed for the purpose of treating diabetes mellitus, and has recently moved from the experimental laboratory to clinical trials. For this purpose the pancreatic islets must be separated from human cadaveric pancreas. The principles adhered to during donor organ retrieval in order to provide pancreatic tissue suitable for islet separation are as follows:

1. Suitable donors should be aged between 20 and 50 years without evidence of pancreatitis or diabetes.
2. The pancreatic blood flow must be maintained during the donor operation to avoid all warm ischaemia (because warm ischaemia is detrimental to islet viability).
3. The gland should be perfused *in situ* with a cold preservation fluid such as hypertonic citrate solution.

4. The pancreas is then rapidly removed, avoiding damage to the surface of the gland. This is extremely important because the technique relies on injection of collagenase enzyme into the pancreatic duct under pressure. Damage to the surface will allow leakage of injected fluid and produce poor distension.
5. As much of the pancreas as possible should be removed – preferably the whole gland – for the obvious reason that the more pancreas that can be processed, the greater the likely yield of islet tissue.
6. Following organ donation the pancreas should be transported to the processing centre as rapidly as possible, preferably keeping the cold ischaemia time to less than 4 h since cold ischaemia times of more than 4 h have been shown to reduce the islet yield.

Operation

Pancreas retrieval

The pancreas is usually retrieved as part of a multi-organ cadaveric donation procedure. The main vessels are prepared for organ perfusion *in situ* in the standard fashion, taking care to maintain the blood flow to the pancreas by keeping the coeliac artery and its splenic branch open throughout. Once the circulation ceases, cold perfusion of the abdominal organs is commenced using a cold preservation solution; hypertonic citrate is the perfusion fluid of choice for islet isolation.

The lesser sac is opened via the greater omentum and saline ice packs are introduced to surface cool the pancreas. This is particularly important if donation of the liver is intended, since the pancreas will remain within the abdomen for some time while the liver is removed, and rewarming of the pancreas from the surrounding tissues is a danger.

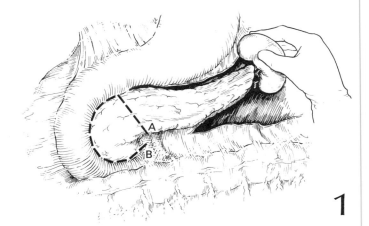

1

1 Once adequate cooling of the pancreas has been assured, it is removed by mobilizing the spleen, followed by the tail of the pancreas using the spleen as a 'handle'. The portal vein is transected and the pancreatic head is dissected from within the duodenal loop (line B).

Although it is possible to remove the pancreatic head intact, clamping the bile duct above the pancreas and at the duodenal papilla to prevent contamination, this dissection takes some time to perform carefully and, to avoid damage to the duodenum by prolonged dissection, it is preferable to leave a cuff of the pancreatic head adherent to the bile duct and duodenum (line A). The removed gland is then separated from the spleen by taking a generous cuff of the splenic hilum to avoid damaging the pancreas, and immersed in iced saline solution.

Preparation of islets

The gland is then packed in three sterile plastic bags containing saline slush and transported to the processing laboratory as rapidly as possible. Within a laminar flow tissue processing hood, the pancreas is dissected free from surrounding fat and attached vessels, again taking care to avoid damaging the surface of the gland.

In the first stage of the islet isolation process the pancreatic duct is cannulated. This may be achieved by cannulating the duct retrogradely from the excised head of the pancreas, but this is often surprisingly difficult

and the cannula will not pass distally. The best technique is to incise across the neck of the pancreas with a scalpel until the duct is seen and opened, tying in two cannulae with purse-string sutures. The duodenal end of the duct is clamped and ligated with a strong ligature. Collagenase enzyme is injected slowly via the cannulae to remove the collagen framework of the pancreas and to allow subsequent dispersion of the tissue.

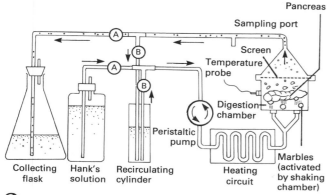

2

2 The distended gland is transferred to an incubation chamber with circulating prewarmed culture medium. The digestion proceeds within the chamber until the pancreas starts to disperse, fragmentation being encouraged by mechanical agitation of the chamber. Once the fragments of pancreas are small enough to pass through the pores (diameter 0.3 mm) of the mesh within the chamber, they are collected from the circulating fluid by centrifugation, cooled and washed several times to remove the enzyme. Finally the islet tissue is purified from the exocrine tissue by density gradient separation which relies on the fact that islet tissue is normally less dense than exocrine tissue.

Donation of islets

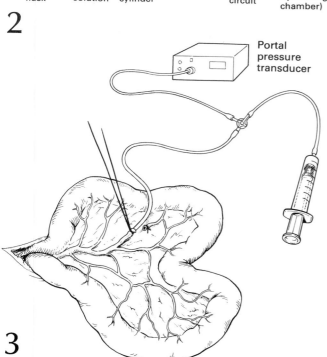

3

3 The transplantation of islets is usually conducted by injection of the islet tissue (ideally less than 5 ml in spun volume) into the portal vein. This may be accessed via a small laparotomy incision, cannulating the obliterated umbilical vein or, perhaps more reliably, cannulating a gut mesenteric vein and threading a 4-Fr cannula up to the main portal vein. Alternatively, and perhaps preferably for the future, a large branch of the portal vein may be cannulated by direct percutaneous puncture under radiological control. Either way, the portal vein pressure is first measured using a water manometer and then the islet tissue is injected slowly via a 4-Fr cannula, stopping intermittently to measure the portal pressure. The normal portal pressure should be around $5\,cmH_2O$ and injection should stop if the portal pressure rises to above $30\,cmH_2O$.

Postoperative care

At present, clinical islet allotransplantation is restricted in application by most centres to patients who have previously undergone kidney transplantation. These patients are already on continuous immunosuppression, but those maintained by cyclosporin and/or azathioprine alone, or those receiving triple therapy with very low dose steroid, are preferred in order to minimize the diabetogenic effects of steroids. The usual practice has been to continue baseline immunosuppression with the addition of a 14-day course of antithymocyte globulin after islet allotransplantation. There is some evidence that hyperglycaemia may impair the early implantation of transplanted islets. Therefore, following the transplant most centres attempt to maintain strict normoglycaemia by an intensive hourly regimen of intravenous insulin, guided by repeated venous blood samples for at least 48–72 h. Some centres continue insulin for long periods (up to 3 months), even in the face of clear evidence of graft function, in the belief that avoidance of hyperglycaemic stress gives the best chance of long-term function by 'resting' the islets during the implantation and stabilization process.

Outcome

The results of human islet allotransplantation have generally been disappointing, with the main problem apparently being insufficient yield of islets in most patients. Some centres have overcome the problem by using islets from several donors, but the yields are gradually improving and most patients given a transplant consisting of more 5000 islets (standardized to an islet diameter of 150 μm)/kg have shown evidence of function, with C peptide production detectable and reduced requirements for insulin. A few patients who had no C peptide production before transplantation have actually become insulin-independent, and at the time of writing there are seven such patients in the world, the longest duration of function being 3 years. One of these patients received islets from only one donor.

Transplantation in chronic pancreatitis

Some centres have performed autotransplantation of islets derived from the pancreas of patients subjected to pancreatectomy for conditions such as chronic pancreatitis. Immunosuppression is not required. In general, the islets derived from such diseased organs have been obtained with minimal purification of exocrine tissue to minimize the tissue loss, and the transplantation of such impure tissue is associated with fairly alarming rises in portal pressure. For this reason the procedure should not be attempted in centres that are unfamiliar with the technique and dealing with the problems that may ensue. Despite this, several centres have reported avoidance of insulin therapy in some patients where total pancreatectomy was thought to have been performed, and evidence of continued function for up to 7 years has been presented.

Acknowledgements

Illustration 2 is reproduced with permission from *Diabetes* 1988; 37: 413 and from *Methods in Cell Transplantation*, C. Ricordi (ed.), 1995, pp. 433–8.

Illustrations by Angela Christie

Pancreatic transplantation: intact organ transplantation

Kenneth L. Brayman MD, PhD
Assistant Professor of Surgery, Department of Surgery, Hospital of the University of Pennsylvania, Philadelphia, USA

Yevgenicy Gincherman MD
Assistant Instructor in Medicine, Department of Medicine, Hospital of the University of Pennsylvania, Philadelphia, USA

Mark M. Levy MD
Assistant Instructor in Surgery, Department of Surgery, Hospital of the University of Pennsylvania, Philadelphia, USA

David E. R. Sutherland MD, PhD
Professor of Surgery, Department of Surgery, University of Minnesota, Minneapolis, Minnesota, USA

History

In 1966 Kelly and Lillehei at the University of Minnesota performed the first transplant of the human pancreas using pancreatic duct ligation to manage pancreatic exocrine secretions. Several variants of the technique were described over the next two decades. In 1973 Gliedman *et al.* described the urinary drainage technique to manage pancreatic exocrine secretions which involved anastomosing the pancreatic duct to the recipient ureter. Nine years later Cook and Sollinger at the University of Wisconsin described a technique for draining pancreatic exocrine secretions directly into the urinary bladder.

Pancreatic transplantation has been performed more frequently in recent years, with over 6500 transplants having been reported to the International Pancreas Transplant Registry by the end of 1995. Approximately two-thirds of all pancreatic transplants have been performed simultaneously with a kidney graft. The remainder are transplanted either after kidney transplantation or alone.

Principles and justification

The objectives of pancreatic transplantation are to improve the quality of life of a diabetic recipient, and to prevent or halt the progression of secondary complications of diabetes by establishing a normoglycaemic, insulin-independent state. Pancreatic transplantation offers the diabetic patient the safest technique to normalize blood glycosylated haemoglobin levels. Numerous studies suggest that only strict glucose control effectively prevents the progression of diabetic retinopathy, nephropathy, polyneuropathy and vasculopathy.

Recipient selection

Pancreatic transplantation is the only treatment for type I diabetes that results in insulin independence. The potential benefits of achieving a normoglycaemic state are weighed against the complications of immunosuppression. Thus, pancreatic transplants are only performed in non-uraemic patients when the potential complications of diabetes are deemed to be more serious than the side effects of anti-rejection medications.

In contrast, diabetic renal allograft recipients are obliged to take immunosuppressive therapy so it has become more routine to perform transplants simultaneously with a kidney graft or after kidney transplantation in these patients. The use of the combined approach results in normoglycaemia in addition to a dialysis-free state. Some centres restrict pancreatic transplantation to young uraemic diabetic recipients without significant cardiovascular disease. Other centres are less restrictive in their recipient selection. Patient data from the University of Minnesota suggest improved clinical outcomes with younger recipients (less than 45 years of age), without cardiovascular disease. Blindness or significant peripheral vascular disease do not represent significant risk factors.

Donor selection: cadaveric versus living-related donor transplants

Although the pancreas was the first extrarenal organ to be transplanted from a living-related donor, most reported pancreatic transplants today use cadaveric donors. However, the need to employ relatively high levels of immunosuppression to maintain the graft has generated interest in using living-related donors. The present indications for living-related donor transplantation to diabetic patients include recipients who are highly sensitized (with a very low probability of obtaining a negative cross-match against a cadaveric organ) and those who choose the living-related donor option because it requires less immunosuppression than with organs of cadaveric origin. The experience at the University of Minnesota demonstrates better long-term graft survival when living-related donor transplants are used.

Preoperative

The potential recipient of a pancreatic transplant undergoes a thorough history and physical examination with particular attention being directed towards detecting the manifestations of diabetes. A routine chest radiograph and electrocardiogram are obtained followed by a stress thalium test to screen for the presence of significant ischaemic heart disease. Preoperative pulse volume recordings help to evaluate the peripheral vasculature, and angiographic evaluation is added if significant disease is documented by non-invasive means. Routine metabolic evaluation includes measurement of serum levels of glucose, C-reactive peptide and insulin. Potential recipients are screened for CMV, HSV and HIV. Preoperative evaluation by an ophthalmologist is recommended to document the degree of diabetic retinopathy. Diabetic neuropathy may be evaluated using electromyelograms and gastric emptying studies. Ultrasonography of the right upper quadrant should be performed to assess the presence of cholelithiasis. Finally, each patient should undergo a psychosocial evaluation to ensure their understanding of the nature of the procedure and to assess their future compliance with the postoperative regimen.

Anaesthesia

Pancreatic transplantation should be carried out under general anaesthesia. Many recipients of pancreatic transplants have compromised cardiovascular and pulmonary reserve so continuous pulse oximetry, blood pressure monitoring and central venous or pulmonary artery pressure monitoring are frequently employed.

Operation

Important technical considerations in pancreatic transplantation include management of pancreatic exocrine secretion, the use of whole organ versus segmental transplants, retroabdominal versus intraperitoneal placement of the graft, and systemic versus portal venous drainage. The majority of the grafts presently performed are whole organ grafts, transplanted intra-abdominally with systemic venous drainage. The most common technique, which entails whole organ intra-abdominal placement with bladder drainage, is described in this chapter. Variations of this technique are briefly discussed in the following sections.

Techniques of pancreatic duct management

1 The three most common techniques used to drain pancreatic exocrine secretions include: (1) injection of the pancreatic duct with a synthetic polymer; (2) enteric drainage from the pancreatic duct or donor duodenum into the recipient bowel; and (3) urinary drainage with a donor duodenum to bladder anastomosis. The latter technique permits the monitoring of pancreatic exocrine function through measurement of urinary amylase levels. During pancreas graft rejection, a decline in urinary amylase levels usually precedes hyperglycaemia. Bladder drainage techniques are most commonly used when pancreatic transplantation is performed simultaneously with a kidney transplant and nearly always when the pancreas is transplanted alone. The major complications specific to this technique are urological and include haematuria, reflux pancreatitis, bladder/duodenal segment leak, recurrent urinary tract infection, urethral strictures and urethritis. Metabolic acidosis may occur secondary to chronic urinary bicarbonate loss. If this complication persists, conversion to enteric drainage may be performed.

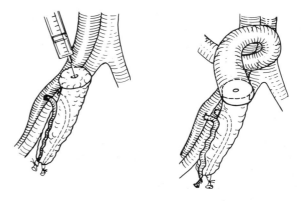

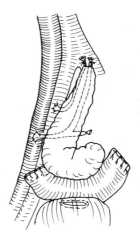

1

DONOR OPERATION

Pancreas procurement techniques

Most transplant centres in the USA now perform combined liver and pancreas procurement. Isolated pancreas procurement should be performed only when the liver cannot be used for transplantation. The multiorgan procurement is performed through either a midline laparotomy or cruciate incision. A systematic exploration of the peritoneal cavity is performed to rule out any pathological processes that would contra-indicate the use of the donor tissue.

2a–c
The arterial blood supply of the pancreas and the liver are carefully dissected and defined, as are the structures of the porta hepatis. Arterial anomalies of the hepatic vasculature are carefully defined. Although priority for procurement is routinely given to the liver, combined liver and pancreas procurement is often feasible. The gastro-duodenal artery is ligated and divided. The common bile duct is ligated and divided proximal to the ligature. The gallbladder fundus is opened and the gallbladder and the biliary system are flushed with normal saline. The lesser sac is entered by dividing the gastrocolic ligament. If the pancreas is deemed suitable for transplantation after a thorough examination, a nasogastric tube is advanced into the duodenum and 300 ml of amphotericin/antibiotic solution are instilled. The proximal duodenum distal to the pylorus is divided with a GIA stapler. Division of the lienophrenic ligament frees the spleen which will remain attached to the pancreas throughout the remainder of the resection. Division of the inferior mesenteric vein at this time will permit later mobilization of the pancreas.

Following isolation of the distal aorta and inferior vena cava, the organ donor is systemically heparinized (70 U/kg). After completion of the necessary thoracic organ dissection, the proximal jejunum is divided at the ligament of Treitz with a GIA stapler, and the distal abdominal aorta is ligated. A perfusion catheter is inserted below the level of the inferior mesenteric artery (ligated) and the proximal thoracic and supra-coeliac aorta are clamped. The aortic flush is started using 2 litres of the University of Wisconsin (UW) solution. The portal vein is promptly divided 1 cm beyond its exit from the pancreas, and 2 litres of the UW solution are flushed through it. Venous drainage is vented by placing a cannula in the inferior vena cava or by draining venous effluent into the chest by dividing the inferior vena cava/right atrial junction.

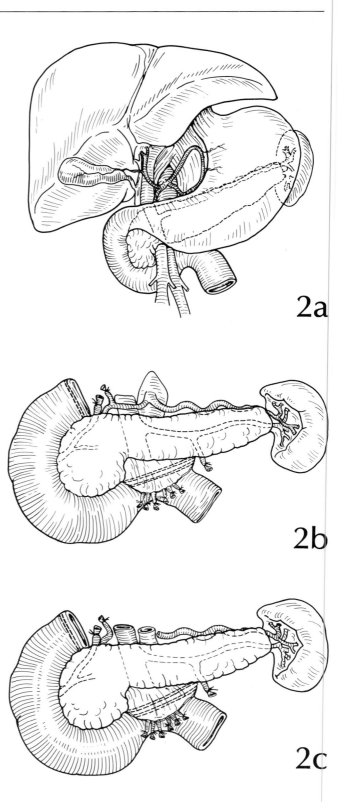

2a

2b

2c

Ex vivo preparation of the pancreaticoduodenal allograft for transplantation

Backbench reconstruction of the pancreas is performed at 4°C.

3 The splenic hilar vessels are isolated, ligated and divided, and the spleen is removed. Attention is directed towards preserving the tail of the pancreas during this step.

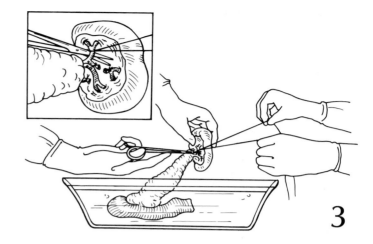

3

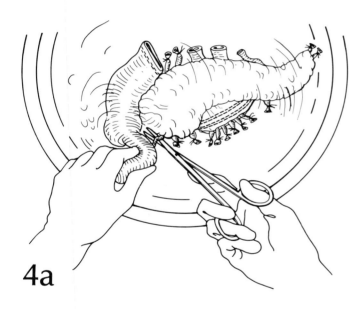

4a

4a,b The distal duodenum is then mobilized to the level of the uncinate process of the pancreas and the proximal and distal duodenal stumps are oversewn in two layers in addition to the staple line.

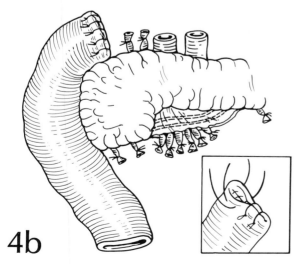

4b

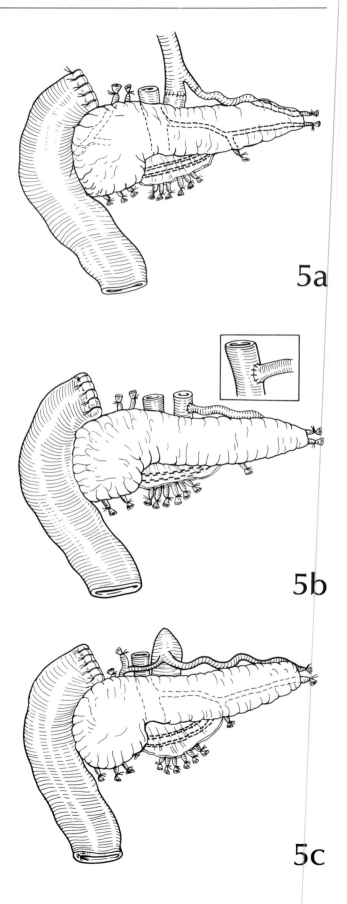

5a

5a–c An iliac artery Y graft is used for vascular reconstruction of the pancreas. The internal iliac artery is anastomosed end-to-end to the splenic artery and the external iliac artery is anastomosed end-to-end to the superior mesenteric artery of the graft. Alternatively, the splenic artery is anastomosed end-to-side to the superior mesenteric artery, creating a single graft arterial inflow. Occasionally, a patch of donor aorta including the coeliac and superior mesenteric arteries will be available (*Illustration 5c*).

Preservation of the pancreas

Reliable preservation of the pancreas is essential for the success of pancreatic transplantation. Most pancreatic transplants performed in the USA are preserved in cold UW solution; the remainder are stored in Collins solution or a plasma based solution. Use of the non-plasma based UW solution, in addition to eliminating the risk of disease transmission, has been correlated with improved graft survival rates in comparison with alternative solutions.

5b

5c

RECIPIENT OPERATION

Incision and exposure

The abdomen is entered through a lower midline incision or through a standard renal transplant incision (authors' preference). Most often, the pancreas is placed on the right side. The caecum is mobilized to create a bed for the pancreaticoduodenal graft, and the right common, external and internal iliac arteries and veins, as well as the right ureter, are mobilized. Lymphatics overlying the iliac vessels are ligated to avoid lymphocoele formation. The gonadal vein can be ligated to avoid impingement on the venous graft anastomosis.

6 Usually all branches of the hypogastric vein are ligated, stick-tied and divided for complete mobilization of the iliac vein from the vena cava to the inguinal ligament.

Dissection is completed by mobilizing the bladder. The lateral attachments of the bladder and the round ligament in women are divided. In men the spermatic cord is preserved. Adequate anterior and lateral mobilization of the bladder eliminates tension on the duodenocystostomy and facilitates distal exposure of the iliac vein.

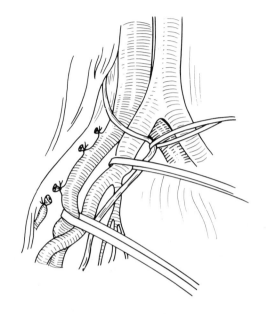

6

Vascular anastomoses

The right iliac vessels are exposed *in situ* with the artery medial to the vein. Intravenous heparin (70 U/kg) can be administered to the recipient before the placement of vascular clamps. The venous anastomosis is performed prior to the arterial anastomosis. After clamping the artery, the ureter should lie medial to the arterial anastomosis. An arteriotomy in the common iliac artery may be created first. Four stay sutures are placed to prepare this arteriotomy for the subsequent anastomosis, and plaques or intimal flaps are tacked down at this time. The venotomy is then created further distal along the external iliac vein. Four 6/0 polypropylene (Prolene) stay sutures expose the sides of the venotomy.

7a,b The donor pancreas is next brought into the operative field. An end-to-side venous anastomosis is constructed from the portal vein to the external iliac vein with a running continuous 6/0 polypropylene suture, and the arterial anastomosis (donor Y graft or superior mesenteric artery to recipient common iliac artery) is completed end-to-side in similar fashion.

Following completion of the arterial anastomosis, 25 g of mannitol are administered to minimize graft reperfusion oedema. Limiting crystalloid infusion during the procedure diminishes the risk of oedematous pancreatitis. Vascular clamps are removed after completing the vascular anastomoses and all bleeding sites are identified and controlled with 5/0 and 6/0 polypropylene sutures.

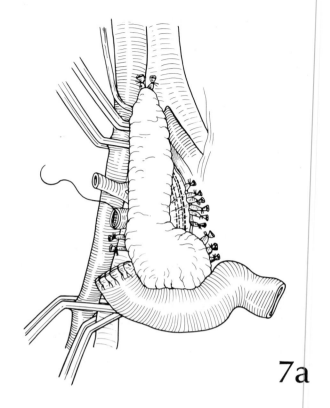

7a

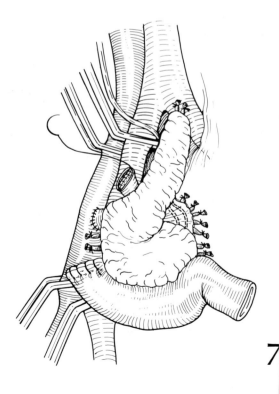

7b

Construction of duodenocystostomy

A pancreaticoduodenocystostomy can be constructed by hand-sewn or EEA stapler techniques. After culturing the duodenal contents, the open distal lumen of the duodenal graft is temporarily clamped to prevent enteric spillage if this has been left open on the back table.

Hand-sewn duodenocystostomy

A horizontal cystostomy is constructed on the postero-superior aspect of the bladder, and a horizontal duodenotomy is made on the antimesenteric side just opposite the ampulla of Vater. A two-layer anastomosis is created between the duodenum and the bladder. The outer posterior layer is constructed first using interrupted 3/0 polypropylene sutures. The inner layer is then constructed using a 3/0 running absorbable suture to appose bladder mucosa to duodenal mucosa. The anastomosis is completed following construction of the anterior outer layer using interrupted 3/0 polypropylene sutures. The distal lumen of the duodenum is closed using the TA55 stapler and reinforced with continuous 4/0 polypropylene sutures followed by interrupted 4/0 Lembert sutures.

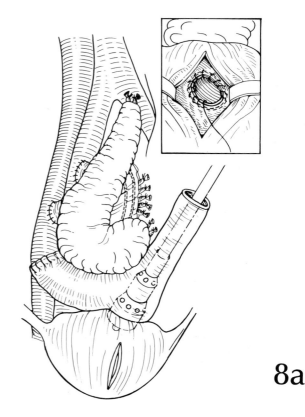

8a

EEA stapler duodenocystostomy

8a,b The curved EEA stapler is inserted into the open distal lumen of the duodenum and passed proximally. With the aid of electrocautery, the rod projecting from within the staple ring is advanced through the antimesenteric wall of the duodenum. If a lateral enterotomy was made at the time of procurement, a stapler rod is passed through this and a purse-string suture is constructed (2/0 polypropylene) to secure the exit. After the bladder is opened anteriorly for exposure, the rod of the EEA stapler is advanced through the posterosuperior wall of the bladder. The EEA anvil is placed on the staple rod from within the bladder. Firing of the stapler creates a circular duodenocystostomy. This anastomosis is oversewn from within the bladder using a 4/0 absorbable suture.

A three-layer closure of the distal duodenal lumen is performed as described previously.

Closure of the bladder and abdomen

If a solitary pancreatic transplant is performed, the anterior cystostomy is closed in three layers following irrigation with antibiotic solution. The mucosa is closed with a 4/0 absorbable suture, the muscularis with a running 3/0 absorbable suture, and the seromuscular layer is closed with an absorbable suture. The graft is examined for evidence of bleeding and pancreatitis. The

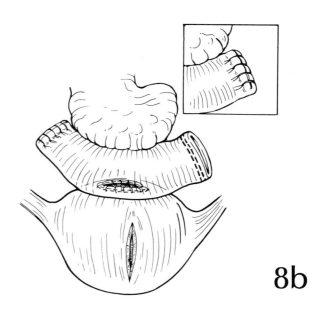

8b

abdomen is irrigated with 4 litres of normal saline treated with amphotericin and antibiotics. The abdominal fascia is closed with interrupted non-absorbable sutures. The subcutaneous tissue is irrigated with antibacterial and antifungal solutions and the skin is approximated with skin staples.

VARIANTS OF THE TECHNIQUE

Simultaneous pancreas and kidney transplants

When transplanting the pancreas and kidney simultaneously, the pancreas is placed on the right side of the pelvis with the kidney on the left. This orientation facilitates the easier construction of a duodenocystostomy, because the sigmoid colon does not interfere with mobilization of the recipient iliac vessel. The kidney is anastomosed to the left external iliac vessels which are mobilized lateral to the sigmoid colon. Transplantation of a left donor kidney to this site is preferred due to the presence of a longer left renal vein. However, the right kidney should be used if multiple left renal arteries are present.

If the pancreatic preservation does not exceed 18 h, the kidney transplant should be performed first. Backbench reconstruction of the pancreatic graft can proceed while the kidney transplant is revascularized. When this is complete, the pancreas is transplanted into the right iliac fossa. The ureteroneocystostomy may be completed using a Litch extravesical approach when the duodenocystostomy is hand-sewn. The Leadbetter–Politano technique of ureteroneocystostomy is preferred when the duodenocystostomy is stapled.

Whole pancreaticoduodenal transplantation on the left side

Transplantation of the pancreas using the left iliac vessels is used if a prior kidney transplant was performed on the right side. Intraperitoneal placement of the pancreatic transplant is preferred. In the left iliac fossa the iliac vein lies medial to the artery distally. The arterial anastomosis is constructed in end-to-side fashion to the external iliac artery. Alternatively, both anastomoses can be placed at the level of the common iliac artery and vein. The duodenocystostomy is constructed in identical fashion regardless of the site of pancreatic transplantation using the same technique as was described for right iliac fossa pancreatic transplantation.

Segmental pancreatic transplantation

The number of segmental pancreatic transplants has decreased dramatically since the introduction of bladder drainage techniques for management of pancreatic exocrine secretions. Segmental grafts are currently used for living-related, living unrelated and split pancreas grafts. When living-related donors are used, only the pancreatic body and tail are transplanted, commonly on the right side of the pelvis. The splenic artery is anastomosed end-to-side to the external iliac artery or end-to-end to the hypogastric artery. The splenic vein is anastomosed distally, end-to-side, to the external iliac vein using 6/0 running sutures.

When a bladder drainage technique is used, a two-layer anastomosis is constructed. The seromuscular layer of the bladder is incised to expose the bladder mucosa. The inner layer of the anastomosis uses absorbable interrupted 7/0 sutures to appose pancreatic duct to bladder mucosa. This anastomosis is routinely stented and the stent is cystoscopically removed 4 weeks after surgery. The outer layer of the anastomosis uses 4/0 polypropylene sutures to appose the seromuscular layer of the bladder to the pancreatic capsule.

Portal venous drainage

Although technically feasible, drainage of the portal vein of the graft to the portal venous system is rarely employed for pancreatic grafts. Systemic venous drainage results in hyperinsulinaemia whereas portal venous drainage eliminates this possible problem by providing normal first-pass metabolism of insulin by the liver. To construct a pancreatic transplant with portal venous drainage, a vascular anastomosis is constructed using splenic or inferior mesenteric vessels in conjunction with one of the following three duct management techniques: pancreatic ductal injection, direct ductogastrostomy, or enteric drainage into a Roux limb of the recipient jejunum. When transplanting a whole pancreaticoduodenal graft, the graft portal vein may be anastomosed to either the recipient superior mesenteric vein or proximal splenic vein. An arterial anastomosis is constructed between the graft inflow vasculature and the aorta. Although theoretically attractive, portal venous drainage has not been found to provide a significant advantage over systemic drainage.

Intra-abdominal drain placement

No surgical drains are routinely employed following pancreatic transplantation. However, if signs of haemorrhagic pancreatitis are present following removal of vascular clamps, drains are placed – one cephalad to the graft to introduce irrigation and others for irrigation drainage (lateral and parallel to iliac vessels, retrocaecally and in the cul-de-sac). The transplant bed is continuously irrigated after the operation until the efflux is transparent.

Conversion from bladder to enteric drainage

When serious metabolic or urological complications arise, conversion from bladder to enteric drainage is beneficial. The most common indications for conversion include chronic intractable metabolic acidosis, cystitis and urethritis, graft pancreatitis as a result of neurogenic bladder dysfunction and haematuria. To convert a graft from bladder to enteric drainage the duodenocystostomy is first divided and the bladder is closed. Graft drainage is re-established by anastomosing the graft duodenum to the recipient jejunum in either a side-to-side fashion or using a Roux-en-Y reconstruction.

Postoperative care

Pancreatic transplant recipients are closely monitored postoperatively with serial haemodynamic evaluations. Foley catheter bladder drainage is maintained for 7–10 days after transplantation and nasogastric decompression is employed until resumption of bowel function. At the University of Minnesota postoperative antibiotic prophylaxis consists of 7 days of treatment with vancomycin and imipenem with cilastatin. Fluconazole is administered prophylactically for 14 days after transplantation. Antiviral prophylaxis consists of 14 days of ganciclovir sodium followed by 3 months of orally administered acyclovir. With the emergence of resistant bacterial strains, limited antibacterial prophylaxis with cephalexin is recommended.

Recipients of pancreatic transplants often receive a regimen of quadruple immunosuppression. Induction consists of an anti-T cell antibody preparation (polyclonal antithymocyte globulin or monoclonal OKT3 antibody) for 10–14 days together with cyclosporin A, azathioprine and prednisone. Maintenance immunosuppression is provided by the latter three agents. Newer immunosuppressive regimens including FK506 (Tacrolimus) and mycophenolate mofetil are under investigation.

Fasting and postprandial blood glucose levels are serially evaluated. If serum glucose levels exceed 150 mg/dl, the transplant recipients are started on an intravenous insulin infusion. Such exogenous insulin therapy may 'rest' the newly transplanted islet population. Less metabolic demand upon the islets immediately after transplantation may be associated with improved long-term graft glucoregulatory ability.

Outcome

Over 6500 pancreatic transplants have been reported to the International Pancreas Transplant Registry since the procedure was first performed in 1966. Patient survival rates between 1987 and 1993 were 94%, 87% and 84% at 1, 2 and 3 years, respectively. Graft survival rates over the same time interval are 81%, 75% and 69% at 1, 2 and 3 years, respectively. Patient survival rates are similar for pancreatic transplants alone or simultaneously with or after kidney transplantation. However, graft survival rates are significantly better for pancreatic transplantation simultaneously with kidney transplantation with 1-year graft survival rates of 76%, compared with 54% graft survival for pancreatic transplantation after a kidney graft and 47% graft survival for pancreatic transplants alone. Multivariate analyses demonstrate that recipient category and age at the time of the pancreatic transplant (less than 45 years) are the most important factors associated with a good outcome.

Further reading

Brayman KL, Gincherman Y, Sutherland DER. Recent studies on pancreas transplantation. *Curr Opin Endocrinol Diabetes* 1995; 2: 56–66.

Brayman KL, Najarian JS, Sutherland DER. Transplantation of the pancreas. In: Cameron JL, ed. *Current Surgical Therapy*, 4th edn. 1992.

Gruessner RWG, Sutherland DER. Pancreas transplantation. Part II: The recipient operation. *Surg Rounds* 1994; 383–91.

Levy MM, Brayman KL, Sutherland DER. Beta cell replacement therapy in the 1990s. In: Braverman MH, Tawes RL, eds. *Surgical Technology International II*, Surgical Technology International, 1993.

Sutherland DER, Gores PF, Farney AC *et al.* Evolution of the kidney, pancreas and islet transplantation for patients with diabetes at the University of Minnesota. *Am J Surg* 1993; 166: 456–91.

Sutherland DER, Moudry-Munns K, Gruessner A. Pancreas transplant results in the United Network for Organ Sharing (UNOS). United States of America Registry with a comparison to non-USA data in the international registry. In: Terasaki PI, ed. *Clinical Transplantation*. Los Angeles: UCLA Tissue Typing Laboratory, 1993.

Pancreaticoduodenal trauma

Charles F. Frey MD, FACS
Professor, Department of Surgery, University of California, Davis Medical Center, Sacramento, California, USA

Hung S. Ho MD
Assistant Professor, Department of Surgery, University of California, Davis Medical Center, Sacramento, California, USA

Trauma to the pancreas and duodenum is relatively uncommon, yet it presents a unique challenge in diagnosis and treatment. Both of these retroperitoneal organs, because of their relatively protected location, account for 3–12% of all abdominal injuries. However, if the index of suspicion is not high and appropriate diagnostic preoperative studies and intraoperative manoeuvres are not done, significant injuries may be missed during exploratory laparotomy. Owing to their intimate relationship and proximity to one another and the biliary tract, it should be a routine practice to investigate thoroughly all three organs should any one be injured.

Principles and justification

Penetrating trauma to the pancreas and duodenum is usually associated with clinical findings that demand exploratory laparotomy and therefore is usually diagnosed during surgery. Blunt trauma is more subtle. When there are no associated intra-abdominal injuries mandating exploration, recognition of blunt pancreaticoduodenal injury may be difficult. The most common mechanism of blunt trauma to these two organs is compression between the vertebral column posteriorly and the offending object impinging on the abdominal wall anteriorly. Typically, pancreaticoduodenal trauma occurs as a result of a violent blow to the abdomen as the victim is thrown against a steering wheel, punched or kicked, in a significant fall, or in any sudden deceleration accident. Children commonly suffer the injury because of bicycle handle bar trauma, a fall against a kerb, or direct, blunt abominal trauma as in child abuse. The direction of the impinging force directed at the vertebral column determines the part of the pancreas or duodenum more likely to be injured. When external injury is localized on the patient's left side, the tail of the pancreas is more likely to be injured. On the other hand, when the right side of the abdomen is hit, the head of the pancreas and the duodenum are at risk. Direct blunt trauma to the mid epigastrium is more likely to produce transection of the neck of the pancreas over the mesenteric vessels. The pancreatic duct is brittle and more rigid than the surrounding vasculature, pancreatic parenchyma and capsule of the pancreas, and may therefore be fractured in the absence of major haemorrhage or capsule disruption. Pancreatic ductal fracture is the main determinant of morbidity associated with pancreatic trauma. Leakage of enzymes leads to severe peripancreatic inflammation. Ductal obstruction causes pancreatic fistula, pseudocysts and pancreatitis. When the duct is intact, the injury is usually not significant.

Preoperative

In patients with penetrating trauma little time should be spent on diagnostic measures to identify specific injuries. The organs should be thoroughly examined during the operation. Evidence of shock or peritoneal irritation should prompt an early exploration. In patients with blunt trauma the pancreas and duodenum are always examined intraoperatively should the patient need an exploratory laparotomy for other intra-abdominal injuries.

Isolated pancreatic or duodenal injury usually does not produce profound shock initially, except for tenderness or guarding over these organs. Patients sometimes may at first have no abnormal abdominal findings. In most instances the abdominal discomfort may be in proportion to the physical findings, an ileus may be present and elevated serum amylase and lipase levels may occur. High levels of serum amylase or lipase are not specific and provide no clues as to the significance of pancreatic injury. Any injury to the upper gastrointestinal tract may result in peritoneal contamination with pancreatic enzymes. Lymphatic absorption of the enzymes in such cases will result in high serum levels. In addition, injury to the parotid gland also results in hyperamylasaemia. On the other hand, a complete fracture of the pancreatic duct may not lead to hyperamylasaemia for 24–48 h after the injury. In principle, exploration is not indicated if there is only one raised amylase reading, or if the initial hyperamylasaemia declines on serial determinations.

Diagnostic peritoneal lavage has not been useful because of the retroperitoneal location of these organs. A contused duodenal wall may progress to necrosis later. In such cases, serial determination of amylase levels is useful to document a persistent or progressive elevation of serum enzyme. Further diagnostic studies including laparotomy are indicated in such instances.

Endoscopic retrograde cholangiography and pancreaticography is the best diagnostic procedure for assessment of pancreatic ductal injury in haemodynamically stable patients. Oesophagogastroduodenoscopy and water-soluble contrast study of the upper gastrointestinal tract may define a duodenal haematoma or identify duodenal extravasation, respectively. Ultrasonography and computed tomographic (CT) scanning may visualize haematoma and peripancreatic swelling. They do not, however, offer information as to the integrity of the pancreatic duct.

The most important point in diagnosing pancreaticoduodenal injury is a high index of suspicion on the part of the examining surgeon. When the results of the clinical examination and mechanism of injury are suggestive, exploration of the abdomen is indicated.

Operation

Exposure

1 The pancreas can be exposed by three main routes. Superiorly, the head can be evaluated via the gastrohepatic ligament. Laterally, an extended Kocher manoeuvre will allow mobilization of the duodenal C-loop and the head of the pancreas for palpation and inspection. Anteriorly, the gastrocolic ligament can be taken down, allowing entrance to the lesser sac and inspection of the body and tail of the pancreas.

A midline incision is made, at least from the xiphoid process to the umbilicus, which may be extended well below the umbilicus if further exposure is needed. The small intestine is eviscerated and retracted downward. Free blood is aspirated and clots are evacuated. All four quadrants of the abdominal cavity are quickly checked for obvious sources of haemorrhage. After ongoing haemorrhage is controlled, a complete review of all other injuries is performed. The retroperitoneum is then inspected. When there is suspicion of injury because of the mechanism of injury, the presence of crepitation, haematoma, bile or gastrointestinal contents, the trajectory of a penetrating injury, or any visceral disruption, a Kocher manoeuvre is performed by incising the peritoneum lateral to the duodenum. The duodenum and pancreatic head are mobilized forwards, and the inferior vena cava is exposed.

Exposure of both sides of the head of the pancreas

2 The hepatic flexure and right transverse colon are mobilized and retracted downward and medially. The transverse mesocolon is followed down to the third portion of the duodenum. The Kocher manoeuvre is then extended upward to the porta hepatis. Dissection between the pancreas and inferior vena cava is carried out. The head of the pancreas can be palpated and inspected.

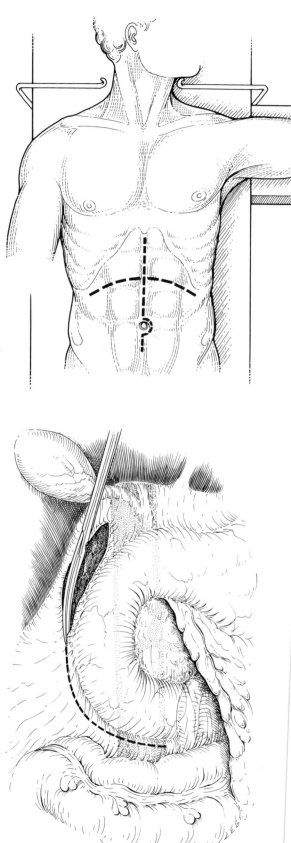

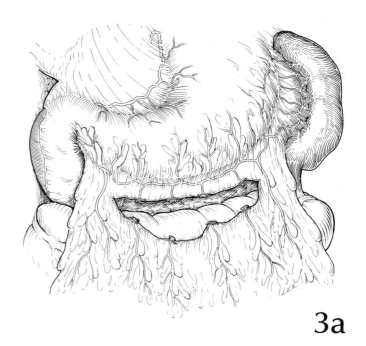

3a

Exposure of the body and tail of the pancreas

3a, b The lesser sac is entered through the gastrocolic omentum. The gastroepiploic arcade along the greater curvature of the stomach is preserved. The middle colic vessels in the transverse colon must be identified and preserved. A wide opening of the lesser sac allows full exposure for complete examination of the body and tail of the pancreas.

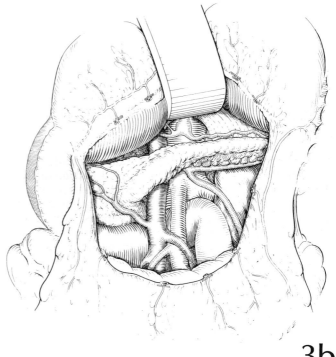

3b

Signs of pancreaticoduodenal injury

4a–f At laparotomy the following signs suggest pancreatic or duodenal injuries: haematoma formation in the lesser sac or duodenum, extravasation of bile or gastric contents, retroperitoneal gas or bile staining. A major pancreatic injury is defined as one in which the main pancreatic duct is completely or partially disrupted. There may be associated enzyme leakage, pancreatic inflammation, or ductal obstruction. When the main pancreatic duct is intact, the injury is not surgically significant. A major duodenal injury is one in which there is full thickness disruption or necrosis of the duodenal wall, with or without associated bile duct injury. A duodenal obstruction due to significant haematoma is usually not a surgical lesion.

Injuries to the pancreas and duodenum can be classified as follows:

A. Pancreatic injury
   Class I: haematoma, contusion, or capsular tear;
   Class II: laceration of pancreatic main duct in body or tail (*Illustration 4b*);
   Class III: laceration of pancreatic main duct in head, or injury to the intrapancreatic common bile duct (*Illustration 4c*).

B. Duodenal injury
   Class I: haematoma, contusion or serosal tear;
   Class II: isolated full thickness injury (*Illustration 4d*);
   Class III: full thickness injury and > 75% circumference involvement, common bile duct injury (*Illustration 4e*)

C. Combined pancreaticoduodenal injury
   Class I: haematoma, contusion or superficial tear to both organs; class II pancreatic or duodenal injury, with a less severe injury to the other organ;
   Class II: class II pancreatic and duodenal injuries;
   Class III: class III pancreatic or duodenal injury with a less severe injury to the other organ;
   Class IV: class III pancreatic and duodenal injuries (*Illustration 4f*).

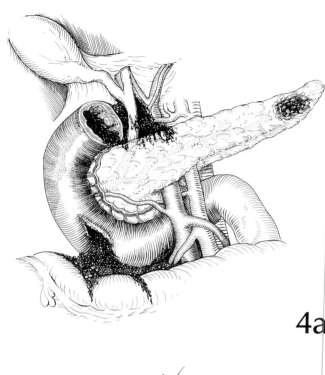

4a

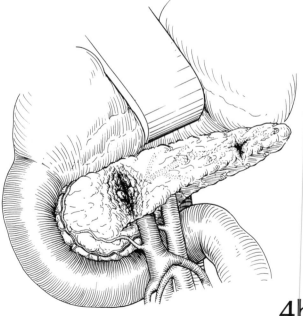

4b

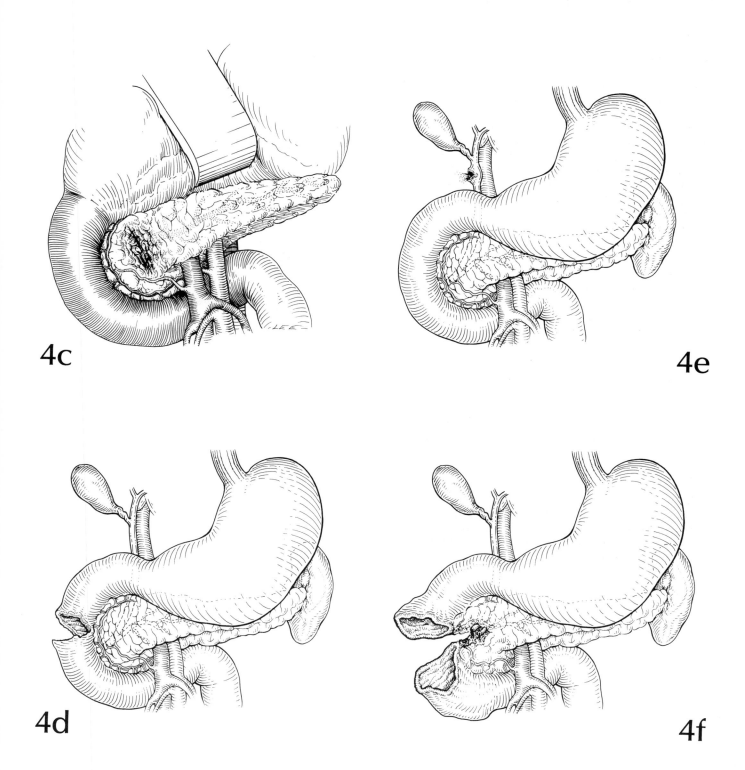

4c

4e

4d

4f

INJURY TO THE BODY AND TAIL OF THE PANCREAS

Distal pancreatectomy

5 The junction of the neck and body of the pancreas is the most common site of injury. The portion distal to this junction constitutes about 60–65% of the pancreatic mass. Resection of the distal pancreas limited to the left of the superior mesenteric vein is not associated with either exocrine or endocrine insufficiency. Distal pancreatectomy is the procedure of choice in any injury to the neck, body or tail of the pancreas with disruption of the main pancreatic duct. Radical distal pancreatectomy (80–95% resection) is rarely indicated and is reserved as a rapid, life-saving solution for injury to the head of the pancreas in patients with multiple other injuries.

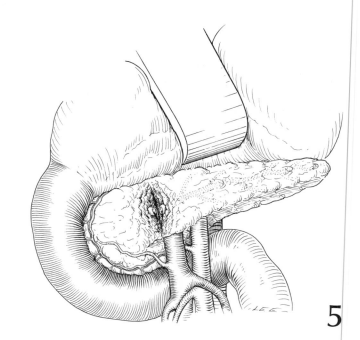

5

6

Distal pancreatectomy: extension of exposure to the tail of the pancreas

6 The gastrocolic ligament is completely taken down and the splenocolic ligament is divided. The stomach is retracted upwards and the transverse colon downwards. Following the middle colic vein to its junction with the superior mesenteric vein, this latter vessel is identified and dissection along the inferior border of the pancreas is continued towards the left side of the abdominal cavity. This dissection separates the inferior border of the pancreas from the retroperitoneal tissue, from the superior mesenteric vein medially and the splenic hilum laterally.

Distal pancreatectomy: dissection and isolation of the splenic artery

7 The splenic artery runs along the superior border of the pancreas. A segment of the artery is dissected out between its origin from the coeliac axis to the superior border of the pancreas where it is divided and suture-ligated. The spleen is mobilized from its spleno-phrenic attachment and splenorenal ligament. The short gastric and left gastroepiploic vessels are divided and ligated.

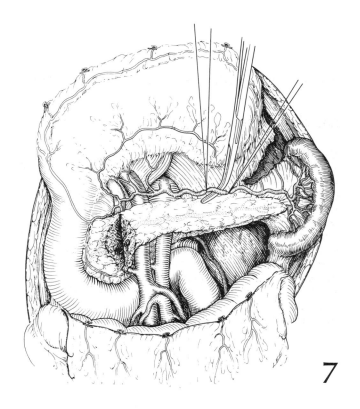

7

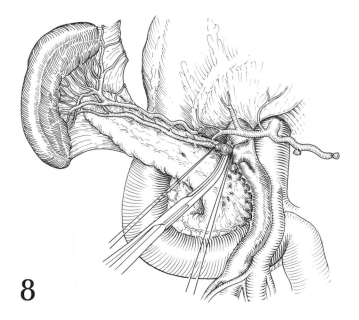

8

Distal pancreatectomy with splenectomy

8 With the splenic pedicle left intact, the spleen and the tail of the pancreas are elevated and reflected medially. The superior border is further mobilized past the point where the splenic artery is ligated. The superior mesenteric, coronary, inferior mesenteric and splenic veins are now clearly identified. The splenic vein is ligated and divided distal to its junction with the inferior mesenteric vein. The pancreas is divided distal to the injury. In 80–95% pancreatectomy the uncinate process must be dissected from the portal and superior mesenteric veins. Small branches of the superior mesenteric artery and vein cross laterally to the uncinate process. These should be ligated in continuity and divided. Both the anterior and posterior pancreaticoduodenal arteries must be preserved to prevent necrosis of the second and third portions of the duodenum. This may be achieved by leaving a cuff of pancreas along the inner aspect of the second and third portions of the duodenum.

Radical distal pancreatectomy: protection of the common bile duct

9 When part of the pancreatic head needs to be resected along with the body and tail, a choledochotomy should be made and a Bake's dilator inserted in the common bile duct to the duodenum in order to clarify its course and prevent injury to the common bile duct. The curvilinear incision is made in the head of the pancreas along the inner aspect of the duodenum, shaped like a C. This dissection is performed by sharp dissection and electrocautery, leaving a rim of pancreatic tissue behind which contains the cannulated common bile duct and both pancreaticoduodenal arterial arcades.

A probe should be passed easily from the open end of the pancreatic duct into the duodenum to ensure proximal ductal patency. Distal pancreatectomy may be associated with pancreatic enzyme leakage, leading to postoperative fistula, fluid collection or pseudocyst. One of the main causes of these complications is the failure to completely tie off the pancreatic duct. With the duct cannulated using an appropriate sized feeding tube, a non-absorbable polypropylene (Prolene) suture ligature is placed. As the suture is tied down, the tube should be withdrawn. If the suture is around the duct the feeding tube should be secured, otherwise the feeding tube would be easily withdrawn. On the final tie, the tube is removed and the knots are completed. If the patient is unstable, time should not be spent searching for the pancreatic duct which is small (2 mm).

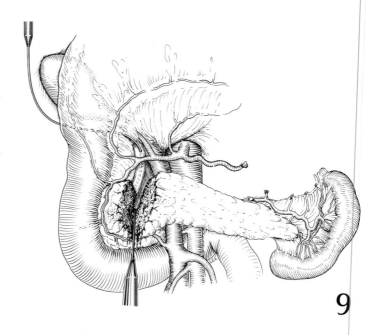

9

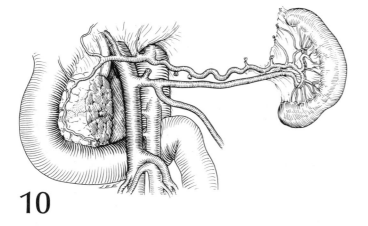

10

Distal pancreatectomy with splenic preservation

10 In isolated pancreatic injury it is possible to preserve the spleen by dissecting out, ligating and dividing the perforating branches of the splenic artery and vein to the tail of the pancreas. Splenic vein preservation is crucial in splenic salvage. Although splenic preservation is encouraged because of the concern over the overwhelming post-splenectomy sepsis syndrome, it is both time consuming and difficult and should only be performed in stable patients with minimal associated injuries. Alternatively, the splenic artery and vein can be ligated and the spleen will remain viable as long as the short gastric vessels are intact.

INJURY TO THE HEAD OF THE PANCREAS

Roux-en- Y pancreaticojejunostomy: preservation of the body and tail

11a, b In a stable patient with trauma to the main pancreatic duct within the head of the pancreas, effort should be expended to preserve the body and tail of the pancreas. This will usually avoid postoperative endocrine insufficiency. A Roux-en-Y limb is fashioned based on the jejunal primary, secondary and tertiary vascular arcades. Good blood supply and no tension after the loop is placed in the lesser sac must be ensured for successful drainage. An end-to-side pancreaticojejunostomy is performed with the end of the jejunum loop closed in two layers. A duct-to-mucosa anastomosis can always be performed even in the presence of a small, normal (2–3 mm) pancreatic duct. The patency of the small pancreatic duct is maintained by intubating the duct with a small polyethylene tube. A posterior row of 3/0 silk Lembert sutures is placed well back from the line of resection, approximating the pancreas and jejunum. An inner circumferential row of 4/0 polypropylene sutures is placed in the intubated pancreatic duct. A small enterotomy is made in the jejunum, opposite the duct. Interrupted 4/0 chromic sutures are used to tack jejunal mucosa to its serosa. The duct-to-mucosa anastomosis is then performed using the previously placed 4/0 polypropylene sutures. The polypropylene tube is placed across the anastomosis and allowed to pass spontaneously postoperatively. An anterior row of 3/0 silk Lembert sutures is placed to bury the pancreas in the jejunum.

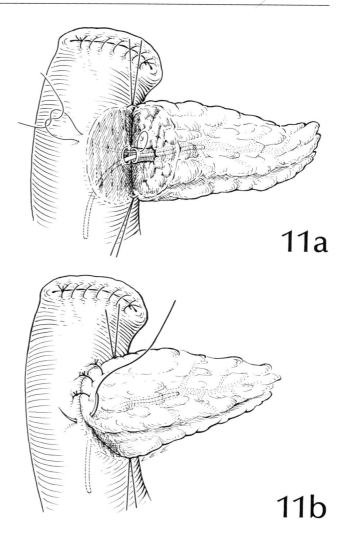

11a

11b

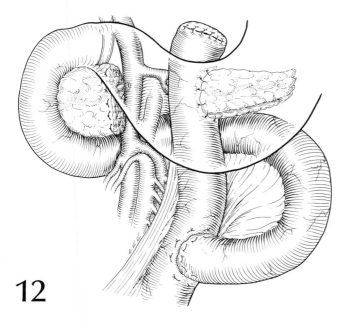

12

Completion of Roux-en-Y pancreaticojejunostomy

12 The proximal end of the pancreas is oversewn with interlocking mattress sutures of 2/0 silk. Treatment of the proximal pancreatic duct and the common bile duct is similiar to that described in distal pancreatectomy. A stapling closure of the proximal pancreas is an acceptable alternative. Gastrointestinal continuity is restored with an end-to-side jejunojejunostomy. The Roux-en-Y jejunal limb should be placed blindly over fresh lacerations or stellate lesions of the pancreas in lieu of the duct-to-mucosa anastomosis. Draining of the proximal pancreas with a Roux-en-Y limb is unnecessary and may increase the incidence of sepsis because of disruption of the suture line.

Choledochojejunostomy or choledochoduodenostomy

13 In the case of combined injury to the pancreatic head and intrapancreatic common bile duct, an end-to-side choledochojejunostomy may be performed 15–20 cm distal to the pancreaticojejunostomy. Similarly, an end-to-side choledochoduodenostomy can be performed. The distal common bile duct is ligated beyond the injury site.

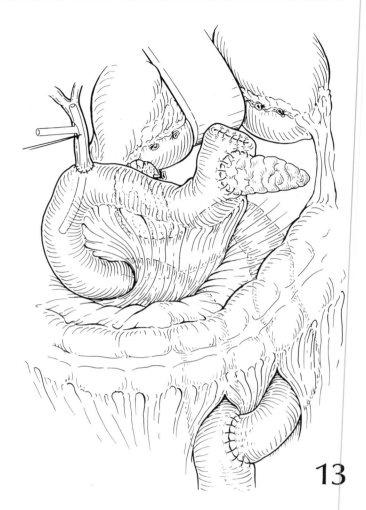

13

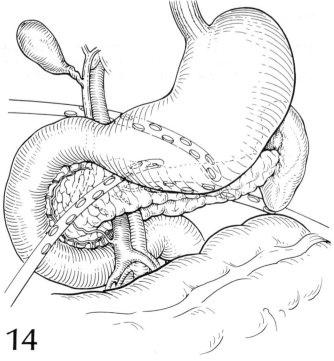

14

Simple drainage

14 In the case of severe pancreatic head injuries in the setting of severe shock, simple drainage is an acceptable alternative. Further attempts at the definitive operative therapy may influence mortality unfavourably in such cases. As a rule, simple drainage for major pancreatic injuries is undesirable. When indicated, it should be generous, wide and directed posteriorly. A pancreatic fistula and its associated morbidity is to be anticipated.

DUODENAL INJURY

Primary repair

15 The site and presence of duodenal injury may be identified by tracking the missile track and signs of active haemorrhage, haematoma, bile staining or crepitation. In penetrating trauma, most duodenal injury is not extensive (usually class II); local debridement and two-layer closure will suffice. Closure should be performed without tension and preferably in a transverse direction.

Blunt trauma is often more extensive, resulting in involvement of more than 75% of the duodenal circumference. Segmental resection and end-to-end anastomosis with a standard two-layer closure is recommended in such cases. This can be performed in all portions of the duodenum. The distal common bile duct should always be intubated with a Bake's dilator placed via a choledochotomy and passed into the duodenum.

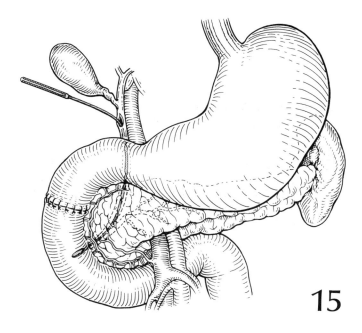

15

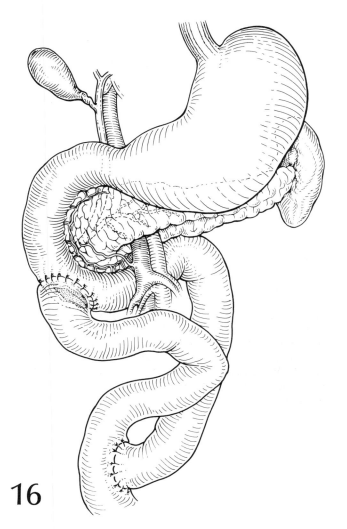

16

Patch duodenojejunostomy

16 On rare occasions, a localized duodenal injury with a large defect may be treated with a jejunal patch or a side-to-end Roux-en-Y duodenojejunostomy.

Resection and duodenojejunal anastomosis

17 In distal duodenal injury with a large segment of devitalized tissue, an end-to-end duodenoduodenostomy may not be feasible because of constraint in mobilization. A Roux-en-Y duodenojejunostomy can be performed. The jejunum is divided 20 cm distal to the ligament of Treitz. The distal limb is brought into the lesser sac via an opening in the transverse mesocolon, and an end-to-end duodenojejunostomy is performed. The proximal jejunal limb is anastomosed end-to-side to the distal jejunum, 30 cm from the duodenojejunostomy. The distal duodenum is oversewn in two layers.

Duodenal diverticulization and pylorus exclusion

18a, b When the victim has more than one duodenal perforation, injury from high velocity missile, extensive loss of duodenal wall, advanced peritonitis or duodenal vascular compromise, diverticulization of the duodenum may be beneficial. The procedure will convert a lateral fistula, should it develop, into an end fistula. The procedure consists of division of the pylorus, gastrojejunostomy, tube duodenostomy, T-tube choledochotomy and oversewing of the duodenal lacerations. A modification, the pylorus exclusion procedure, includes oversewing the pylorus with absorbable sutures through the gastrostomy before completion of the gastrojejunostomy.

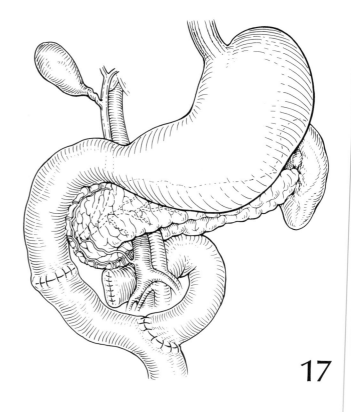

17

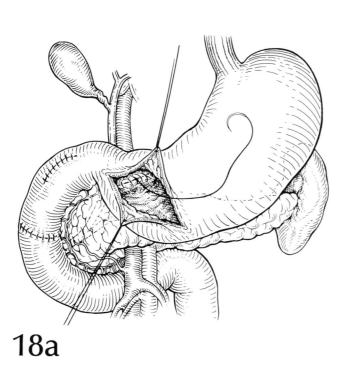

18a

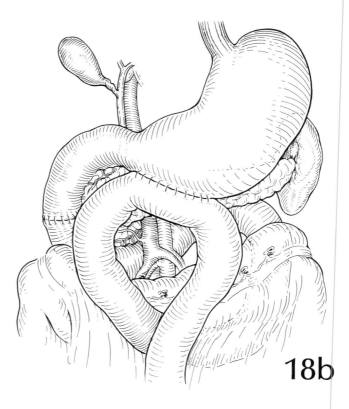

18b

Combined duodenal and biliary injury

19 About 5% of duodenal injuries also involve the bile duct. In most patients, addition of an end-to-side choledochojejunostomy using a Roux-en-Y jejunal limb to the appropriate duodenal repair is usually adequate. Intraoperative pancreaticography should be utilized to rule out injury to the main pancreatic duct. Patients with major duodenal injury and associated biliary trauma may need pancreatico-duodenectomy.

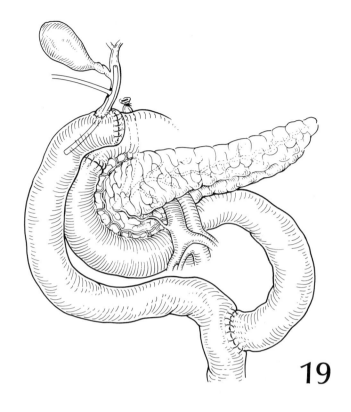

19

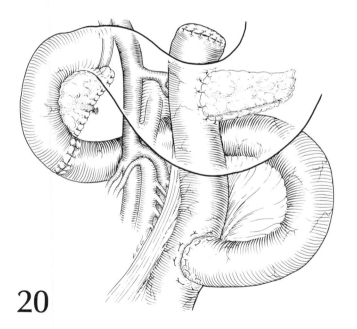

20

COMBINED PANCREATICODUODENAL INJURY

Primary duodenal repair, pancreatic resection and Roux-en-Y pancreaticojejunostomy

20 In patients with main pancreatic ductal disruption within the head of the pancreas and associated duodenal lacerations, neither radical distal pancreatectomy nor pancreaticoduodenectomy is indicated. Segmental resection and end-to-end reanastomosis of the duodenum is adequate and safe. The ampulla of Vater is intubated through the duodenal laceration, an on-table pancreaticogram is obtained, and the integrity of the pancreatic duct assessed. When injury to the duct within the head of the pancreas is confirmed, the injured portion of the pancreas is resected, the proximal end of the pancreas oversewn and Roux-en-Y jejunal drainage of the distal pancreas performed.

Pancreaticoduodenectomy

21 Severe injury to the duodenum, the common bile duct and the main pancreatic duct is best treated by pancreaticoduodenectomy. Although pancreaticoduodenectomy following trauma is associated with a mortality rate as high as 30%, drainage alone for severe combined biliary tract and pancreaticoduodenal injury is usually fatal. Diverticulization or pylorus exclusion procedures are not adequate.

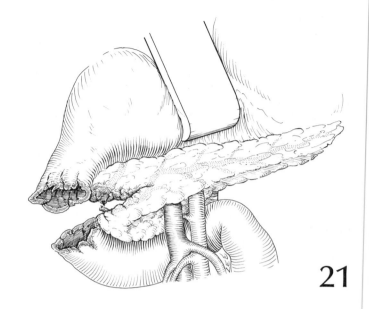

21

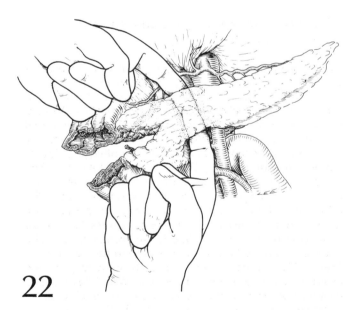

22

Mobilization of the neck of the pancreas

22 After completion of the abdominal exploration and assessment of the injury, a generous Kocher manoeuvre is performed, the gastrocolic ligament is divided, and the superior mesenteric vein and porta hepatis are identified. The common bile duct is then dissected off the hepatic artery, encircled with a tape and the portal vein is carefully exposed. A plane can be developed safely between the neck of the pancreas anteriorly and the portal and superior mesenteric veins posteriorly. There are no venous tributaries between the neck of the pancreas and the anterior surface of these two veins.

Mobilization of the body and tail of the pancreas

23 The splenic artery is traced by palpation from its origin at the coeliac axis to its contact with the superior border of the pancreas. This junction is usually 3–6 cm to the left of the portal vein. Perforating branches from the splenic artery to the superior aspect of the pancreas are taken down up to the site of pancreatic division. The inferior border of the pancreas is freed from the retroperitoneal tissues, from the superior mesenteric vein medially to the splenic hilum laterally. This portion of dissection is usually avascular. The body of the pancreas is rotated upwards around the splenic vein. The small venous tributaries from the pancreas to the splenic vein are doubly ligated in continuity and divided until the pancreas can be separated from the splenic vein for 2–4 cm at the point of division.

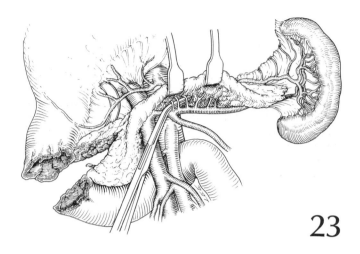

23

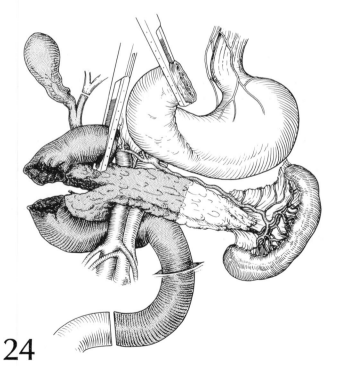

24

Division of the injured duodenum and common bile duct

24 Branches of the left gastric artery supplying the lesser curvature of the stomach and the duodenum in the line of resection are ligated and divided. If the first portion of the duodenum is intact, the pylorus is preserved. The dorsal pancreatic and gastroduodenal arteries are divided and suture ligated. Cholecystectomy is performed because the absence of a biliary sphincter would prevent normal filling of the gallbladder. The common bile duct is divided with its proximal end occluded with a paediatric Satinsky vascular clamp. The third and fourth portions of the duodenum are mobilized from the superior mesenteric vessels by sharp dissection of the surrounding loose areolar tissue. The jejunum is divided just distal (10 cm) to the ligament of Treitz. The short jejunal vasculature supplying the proximal cut end of jejunum is divided and ligated. The ligament of Treitz is released and the proximal jejunum is brought out to the right beneath the mesenteric vessels.

Division of the injured pancreas

25 To prepare for division of the pancreas, haemostatic sutures are placed on both sides of the division line in the superior and inferior border of the pancreas. The pancreas is divided by a sharp scalpel. Further haemostatic mattress sutures are placed along the cut edges. The distal pancreatic duct is identified and avoided when placing these sutures. Patency of the duct is ensured by intubating it with a splint of polyethylene feeding tube when the haemostatic sutures are placed above and below it on the pancreatic parenchyma.

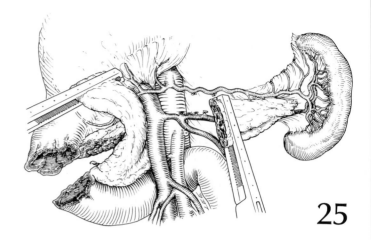

25

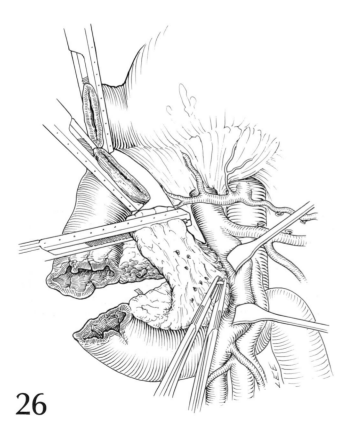

26

Dissection of the uncinate process

26 After division of the pancreas, the proximal pancreas is lifted and rotated to the right, exposing the arterial and venous branches to the uncinate process from the superior mesenteric vessels. The dissection to separate the uncinate process from the superior mesenteric vein is begun inferiorly by division and ligation of the inferior pancreaticoduodenal vessel. The superior mesenteric vein is retracted to the patient's left. The small vessels to the uncinate process are further exposed and stretched; these should be ligated in continuity and divided. After complete division of the blood vessels coursing between the superior mesenteric vessels and the uncinate process, the entire specimen is removed *en bloc*.

Restoration of gastrointestinal continuity

27 Reconstruction following pancreaticoduodenectomy is begun with an end-to-side pancreaticojejunostomy using a duct-to-mucosa anastomosis. A choledochojejunostomy is performed with interrupted 4/0 polydioxanone in a single layer. A T tube is placed in the common bile duct to facilitate the anastomosis. The jejunal mucosa is tacked down to the serosa to ensure a duct-to-mucosa anastomosis. The distal limb of the T tube is passed into the jejunum to serve as a splint. When there is insufficient space to place a T tube between the anastomosis and the junction of the left and the right hepatic ducts, a Robinson catheter with extra holes placed within it may be inserted retrograde through the anastomosis from the jejunal limb.

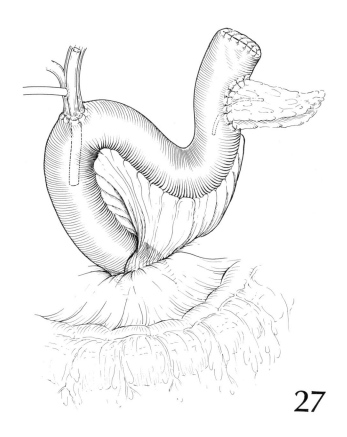

27

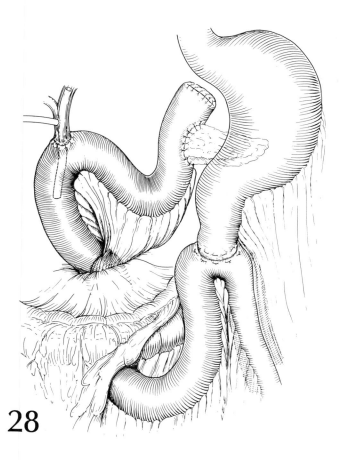

28

Completed procedure

28 An antecolic two-layer duodenojejunostomy consisting of an inner running layer of 3/0 polydioxanone sutures and an outer layer of interrupted, inverting Lembert sutures of 3/0 silk completes the reconstruction. Appropriate drains are placed and secured in the abdominal wall. Consideration should be given to placing a needle feeding jejunostomy for postoperative enteral feeding. The abdomen is closed.

Exteriorization procedures

29 In the most severe combined biliary tract and pancreaticoduodenal injury with other life-threatening injuries a series of exteriorization procedures can be quickly performed. The abdominal cavity is adequately drained. The patient is allowed to stabilize and recover before ductal and enteric continuity of the gastrointestinal tract is restored.

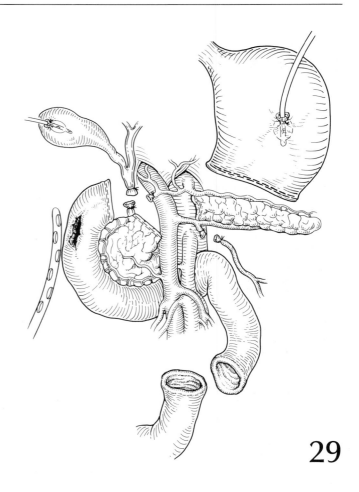

29

Postoperative care

The patient may have a prolonged ileus. Nasogastric decompression will prevent acid entering the duodenum, stimulating pancreatic secretion of bicarbonate. Total parenteral nutrition may be needed 4–5 days after surgery. In cases of duodenal diverticulization, pylorus exclusion or pancreaticoduodenectomy, total parenteral nutrition may be started as soon as the circulation becomes stable. In patients in whom a feeding jejunostomy has been placed, enteral feeding is an option once the ileus has resolved. Oral feeding is started slowly and cautiously if clinically indicated by the seventh postoperative day. In patients with sepsis, intra-abdominal infection should always be anticipated and ruled out. An abdominal CT scan or exploratory laparotomy may be necessary. The timing of drain removal is dictated by clinical status and the volume and composition of the drainage fluid. A concentration of 100 000 units/l amylase persisting in the drainage fluid for 1 week after the injury indicates the presence of a pancreatic fistula. Persistent high pancreatic drainage without ductal injury can be managed by total bowel rest, total parenteral nutrition and treatment with H_2 receptor antagonists and somatostatin analogue. The majority of these pancreatic fistulas will close spontaneously within 4–6 weeks during which time the drains should be left in place.

Further reading

Heimansohn DA, Canal DF, McCarthy MC, Yaw PB, Madura JA, Broadie TA. The role of pancreaticoduodenectomy in the management of traumatic injuries to the pancreas and duodenum. *Am Surg* 1990; 56: 511–4.

Ivatury RR, Nallathambi M, Rao P, Stahl WM. Penetrating pancreatic injuries: analysis of 103 consecutive cases. *Am Surg* 1990; 56: 90–5.

Jurkovich GJ, Carrico CJ. Pancreatic trauma. *Surg Clin North Am* 1990; 70: 575–93.

Wisner DH, Wold RL, Frey CF. Diagnosis and treatment of pancreatic injuries: an analysis of management principles. *Arch Surg* 1990; 125: 1109–13.

Index